# PROGRESS IN BRAIN RESEARCH

## VOLUME 34

## HISTOCHEMISTRY OF NERVOUS TRANSMISSION

# PROGRESS IN BRAIN RESEARCH

PROGRESS IN BRAIN RESEARCH

VOLUME 34

# HISTOCHEMISTRY
# OF
# NERVOUS TRANSMISSION

EDITED BY

OLAVI ERÄNKÖ

*Department of Anatomy,
University of Helsinki (Finland)*

ELSEVIER PUBLISHING COMPANY

AMSTERDAM / LONDON / NEW YORK

1971

ELSEVIER PUBLISHING COMPANY
335 JAN VAN GALENSTRAAT,
P.O. BOX 211, AMSTERDAM, THE NETHERLANDS

AMERICAN ELSEVIER PUBLISHING COMPANY, INC.
52 VANDERBILT AVENUE, NEW YORK, N.Y. 10017

LIBRARY OF CONGRESS CARD NUMBER 70–168912

ISBN 0-444-40951-3

PRINTED IN THE NETHERLANDS

# List of Contributors

LIISA AHTEE, Department of Pharmacology, University of Helsinki, Siltavuorenpenger Helsinki (Finland).

K. AKERT, Brain Research Institute, University of Zürich, Zürich (Switzerland).

U. ATTILA, Department of Anatomy and Embryology, Veterinary College, Helsinki (Finland).

P. BANKS, Departments of Human Biology & Anatomy and Biochemistry, University of Sheffield, Sheffield (England).

R. J. BARRNETT, Department of Anatomy, Yale University School of Medicine, New Haven, Conn. (U.S.A.).

A. BJÖRKLUND, Institute of Anatomy and Histology, University of Lund, Lund (Sweden).

H. BLASCHKO, University Department of Pharmacology, Oxford (England).

D. F. BOGDANSKI, Laboratory of Chemical Pharmacology, National Heart and Lung Institute, National Institutes of Health, Bethesda, Maryland 20014 (U.S.A.).

G. BURNSTOCK, Department of Zoology, University of Melbourne, Melbourne, Parkville, Victoria (Australia).

A. M. BURT, Department of Anatomy, Vanderbilt University School of Medicine, Nashville, Tennessee (U.S.A.)

R. E. COUPLAND, Department of Human Morphology, University of Nottingham, Nottingham (England).

B. CSILLIK, Department of Anatomy, University Medical School, Szeged (Hungary).

R. DAVIS, Department of Pharmacology, Medical School, University of Pennsylvania, Philadelphia, Pa. (U.S.A.).

LIISA ERÄNKÖ, Department of Anatomy, University of Helsinki, Siltavuorenpenger, Helsinki (Finland).

O. ERÄNKÖ, Department of Anatomy, University of Helsinki, Siltavuorenpenger, Helsinki (Finland).

ISABELLE FAEDER, Department of Anatomy, Duke University Medical College, Durham, North Carolina (U.S.A.).

B. FALCK, Institute of Anatomy and Histology, University of Lund, Lund (Sweden).

K. FUXE, Department of Histology, Karolinska Institutet, Stockholm (Sweden).

J. R. GARRETT, Department of Oral Pathology, The Dental School, King's College Hospital Medical School, London (England).

E. GIACOBINI, Department of Pharmacology, Karolinska Institutet, Stockholm (Sweden).

M. GOLDSTEIN, Department of Psychiatry, New York University Medical Center, New York (U.S.A.)

J. A. GOSLING, Department of Medical Pharmacology and Therapy, University of California, Irvine, California (U.S.A.).

E. G. GRAY, Department of Anatomy, University College London, London (England),

ROSANNE GRIGAS, Departments of Human Biology & Anatomy and Biochemistry, University of Sheffield, Sheffield (England).

R. GUEUDET, Instituto de Anatomía General y Embriología, Facultad de Medicina, Buenos Aires (Argentina).

P. H. HASHIMOTO, Department of Anatomy, Osaka University Medical School, Osaka (Japan).

A. HERVONEN, Department of Anatomy, University of Helsinki, Siltavuorenpenger, Helsinki (Finland).

T. HÖKFELT, Department of Histology, Karolinska Institutet, Stockholm (Sweden).

T. HYUB JOH, Department of Psychiatry, New York University Medical Center, New York (U.S.A.).

S. ISHII, The Center for Adult Disease and Department of Neuroanatomy, Osaka University Medical School, Osaka (Japan).

T. IWAYAMA, Department of Zoology, University of Melbourne, Melbourne, Parkville, Victoria (Australia).

S.-E. JANSSON, Department of Anatomy, University of Helsinki, Siltavuorenpenger, Helsinki (Finland).

G. JONSSON, Department of Histology, Karolinska Institutet, Stockholm (Sweden).

L. KANERVA, Department of Anatomy, University of Helsinki, Silvatuorenpenger, Helsinki (Finland)

P. KÁSA, Department of Anatomy, University Medical School, Szeged (Hungary).

E. KAWANA, Brain Research Institute, University of Tokyo (Japan).

M. KEKKI, Department of Anatomy and Embryology, Veterinary College, Helsinki (Finland).

E. KLINGE, Department of Pharmacology, University of Helsinki, Siltavuorenpenger, Helsinki (Finland).

G. B. KOELLE, Department of Pharmacology, Medical School, University of Pennsylvania, Philadelphia, Pennsylvania (U.S.A.).

A. KOKKO, Department of Anatomy, Yale University School of Medicine, New Haven, Conn. (U.S.A.).

J. D. LEVER, Department of Anatomy, University College, Cardiff (England).

Å. LJUNGDAHL, Department of Histology, Karolinska Institutet, Stockholm (Sweden).

A. B. M. MACHADO, Institute of Biological Sciences, University of Minas Gerais, Belo Horizonte (Brazil).

T. MALMFORS, Department of Histology, Karolinska Institutet, Stockholm (Sweden).

LUCIA MASTROLIA, Instituto di Zoologia Dell'Universita, Roma (Italy).

D. MASUOKA, Neuropharmacology Research Laboratory, Veterans Administration Hospital, Sepulveda, California (U.S.A.).

D. MAYOR, Departments of Human Biology & Anatomy and Biochemistry, University of Sheffield, Sheffield (England).

P. K. NAKANE, Department of Pathology, School of Medicine, University of Colorado, Denver, Colorado (U.S.A.)

L. OLSON, Department of Histology, Karolinska Institutet, Stockholm (Sweden).

M. K. PAASONEN, Department of Pharmacology, University of Helsinki, Silta-vuorenpenger, Helsinki (Finland).

A. PALKAMA, Department of Anatomy, University of Helsinki, Siltavuorenpenger, Helsinki (Finland).

AMANDA PELLEGRINO DE IRALDI, Instituto de Anatomía y Embriología, Facultad de Medicina, Buenos Aires (Argentina).

G.-F. PLACIDI, Department of Medical Pharmacology and Therapy, University of California, Irvine, California (U.S.A.)

P. POHTO, Department of Pharmacology, University of Helsinki, Siltavuorenpenger, Helsinki (Finland).

R. PRESLEY, Department of Anatomy, University College, Cardiff (England).

LEENA RECHARDT, Department of Anatomy, University of Helsinki, Siltavuoren-penger, Helsinki (Finland).

PETER M. ROBINSON, Department of Anatomy, University of Melbourne, Victoria (Australia).

D. A. SAKHAROV, Institute of Developmental Biology, Academy of Sciences, Moscow (U.S.S.R.).

A. V. SAKHAROVA, Institute of Neurology, Academy of Medical Sciences, Moscow (U.S.S.R.).

MIRIAM SALPETER, Department of Applied Physics, Cornell University, Ithaca, New York (U.S.A.).

CLARA SANDRI, Brain Research Institute, University of Zürich, Zurich (Switzerland).

T. H. SCHIEBLER, Department of Anatomy, University of Würzburg, Würzburg (Germany).

ANN SILVER, Institute of Animal Physiology, Agricultural Research Council, Babra-ham, Cambridge (England).

ELOISE G. SMYRL, Department of Pharmacology, Medical School, University of Pennsylvania, Philadelphia, Pennsylvania (U.S.A.).

E. SOLATUNTURI, Department of Pharmacology and Electron Microscope Laboratory, University of Helsinki, Siltavuorenpenger, Helsinki (Finland).

U. STENEVI, Institute of Anatomy and Histology, University of Lund, Lund (Sweden).

L. STJÄRNE, Department of Physiology, Karolinska Institutet, Stockholm (Sweden).

ANGELA M. SUBURO, Instituto de Anatomía General y Embriología, Facultad de Medicina, Buenos Aires (Argentina).

S. TALANTI, Department of Anatomy and Embryology, Veterinary College, Helsinki (Finland).

H. THOENEN, Department of Experimental Medicine, F. Hoffmann-La Roche & Co. Ltd., Basle (Switzerland).

ANJA TISSARI, Department of Pharmacology, University of Helsinki, Siltavuoren-penger, Helsinki (Finland).

D. R. TOMLINSON, Departments of Human Biology & Anatomy and Biochemistry, University of Sheffield, Sheffield (England).

J. P. TRANZER, Department of Experimental Medicine, F. Hoffmann-La Roche & Co. Ltd., Basle (Switzerland).

R. Uusitalo, Department of Anatomy, University of Helsinki, Siltavuorenpenger, Helsinki (Finland).

Marthe Vogt, Institute of Animal Physiology, Agricultural Research Council, Babraham, Cambridge (England).

Brenda Weakley, Department of Anatomy, University of Dundee, Dundee (England).

J. Winckler, Department of Anatomy, University of Würzburg, Würzburg (Germany).

*Other volumes in this series:*

Volume 1: *Brain Mechanisms*
*Specific and Unspecific Mechanisms of Sensory Motor Integration*
Edited by G. Moruzzi, A. Fessard and H. H. Jasper

Volume 2: *Nerve, Brain and Memory Models*
Edited by Norbert Wiener† and J. P. Schadé

Volume 3: *The Rhinencephalon and Related Structures*
Edited by W. Bargmann and J. P. Schadé

Volume 4: *Growth and Maturation of the Brain*
Edited by D. P. Purpura and J. P. Schadé

Volume 5: *Lectures on the Diencephalon*
Edited by W. Bargmann and J. P. Schadé

Volume 6: *Topics in Basic Neurology*
Edited by W. Bargmann and J. P. Schadé

Volume 7: *Slow Electrical Processes in the Brain*
by N. A. Aladjalova

Volume 8: *Biogenic Amines*
Edited by Harold E. Himwich and Williamina A. Himwich

Volume 9: *The Developing Brain*
Edited by Williamina A. Himwich and Harold E. Himwich

Volume 10: *The Structure and Function of the Epiphysis Cerebri*
Edited by J. Ariëns Kappers and J. P. Schadé

Volume 11: *Organization of the Spinal Cord*
Edited by J. C. Eccles and J. P. Schadé

Volume 12: *Physiology of Spinal Neurons*
Edited by J. C. Eccles and J. P. Schadé

Volume 13: *Mechanisms of Neural Regeneration*
Edited by M. Singer and J. P. Schadé

Volume 14: *Degeneration Patterns in the Nervous System*
Edited by M. Singer and J. P. Schadé

Volume 15: *Biology of Neuroglia*
Edited by E. D. P. De Robertis and R. Carrea

Volume 16: *Horizons in Neuropsychopharmacology*
Edited by Williamina A. Himwich and J. P. Schadé

x

Volume 17: *Cybernetics of the Nervous System*
Edited by Norbert Wiener† and J. P. Schadé

Volume 18: *Sleep Mechanisms*
Edited by K. Akert, Ch. Bally and J. P. Schadé

Volume 19: *Experimental Epilepsy*
by A. Kreindler

Volume 20: *Pharmacology and Physiology of the Reticular Formation*
Edited by A. V. Valdman

Volume 21A: *Correlative Neurosciences. Part A: Fundamental Mechanisms*
Edited by T. Tokizane and J. P. Schadé

Volume 21B: *Correlative Neurosciences. Part B: Clinical Studies*
Edited by T. Tokizane and J. P. Schadé

Volume 22: *Brain Reflexes*
Edited by E. A. Asratyan

Volume 23: *Sensory Mechanisms*
Edited by Y. Zotterman

Volume 24: *Carbon Monoxide Poisoning*
Edited bij H. Bour and I. McA. Ledingham

Volume 25: *The Cerebellum*
Edited by C. A. Fox and R. S. Snider

Volume 26: *Developmental Neurology*
Edited by C. G. Bernhard

Volume 27: *Structure and Function of the Limbic System*
Edited by W. Ross Adey and T. Tokizane

Volume 28: *Anticholinergic Drugs*
Edited by P. B. Bradley and M. Fink

Volume 29: *Brain Barrier Systems*
Edited by A. Lajtha and D. H. Ford

Volume 30: *Cerebral Circulation*
Edited by W. Luyendijk

Volume 31: *Mechanisms of Synaptic Transmission*
Edited by K. Akert and P. G. Waser

Volume 32: *Pituitary, Adrenal and the Brain*
Edited by D. de Wied and J. A. W. M. Weijnen

Volume 33: *Computers and Brains*
Edited by J. P. Schadé and J. Smith

# Preface

Nervous transmission, which some time ago was a subject reserved mainly for neuro-physiologists and pharmacologists, has recently attracted an ever-increasing number of investigators using histochemical methods. The expanding work in the field of histochemistry has, indeed, made it possible to localize at the cellular and sub-cellular level the transmitter substances and the enzymes synthetizing or hydrolyzing them with a precision not attainable by other means.

During the International Congress of Histochemistry in August 1968 in New York, several prominent histochemists, among them the President of the American Histo-chemical Society, Professor R. L. Hunter, proposed that a neurohistochemical symposium should be held in Helsinki. As a result of this encouragement and further endorsement by the Histochemical Society of Finland and the Societas Biochemica, Biophysica et Microbiologica Fenniae, an Organizing Committee was formed con-sisting of Liisa Eränkö, O. Eränkö (Chairman), A. Hervonen, L. Kanerva, J. Karkamo, Anneli Laitinen (Managing Secretary), A. Palkama (General Secretary), and Leena Rechardt, all members of the staff of the Department of Anatomy, University of Helsinki. The subject was limited to nervous transmission, because preliminary con-siderations made it clear that the field of neurohistochemistry would cover too large an area for a symposium.

The meeting was planned to include all aspects of the histochemistry of nervous transmission in such a way as to provide for a well-balanced programme. A list was then prepared of about 45 distinguished investigators, and invitations were sent to them. Almost all invited speakers responded enthusiastically and attended the meeting, which was held in the Nokkala Congress Center near Helsinki on August 11–14, 1970. The original aim was achieved better than the Organizing Committee ever dared to dream, and the present volume is composed of the 41 papers read at the Symposium and the 3 papers submitted by investigators who were not able to come. We believe that it represents a valid summary of the latest developments in the histochemistry of nervous transmission.

The organizers and members of the Symposium noted with pleasure that the Pre-sident of Finland, Doctor Urho Kekkonen, agreed to function as the Patron of the Symposium. The meeting was sponsored by the International Committee of Histo-chemistry and Cytochemistry, whose General Secretary, Professor T. H. Schiebler, took part in the Symposium. The City of Helsinki welcomed the participants by holding a reception in the heart of the city.

Our thanks for financial support are due to the Ministry of Education of Finland, The Sigrid Jusélius Foundation, The Finnish Medical Society Duodecim, The Fin-nish Medical Association, Oy Astra Ab, G. W. Berg & Co., Havulinna Oy, F. Hoffmann–La Roche & Co. AG., A. Ilmonen Oy, Oy Christian Nissen Ab and Oy

Philips Ab. Thanks are also due to the many members of the medical profession who took part in the meetings as local observers and helped the Organizing Committee to entertain the foreign visitors.

Olavi Eränkö

# Contents

List of Contributors . . . . . . . . . . . . . . . . . . . . . . . V
Preface. . . . . . . . . . . . . . . . . . . . . . . . . . . . . XI

Opening address: Functional aspects of the localization of transmitter substances
  Marthe Vogt (Cambridge) . . . . . . . . . . . . . . . . . . . . 1

**I. Light Microscopic Histochemistry of Monoamine Transmitters**     9

Visualization of intraneuronal monoamines by treatment with formalin solutions
  A. V. Sakharova and D. A. Sakharov (Moscow) . . . . . . . . . . . . . . . . . 11
The microscopic differentiation of the colour of formaldehyde induced fluorescence
  J. S. Ploem (Leiden) . . . . . . . . . . . . . . . . . . . . . . . . . 27
Small, intensely fluorescent, granule-containing cells in the sympathetic ganglion of the rat
  O. Eränkö and Liisa Eränkö (Helsinki). . . . . . . . . . . . . . . . . . . . 39
Quantitation and differentiation of biogenic monoamines demonstrated with the formaldehyde
  fluorescence method
  G. Jonsson (Stockholm) . . . . . . . . . . . . . . . . . . . . . . . 53
Microspectrofluorometric characterization of monoamines in the central nervous system:
  evidence for a new neuronal monoamine-like compound
  A. Björklund, B. Falck and U. Stenevi (Lund) . . . . . . . . . . . . . . . . 63

**II. Autoradiography and Immunohistochemistry**     75

Histochemical fluorescence microscopy and micro-autoradiography techniques combined for
  localization studies
  D. T. Masuoka, G.-F. Placidi and J. A. Gosling (Sepulveda and Irvine) . . . . . . . . 77
Uptake of [³H]noradrenaline and γ-[³H]aminobutyric acid in isolated tissues of rat: an
  autoradiographic and fluorescence microscopic study
  T. Hökfelt and Å. Ljungdahl (Stockholm) . . . . . . . . . . . . . . . . 87
The role of sheath cells in glutamate uptake by insect nerve muscle preparations
  Miriam M. Salpeter and Isabelle R. Faeder (Ithaca and Durham) . . . . . . . . . . . 103
On the kinetics of ³⁵S-labelled L-cysteine in the hypothalamic–hypophyseal neurosecretory
  system of the rat: an experimental study by autoradiography
  S. Talanti, U. Attila and M. Kekki (Helsinki) . . . . . . . . . . . . . . . 115
Cellular localization of dopamine-β-hydroxylase and phenylethanolamine-N-methyl transferase
  as revealed by immunohistochemistry
  K. Fuxe, M. Goldstein, T. Hökfelt and T. Hyub Joh (Stockholm and New York) . . . . . 127
Effect of thyrotropin-releasing factor on thyrotropic cells *in vitro*
  P. K. Nakane (Denver) . . . . . . . . . . . . . . . . . . . . . . . . 139

**III. Electron Microscopic Histochemistry of Monoamine Transmitters**     147

The fine structural characterization of different types of synapses
  E. G. Gray (London) . . . . . . . . . . . . . . . . . . . . . . . . 149
Differentiation between 5-hydroxytryptamine and catecholamines in synaptic vesicles
  Amanda Pellegrino de Iraldi, R. Gueudet and Angela M. Suburo (Buenos Aires) . . . . . 161
Electron microscopy of developing sympathetic fibres in the rat pineal. The formation of granular
  vesicles
  A. B. M. Machado (Belo Horizonte) . . . . . . . . . . . . . . . . . . . 171

Morphological studies on the mechanism of adrenergic transmission in the central nervous system I. Granulated vesicles
S. Ishii (Osaka) . . . . . . . . . . . . . . . . . . . . . . 187
Morphological studies on the mechanism of adrenergic transmission in the central nervous system II. Minute vesicles
P. H. Hashimoto (Osaka) . . . . . . . . . . . . . . . . . . . 207
Ultrastructural localization of intraneuronal monoamines — some aspects on methodology
T. Hökfelt (Stockholm) . . . . . . . . . . . . . . . . . . . . 213
Functional importance of subcellular distribution of false adrenergic transmitters
H. Thoenen and J. P. Tranzer (Basle) . . . . . . . . . . . . . . . 223


IV. Release, Uptake, Storage and Metabolism of Transmitter Substances 237

Observations on chromogranins, the satellite proteins of the catecholamines in chromaffin cells and adrenergic neurones
H. Blaschko (Oxford) . . . . . . . . . . . . . . . . . . . . 239
Molecular mechanisms of nervous transmission and synaptic plasticity
E. Giacobini (Stockholm) . . . . . . . . . . . . . . . . . . . 243
Preferential secretion of newly formed catecholamines: comparison between sympathetic nerves and adrenal medulla
L. Stjärne (Stockholm) . . . . . . . . . . . . . . . . . . . . 259
Blood platelet as a model for monoaminergic neurones
M. K. Paasonen, Liisa Athee and E. Solatunturi (Helsinki) . . . . . . . . . . . . 269
Mast cell as a model for uptake and storage of 5-hydroxytryptamine
S.-E. Jansson (Helsinki) . . . . . . . . . . . . . . . . . . . 281
Effects of inorganic electrolytes on the membrane transport and metabolism of serotonin and norepinephrine by synaptosomes
Anja H. Tissari and D. F. Bogdanski (Helsinki and Bethesda) . . . . . . . . . . 291


V. Histochemistry of Cholinergic Nervous Transmission 303

ZIO-positive and ZIO-negative vesicles in nerve terminals
K. Akert, E. Kawana and Clara Sandri (Zürich and Tokyo) . . . . . . . . . . . 305
Dense contents in synaptic vesicles produced by sequential cation binding, alcohol treatment and osmium tetroxide fixation
A. Kokko and R. J. Barrnett (New Haven) . . . . . . . . . . . . . . . 319
The histochemical localization of choline acetyltransferase
A. M. Burt (Nashville) . . . . . . . . . . . . . . . . . . . . 327
Ultrastructural localization of choline acetyltransferase and acetylcholinesterase in central and peripheral nervous tissue
P. Kása (Szeged) . . . . . . . . . . . . . . . . . . . . . . 337
The significance of cholinesterase in the developing nervous system
Ann Silver (Cambridge) . . . . . . . . . . . . . . . . . . . . 345
The demonstration of acetylcholinesterase in autonomic axons with the electron microscope
P. M. Robinson (Melbourne) . . . . . . . . . . . . . . . . . . 357
New findings concerning the localization by electron microscopy of acetylcholinesterase in autonomic ganglia
G. B. Koelle, R. Davis and Eloise G. Smyrl (Philadelphia) . . . . . . . . . . . 371
Spatial relations between acetylcholinesterase and the acetylcholine-synthesizing system in a cholinergic neuron
B. Csillik (Szeged) . . . . . . . . . . . . . . . . . . . . . 377


VI. Autonomic Innervation Patterns 387

Fine-structural identification of autonomic nerves and their relation to smooth muscle
G. Burnstock and T. Iwayama (Melbourne) . . . . . . . . . . . . . . . 389
On the vegetative cardiac innervation
T. H. Schiebler and J. Winckler (Würzburg) . . . . . . . . . . . . . . 405

Innervation of bull retractor penis muscle and peripheral autonomic mechanism of erection
  E. Klinge and P. Pohto (Helsinki) . . . . . . . . . . . . . . . . . . . . . . . 415
Observations on the nerve terminals in the neural lobe of the hypophysis of the rat
  Leena Rechardt (Helsinki) . . . . . . . . . . . . . . . . . . . . . . . . . . 423
The postnatal development of monoamines and cholinesterases in the paracervical ganglion
  of the rat uterus
  L. Kanerva (Helsinki) . . . . . . . . . . . . . . . . . . . . . . . . . . . 433
On the innervation and differentiation of human fetal chromaffin tissue
  A. Hervonen (Helsinki) . . . . . . . . . . . . . . . . . . . . . . . . . . . 445
Localization of acid phosphatase in the adrenal medulla of the albino rat
  R. E. Coupland, Lucia Mastrolia and Brenda S. Weakley (Nottingham, Roma and Dundee) 455


**VII. Experimental Histochemistry of Autonomic Innervation**                         465

Sympathetic reinnervation of anterior chamber transplants
  T. Malmfors and L. Olson (Stockholm) . . . . . . . . . . . . . . . . . . . 467
Changes in autonomic nerves of salivary glands on degeneration and regeneration
  J. R. Garrett (London) . . . . . . . . . . . . . . . . . . . . . . . . . . 475
Noradrenaline transport in sympathetic nerves
  D. Mayor, P. Banks, D. R. Tomlinson and Rosanne Grigas (Sheffield) . . . . . . . . . 489
Studies on the sympathetic neurone *in vitro*
  J. D. Lever and R. Presley (Cardiff) . . . . . . . . . . . . . . . . . . . . . 499
Evidence for the nervous control of secretion in the ciliary processes
  R. Uusitalo and A. Palkama (Helsinki) . . . . . . . . . . . . . . . . . . . 513
Author index . . . . . . . . . . . . . . . . . . . . . . . . . . . . . . . 522
Subject index . . . . . . . . . . . . . . . . . . . . . . . . . . . . . . . 523

# Functional Aspects of the Localization of Transmitter Substances

MARTHE VOGT

*Agricultural Research Council Institute of Animal Physiology, Babraham, Cambridge (England)*

When substances of high biological activity are found in the brain, the question of their possible function immediately comes to mind. If, furthermore, such a compound is found to be unevenly distributed, this fact suggests that the compound may take part in some specialized function attached to those regions which are particularly rich in it. It is with this reasoning in mind that the monoamines were first mapped in the brain, noradrenaline (NA) and 5-hydroxytryptamine (5-HT) in 1954 (Vogt; Amin *et al.*) and dopamine (DA) in 1959 (Carlsson). In the course of the last 10 years, the view has been strengthened that the monoamines act as transmitters (or modulators of transmission) in the brain. This view was not difficult to accept for NA which is known to be a transmitter at adrenergic synapses in the periphery, but often doubted for 5-HT or DA since transmission by 5-HT or DA is unknown in vertebrate peripheral nerves; such transmission has, however, been demonstrated for invertebrates.

The evidence for the transmitter nature of cerebral monoamines is based (1) on fluorescence microscopy (Carlsson *et al.*, 1962), which shows the localization within the entire neurone; (2) on electron microscopy, which makes it likely that all monoamines are stored in axonal vesicles: many papers in this symposium are going to deal with this aspect; (3) on the fact that release of some of these substances can be obtained as a response of the brain to suitable stimuli. Thus DA or one of its metabolites is released from the striatum on stimulation of the substantia nigra (McLennan, 1965; Portig and Vogt, 1969), and release of 5-HT from cortex and subcortical regions is seen on stimulation of the raphe nuclei (Eccleston *et al.*, 1969; Holman and Vogt, 1970); (4) on electrophysiological evidence: York (1970) recorded potentials from cells in the cat's putamen and compared the changes produced by local application of DA with those following electrical stimulation of the substantia nigra. The changes were identical in 77% of the excited cells. In similar experiments carried out by Connor (1970) on the caudate nucleus, correlation was complete for inhibitory effects, but only about half the neurones excited by electrical stimulation were facilitated by DA.

Thus the monoamines, like acetylcholine, are formed and contained in groups of neurones which appear to transmit their impulses with the help of these amines. Therefore the question of the function of these substances becomes the question of the action of these systems of neurones, a problem which can only be attacked by a combination of physiological and anatomical methods. Histologically, the axons of 'monoaminergic' neurones have in common to be thin and unmyelinated, by far the finest fibres, according to both electrophysiological and anatomical data, being those containing DA. Therefore these neurones are difficult to identify with conventional neuroanatomical methods. Some myelinated fibres use acetylcholine as transmitter, but the transmitters serving the majority of myelinated fibres have still to be established.

The first question one tends to ask is whether a neuronal system making use of a particular transmitter subserves an excitatory or an inhibitory function. In some cases this is easy to answer. Thus it has become very likely that certain amino acids, such as γ-aminobutyric acid (GABA), glycine and glutamic acid play, in addition to their metabolic role, the role of transmitters of impulses. If this view is confirmed, there is little doubt that the first two amino acids, which hyperpolarize cells, will form part of inhibitory pathways, whereas glutamic acid, known to accelerate or evoke cell discharge, could only be a transmitter of excitatory impulses. No such simple answer exists for neurones using acetylcholine or the monoamines as transmitters; depending on circumstances, these substances when applied locally by iontophoresis can inhibit or excite nerve cells, as has been shown for acetylcholine (Randic et al., 1964; Phillis and York, 1967), NA and 5-HT (Bradley and Wolstencroft, 1962; Phillis and Tebecis, 1967; Johnson et al., 1968) and DA (York, 1970).

There are several ways of obtaining information on the role in brain function of neurones containing a particular transmitter: apart from applying the substance locally or systemically, drugs can be used to cause accumulation or disappearance of a single transmitter, and a study made of functional disturbances thus elicited. Occasionally, neuronal degeneration in man can be sufficiently selective to allow conclusions to be drawn about the function of one type of neurone.

## ACETYLCHOLINE

Shute and Lewis (1967) and Krnjević and Silver (1965, 1966) have traced many of the cerebral cholinergic neurones histologically by staining the tissue for cholinesterase. A good example of a system of cholinergic neurones appearing to subserve a particular function is the ascending activating system of the reticular formation. Thus hemisection of the midbrain in front of the activating reticular formation produces an EEG characteristic of sleep and an accumulation of acetylcholine in the inactive hemisphere (Pepeu and Mantegazzini, 1964). Anticholinesterases or acetylcholine given intravenously, or applied to the ventricular surfaces in moderate doses, cause arousal which can be suppressed by atropine (Freedman et al., 1949). Electrical stimulation of the reticular formation not only causes arousal which also is atropine sensitive, but simultaneously increases the amount of acetylcholine released from the surface of the cortex (Kanai and Szerb, 1965; Phillis, 1968). One is tempted to conclude that arousal is the result of the stimulation of cholinergic neurones in the reticular formation. However, two disturbing observations were made by Desmedt (1956) and Desmedt and La Grutta (1957). Desmedt found that inhibitors of pseudo-cholinesterases were much more potent than inhibitors of acetyl-cholinesterases in producing arousal; and he and La Grutta saw arousal by anticholinesterases in preparations in which the whole of the reticular formation had been removed. This need only mean that the alert pattern of the EEG can also be obtained by stimulating cholinergic neurones situated in the cortex, but it emphasizes the shaky nature of evidence obtained on a structure as complex as the brain.

The second site worthy of discussion is the corpus striatum, well known for its richness in acetylcholine, choline acetylase and choline esterase. In this region, acetyl-choline esterase is found both in cells and in terminals. Iontophoretic application of acetylcholine in the unanaesthetized decerebrate cat increases the rate of firing of many striatal neurones (Bloom et al., 1965). Furthermore, as shown by Portig and Vogt (1969), a multitude of afferent stimuli causing evoked potentials in the caudate nucleus increases the release of acetylcholine from the ventricular surface of the caudate nucleus, provided anticholinesterases are present. Atrophy of the striatum leads to different forms of chorea, such as the hereditary Huntington's chorea, and overactivity of its cholinergic neurones, as will be discussed later, appears to be causally related to some signs of Parkinson's disease. This causal relation is probably the basis for the beneficial effect of atropine-like drugs in this disease. It is thus possible to allocate specific motor dysfunctions to the overactivity of striatal cholinergic neurones, but a positive statement about the way in which they keep motility normal is not possible at the present state of physiological knowledge of the interaction of motor pathways.

## NORADRENALINE

Early experiments by Bonvallet, Dell and Hiebel (1954) in which arousal was seen to follow intravenous injections of adrenaline and noradrenaline, were interpreted as a direct central stimulatory effect of these amines on the reticular formation. This inter-pretation had to be revised, and the present view is inclined to attribute the arousal to direct or indirect stimulation of afferents in the periphery. One reason for this view is that, unless the doses used are extremely large, very little amine penetrates the blood–brain barrier.

A clear correlation, however, exists between accelerated turnover of endogenous NA in hypothalamus and midbrain and increased central sympathetic activity. This may be produced by drugs (Vogt, 1954), by stress (Maynert and Levi, 1964, and many others), or by stimulation of the amygdala (Reis and Gunne, 1965). These last experi-ments confirmed that noradrenaline turnover was only enhanced if the stimulation elicited a defence reaction, in other words, when the hypothalamus was activated. It is important to remember, however, that excitement and motor activity may accompany, but are no integral part of increased central sympathetic activity; in some circum-stances it is accompanied by so-called 'freezing', and in others it is completely lacking in behavioural counterparts, as when it is caused by, say, insulin.

In contrast to the manifestations of enhanced sympathetic activity which are accompanied by increased turnover of endogenous NA, administration of this compound in a way that reaches the brain causes general depressant effects or sleep. The effect is seen when NA is applied to ventricle-near structures by intraventricular injection (Feldberg and Sherwood, 1954), or applied to the whole brain, either by

giving the NA precursor dihydroxyphenylserine parenterally (Havlicek and Sklenovsky, 1967), or by injecting NA intravenously into small chicks in which the blood–
brain barrier is undeveloped (Dewhurst and Marley, 1965). The site of this action is
not known, but it may be relevant that according to Roussel (1967) the destruction of
pontine nuclei rich in adrenergic neurones (Locus coeruleus) abolishes paradoxical
sleep.

Interpretation (in terms of physiological events) of experiments in which a transmitter substance is applied to the brain is complicated by the fact that cells may have
receptors for the transmitter and yet may not be innervated by terminals releasing that
transmitter. Bearing that difficulty in mind, those experiments are most relevant in
which effects are obtained by micro-injection of substances into the vicinity of terminals known to act by releasing these substances. Thus, Feldberg and Myers (1964)
injected NA into the hypothalamus and reported changes in body temperature of cats,
and Grossman (1960, 1964), injecting a few $\mu$g of solid drug into the lateral hypothalamus of rats, saw compulsive eating when he applied NA, and drinking when the
NA was replaced by acetylcholine. In view of the presence of both adrenergic and
cholinergic neurones in the hypothalamus, the chances are good that physiological
events make use of the same transmitters.

## DOPAMINE

Flooding of the brain with DA, either by intracarotid injection of its precursor,
DOPA (Mantegazzini and Glässer, 1960), or by following the administration of an
inhibitor of MAO with that of DOPA, causes arousal, or increased irritability and
motor activity (Everett, 1961). In man, choreiform movements may develop on
repeated oral administration of L-DOPA. There are good reasons for attributing these
effects of injected DOPA to the formation of DA and not of NA. Chemical estimation
of the amines at the time of appearance of arousal after intracarotid injection showed
NA concentrations to be unchanged, whereas DA concentrations were elevated
(Dagirmanjian et al., 1963) and had risen by the same proportion in the DA-rich
caudate nucleus and in the DA-poor hypothalamus. The justification for attributing
the arousal under these conditions to the rise in DA is supported by the experiments
with dihydroxyphenylserine referred to above (Havlicek and Sklenovsky, 1967),
which demonstrate that an increase in catecholamines limited to NA causes prolonged
sleep in rats, not enhanced excitability. Different responses are, however, obtained in
birds. In the young chick DA and NA both cause sleep (Dewhurst and Marley, 1965),
whereas DOPA does not (Spooner and Winters, 1967); furthermore, the injection of
DOPA in adult pigeons fails to produce excitement (Jurio and Vogt, 1967). It may be
that the enzymatic transformation of DA to NA is more rapid in the bird than in the
mammal so that less DA accumulates in the brain.

A selective loss of DA from the human striatum is known to be at least part of the
biochemical basis of Parkinson's disease; it comes about through degeneration of
what are considered to be dopaminergic axons originating in cells of the substantia
nigra. These cells are destroyed in Parkinsonism, and this knowledge should provide

an unique opportunity to discover the function of striatal dopamine. As pointed out earlier, some of the signs of Parkinson's disease are believed to result from uninhibited action of striatal cholinergic neurons, and DA is held to be the transmitter which normally keeps this activity in check. A model for this interaction is found in experiments by Bloom *et al.* (1965) in the cat. By applying acetylcholine and DA electrophoretically to neurones of the caudate nucleus, these authors observed a suppression by DA of the rapid discharge elicited by acetylcholine. Of the different signs of Parkinson's disease, such as akinesia, rigidity and tremor, the first two, and particularly the akinesia, are the more likely ones to be produced by lack of dopaminergic activity.

A small isolated group of dopamine-containing cells is found in the hypothalamus where it forms part of the nucleus arcuatus. Since injection of DA into the third ventricle of rats causes the release of luteinizing hormone (LH), this release is also supposed to be the normal function of the nucleus arcuatus. The release of LH probably takes place through the intermediary of the so-called releasing factor LRF (Schneider and McCann, 1970; Kamberi *et al.*, 1970).

I cannot leave the subject of DA without raising the question of the interrelation between catecholamine-containing neurones and mood. The fact that antidepressive drugs affect metabolism or uptake of monoamines, and that all phenothiazine derivatives useful in schizophrenia interfere with DA metabolism suggests that monoaminergic neurones must play some role in the clinical picture of psychoses. There is, however, not a shred of evidence that these are the nigro-striatal dopaminergic neurones. Yet, just as the motor disability accompanying the disappearance of DA-containing terminals from the striatum is improved by giving atropine, the deleterious effect on conditioned avoidance reflexes of drugs such as the phenothiazines which interfere with DA metabolism is antagonized by atropine and its congeners (Hanson *et al.*, 1970). It may be that the effect of the phenothiazines which is responsible for the disruption of the conditioned avoidance response is completely divorced from their effect on DA metabolism, but since this disruption is antagonized by atropine, it is likely to involve excessive or unchecked activity of cholinergic neurones somewhere in the brain.

## 5-HYDROXYTRYPTAMINE

Views about the function of 5-HT-containing neurones have recently made some spectacular progress. Not that we are any nearer an understanding of their possible role in psychoses, but their importance in some fundamental nervous processes is becoming clearer. The cruder methods of flooding the brain with 5-HT, either by arterial injection of its precursor amino acid (Glässer and Mantegazzini, 1960), or by intraventricular injection of the base (Feldberg and Sherwood, 1954), produce a state of sleep in the EEG of the cerveau isolé, and cause lethargy in the intact conscious cat.

Participation in certain brain functions by neurones transmitting their impulses with 5-HT has now been shown in four fields. First, Feldberg and Myers (1964) found that injection of 5-HT into the anterior hypothalamus raised the body temperature of cats, and suggested that this may mimic the natural function of 5-HT-releasing synapses in that region. Work with inhibitors of MAO and with *p*-chlorophenyl-alanine confirmed this view. The importance of 5-HT for temperature regulation is also indicated by experiments in which Sheard and Aghajanian (1967, 1968) showed that stimulation of the 5-HT-containing caudal raphe nuclei in the rat increased both body temperature and forebrain concentration of 5-hydroxyindole acetic acid, the main metabolite of 5-HT. Furthermore, a rise in ambient temperature increased, and a fall decreased the turnover of 5-HT (Corrodi *et al.*, 1967), a temperature dependence which was not found for the catecholamines. Aghajanian and Weiss (1965) showed that this temperature dependence was abolished by LSD. Since LSD also inhibited the firing of 5-HT-containing neurones (Aghajanian *et al.*, 1968), the findings support the idea of a connection between temperature regulation and the activity of such neurones.

The next advance was the demonstration that the 5-HT-rich raphe nuclei of the lower midbrain and anterior medulla are necessary for sleep. Work by Jouvet (1962) and his colleague Renault (1967) has shown that surgical destruction of these nuclei, or serious reduction of their 5-HT content by the drug *p*-chlorophenylalanine, render the animals incapable of sleep; restoration can be obtained by giving 5-HTP, the precursor of 5-HT, to such sleepless animals. It appears that the raphe nuclei are directly responsible for the production of slow-wave sleep, whereas their influence on the noradrenaline-rich region of the nucleus coeruleus is controlling paradoxical sleep.

A third cerebral function in which 5-HT carrying neurones have recently been found to be involved is pain sensation. Rats treated with *p*-chlorophenylalanine develop hyperalgesia, so that they can be trained more easily than normal rats to avoid electric shocks to their feet (Tenen, 1967). Morphine and other analgesics have much reduced effects on the pain threshold of such animals (Tenen, 1968). The site of this action might again be the raphe nuclei and these would act by sending impulses into the cord which could modulate the sensory input from the periphery (Melzack and Wall, 1965). Recently, Sparkes and Spencer (1969) reported that the well-known loss of analgesic effect of morphine which is elicited in the rat by giving reserpine can be restored by intraventricular injection of 5-HT. However, I would be negligent of my duties if I would conceal that the analgesic effect of morphine is also adversely affected by inhibiting the synthesis of catecholamines by means of α-methyl-DOPA (Verri *et al.*, 1968). There are obviously more than one mechanisms controlling pain perception.

Finally, experiments with *p*-chlorophenylalanine (PCPA) on rats and cats have shown that manifestations of sexual activity are under control of cerebral 5-HT. Shillito (1969, 1970a) treated young male rats with doses of PCPA which reduced the cerebral 5-HT content by over 80%. She found that the animals groomed each other excessively to the extent of producing bald patches on rats with which they shared the cage, whereas adult males showed misdirected sexual activity by mounting each other; female rats were not affected. In cats, mounting behaviour was seen in both young and adult males, and young and adult animals of both sexes exhibited postures adopted by normal oestrous females (Shillito, 1970b; Hoyland *et al.*, 1970). Injection of the precursor of 5-HT, 5-hydroxytryptophan, arrested all abnormal behaviour in both species for a few hours while the 5-HT content of the brain was temporarily raised.

My last reference will again have to be to Parkinson's disease. There are not only acetylcholine and DA in the striatum, but also 5-HT; its concentration is lowered in the brain of Parkinsonian patients (Hornykiewicz, 1963). In monkeys in which hypokinesia and tremor were produced by ventromedial tegmental lesions, the administration of 5-HTP relieved the tremor (Goldstein *et al.*, 1969). Thus all three transmitters known to occur in the striatum appear to contribute to the control of motor function exerted by that region.

## REFERENCES

AGHAJANIAN, G. K., FOOTE, W. E. AND SHEARD, M. H., (1968) *Science*, **161**, 706.
AGHAJANIAN, G. K. AND WEISS, B. L. (1965), *Nature*, **220**, 795.
AMIN, A. H., CRAWFORD, T. B. B. AND GADDUM, J. H. (1954), *J. Physiol.*, **126**, 596.
BLOOM, F. E., COSTA, E. AND SALMOIRAGHI, G. C. (1965), *J. Pharmacol.*, **150**, 244.
BONVALLET, M., DELL, P. AND HIEBEL, G. (1954), *Electroencephalog. clin. Neurophysiol.*, **6**, 119.
BRADLEY, P. B. AND WOLSTENCROFT, J. H. (1962) *Nature*, **196**, 840.
CARLSSON, A. (1959), *Pharmacol. Rev.*, **11**, 490.
CARLSSON, A., FALCK, B. AND HILLARP, N.-Å. (1962), *Acta physiol. scand.*, **56**, suppl. 196.
CONNOR, J. D. (1970), *J. Physiol.*, **208**, 691.
CORRODI, H., FUXE, K. AND HÖKFELT, T. (1967), *Acta physiol. scand.*, **71**, 224.
DAGIRMANJIAN, R., LAVERTY, R., MANTEGAZZINI, P., SHARMAN, D. F. AND VOGT, M. (1963), *J. Neurochem.*, **10**, 177.
DESMEDT, J. E. (1956), *Electroencephalog. clin., Neurophysiol.*, **8**, 701.
DESMEDT, J. E. AND LA GRUTTA, G. (1957), *J. Physiol.*, **136**, 20.
DEWHURST, W. Q. AND MARLEY, E. (1965), *Brit. J. Pharmacol. Chemotherap.*, **25**, 705.
ECCLESTON, D., RANDIĆ, M., ROBERTS, M. H. T. AND STRAUGHAN, D. W., *Metabolism of Amines in the Brain*, in G. HOOPER (Ed.), Macmillan, London, 1969, p. 29.
EVERETT, G. (1961), *Neuro-psychopharmacology*, **2**, 479.
FELDBERG, W. AND MYERS, R. D. (1964), *J. Physiol.*, **173**, 25P.
FELDBERG, W. AND SHERWOOD, S. L. (1954), *J. Physiol.*, **123**, 148.
FERGUSON, J., HENRIKSEN, S., COHEN, H., MITCHELL, G., BARCHAS, J. AND DEMENT, W. (1970), *Science*, **168**, 499.
FREEDMAN, A. M., BALES, P. D., WILLIS, A. AND HIMWICH, H. E. (1949), *Am. J. Physiol.*, **156**, 117.
GLÄSSER, A. AND MANTEGAZZINI, P. (1960), *Arch. Ital. Biol.*, **98**, 351.
GOLDSTEIN, M., BATTISTA, A. F., NAKATANI, S. AND ANAGNOSTE, B. (1969), *Proc. Natl. Acad. Sci. U.S.*, **63**, 1113.
GROSSMAN, S. P. (1960), *Science*, **132**, 301.
GROSSMAN, S. P. (1964), *Intern. J. Neuropharmacol.*, **3**, 45.
HANSON, H. M., STONE, C. A. AND WITOSLAWSKI, J. J. (1970), *J. Pharmacol.*, **173**, 117.
HAVLICEK, V. AND SKLENOVSKY, A. (1967), *Brain Res.*, **4**, *345*.
HOLMAN, R. B. AND VOGT, M. (1970), *J. Physiol.*, **210**, 163.
HORNYKIEWICZ, O. (1963), *Wien. klin. Wochschr.*, **75**, 309.
HOYLAND, V., SHILLITO, E. AND VOGT, M. (1970), *Brit. J. Pharmac.*, in the press.
JOHNSON, E. S., ROBERTS, M. H. T., SOBIESZEK, A. AND STRAUGHAN, D. W. (1968), *Brit. J. Pharmac.*, **34**, 221 P.
JOUVET, M. (1962), *Arch. Ital. Biol.*, **100**, 125.
JUORIO, A. V. AND VOGT, M. (1967), *J. Physiol.*, **189**, 489.
KAMBERI, I. A., MICAL, R. S. AND PORTER, J. C. (1970), *Endocrinology*, **87**, 1.
KANAI, T. AND SZERB, J. C. (1965), *Nature*, **205**, 80.
KRNJEVIĆ, K. AND SILVER, A. (1965), *J. Anat.*, **99**, 711.
KRNJEVIĆ, K. AND SILVER, A. (1966), *J. Anat.* **100**, 63.
LEWIS, P. R. AND SHUTE, C. C. D. (1967), *Brain*, **90**, 521.
MCLENNAN, H. (1965), *Experientia*, **21**, 725.
MANTEGAZZINI, P. AND GLÄSSER, A., (1960), *Arch. Ital. Biol.*, **98**, 367.

MAYNERT, E. W. AND LEVI, R. (1964), *J. Pharmacol.*, **143**, 95.

MELZACK, R. AND WALL, P. D. (1965), *Science*, **150**, 971.

PEPEU, G. AND MANTEGAZZINI, P., (1964) *Science*, **145**, 1069.

PHILLIS, J. W. (1968), *Brain Res.*, **7**, 378.

PHILLIS, J. W. AND TEBĒCIS, A. K. (1967), *J. Physiol.*, **192**, 715.

PHILLIS, J. W. AND YORK, D. H. (1967), *Brain Res.*, **5**, 517.

PORTIG, P. J. AND VOGT, M. (1969), *J. Physiol.*, **204**, 687.

RANDIĆ, M., SIMINOFF, R. AND STRAUGHAN, D. W. (1964), *Exp. Neurol.*, **9**, 236.

REIS, D. J. AND GUNNE, L.-M. (1965), *Science*, **149**, 450.

RENAULT, J., *Monoamines et Sommeils III.* (Thèse), Tixier et fils, Lyon, 1967.

ROUSSEL, B., *Monoamines et Sommeils IV.* (Thèse), Tixier et fils, Lyon, 1967.

SCHNEIDER, H. P. G. AND McCANN, S. M. (1970), *Endocrinology*, **86**, 1127.

SHEARD, M. A. AND AGHAJANIAN, G. K. (1967), *Nature*, **216**, 495.

SHEARD, M. A. AND AGHAJANIAN, G. K. (1968), *J. Pharmacol.*, **163**, 425.

SHILLITO, E. (1969), *Brit. J. Pharmac.*, **36**, 193 P.

SHILLITO, E. (1970a), *Brit. J. Pharmac.*, **38**, 305.

SHILLITO, E. (1970b), *J. Physiol.*, **210**, 162.

SHUTE, C. C. D. AND LEWIS, P. R. (1967) *Brain*, **90**, 497.

SPARKES, C. G. AND SPENCER, P. S. J. (1969), *Brit. J. Pharmacol.*, **35**, 362 P.

SPOONER, C. E. AND WINTERS, W. D. (1967), *Brain Res.*, **4**, 189.

TENEN, S. S. (1967), *Psychopharmacologia (Berl.)*, **10**, 204.

TENEN, S. S. (1968), *Psychopharmacologia (Berl.)*, **12**, 278.

VERRI, R. A., GRAEFF, F. G. AND CORRADO, A. P. (1968), *Intern. J. Neuropharmacol.*, **7**, 283.

VOGT, M. (1954), *J. Physiol.*, **123**, 451.

YORK, D. A. (1970), *Brain Res.*, **20**, *233*.

# I. LIGHT MICROSCOPIC HISTOCHEMISTRY OF MONOAMINE TRANSMITTERS

# Visualization of Intraneuronal Monoamines by Treatment with Formalin Solutions

A. V. SAKHAROVA AND D. A. SAKHAROV

*Institute of Neurology, Academy of Medical Sciences, and Institute of Developmental Biology, Academy of Sciences, Vavilowstr. 26, Moscow (U.S.S.R.)*

## INTRODUCTION

For a long time, the only method available for demonstrating intraneuronal monoamines was the gaseous formaldehyde (F) condensation technique developed by Falck and Hillarp (1962; Falck and Owman, 1965; Corrodi and Jonsson, 1967). Aqueous F, which had been used in the early days of fluorescence histochemistry of biogenic amines (Erös, 1932; Eränkö, 1955), at first found no favour among neurohistochemists. It was generally accepted that the procedure involving the incubation of pieces of tissue in formalin solutions, though suitable for inducing catecholamine fluorescence in the adrenal medulla, was not sensitive enough to visualize catecholamines of adrenergic nerves.

However, contrary to this view, Eränkö and Räisänen (1966) were able to demonstrate noradrenaline (NA) of sympathetic fibres in the stretch preparation of rat iris after incubation in an aqueous F solution. This observation was followed by attempts to apply the aqueous technique to cryostat sections and successful visualization of intraneuronal NA (Laties *et al.*, 1967; El-Badawi and Schenk, 1967; Sakharova and Sakharov, 1968b), dopamine (DA) and 5-hydroxytryptamine (5-HT) (Sakharova and Sakharov, 1968a) was reported.

From 1967 on, we used the aqueous F method routinely in continuing studies of adrenergic nerves in the rat (A.V.S.) and of monoaminergic neurones in gastropod molluscs (D.A.S.). The method, in our hands, gives reproducible results supporting the idea that the aqueous and gaseous techniques, when properly used, have essentially the same specificity and sensitivity while differing in their respective restrictions. Our purpose here is to report the methodology of the aqueous technique and to discuss some of its advantages and limitations.

## ABBREVIATIONS

| | | | | |
|---|---|---|---|---|
| CA | = catecholamine | | F | = formaldehyde |
| CNS | = central nervous system | | NA | = noradrenaline |
| DA | = dopamine | | 5-HT | = 5-hydroxytryptamine |

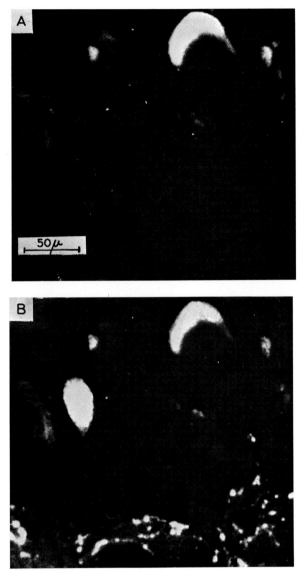

Fig. 1. Cryostat section of the cerebral ganglion of a pulmonate snail, *Caucasotachea*. Incubation in 0.5% formalin for 30 min, drying in air at room temperature for 40 min. A — just after mounting in paraffin oil: autofluorescence in some nerve cells. B — the same area after heating at 80° for 10 min: a single perikaryon and numerous axonal varicosities show specific fluorescence.

## DISTINCTIVE FEATURES OF THE AQUEOUS TECHNIQUE

Outlined schematically, the procedure used is as follows (Sakharova and Sakharov, 1968b). Pieces of tissue are incubated in ice-cold formalin–saline solution, then frozen with $CO_2$ and sectioned in a cryostat. Sections placed on slides are dried in air and mounted under a coverslip in mineral (paraffin) oil. After noting, and if necessary recording photographically the autofluorescence present (Fig. 1A), the mounts are heated to induce the specific fluorescence (Fig. 1B). Whole mounts are processed in the same way. Details are given and discussed below.

The obvious difference of this procedure from the gaseous one does not mean that the two procedures differ in their basic chemistry. On the contrary, there is little doubt that the reaction products are the same. The colour of the specific fluorescence is identical in identical cells treated with gaseous or aqueous F. We have studied spectral characteristics of the fluorescence induced by a formalin solution in rat meninges. The fluorescent product of NA (sympathetic fibres) was shown to have an emission peak at about 480 nm and the product of 5-HT (mast cells) at 525–528 nm. The velocity of photodecomposition of the fluorescence was much greater in mast cells and identifiable serotoninergic nerve cells of molluscs than that in DA- and NA- containing cells and fibres. The fluorescence induced by formalin is quenched by water. It can be also quenched by sodium borohydride in alcoholic solutions and then be regenerated by F gas.

The identity of the reaction products suggests that the two methods, gaseous and aqueous, have an identical chemical background.

The mechanism underlying the gaseous method of Falck and Hillarp is known to involve the condensation of an amine with F, and the subsequent dehydrogenation of the condensed compound by F (Corrodi and Jonsson, 1967). In the gaseous method, the two reactions are carried out simultaneously when the tissue is exposed to the hot F gas. As to the aqueous technique, our working hypothesis is that the condensation reaction occurs during the incubation of tissue samples in aqueous F solution, while the final step of the procedure, heating in oil, corresponds to the dehydrogenation reaction.

Actually, water is known to be an adequate medium for the condensation reaction (see Corrodi and Jonsson, 1967). Immediately after drying, sections show no specific fluorescence. This fact clearly indicates that the dehydrogenation reaction does not take place during the incubation of tissue in a cold F solution. The fluorescence develops in dried sections owing to a spontaneous reaction which is facilitated by covering sections with oil. This reaction is temperature dependent and requires F.

Although supported by these facts, our working hypothesis so far is without direct experimental justification. The role of water at the final step of the procedure also remains to be elucidated. Available data in this respect are controversial.

Lacking firm chemical data, we can nevertheless emphasize the most important difference between the gaseous and the aqueous F methods. In the former the reactions are inseparable and provided with a uniform set of reaction conditions. In the latter the reaction conditions are different at two steps of the chemical process. As a result of this separation, the aqueous method is highly flexible compared with the gaseous one.

### INCUBATION

We prepare the incubation medium by the dilution of commercial formalin (approximately 40% w/v F solution) with a corresponding Ringer's solution or with a solution

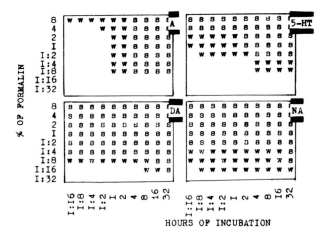

Fig. 2. The effect of the time of incubation and of formalin concentration on development of specific fluorescence in model experiments. w — weak fluorescence, s — strong fluorescence; A — adrenaline, other abbreviations as in the text.

of a neutral salt, usually sodium chloride. It appears that solutions prepared from paraformaldehyde do not offer significant advantage. Since the incubation is carried out at about 0°, there is no need to use complex media containing metabolic substrates. The cooling is believed to prevent the dislocation of cellular monoamines; it also arrests cytolytic changes, providing preservation of tissue structure.

Studies involving model experiments were undertaken to determine more precisely the time of incubation and concentration of formalin required for the formation of fluorophores. The following substances were used: L-adrenaline (Fluka), dopamine chlorhydrate (Fluka), serotonin creatinine phosphate (Reanal), DL-noradrenaline hydrochloride (Winthrop Lab.).

The procedure for the model experiments was an imitation of the histochemical method. Two ml of ice-cold aqueous solution of the substance to be examined in a concentration of 4 mg/ml was added to 2 ml of ice-cold formalin solution and incubated at about 0°. From time to time, a drop was taken from the mixture and spread over the cooled slide covered with the dry protein film. The smear was then dried in a stream of cold air, covered with paraffin oil and heated at 80° for 15 min.

In these experiments, the concentration of formalin varied from 1:32 to 16% and the time of incubation from 4 min to 32 h.

Model experiments have shown that formalin is capable of inducing fluorescence even in very dilute solutions. Moreover, the actual time of incubation can be very short, adrenaline being an exception in this respect (Fig. 2). A small decrease in F concentration can be compensated for by increased reaction time, and vice versa; for adrenaline, however, the time of incubation seems to be a more important factor than the concentration of F.

Model experiments thus demonstrate that reaction conditions are specific for each of the transmitter amines in question. They can be selected within a fairly wide area

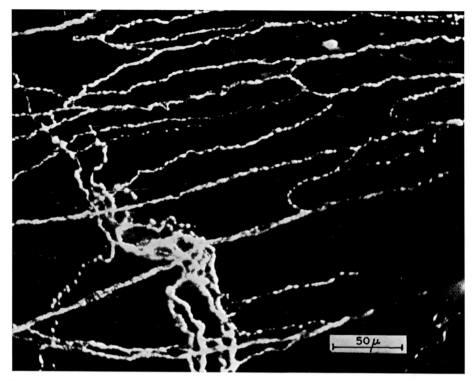

Fig. 3. Whole mount preparation of the rat meninges. Incubation in 0.5% formalin for 135 min. Fluorescence of NA in perivascular and free sympathetic fibres.

which, in fact, is not so wide when tissue monoamines are revealed. In the latter case, the threshold concentrations of F are higher than those in model experiments since F takes part in reactions other than condensation with transmitter amines. For example, DAergic nerve cells and fibres in snails can be effectively visualized after incubation in 0.5% formalin, while a 0.25% solution induces barely visible fluorescence. For visualization of sympathetic NA in rat, the lowest actual concentration of formalin is of the same order (Figs. 1, 3). To induce maximal fluorescence of cellular 5-HT the concentration should be 4% or even higher.

The time of incubation with a thin tissue, such as rat meninges can be as short as with chemical models. If a piece of tissue is incubated, the incubation time should be sufficient for formalin to penetrate the block. We usually incubate small pieces of tissue for 20–30 min.

Diffusion of amines from cells is the main factor limiting the time of incubation. Systematic experiments performed on rat meninges have shown that, in adrenergic fibres, diffusion of fluorescence can be marked after 2–4 h of incubation. In the same tissue, 5-HT of mast cells can still be seen fairly sharply in its characteristic granule localization after 16 h of incubation (Fig. 4), but after 32 h the fluorescence disappears. However, in mollusc nerve cells, 5-HT is diffused more readily than a primary catechol-

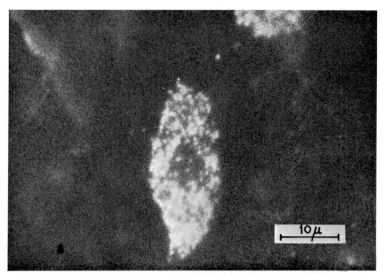

Fig. 4. Preparation as in Fig. 3. Incubation in 1 % formalin for 22.5 h. Practically no NA in sympathetic fibres while 5-HT still shows granular localization in mast cells.

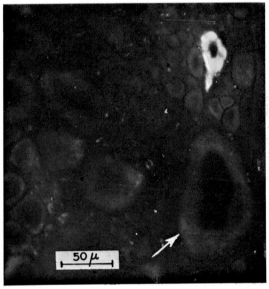

Fig. 5. Section from the same block as in Fig. 1. An identifiable DA-containing neurone in the vicinity of the dorsal giant metacerebral cell (arrow). No diffusion of DA from the neurone or into the nucleus.

amine, DA, 4 h being too long an incubation time for serotoninergic neurones.

One must agree that the time of incubation required for the reaction is much shorter than the period during which the risk of diffusion appears as far as DA, NA and 5-HT are concerned (Fig. 5). The situation seems to be different with regard to adrenaline. In frogs pretreated with adrenaline (McLean and Burnstock, 1966), the intensity of specific fluorescence of adrenergic nerves was markedly higher than in control animals when reaction conditions were as follows: incubation in 8% formalin for 3 h plus heating in oil at 80° for 90 min. It appears that the aqueous method in the present form cannot be recommended for the demonstration of adrenaline since the risk of diffusion is too obvious in this case.

In summary, the reaction conditions at this step may be varied according to the aim of the investigation. It is possible to reveal primary catecholamines only, since 5-HT requires a higher concentration of formalin. More delicate methods for differentiation between amines can be elaborated based on the addition to the incubation solution of factors influencing its pH, redox potential, etc.

Of special interest is the fact that formalin is histochemically effective in concentrations lower than those used for fixing. This enables one to select reaction conditions so as not to inactivate formalin-sensitive enzymes. These can then be revealed histochemically in the same sections. We did not pay much attention to the methodology of consecutive demonstration of monoamines and enzymes. In general, the following steps of the procedure can affect the enzymatic activity: incubation, mounting in oil, heating, and washing the oil out. Enzymes to be demonstrated differ in their relative sensitivity to these factors. Preliminary tests may indicate which of the factors demand special attention in each case. Our incidental attempts in this direction gave satisfactory results. Monoamine oxidase and glucose-6-phosphate dehydrogenase were among the enzymes which we could visualize, though with somewhat depressed activity, after the demonstration of primary catecholamines.

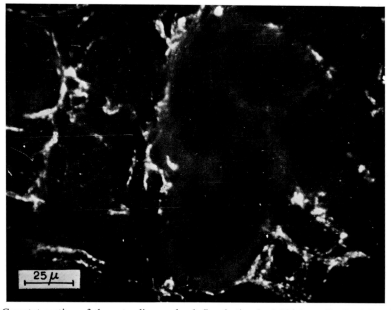

Fig. 6. Cryostat section of the rat salivary gland. Incubation in 0.8% formalin for 1 h, air-dried section was treated with paraformaldehyde–paraffin oil mixture at 80° for 10 min. Sympathetic innervation of acinar cells.

TABLE 1

RESULTS OF TESTING OF THE AQUEOUS FORMALDEHYDE TECHNIQUE ON REPRESENTATIVE ANIMAL SPECIES

| Species | Ref.[a] | Organs examined | Aqueous technique | | |
|---|---|---|---|---|---|
| | | | Prep.[b] | Res.[c] | Comments |
| Coelenterata Anthozoa | | | | | |
|   Metridium senile (sea anemone) | Dahl et al., 1963 | Tentacles | S | + | |
| Plathyhelminthes Turbellaria | | | | | |
|   Dendrocoelum lacteum (planarian) | Plotnikova and Kuzmina 1968 | Total | S | + | |
| Annelida Oligochaeta | | | | | |
|   Lumbricus terrestris (earth worm) | Rude, 1966; Myhrberg, 1967; Plotnikova and Govyrin, 1967 | CNS | S, WM | + | |
| Arthropoda Crustacea | | | | | |
|   Astacus leptodactylus (crayfish) | Elofsson et al., 1966 | CNS, head ganglia | S | − | |
| | | CNS, ventral cord | S | ± | |
| Arthropoda Insecta | | | | | |
|   Blatta orientalis (cockroach) | Frontali, 1968 | CNS, head ganglia | S | − | |
|   Eurigaster sp. (bug) | | CNS, head ganglia | S | − | |
|   Corethra crystallinus, larvae | | Total | S | − | |
|   Chironomus sp. (midges), larvae | | Total | S | − | |
| Mollusca Pelecypoda | | | | | |
|   Sphaerium corneus (orb shell) | Sweeney, 1968 | Total | S | + | |
| Mollusca Gastropoda Prosobranchia | | | | | |
|   Acmaea testudinalis (limpet) | | CNS; foot; pharynx | S | + + | |
|   Pomatias elegans | | CNS | S | + + | |
| Mollusca Gastropoda Opisthobranchia | | | | | |
|   Dendronotus frondosus (sea slug) | | CNS; foot; penis | S | + | |
| Mollusca Gastropoda Pulmonata | | | | | |
|   Lymnaea stagnalis (pond snail) | Sakharov and Zs.-Nagy, 1968 | CNS; foot; heart | S, WM | + | |
|   Helix pomatia (edible snail) | Dahl et al., 1966; Sedden et al., 1968 | CNS; heart; etc. | S, WM | + | Positive results also on 5 other species of land snails |
|   Limax maximus (slug) | Cottrell and Osborne, 1970 | CNS; tentacles; etc. | S | + | Positive results also on 3 other species of slugs |
|   Agriolimax reticulatus (slug), late embryos | | Total | S | + | Green and yellow fluorescence in unidentified cells |
| Echinodermata Holothurioidea | | | | | |
|   Cucumaria frondosum (sea cucumber) | Cobb, 1969; Hehn, 1970; Cottrell and Pentreath, 1970 | pharynx | S | + | Primary catecholamine in ecto-neural system |

| Species | Reference | Tissue | Mode | Result | Remarks |
|---|---|---|---|---|---|
| **Echinodermata Echinoidea** | | | | | |
| *Strongylocentrotus dröbachiensis* (sea urchin), developing eggs | | Total | WM | + | Yellow fluorescence in cells of primary gut |
| **Vertebrata Cyclostomata** | | | | | |
| *Lampetra fluviatilis* (lamprey) | Leontieva, 1966 | Perivascular fibres | WM | + | |
| **Vertebrata Pisces** | | | | | |
| *Misgurnus fossilis* (freshwater mudfish) | Leontieva, 1966 | Perivascular fibres | WM | + | |
| **Vertebrata Amphibia** | | | | | |
| *Rana temporaria* (frog) | Leontieva, 1966; Mc Lean and Burnstock, 1966 | Mesentery | WM | + | Special reaction conditions (see text) |
| | | Chromaffin tissue | S | + | Primary catecholamine |
| **Vertebrata Aves** | | | | | |
| *Gallus domesticus* (fowl) | Bennett and Malmfors, 1970 | Brain | S | — | |
| | | Meninges; heart; glands; etc. | WM, S | + | |
| **Vertebrata Mammalia** | | | | | |
| *Rattus rattus* (rat) | see in Corrodi and Jonsson, 1967 | Brain | S | — | |
| | | Meninges; heart; glands; spleen; vas deferens; etc. | WM, S | + | |
| *Mus musculus* (mouse) | see in Corrodi and Jonsson, 1967 | Brain | S | — | |
| | | Heart; glands; etc. | S | + | |
| *Ovis aries* (sheep) | Falck et al. 1964 | Mesentery; lungs | WM, S | + | |

a. Reference source to results obtained with the aid of Falck–Hillarp method on the same or allied animals.

b. Mode of preparation: S = cryostat sections, WM = whole mounts.

c. Results: + = comparable with those obtained with the aid of Falck-Hillarp method, ± = of inferior fluorescence intensity, — = no specific fluorescence.

References p. 25

## STEPS FOLLOWING THE INCUBATION

In practice, the problem of dislocation of monoamines arises just after sections are cut. We prefer therefore to place sections on cooled slides. Gentle warming of the mounts prior to removing them from the cryostat prevents condensation of water from air on the sections (Hamberger and Norberg, 1964). These simple precautions make it possible to avoid diffusion artifacts at this step of the procedure.

Drying the sections over $P_2O_5$ or in cold dehydrating fluids such as acetone or an acetone–chloroform mixture gives quite good results. Drying in air is also suitable and much simpler. We dried sections in a stream of cold air or for 30–60 min at room temperature and then for a few minutes at 60–80°. However freeze-drying is unavoidable in some special cases discussed in the next paragraph.

Regardless of the method of drying, the sections should then be mounted in paraffin oil. We wish to emphasize that this is a necessary requirement for obtaining a high intensity of fluorescence, which is especially important when relatively low concentrations of formalin are used. At the final step of the procedure when a temperature-dependent reaction occurs, the oil is believed to prevent evaporation of free F which thus becomes available for the reaction. The temperature-dependent reaction can be carried out in some liquid medium other than paraffin oil, for example in chloroform. Entellan gives inferior results compared with paraffin oil.

The final heating is performed after examining the autofluorescence. Thus the differentiation between specific and nonspecific fluorescence is quite simple in the method used. It might be added that when the concentration of primary catecholamines is high (chromaffin tissue), specific fluorescence may easily appear at room temperature. Such sections must be handled at a low temperature prior to examining for autofluorescence.

In routine practice, we heat the mounts at 75–85°. To induce the fluorescence of primary catecholamines, a few minutes of heating is usually enough although 5-HT requires some minutes more. At 30–40° the fluorescence develops much more slowly but such conditions should be selected if enzymes are to be revealed.

When specific fluorescence is too strong so that details of its localization are difficult to recognize, it can be differentiated by remounting in glycerin. On the other hand, when the fluorescence is poor due to insufficient treatment with F at the aqueous step of the procedure, it can be improved by adding exogenous F. For this purpose, we introduced a simple procedure which is actually a modification of the method of Falck and Hillarp (Sakharova and Sakharov, 1971). Sections are remounted in paraffin oil mixed with a small amount of paraformaldehyde powder. When the slide is heated in an 80° oven (coverslip down), depolymerization of the aldehyde occurs and the gaseous monomeric product is taken up by sections. Such mounts can be examined under low power and after monoamines develop maximum fluorescence, the sections may be remounted in liquid paraffin. Fig. 6 shows the result of the reaction performed in this way.

This modification, in general, is suitable for air-dried cyrostat sections of fresh tissue. In such cases, the suspension should be prepared from paraformaldehyde of a proper humidity (Hamberger, 1967). Our observations confirm and extend the findings of Laties *et al.* (1967) in that the F gas gives better results when applied to tissues previously treated with aqueous F than to fresh ones.

## LIMITATIONS OF THE PRESENT TECHNIQUE

We failed to demonstrate monoamines by the aqueous method in cryostat sections of rat brain (Sakharova and Sakharov, 1968b). This fact indicated that the procedure used had restricted applicability. To learn the limits of the method, a series of tissue samples has been examined with this procedure. The representative animals used are listed in Table 1 which also contains references to studies performed by other workers using the Falck and Hillarp method on the same or allied species.

Results of the examination summarized in Table 1 show that with most of the species and tissues listed, the techniques give comparable results. However, we regularly were unable to obtain satisfactory fluorescence with central nervous system (CNS) preparations of mammals, birds and arthropods. Although the CNS of lower vertebrates and of cephalopods have not yet been examined, the area of application of the present aqueous technique in neurohistochemistry is fairly well outlined. It includes peripheral nervous systems of lower and higher vertebrates and seemingly all monoaminergic neurones, central and peripheral, of invertebrate phyla other than arthropods (Figs. 7–10).

At the present time it is difficult to satisfactorily explain the failure of the aqueous

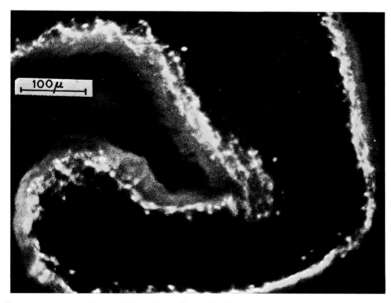

Fig. 7. Cryostat section of a nudibranch mollusc, *Dendronotus*. Incubation of the fore-part of the animal in 6% formalin for 40 min. Plexus of nerve fibres containing a primary catecholamine in the muscular wall of penis.

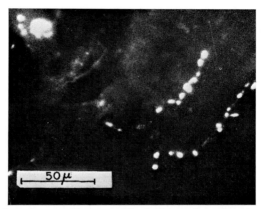

Fig. 8. Section from the same block as in Fig. 7. Fine varicose fibres in the foot muscle.

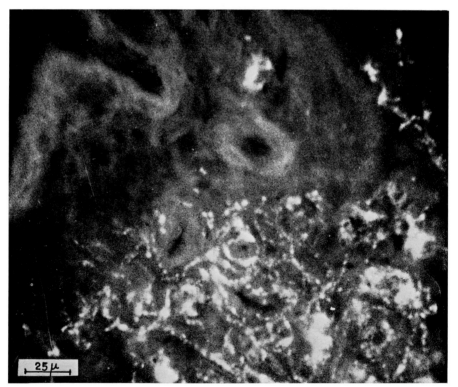

Fig. 9. Cryostat section of the carotid bifurcation region of the rat. Incubation in 0.8 % formalin for 2 h. The supplying artery of the carotid body and specific fluorescence in chromaffin cells and adrenergic fibres can be seen.

technique to yield fluorescence in some nervous tissues. The CNS of mammals and of arthropods is known to contain intraneuronal monoamines which can be revealed by the method of Falck and Hillarp. The concentration of catecholamines in presynaptic varicosities in the rat brain is reported to be of the same order of magnitude as that in

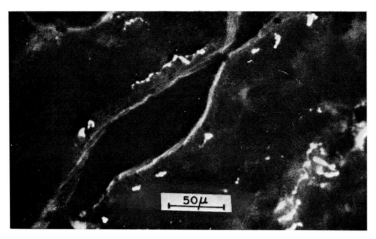

Fig. 10. Section from the same block as in Fig. 9. Relatively loose adrenergic innervation of a large vessel.

peripheral adrenergic endings (Corrodi and Jonsson, 1967). Thus, it is not the sensitivity which is the limiting factor of the aqueous technique. In rat brain treated with aqueous F and then freeze-dried *in vacuo*, intraneuronal catecholamines may develop fluorescence without any additional treatment with F gas (Laties *et al.*, 1967 and personal observations). This finding suggests that neither diffusion during the incubation nor the aqueous form of application of the aldehyde is the cause of the limitations discussed.

Actually, the aqueous and the gaseous F methods share these limitations. Like the formalin solutions, hot F gas is not capable of inducing fluorescence in cryostat section of the brain dried in air or over $P_2O_5$, whereas the same procedure is useful in the study of peripheral adrenergic fibres.

It appears that the CNS of some animals, unlike other nervous tissues, contains a factor inhibiting the histochemical reaction. It may be some fraction of 'bound' water or another chemical peculiarity which disappears *in vacuo*. Since the freeze-drying procedure is effective when used both prior to treatment with gaseous F and after treatment with aqueous F, it seems that the supposed inhibitory factor affects the final reaction which, in the aqueous method, occurs in sections mounted in oil.

### CONCLUSION

It is impossible to overestimate the effect of the method of Falck and Hillarp upon the progress and practice of neurohistochemistry. One must agree, however, that the method in its original form is rather complicated and time consuming. Therefore rapid modifications were developed which permit the study of intraneuronal monoamines in fresh-frozen sections (Hamberger and Norberg, 1964), slices (Ehinger *et al.*, 1969), smears (Olson and Ungerstedt, 1970), etc.

An alternative approach discussed in this paper makes use of aqueous F solution, which is believed to be an adequate medium for the initial stage of the histochemical reaction. Its final stage takes place in dried sections and is facilitated by the mounting medium, mineral oil. Thus, the negative effects of unification of reaction conditions seem to be eliminated.

The aqueous procedure is rapid and simple. It does not need special effort for differentiation between specific and nonspecific fluorescence. The histochemical reaction is more easily controled and much less destructive of enzymatic activity than that in the gaseous method. Reaction conditions can be selected within a fairly wide range according to the aim of the investigation.

The results of the present investigation reinforce doubts regarding the assumptions on which the uselessness of aqueous F in fluorescence histochemistry of monoamines is generally based.

It is customary to state that it is not possible to visualize intraneuronal monoamines by treatment with aqueous F since they must have diffused away from nerve cells and fibres into the fluid. We have succeeded in disproving this assumption and showing that, in ice-cold solutions, the time required for the reaction to be carried out is shorter than the period after which the dislocation of amines becomes visible.

Further, it is stated that the extreme sensitivity of the F condensation method relies upon the fact that the aldehyde is used in gaseous form. This seems to be a misinterpretation of the excellent results obtained with the Falck and Hillarp method. An aqueous F procedure can be highly sensitive as well. It should be repeated that the high sensitivity of the present technique relies mainly upon the use of a mounting medium which facilitates the final stage of the histochemical reaction.

Finally, the limitations of the present aqueous technique are seemingly connected with chemical peculiarities of some nervous tissues rather than with specificity and sensitivity of the method. The disadvantages offered by these limitations are obvious. One must remember, however, that the aqueous F method as applied to neurohistochemistry is still at an early stage of its development. We hope that this report will stimulate other workers to engage in further research which may help to elucidate some of the methodological problems.

### ACKNOWLEDGEMENTS

The authors are grateful to the chief of the Department of Pathological Anatomy, Institute of Neurology, Dr. A. N. Koltover, for her continuous interest and support during the course of this study. The microspectrofluorometer used in the study was kindly provided by Dr. V. N. Karnaukhov and Dr. V. N. Zinchenko, Institute of Biophysics, Pushchino. We are also indebted to Dr. G. A. Buznikov and Dr. G. N. Korobtsov, Institute of Developmental Biology, for the supply of marine animals, and to Dr. Imre Zs.-Nagy, Institute of Biology, Tihany, for his helpful criticism of the manuscript.

## REFERENCES

BENNETT, T. AND MALMFORS, T. (1970) *Z. Zellforsch. Mikrosk. Anat.*, **106**, 22.

COBB, J. L. (1969) *Comp. Biochem. Physiol.*, **28**, 967.

CORRODI, H. AND JONSSON, G. (1967) *J. Histochem. Cytochem.*, **15**, 65.

COTTRELL, G. A. AND OSBORNE, N. N. (1970) *Nature*, **225**, 470.

COTTRELL, G. A. AND PENTREATH, V. W. (1970) *Comp. Gen. Pharmacol.*, **1**, 73.

DAHL, E., FALCK, B., MECKLENBURG, C. VON AND MYHRBERG, H. (1963) *Quart. J. Microscop. Sci.*, **104**, 531.

DAHL, E., FALCK, B., MECKLENBURG, C. VON, MYHRBERG, H. AND ROSENGREN, E. (1966) *Z. Zellforsch. Mikroskop. Anat.*, **71**, 489.

EHINGER, B., FALCK, B. AND STENEVI, U. (1969) *J. Histochem. Cytochem.*, **17**, 351.

EL-BADAWI, A. AND SCHENK, E. A. (1967) *J. Histochem. Cytochem.*, **15**, 580.

ELOFSSON, R., KAURI, T., NIELSEN, S.-O. AND STRÖMBERG, J.-O. (1966) *Z. Zellforsch. Mikroskop. Anat.*, **74**, 464.

ERÄNKÖ, O. (1955) *Acta Endocrinol.*, **18**, 174.

ERÄNKÖ, O. AND RÄISÄNEN, L. (1966) *J. Histochem. Cytochem.*, **14**, 690.

ERÖS, G. (1932) *Zentr. Allg. Pathol.*, **54**, 385.

FALCK, B., HILLARP, N.-Å., THIEME, G. AND TORP, A. (1962) *J. Histochem. Cytochem.*, **10**, 348.

FALCK, B., NYSTEDT, T., ROSENGREN, E. AND STENFLO, J. (1964) *Acta Pharmacol. Toxicol.*, **21**, 51.

FALCK, B. AND OWMAN, C. (1965) *Acta Univ. Lund, Sect. II*, No. **7**, 1.

FRONTALI, N. (1968) *J. Insect Physiol.*, **14**, 881.

HAMBERGER, B. (1967) *Acta Physiol. Scand.*, Suppl. **295**, 1.

HAMBERGER, B. AND NORBERG, K.-A. (1964) *J. Histochem. Cytochem.*, **12**, 48.

HEHN, G. VON (1970) *Z. Zellforsch. Mikroskop. Anat.*, **105**, 137.

LATIES, A. M., LUND, R. AND JACOBOWITZ, D. (1967) *J. Histochem. Cytochem.*, **15**, 535.

LEONTIEVA, G. R. (1966) *Zh. Evol. Biokhim. Fiziol.*, **2**, 31 (in Russian).

MCLEAN, J. R. AND BURNSTOCK, G. (1966) *J. Histochem. Cytochem.*, **14**, 538.

MYHRBERG, H. E. (1967) *Z. Zellforsch. Mikroskop. Anat.*, **81**, 311.

OLSON, L. AND UNGERSTEDT, U. (1970) *Brain Res.*, **17**, 343.

PLOTNIKOVA, S. I. AND GOVYRIN, V. A. (1967) *Zh. Evol. Biokhim. Fiziol.*, **3**, 226 (in Russian).

PLOTNIKOVA, S. I. AND KUZMINA, L. V. (1968) *Zh. Evol. Biokhim. Fiziol.*, Suppl. 23 (in Russian).

RUDE, S., (1966) *J. Comp. Neurol.*, **128**, 397.

SAKHAROV, D. A. AND ZS.-NAGY, I. (1968) *Acta Biol. Hung.*, **19**, 145.

SAKHAROVA, A. V., In V. V. MEN'SHIKOV (Ed.), *Dopamine*, 1st Medical Institute, Moscow, 1969, p. 130. (in Russian).

SAKHAROVA, A. V. AND SAKHAROV, D. A. (1968a) *Tsitologiya*, **10**, 389 (in Russian).

SAKHAROVA, A. V. AND SAKHAROV, D. A. (1968b) *Tsitologiya*, **10**, 1460 (in Russian).

SAKHAROVA, A. V. AND SAKHAROV, D. A. (1971) *Arkh. Pathol.* (in press).

SEDDEN, C. B., WALKER, R. G. AND KERKUT, G. A. (1968) *Symp. Zool. Soc. (London)*, **22**, 19.

SWEENEY, D. C. (1968) *Comp. Biochem. Physiol.*, **25**, 601.

# The Microscopic Differentiation of the Colour of Formaldehyde-induced Fluorescence

J. S. PLOEM

*Histochemical Laboratory, University of Leiden (Netherlands)*

## INTRODUCTION

Biogenic amines such as catecholamines (CA) and 5-hydroxytryptamine (5-HT) can be converted into highly fluorescent products by treating dried tissues with formaldehyde vapour (Falck *et al.*, 1962; Eränkö, 1964; Corrodi and Jonsson, 1967). The fluorophores obtained in this way can often be differentiated on the basis of a characteristic fluorescence colour. A full characterization leading to an identification of the fluorophores can nearly always be achieved with a microspectrofluorometer enabling the recording of the excitation and emission spectrum of the fluorophore (Caspersson *et al.*, 1965; Thieme, 1966; Björklund *et al.*, 1968). With such an instrument the excitation and fluorescence spectra of the CA fluorophore were found to be at 410 nm and 480 nm, and of the 5-HT fluorophore at 410 nm and 530 nm, respectively (Caspersson *et al.*, 1966). Microspectrofluorometric studies are, however, not suited as a routine technique in fluorescence microscopy.

To enable an optimal characterization of fluorophores in routine fluorescence microscopy, the primary filter should select light with a wavelength as close as possible to the excitation maximum of the fluorophore. The secondary filter should transmit the full fluorescence spectrum, thus facilitating the recognition of the fluorophore on the basis of its typical fluorescence colour. If only a part of the fluorescence spectrum is observed, as is the case when a yellow coloured barrier filter (*e.g.* K 510) is used, the identification of the fluorophore will be much more difficult.

Several types of filters are at present available for the excitation of formaldehyde-induced fluorescence (FIF): coloured glass filters, band- and double-band interference filters and a new type of short-wave pass-interference filter to be described in this paper.

The coloured glass filters of the Schott (BG 3, BG 12) or Corning (5113) type have a satisfactory transmittance at the excitation peak (410 nm) of the CA or 5-HT fluorophores, but they require the use of secondary filters like the K 510, OG 515 or 3384 to absorb all light with a wavelength shorter than 500 nm in order to exclude the unwanted excitation light from observation. Such barrier filters absorb the blue component of the fluorescence of the CA fluorophores, and only permit the observation of a relatively small (green) part of the CA fluorescence spectrum. When an ultraviolet-transmitting filter like an UG 1 is employed, a barrier filter with an absorption below 430 nm (K 430 or GG 435) can be used to absorb the unwanted ultraviolet excitation light, thus enabling the visualization of the total fluorescence spectrum of the CA fluorophore. Ultraviolet light, however, often causes an undesirable strong autofluorescence of tissue components, leading to a reduced image contrast.

Eränkö (1967) has discussed the practical results obtained with some commonly used glass filters. He concluded that the UG 1 filter can be recommended when it is desirable to study the fluorescence colour of a fluorophore. But since the UG 1 filter is not very efficient in exciting FIF, he and most other investigators recommended the BG 12 filter as the best all-round filter for FIF excitation, although the colour differentiation between the green fluorescence of the CA fluorophore and the yellow fluorescence of the 5-HT fluorophore is not very striking with the BG 12 filter.

Efforts were made to improve colour contrast in fluorescence microscopy. Angela-kos (1964) employed narrow-band excitation with a double-band interference filter (half width 20 nm) with a maximal transmittance at 405 nm. By excluding ultraviolet excitation light from the exciting light, he could visualize blue CA and yellow 5-HT fluorophores and achieve a relatively low level of autofluorescence of tissue components. The high level of autofluorescence of tissue components resulting from the use of an ultraviolet broad-band glass filter like an UG 1 often limited the observation of weak blue FIF. Unfortunately double-band interference filters have relatively low transmittances.

Gillis and coworkers (1966) also obtained satisfactory results by employing inter-ference filters for the excitation of FIF. The present author described a TAL 405 interference filter for excitation of CA and 5-HT fluorophores with a relatively high transmittance at 405 nm (1969a). This filter has a half width of about 20 nm and transmits therefore a relatively narrow band as compared to the coloured glass filters UG 1 and BG 12, which have a half width of more than 50 nm. If used in epi-illumination with objectives of high numerical aperture and in combination with a dichroic mirror which reflects the violet excitation light (Ploem, 1969b), an effective visualization of FIF could be achieved. The TAL 405 filter permits the use of the barrier filters K 460 or OG 455 which transmit blue FIF. Excitation with the TAL 405 filter gave in many applications a relatively weak autofluorescence of tissue com-ponents and since a relatively strong FIF fluorescence was obtained, a satisfactory image contrast resulted.

In this paper a new type of excitation filter for the excitation of FIF will be de-scribed. This filter has a particularly high transmittance for violet light.

## MATERIALS AND METHODS

### *Instrumentation*

A Leitz Orthoplan fluorescence microscope equipped with a vertical illuminator was used (Ploem, 1969b). The vertical illuminator was provided with a revolver adapting four excitation filters of 18 mm diameter. The fifth position of this filter revolver was kept empty in order to allow excitation with filters mounted in the lamp housing.

### Light source

As a light source a high-pressure mercury lamp HBO 100 (Osram, Berlin, Germany) was used. This lamp was operated on a stabilized direct current supply (E. Leitz, Wetzlar, Germany). The HBO 100 lamp has a small arc ($0.25 \times 0.25$ mm) of relatively high luminance (170 000 cd/cm$^2$) and can effectively fill the relatively small entrance pupil of most objectives used for epi-illumination.

### Filters

For the studies described in this paper two different filters for "narrow-band" excitation with violet light (405 nm) were mounted in the filter revolver: (1) A TAL 405 (Schott and Gen., Mainz, Germany) interference filter with about 50% transmittance (T) at 405 nm and 0.002% T at 480 nm. (2) A new type of short-wave pass-interference filter for excitation with violet light (KP 425, E. Leitz, Wetzlar). The KP 425 filter we tested had about 85% T at 405 nm and about 0.001%, at 480 nm. The transmittance of red light by the KP 425 filter can be eliminated by combining this filter with a 3-mm BG 3 coloured glass filter. This filter combination still transmits a considerable amount of ultraviolet light (365 nm). To eliminate this light, these filters must be used in combination with a 3 mm Schott GG 400 filter as an additional excitation filter to absorb ultraviolet light below 400 nm. The filters combined (KP 425 + 3 mm BG 3 + 3 mm GG 400) will have a half width of about 25 nm. The KP 425 is especially designed for FIF excitation and can be used in combination with barrier filters having a cutoff value (50% T) at 460 nm. Both (TAL 405 and KP 425) excitation filters were used in combination with a dichroic mirror with $\lambda$H at 450 nm (50% reflectance and 50% transmittance at 450 nm) in position two of the internal turret of the vertical illuminator. A Schott 2-mm UG 1 or 5-mm BG 12 glass filter (in the filter compartment of the lamp housing) were used in combination with the positions one and three of the internal turret of the vertical illuminator, containing the dichroic mirrors with $\lambda$H's at 400 and 495 nm, respectively.

Slides with Leitz barrier filters K 430, K 460 and K 510 (50% T at 430, 460 and 510 nm respectively) and Schott fluorescence selection filters (Ploem, 1969b) SAL 480 and SAL 530 were brought in the light path above the vertical illuminator. A Schott neutral density filter NG 9 with a transmittance of 10% could also be used as a secondary filter.

### Objectives and eyepieces

For epi-illumination in fluorescence microscopy, only objectives of relatively high numerical aperture (NA) are suitable. Both the illumination of the microscopic preparation and the observation of the fluorescence obtained from a fluorophore are proportional to the square power of the NA of the objective. The final intensity of the fluorescence thus depends on the fourth power of the NA of the objective. Immersion

*References pp. 36–37*

objectives are preferred for epi-illumination, since the reflectance of unwanted excitation light by the cover glass is strongly reduced if water-, glycerol or oil-immersion fluid is used. Low-power dry objectives are not suitable for epi-illumination.

The objectives used for this study were: Leitz oil–water immersion achromate 22x/NA 0.65; C. Zeiss (Oberkochen) oil immersion apochromate 40x/NA 1.00; Leitz water immersion achromate 50x/NA 1.00; oil immersion fluorites Leitz 54x/NA 0.95, C. Zeiss 63x/NA 1.25 and Leitz 95x/NA 1.32.

We used 6.3x or 5x eyepieces for most work, but in some cases when only weakly fluorescent structures were present in the microscopic preparation, 4x or 3.2x projectives were employed. The latter type of eypiece is somewhat difficult in use due to its high exit pupils.

When the total microscopic magnification has to be kept low, it is more efficient to use moderate-power objectives of high NA with low-power eyepieces than low-power objectives of low NA combined with high-power eyepieces. This can be understood from the fact that the numerical aperture of the objective strongly determines the intensity of the fluorescence observed.

*Photography*

FIF must be photographed before it has faded under the influence of the irradiation. Since fading of fluorescence occurs more rapidly when the intensity of irradiation is increased, it is often not possible to shorten the exposure time in this way. Shortening of the exposure time can, however, most times be achieved by using objectives of the same magnification but with higher NA. In order to photograph weak FIF before it has faded, we employed sensitive black and white films like Kodak Tri X. For colour photography we used Kodak Ektachrome artificial light film, since the blue and yellow colours obtained with this film corresponded better to the fluorescence colours observed with the eye than the colours obtained with a more rapid daylight film like Anscochrome 500.

*Formaldehyde condensation*

Stretch preparations of the rat mesentery and iris, and "delamination" preparations obtained by microdissection from the guinea pig intestinal wall were made on microscopic slides at room temperature and quickly dried with a fan. After drying, fat tissue was removed from the mesentery with a razor blade. The dried preparations were then treated with formaldehyde vapour (obtained from paraformaldehyde of 50% humidity) during one and a half hour at 80°C. The preparations were embedded in Fluormount (E. Gurr, London, England) under a cover glass, and flattened during the night under a weight of two kg. The fluormount pressed out under the cover glass was removed with a razor blade. If not directly examined in the fluorescence microscopy, the slides were kept in a deepfreezer at —25°C. Under these conditions a satisfactory level of fluorescence could be maintained for at least some weeks.

Preparations of the ductus deferens of the rat, and of the intestinal wall and pancreas of the guinea pig were made by dipping the fresh tissue pieces in talcum powder and immersing them in liquid nitrogen. The preparations were then freeze-dried, embedded in paraffin wax, and cut as described elsewhere (Eränkö, 1967).

*Specificity tests*

Stretch preparations of the rat mesentery were air-dried and then kept at 80°C during one and a half hour in an environment free from formaldehyde vapour. As a second test, preparations already treated with formaldehyde vapour and showing FIF, were treated with 0.02% sodium borohydride ($NaBH_4$) in 90% isopropanol (Corrodi *et al.*, 1964). After disappearance of the specific fluorescence, the preparations were again treated with formaldehyde vapour for a test of reappearance of the specific fluorescence.

## RESULTS

Since colour figures are not used in this volume, the results cannot be adequately illustrated and the reader must rely on written description of the colours. For colour photomicrographs taken with narrow-band excitation, reference is made to the author's recent paper (1969b).

In stretch preparations of the rat mesentery treated with formaldehyde vapour and excited with violet light (TAL 405 or KP 425 + 3 mm BG 3), using epi-illumination (dichroic mirror Nr. 2) and a K 460 barrier filter, a blue fluorescence of the nerve fibres of the adrenergic plexus and a yellow fluorescence of the mast cells was observed. Before concluding that the observed fluorescence was formaldehyde induced, control preparations were air dried and heated during one and a half hour at 80°C in an environment free from formaldehyde vapour. Other preparations already treated with formaldehyde vapour, were exposed to a treatment with borohydride followed by a retreatment with formaldehyde vapour. From these experiments could be concluded that the FIF was monoamine fluorescence.

The blue fluorescence colour observed from the adrenergic plexus corresponds fairly well with the colour of the blue light seen through a band-interference filter (SAL 480) with a maximal transmittance at 480 nm (= fluorescence peak of the CA fluorophore). In those places where relatively high concentrations of the CA fluorophores might be present, the fluorescence appeared blue-white rather than blue to the eye. In general the visual observations of the CA fluorophore are in accordance with the spectral data obtained in microspectrofluorometric studies. The yellow fluorescence observed from the mast cells, however, seemed to differ from the green light seen through a band-interference filter (SAL 530) with a maximal transmittance at 530 nm (= fluorescence peak of 5-HT). The mast cells appeared much more yellow (about 570 nm). This is probably not due to a shift in the colour appreciation of the eye occurring with observation of fluorescence light of relatively high intensity, since the mast cells still appeared yellow through a NG 9 neutral density filter with a transmittance of only 10%. Probably the rather broad fluorescence spectrum of the 5-HT fluorophore that reaches into the orange-red wavelength range is appreciated by the eye as yellow.

*References pp. 36–37*

The large colour contrast between the blue fluorescence of the CA fluorophore and the yellow fluorescence of the 5-HT fluorophore, obtained with the new filter combination described in this paper, permits an easy distinction between these fluorophores. Fine blue fluorescent nerve fibres could, *e.g.*, be distinguished within patches — in some areas of the rat mesentery — consisting of numerous closely packed yellow fluorescent mast cells. The colour contrast obtained in this preparation with "broad-band" excitation using a BG 12 filter was insufficient for the distinction of these weakly blue fluorescent nerve fibres.

A relatively low level of autofluorescence of the components of the vessel wall of small arteries resulted from "narrow-band" violet light excitation (Fig. 1). Adrenergic nerve fibres running across the vessel walls could be clearly distinguished. Other tissue components in the mesentery like the elastic fibres and cells not containing CA or 5-HT fluorophores also showed little autofluorescence and, even with the moderate levels of FIF obtained with the rather mild condensation conditions used, a satisfactory contrast resulted (Fig. 2). This large image contrast permitted the observation of weakly fluorescent nerve fibre bundles with a much lower level of fluorescence than the terminal nerve fibres running along the vessels (Fig. 3). The rather large difference in CA fluorescence in the various nerve bundles was often striking. The microscopic resolution was, however, not always sufficient to detect whether this

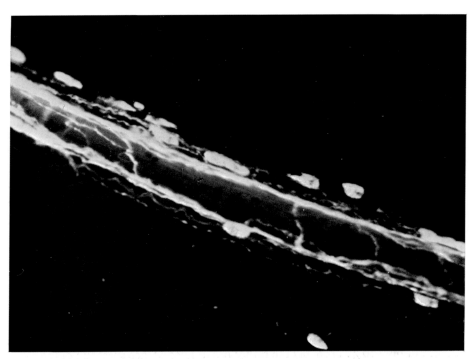

Fig. 1. Stretch preparation of the rat mesentery showing FIF. A small artery surrounded by an adrenergic nerve plexus is shown. Note the low level of autofluorescence of the vessel wall. Some shades of erythrocytes can be seen. Yellow fluorescent mast cells are lying close to the vessel.

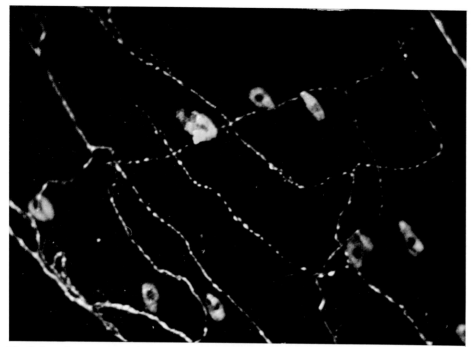

Fig. 2. Stretch preparation of the rat mesentery showing FIF. Elastic and collagenous fibres and non-nerve cells lying in the background are hardly visible due to their weak autofluorescence. Moderate FIF is visualized by slight over-exposure of the picture.

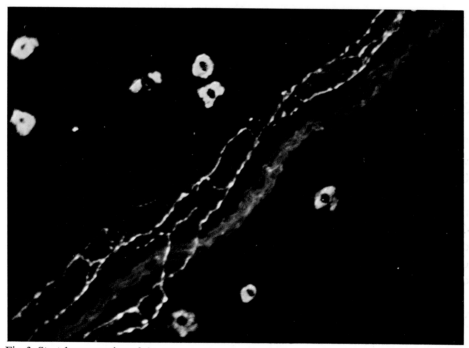

Fig. 3. Stretch preparation of the rat mesentery showing FIF. A bundle of weakly fluorescent (blue) fibres is visible along a small vessel surrounded by terminal axons. Note the large image contrast.

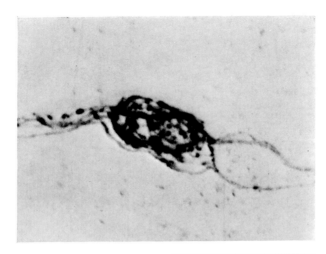

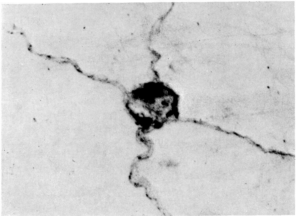

Fig. 4. Stretch preparations of the rat mesentery showing FIF. Negative copies made from colour slides. Weakly fluorescent (blue) fibres lead to a plexus of strongly fluorescent (blue-white) elements.

was caused by differences in the number of individual axons, running together in one bundle or by differences in the CA content of one axon.

Typical intensely blue-white fluorescent cells were incidentally observed in the rat mesentery. The cells appeared blue-white as long as a barrier filter with a cutoff at 460 nm (K 460) was used. When, however, a yellow-coloured barrier filter was employed with a cutoff at 510 nm (K 510), these intensely fluorescent cells were observed as yellow. The exact fluorescence spectrum of these cells could not be established, since no microspectrofluorometric studies were performed.

Another structure which was found incidentally in the rat mesentery consisted of very weakly fluorescent fibres — just distinguishable from the background — with locally a small plexus of intensely blue fluorescent fibres (Fig. 4). A low level of autofluorescence as can be obtained with narrow-band excitation with violet light, facilitated the observation of such structures.

In delamination preparations of the guinea pig intestinal wall, we could observe blue-white fluorescent fibres around unstained ganglion cells (dark spaces) in the mesenteric plexus. Also in freeze-dried tissue sections of *e.g.* the ductus deferens of the rat and the pancreas of the guinea pig, both prepared in the usual way for FIF (Eränkö, 1967), CA fluorescence of terminal fibres of the adrenergic plexus could be visualized as blue. In a few freeze-dried preparations the fluorescence appeared blue-green rather than blue. The exact spectra of these preparations should be studied with a microspectrofluorometer.

In sections of the guinea pig pancreas we observed blue and yellow fluorescent cells in the pancreatic islets indicating the presence of cells with CA fluorophores and cells with 5-HT-like fluorophores.

The level of autofluorescence of tissue components was comparatively low in most of the tissue sections we studied. Elastic fibres and cytoplasm granules in nerve cells show a considerably weaker autofluorescence on excitation with narrow-band TAL 405 or KP 425 + GG 400 filters than with the broad-band filters like UG 1 or BG 12 in relation to the FIF obtained with these filters. This is of considerable importance for quantitative fluorescence microscopy, since the possibility to detect very weak FIF is mainly determined by the image contrast that can be obtained. The present high-gain multipliers are capable to detect minute concentrations of the fluorophore as long as the background is dark enough.

## DISCUSSION

The new interference filters TAL 405 and KP 425 + GG 400 have relatively high transmittances, but since they are narrow-band filters the total transmitted energy is rather limited as compared to the total energy transmitted by the wide-band UG 1 and BG 12 coloured-glass filters. If they are used for epi-illumination through objectives of high NA in combination with low-power eyepieces, they can provide a sufficiently strong FIF. The possibility provided by the TAL 405 and the KP 425 filter to visualize CA and 5-HT fluorophores in their "true" colours could be demonstrated in the pancreatic islets of the guinea pig where the colour differentiation between the various cellular elements has always been somewhat difficult with the commonly used coloured glasses. With these filters, difficulties in colour differentiation have also been encountered in other applications, such as strongly fluorescent nerve cells containing high concentrations of the CA fluorophore. They appeared yellow to the eye whereas microspectrofluorometric studies revealed an emission spectrum of the fluorophore at 480 nm (Norberg *et al.*, 1966). This discrepancy is probably due to differences in sensitivity of the eye at various parts of the spectrum and at various light intensities. The sensitivity of the eye is shifted towards longer wavelengths with increasing intensity of light. This phenomenon has also been noticed in other fluorescence histochemical applications such as immunofluorescence where high concentrations of fluorescein isothiocyanate (FITC) appear yellow to the eye instead of green (525 nm = fluorescence peak of FITC). An interesting advantage of narrow-band excitation with violet light lies in the fact that a relatively high concentration of

CA fluorophore seems to present itself as blue-white to the eye, and is easily distinguished from the yellow 5-HT fluorophore. We did, however, up till now examine only a limited number of tissues and cells and used for our studies rather mild reaction conditions (1½ hour exposure at 80°C to formaldehyde vapours equilibrated at 50% humidity).

In our opinion mild reaction conditions are desirable for several reasons: (1) The fluorescence of the CA fluorophore can under certain conditions exhibit a shift of the emission peak from 480 nm to 500–540 nm (Caspersson et al., 1966; Jonsson, 1967), but this reaction can often be prevented by using drier formaldehyde gas and shorter condensation times. (2) High concentrations of the fluorophore might cause a non-linearity between the fluorescence and the concentration of the fluorophore as is suggested by Jonsson (1969). (3) Milder reaction conditions facilitate cytochemical procedures like, e.g., the demonstration of cholinesterases in the same section (Eränkö, 1966).

Lower concentrations of fluorophores will, however, result in a lower fluorescence intensity and require a correspondingly darker background to maintain a satisfactory image contrast. Autofluorescence of tissue components must therefore be kept minimal. This can be achieved with narrow band excitation with violet light described in this paper. Lower concentrations of fluorophores require either stronger excitation light or a more effective collection by the objective of the fluorescence emitted in order to obtain a sufficiently bright microscopic image. More intense excitation light that is transmitted by a TAL 405 or KP 425 filter — maintaining the principle of narrow-band excitation in order to avoid autofluorescence — is at present not available at a reasonable cost.

Moreover, very intense excitation light is undesirable, since it will cause a more rapid fading of the fluorophores and may destroy enzymes that should be preserved for subsequent cytochemical staining procedures (Eränkö, 1966). A better solution is provided by the use of objectives at maximal NA — using bright-field epi-illumination — in combination with low-power eye pieces. This combination provides the practical optimum for excitation and observation of fluorescence.

## ACKNOWLEDGEMENTS

The author is grateful to Mr. R. Schläfer at Schott and Gen., Mainz (Germany) for his aid in the development of the TAL 405 interference filter. The author is indebted to Mr. W. Kraft at Leitz, Wetzlar (Germany), for his important contribution to the development of the KP 425 filter.

## REFERENCES

ANGELAKOS, E. T. (1964) J. Histochem. Cytochem., 12, 929.
BJÖRKLUND, A., EHINGER, B. AND FALCK, B. (1968) J. Histochem. Cytochem., 16, 252.
CASPERSSON, T., HILLARP, N. A. AND RITZÉN, M. (1966) Exp. Cell Res., 42, 415.
CASPERSSON, T., LOMAKKA, G. AND RIGLER, R. JR. (1965) Acta Histochem., Suppl. 6, 123.
CORRODI, H., HILLARP, N. A. AND JONSSON, G. (1964) J. Histochem. Cytochem., 12, 582.

CORRODI, H. AND JONSSON, G. (1967) *J. Histochem. Cytochem.*, **15**, 65.

ERÄNKÖ, O. (1964) *J. Histochem. Cytochem.*, **12**, 487.

ERÄNKÖ, O. (1966) *Pharmacol. Rev.*, **18**, 353.

ERÄNKÖ, O. (1967) *J. Roy. Microscop. Soc.*, **87**, 259.

FALCK, B., HILLARP, N. A., THIEME, G. AND TORP, A. (1962) *J. Histochem. Cytochem.*, **10**, 348.

GILLIS, C. N., SCHNEIDER, F. H., VAN ORDEN, L. S. AND GIARMAN, N. J. (1966) *J. Pharmacol. Exp. Therap.*, **151**, 466.

JONSSON, G. (1967) *Histochemie*, **26**, 379.

JONSSON, G. (1969) *J. Histochem. Cytochem.*, **17**, 714.

NORBERG, K. A., RITZÉN, M. AND UNGERSTEDT, U. (1966) *Acta Physiol. Scand.*, **67**, 260.

PLOEM, J. S. (1969a) *Arch. Intern. Pharmacodyn.*, **182**, 421.

PLOEM, J. S. (1969b) *Leitz Mitt. Wiss. u. Techn.*, **4**, 225.

THIEME, G. (1966) *Acta Physiol. Scand.*, **67**, 514.

# Small, Intensely Fluorescent Granule-containing Cells in the Sympathetic Ganglion of the Rat

OLAVI ERÄNKÖ AND LIISA ERÄNKÖ

*Department of Anatomy, University of Helsinki, Siltavuorenpenger, Helsinki (Finland)*

In an early study on histochemical demonstration of catecholamines in the sympathetic superior cervical ganglion of the rat (Eränkö and Härkönen, 1963), a diffuse formaldehyde-induced fluorescence due to noradrenaline was reported in all ganglion cells, as well as brilliantly fluorescent small granules in the cytoplasm of many cells and in fibres between the cells. However, amongst typical ganglion cells, occasional small cells were observed to exhibit an extremely bright yellow fluorescence. It was later shown (Eränkö and Härkönen, 1965a) that the fluorescence of these cells, called 'small intensely fluorescent cells' (SIF cells) remained essentially unchanged after division of pre- or postganglionic nerves close to the ganglion, although the latter caused an almost complete disappearance of histochemically demonstrable catecholamines from the cytoplasm of the ordinary ganglion cells.

Since noradrenaline-containing chromaffin cells of the adrenal medulla were known to exhibit an intense formaldehyde-induced fluorescence (Eränkö, 1955b) and since chromaffin cell clusters had been reported in the mesenteric ganglion of the dog (Muscholl and Vogt, 1964), the possibility appeared likely that the SIF cells were, in fact, chromaffin cells. Therefore, in a further study (Eränkö and Härkönen 1965b) complete series of sections were prepared from ganglia fixed in 3.5% potassium dichromate. No or few chromaffin cells were found in the superior cervical ganglion, although numerous small cells were detected in it with formaldehyde-induced fluorescence. However, in the same paper it was also stated that 'cells of the same size and shape as the strongly fluorescent ones were electron microscopically observed to closely resemble the chromaffin cells of the adrenal medulla, containing, like these, numerous intensely osmiophilic granules'. The small cells were therefore considered a new variety of non-chromaffin amine-storing cells, and because the colour of the fluorescence was yellow, 'a monoamine, perhaps 5-hydroxytryptamine', was thought to be stored in the secretory granules of the SIF cells in the same manner as catecholamines in the adrenal medulla.

Soon after our first report on the SIF cells in the superior cervical ganglion of the rat, the presence of SIF cells was confirmed not only in the superior cervical ganglion of the rat but in other sympathetic ganglia and other species as well (Norberg and Hamberger, 1964; Owman and Sjöstrand, 1965; Norberg and Sjöqvist, 1966; Csillik, Kalman and Knyihar, 1967; Jacobowitz, 1967; Olson, 1967). Subsequent

*References pp. 50–51*

electron microscopic studies also confirmed the presence of granules resembling those in the chromaffin cells in small cells of a shape similar to the SIF cells, and there is little doubt at present that these granular cells are indeed identical with the SIF cells (Grillo, 1966; Williams, 1967; Elfvin, 1968; Siegrist *et al.*, 1968; Hökfelt, 1969; Matthews and Raisman, 1969; Williams and Palay, 1969; Watanabe, 1970). Electron microscopic evidence has further indicated that these small cells receive afferent, apparently non-adrenergic synapses from preganglionic fibres and send efferent synapses to dendrites of sympathetic ganglion cells (Siegrist *et al.*, 1968; Matthews and Raisman, 1969; Williams and Palay, 1969). Close contacts with blood vessels have also been reported (Siegrist *et al.*, 1968; Matthews and Raisman, 1969).

Data on the nature of the monoamines contained in the SIF cells are somewhat confusing. Muscholl and Vogt (1964) found adrenaline and noradrenaline in the chromaffin-cell-containing inferior mesenteric ganglion of the dog, and Owman and Sjöstrand (1965) found a correlation between the occurrence of small cells and adrenaline in the pelvic ganglia of some species. Our early, expressly tentative guess of 5-hydroxytryptamine in the superior cervical ganglion (Eränkö and Härkönen, 1965b) was rejected by Norberg, Ritzén and Ungerstedt (1966), who reported that dopamine or noradrenaline is responsible, as judged by microspectrofluorimetry. Recently, Björklund *et al.*, (1970), who used hydrochloric acid vapour to differentiate between dopamine and noradrenaline (Björklund *et al.*, 1968), reported that the amine of the SIF cells of the sympathetic ganglia of the pig, the cat and the rat is dopamine.

Few reports are available on the development, number and distribution of the SIF cells. Norberg and Sjöqvist (1966) considered that the 'small number and scattered distribution of these cells would indicate that they are of no major physiological importance' and Norberg *et al.* (1966) counted 568 SIF cells in 39 sections of 8 serially sectioned superior cervical ganglia of the rat, while Matthews and Raisman (1969) found in a single superior cervical ganglion of the rat 30 clusters of small cells, including 6 larger groups.

The present study was undertaken to study the constancy, number and distribution of the SIF cells, as yet almost unexamined, as well as the problem of the amine responsible for their intense formaldehyde-induced fluorescence.

MATERIAL AND METHODS

Rats of the Sprague–Dawley strain were briefly anaesthetized with ether and killed by cutting the vertebral column and the aorta with scissors. The superior cervical ganglia were removed and spread on an aluminium foil marked to show the distal and proximal end of the ganglion. The ganglia were frozen by immersion in isopropane precooled with liquid nitrogen and dried under vacuum at —50°C. After complete drying the temperature was increased gradually to about plus 40°C, the vacuum was broken and the ganglia transferred to a Petri dish for exposure to formaldehyde vapour. This was generated from paraformaldehyde powder equilibrated with 60% relative humidity, using different temperatures of exposure. For details of the technique see Eränkö (1967).

For serial sectioning, the ganglia exposed to formaldehyde vapour were directly transferred in the following mixture of epoxy resin: Araldite 502, 15 ml; Epon 812, 25 ml; dibutyl phthalate, 4 ml. To 1.8 ml of this mixture was added 2.2 ml of dodecinyl succinic anhydride and 8 drops of benzyl dimethylamine. They were then poured into flat dishes made of aluminium foil, and the resin was hardened by incubation at 45°C overnight. Serial sections were cut at 5 $\mu$m with the LKB pyramitome, using a glass knife. The sections were transferred dry onto slides, 24 sections on each slide, and mounted in Entellan (E. Merck). All sections were examined in a fluorescence microscope using a 3-mm BG 3 and a TAL 403 nm interference filter by Schott for excitation and Leitz K 470 filter for emission. The number of SIF cells was counted in each section, denoting their location in the ganglion and the number of cells in each group. The error due to section thickness was compensated for by using the Floderus formula (see Eränkö, 1955a).

For microspectrofluorimetric analysis, freeze-dried ganglia exposed to formaldehyde vapour were quickly embedded in paraffin wax through xylene. Sections cut at 5 $\mu$m were transferred dry onto slides. The paraffin wax was removed with toluene and the sections were mounted in paraffin oil. Excitation and emission spectra were recorded before and after exposure for 5 seconds – 30 minutes to hydrochloric acid vapour generated at room temperature from concentrated hydrochloric acid, density 1.19 g/ml, following the spectral changes in the same cell groups between exposures.

The microspectrofluorimeter is described elsewhere (Eränkö, 1971). It features two Farrand grating monochromators for excitation and emission, respectively, in front of and behind a Zeiss Jena microscope fitted with a Reichert dichroic mirror illuminator to reflect the exciting ultraviolet light on the specimen through the objective yet allowing most of the fluorescent light to pass through to the ocular. A Zeiss 40 × aprochromatic objective was used. A battery-fed RCA 1P28 photomultiplier tube was connected with the $y$ axis of a Moseley $x - y$ recorder, the $x$ axis being run by the wavelength potentiometer.

## RESULTS

A typical cluster of SIF cells amongst the larger, less intensely fluorescent, 'ordinary' sympathetic ganglion cells is illustrated in Fig. 1. As in this cell group, the SIF cell profiles were often elongated and sent thin intensely fluorescent processes some distance away from the cell body. Processes originating from individual SIF cells were close to each other and often reached the surface of ordinary sympathetic ganglion cells. Sometimes the SIF cell processes surrounded ganglion cells in intimate contact with them, and their beadings were impinging on the ganglion cell cytoplasm (Fig. 2). Clusters of SIF cells were also observed amongst nerve tracts inside the ganglion (Fig. 3), in preganglionic or postganglionic nerve trunks near the ganglion (Fig. 4), and sometimes directly on ganglion cell bodies (Fig. 7).

The SIF cells were very often grouped around small blood vessels (Figs. 5–8), and if a blood vessel was not visible near or within a group of SIF cells in a section, it was usually possible to find such a vessel in nearby sections cut through the same

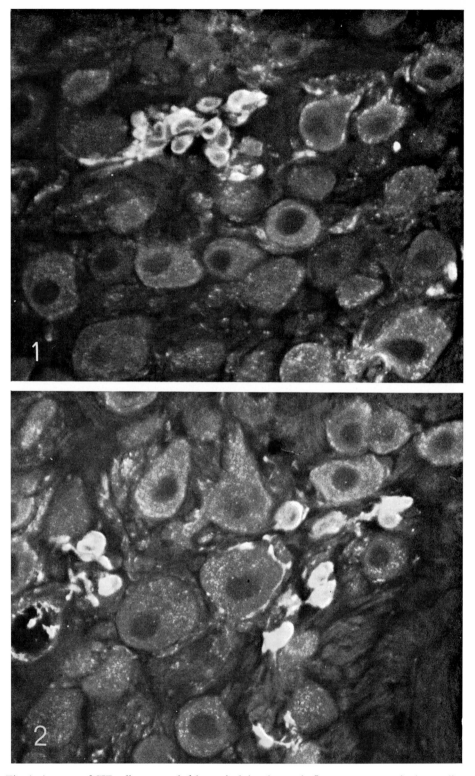

Fig. 1. A group of SIF cells surrounded by typical, less intensely fluorescent sympathetic ganglion cells in the superior cervical ganglion of an adult rat. Magnification 470 ×.

Fig. 2. SIF cells amongst ordinary ganglion cells. The ganglion cell in the centre is surrounded by a slender SIF cell process with beadings. Magnification 470 ×.

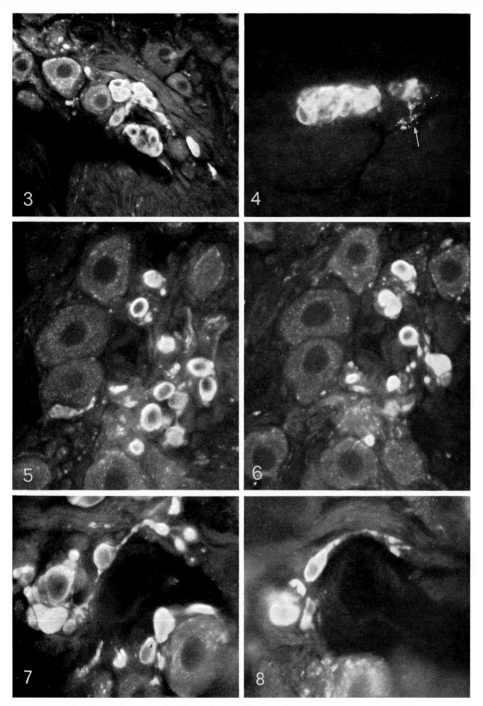

Fig. 3. Blood vessel surrounded by a cluster of SIF cells amongst nerve tracts. 310 ×.
Fig. 4. Typical, dense SIF cell cluster in a postganglionic nerve trunk. Arrow indicates a mast cell. 310 ×.
Fig. 5. Blood vessel surrounded by SIF cells and their processes. On the left a SIF cell in close contact with a ganglion cell. 490 ×.
Fig. 6. Neighbouring section to that shown in Fig. 5. Processes originating from cell bodies in Fig. 5 are seen. 490 ×.
Fig. 7. A SIF cell riding on a blood vessel and sending beaded processes to two directions. On lower right, SIF cells on a ganglion cell. 490 ×.
Fig. 8. Neighbouring section to that shown in Fig. 7. Another SIF cell riding on the same vessel sends a branching process in the nearby neuropil. 490 ×.

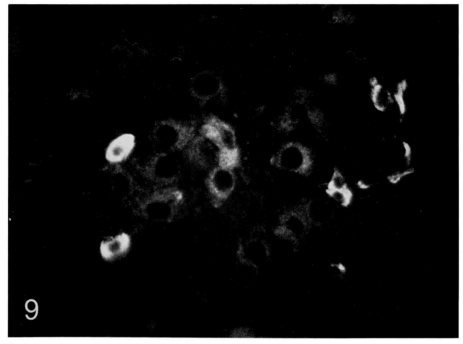

Fig. 9. Superior cervical ganglion of a newborn rat. The ganglion cells are still small and show a weak, even, cytoplasmic fluorescence. On the left, two solitary SIF cells can be seen. On the right, a loose cluster of SIF cells. 490 ×.

cluster of SIF cells. The processes of the SIF cells were often in close proximity to the vessel walls, and sometimes the SIF cells themselves were on a blood vessel (Figs. 7 and 8).

In the sympathetic ganglia of newborn rats and those a few days old, the ordinary ganglion cells were smaller and showed a diffuse cytoplasmic fluorescence. The SIF cells observed in each section were often solitary (Fig. 9, left), in contrast to the SIF cells of adult rats, which formed groups as a rule. As can be seen on the right in Fig. 9, groups of SIF cells were also to be found in young ganglia, although the cells were not usually as close to each other as in the adult ganglia.

The grouping and distribution of the SIF cells in the superior cervical ganglion is schematically illustrated in Fig. 10 in which the number of SIF cells in each cluster is given by the figure nearby. Table 1 gives the number of grouped and individual SIF cells in the left superior cervical ganglion of 5 adult male rats and 3 young rats. The number of individual SIF cells, of SIF cell groups and of grouped SIF cells was reasonably constant in adult animals. In the young ganglia, the total number of SIF cells was almost the same as that in adult ganglia, while only a small part of these cells were observed to form groups.

Emission and excitation spectra of ordinary ganglion cells and SIF cells are compared in Fig. 11 with similar spectra obtained from noradrenaline- and dopamine-incubated iris used as references (Eränkö and Eränkö, 1971). It is obvious that all

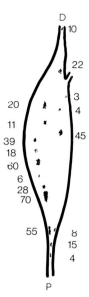

Fig. 10. Drawing illustrating the grouping of SIF cells in an adult superior cervical ganglion. The number of cells in each group is indicated by the figure beside it. D, distal, P, proximal end of the ganglion.

TABLE I

NUMBER OF SIF CELL GROUPS AND SIF CELLS IN THE SUPERIOR CERVICAL GANGLION OF YOUNG AND ADULT RATS

| Age (days) | Cell groups in the ganglion | | | | | | Solitary cells | Total cells |
|---|---|---|---|---|---|---|---|---|
| | Distal | | Central | | Proximal | | | |
| | Groups | Cells | Groups | Cells | Groups | Cells | | |
| Newborn | 0 | 0 | 5 | 160 | 1 | 13 | 199 | 372 |
| 1 | 1 | 18 | 6 | 180 | 2 | 61 | 174 | 433 |
| 3 | 0 | 0 | 5 | 222 | 0 | 0 | 326 | 548 |
| 90 | 9 | 281 | 10 | 231 | 2 | 51 | 15 | 578 |
| 90 | 12 | 283 | 6 | 170 | 1 | 40 | 10 | 503 |
| 90 | 14 | 566 | 2 | 19 | 8 | 195 | 14 | 794 |
| 90 | 5 | 62 | 5 | 86 | 13 | 262 | 19 | 429 |
| 90 | 8 | 338 | 7 | 192 | 14 | 442 | 14 | 986 |

spectra are essentially similar, indicating that catecholamines are responsible for the formaldehyde-induced fluorescence of the SIF cells. It should be noted that 5-hydroxytryptamine produced an entirely different spectrum (not illustrated here), in accordance with previous observations, by Corrodi and Hillarp (1964).

The effect of hydrochloric acid vapour on the excitation spectra of the fluorescent compounds formed from noradrenaline and dopamine is shown in Fig. 12, which

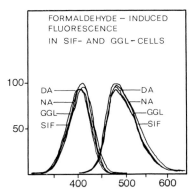

Fig. 11. Excitation (left) and emission (right) spectra of the formaldehyde-induced fluorescence in ganglion (GGL) and SIF cells, as well as in nerve fibres of iris containing noradrenaline (NA) or dopamine (DA).

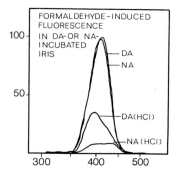

Fig. 12. Excitation spectra of formaldehyde-induced fluorescence in nerve fibres of iris containing noradrenaline (NA) or dopamine (DA) before and after exposure to hydrochloric acid (HCl) vapour

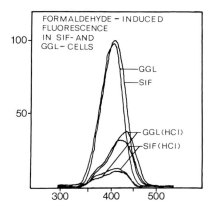

Fig. 13. Excitation spectra of formaldehyde-induced fluorescence in ganglion (GGL) and SIF cells before (high curves) and after exposure for 30 sec (middle curves) or 2 min (lowest curves) to hydrochloric acid (HCl) vapour. The spectra obtained after HCl treatment are in both cases similar to those obtained with noradrenaline.

illustrates the typical difference between these two amines: hydrochloric acid caused a rapid weakening of the noradrenaline fluorophore, while the intensity of the dopamine fluorophore was less affected, the excitation maximum shifting towards shorter wavelengths. The effect of hydrochloric acid on the excitation spectra of the formaldehyde-induced fluorescence of the SIF cells and ordinary ganglion cells is shown in Fig. 13. It is obvious that the spectra are closely similar for both cell types before and after exposure to hydrochloric acid. Since the spectrum continually changed upon exposure, two sets of spectra are shown, after 30 seconds' and 2 minutes' exposure to hydrochloric acid of the same cell groups. Comparison with Fig. 12 shows that the spectra obtained after the 2-minute exposure to hydrochloric acid from the ganglion cells and from the SIF cells were both similar to the spectrum of similarly treated noradrenaline in Fig. 12.

It is important to note in this connection that exposure to hydrochloric acid causes a sequence of changes in the excitation spectra of both noradrenaline and dopamine: first a shift of the excitation maximum to the left and a decrease in the fluorescence intensity, then a shift in the excitation maximum back towards the longer wavelengths and a new increase in the fluorescence intensity (Eränkö and Eränkö, 1970) However, these changes occur more rapidly with noradrenaline than with dopamine, thus allowing discrimination between these amines, but only if other factors, which also affect the rapidity of these changes, are kept constant. Therefore, it is essential to follow, in the same structure, changes induced by consecutive short exposures to hydrochloric acid in the excitation spectra. In the present case this was easy because the SIF cells and the ganglion cells were in the same section and they were thus necessarily exposed to hydrochloric acid and otherwise treated in an identical way. The spectra of the SIF cells treated with hydrochloric acid after formaldehyde clearly showed that the amine they contained was not dopamine.

Since the fluorescence intensity of the SIF cells reached its normal level after just a 10-min exposure to formaldehyde vapour from paraformaldehyde powder equilibrated with 60% relative humidity at 50°C, it seems apparent that noradrenaline is responsible instead of adrenaline, which reacts more slowly (see Eränkö, 1964, 1967).

DISCUSSION

Microspectrofluorimetric observations of the present study clearly indicated that the SIF cells of the superior cervical ganglion of our rats contained noradrenaline rather than dopamine. This observation is at variance with the only previous study in which dopamine and noradrenaline have been differentiated microspectrofluorimetrically (Björklund et al., 1970). Methodological differences are not likely to be responsible because the typically different spectral changes due to hydrochloric acid in noradrenaline and dopamine fluorophores were clearly enough observed in both studies (Björklund et al., 1970; Eränkö and Eränkö, 1971). The main part of the study by Björklund et al. (1970) was apparently done with the pig and the cat, with only a passing note on the rat. The presence of dopamine in the SIF cells of one species does not rule out the presence of noradrenaline or even adrenaline (cf. Muscholl and

Vogt, 1964; Owman and Sjöstrand, 1965) in the SIF cells of another species, or perhaps even of a different strain of the same species. Moreover, it is not impossible that there might be different types of SIF cells with different amines in different ganglia of the same individual animal, just as there are different types of mast cells containing either dopamine, 5-hydroxytryptamine or histamine (Adams-Ray et al., 1964; Eränkö and Kauko, 1965), or that functional changes may interfere with the beta-hydroxylation or N-methylation mechanisms of these cells, resulting in failure of dopamine to be converted into noardrenaline or adrenaline. It would not be surprising to find even 5-hydroxytryptamine in some SIF cells, even if our early, expressly tentative, suggestion that the rat SIF cells might perhaps contain 5-hydroxytryptamine (Eränkö and Härkönen, 1965b) did not prove to be correct. Such a possibility is obvious in view of the observation that not only mast cells but also the sympathetic fibres of the pineal gland originating from the superior cervical ganglion contain appreciable concentrations of 5-hydroxytryptamine (Owman, 1964).

Our earlier observation (Eränkö and Härkönen, 1965b) that the chromaffin reaction is negative in the SIF cells of the superior cervical ganglion of the rat has been confirmed (Norberg et al., 1966). The negative chromaffin reaction is at first sight somewhat surprising considering that noradrenaline was demonstrated in these cells, an amine which readily gives the chromaffin reaction in the adrenal medulla (e.g. Coupland, 1965). However, the discrepancy is probably more apparent than real. For the chromaffin reaction to be positive it is necessary that the reactive amine remain in situ until dichromate dissolved in water has formed a precipitate with it. The reaction is therefore positive only in those cells in which the amine is relatively firmly bound, such as is the case in the adrenal medulla and in the enterochromaffin cells, while noradrenaline-containing structures with smaller storage granules, such as the sympathetic nerve terminals, do not exhibit a positive chromaffin reaction, even if the local concentration of noradrenaline in itself should be sufficient for the reaction. The explanation lies in the fine structural differences of the granular vesicles in which the amines are bound.

In agreement with the observation from our laboratory that the SIF cells contain granules resembling those in the adrenal medullary cells (Eränkö and Härkönen, 1965b), several authors have observed typical granular vesicles in the SIF cells (Grillo, 1966; Williams, 1967; Elfvin, 1968; Siegrist et al., 1968; Hökfelt, 1969; Matthews and Raisman, 1969; Williams and Palay, 1969; Watanabe, 1970). However, as was pointed out by Matthews and Raisman (1969), the granular vesicles of the small cells of the superior cervical ganglion of the rat are much smaller, about 100 nm, than those of the adrenal medullary cells but much larger than the granular vesicles in ordinary sympathetic ganglion cells. Thus, the SIF cells are in this respect intermediate between sympathetic ganglion cells and adrenal medullary chromaffin cells. Very likely there are differences dependent on the species and on the ganglion concerned in the size of the granular vesicles in the SIF cells. Although no chromaffin cells can be normally found in the rat sympathetic ganglia (Lempinen, 1964; Eränkö and Härkönen, 1965b; Coupland, 1965; Norberg et al., 1966), which contain numerous SIF cells, this does not apply to all species: groups of chromaffin cells have been reported in sympathetic ganglia of several species (Kohn, 1903; Iwanow, 1932; Muscholl and Vogt, 1964). However, loose usage of the term 'chromaffin' can be confusing. While Siegrist *et al.* (1968) felt that 'with the electron microscope there can be no doubt about the presence of chromaffin cells' in the superior cervical ganglion of the adult rat, this is not so; and Williams and Palay (1969) rightly maintain that 'the term cannot be used properly on the basis of electron microscopic appearances,' when this reaction is not carried out, or proves negative. It remains to be examined whether the true chromaffin cells observed in the sympathetic ganglia have similar ultrastructural features to the SIF cells of the rat.

In adult rats, the SIF cells were almost always grouped into clusters near blood vessels. The close relation to blood vessels has previously led to the assumption that these cells might serve an endocrine function (Eränkö and Härkönen, 1965b). Such a function would indeed be compatible with the electron microscopic observation that fenestrated capillaries similar to those of the adrenal medulla are often seen close to the small granular cells (Siegrist *et al.*, 1968; Matthews and Raisman, 1969).

On the other hand, the close association of the SIF cell processes with the ganglion cell bodies and the intercellular neuropil strongly suggests interaction of a nervous nature, also in cells located close to blood vessels. Indeed, efferent synapses have been clearly demonstrated electron microscopically in these cells (Siegrist *et al.*, 1968; Matthews and Raisman, 1969; Williams and Palay, 1969). The efferent synaptic contacts from the small granular cells have been reported mainly in contact with the dendrites of sympathetic ganglion cells (Matthews and Raisman, 1969; Williams and Palay, 1969), which fits in well with the present observation of fluorescent SIF cell processes in the intercellular neuropil, in which the dendrites lie. However, it is of interest that the long, slender processes of the SIF cells were in the present study observed frequently to be in contact with the ganglion cell body, a phenomenon not described with the electron microscope.

Since afferent synapses, apparently from preganglionic fibres, have also been observed on the small granular cells (Williams, 1967; Siegrist *et al.*, 1968; Matthews and Raisman, 1969; Williams and Palay, 1969), these cells have been presumed to function as interneurons, presumably mediating intraganglionic inhibitory processes, formerly postulated by Eccles and Libet (1961) without morphological evidence to be due to liberation of adrenaline from intraganglionic chromaffin cells.

An inhibitory effect can be caused (1) if the SIF cells release catecholamine into the blood which subsequently reaches ganglion cells or (2) if the SIF cells send inhibitory impulses through their efferent adrenergic synapses to the ordinary ganglion cells. While the second effect can reach but a limited number of ganglion cells because of relatively short processes of the SIF cells and their cluster formation, a large number of ganglion cells could be affected through the blood circulation (*cf.* adrenal medulla).

The present study showed that the number of SIF cells is reasonably constant in the superior cervical ganglion of the rat, as are grouping of the cells into clusters and distribution of these clusters in the ganglion. Moreover, it was shown that almost as many SIF cells can be seen in the ganglion of newborn rats, although mainly scattered individually in the ganglion with smaller and looser clusters, as in the adult ganglion. The superior cervical ganglion of a newborn rat is at a very immature stage, and clustering may be an essential feature connected with the SIF cell function which develops later.

Grouping of the SIF cells along blood vessels certainly facilitates their eventual endocrine function. However, light microscopic observations of the present study and electron microscopic description of afferent and efferent synapses, as well as attachment plaques, connecting with other small cells and ganglion cells those small cells which are at the same time in close contact with blood vessels (Matthew and Raisman, 1969), suggests rather that the small organ formed by several SIF cells might perform even more sophisticated functions. Could it be possible that the SIF cell clusters take part in the hormonal regulation of the nervous function of the ganglion by sensing the blood composition? In view of the presence of granular vesicles in the chemoreceptor cells of the carotid body this might be a possibility.

While the grouping of the SIF cells around blood vessels can be due to their endocrine or chemoreceptor function, closeness to blood circulation providing for a suitable hormonal milieu may also be a condition for the formation and survival of these cells. Extra-adrenal chromaffin cells which normally degenerate after birth in the rat, surviving only inside adrenocortical tissue, fail to disappear and hypertrophy if hydrocortisone is administered to the animal in the first few days after birth (Lempinen, 1964). Moreover, adrenaline is already found in these cells during the prenatal period if hydrocortisone is given, although normally only noradrenaline can be found in the extra-adrenal chromaffin tissue of the rat (Eränkö, Lempinen and Räisänen, 1967). Such hormonal effects would perhaps not only explain the perivascular location of the SIF cells but also make possible the later humoral modulation of their nervous and endocrine functions.

### ACKNOWLEDGEMENTS

The present work was supported by a personal grant to O. E. from the Sigrid Jusélius Foundation and by a grant to the neurohistochemistry group of the Department of Anatomy from the Medical Research Council of Finland. The skilful technical assistance of Mrs. Tuula Stjernvall and Mr. Jarmo Seppänen is gratefully acknowledged.

### REFERENCES

ADAMS-RAY, J., DAHLSTRÖM, A., FUXE, K. AND HILLARP, N.-Å. (1964) *Experientia (Basel)*, **20**, 80.
BJÖRKLUND, A., CEGRELL, L., FALCK, B., RITZÉN, M. AND ROSENGREN, E. (1970) *Acta Physiol. Scand.*, **78**, 334–338.
BJÖRKLUND, A., EHINGER, B. AND FALCK, B. (1968) *J. Histochem. Cytochem.*, **16**, 263–270.
CORRODI, H. AND HILLARP, N.-Å. (1964) *Helv. Chim. Acta*, **47**, 911–918.
COUPLAND, R. E. (1965) *The Natural History of the Chromaffin Cell*, Longmans, London.
CSILLIK, B., KALMAN, G. AND KNYIHAR, E. (1967) *Experientia (Basel)*, **23**, 477–478.
ECCLES, R. M. AND LIBET, B. (1961) *J. Physiol. (Lond.)*, **157**, 484–503.
ELFVIN, L. (1968) *J. Ultrastruct. Res.*, **22**, 37–44.

ERÄNKÖ, O. (1955a) *Quantitative Methods in Histology and Microscopic Histochemistry.* Karger, Basel; Little, Brown & Company, Boston.

ERÄNKÖ, O. (1955b) *Acta Endocrinol.*, **18**, 174–179.

ERÄNKÖ, O. (1964) *J. Histochem. Cytochem.*, **12**, 487–488.

ERÄNKÖ, O. (1967) *J. Roy. microscop. Soc.*, **87**, 259–276.

ERÄNKÖ, O. (1971) (In the course of publication).

ERÄNKÖ, O. AND ERÄNKÖ, L. (1971) *J. Histochem. Cytochem.*, in press.

ERÄNKO, O. AND HÄRKÖNEN, M. (1963) *Acta Physiol. Scand.*, **58**, 285–286.

ERÄNKÖ, O. AND HÄRKÖNEN, M. (1965a) *Acta Physiol. Scand.*, **63**, 411–412.

ERÄNKÖ, O. AND HÄRKÖNEN, M. (1965b) *Acta Physiol. Scand.*, **63**, 511–512.

ERÄNKÖ, O. AND KAUKO, L. (1965) *Acta Physiol. Scand.*, **64**, 283–284.

ERÄNKÖ, O., LEMPINEN, M. AND RÄISÄNEN, L. (1967) *Acta Physiol. Scand.*, **69**, 255–256.

GRILLO, M. A. (1966) *Pharmacol. Rev.*, **18**, 387–399.

HÖKFELT, T. (1969) *Acta Physiol. Scand.*, **76**, 427–440.

IWANOW, G. (1932) *Ergeb. Anat. Entwickl.-Gesch.*, **29**, 87–280.

JACOBOWITZ, D. (1967) *J. Pharmacol. Exp. Therap.*, **158**, 227–240.

KOHN, A. (1903) *Arch. Mikroskop. Anat.*, **62**, 263–365.

LEMPINEN, M. (1964) *Acta Physiol. Scand.*, **66**, suppl. **231**, 1–91.

MATTHEWS, M. R. AND RAISMAN, G. (1969) *J. Anat. (Lond.)*, **105**, 255–282.

MUSCHOLL, E. AND VOGT, M. (1964) *Brit. J. Pharmacol.*, **22**, 193–203.

NORBERG, K.-A. AND HAMBERGER, B. (1964) *Acta Physiol. Scand.*, **63**, suppl. **238**, 1–42.

NORBERG, K.-A., RITZÉN, M. AND UNGERSTEDT, U. (1966) *Acta Physiol. Scand.*, **67**, 260–270.

NORBERG, K.-A. AND SJÖQVIST, F. (1966) *Pharmacol. Rev.*, **18**, 743–751.

OLSON, L. (1967) *Z. Zellforsch.*, **81**, 155–173.

OLSON, L. (1970) *Histochemie*, **22**, 1–7.

OWMAN, C. (1964) *Acta Physiol. Scand.*, **63**, suppl. **240**, 1–40.

OWMAN, C. AND SJÖSTRAND, N. O. (1965) *Z. Zellforsch.*, **66**, 300–320.

SIEGRIST, G., DOLIVO, M., DUNANT, Y., FOROGLOV-KERAMEUS, C., DE RIBAUPIERRE, F. AND ROULLIER, C. (1968) *J. Ultrastruct. Res.*, **25**, 381–407.

WATANABE, H. (1970) *Experientia*, **26**, 69–70.

WILLIAMS, T. H. (1967) *Nature (Lond.)*, **214**, 309–310.

WILLIAMS, T. H. AND PALAY, S. L. (1969) *Brain Res.*, **15**, 17–34.

# Quantitation and Differentation of Biogenic Monoamines Demonstrated with the Formaldehyde Fluorescence Method

GÖSTA JONSSON

*Department of Histology, Karolinska Institutet, Stockholm (Sweden)*

## INTRODUCTION

The formaldehyde vapour technique for the histochemical demonstration of biogenic monoamines, introduced by Falck and Hillarp in the early sixties, has come to be extensively used, not only in purely morphological work but also in studies on transmitter mechanisms such as synthesis, transport, uptake, storage, release and catabolism of neuronal and extraneuronal monoamines. The technique is furthermore frequently used for studies on the action of certain drugs on monoaminergic transmitter mechanisms. In all these types of studies very often the following questions arise: (a) Specificity of the observed fluorescence? (b) What compound is the fluorescence due to? (c) To what extent does the fluorescence intensity really reflect the amount of monoamine present in the tissue structures that are studied? The purpose of the present paper is to review the basic chemistry of the reaction between monoamines and formaldehyde and to discuss some problems concerning limitations and pitfalls in differentiation and quantitation of biogenic monoamines demonstrated with the Falck–Hillarp technique.

## CHEMISTRY

The method is based on the principle that certain monoamines condense with formaldehyde in the presence of proteins to yield strongly fluorescent products (Falck *et al.*,

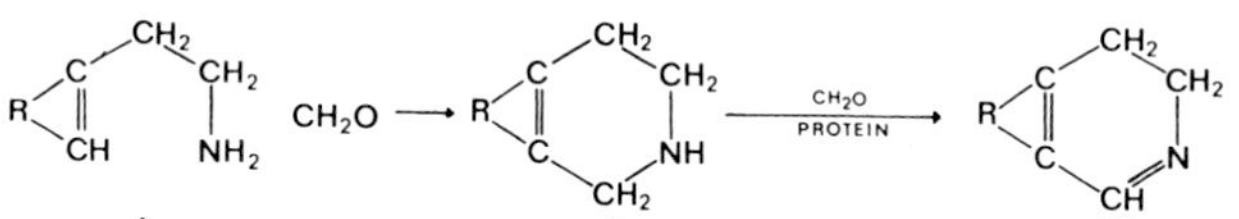

Fig. 1. The reaction between a $\beta$-arylethylamine (I) enclosed in a protein layer and formaldehyde.

---

Abbreviations used: A = adrenaline; CA = catecholamine(s); DA = dopamine; DOPA = 3,4-dihydroxyphenylalanine; 5-HT = 5-hydroxytryptamine; 6-HT = 6-hydroxytryptamine; 5,6-diHT = 5,6-dihydroxytryptamine; 5-HTP = 5-hydroxytryptophan; MTA = 3-methoxytyramine; NA = noradrenaline; $\alpha$-m-NA = $\alpha$-methyl-noradrenaline; NM = normetanephrine; T = tryptamine; Try = tryptophan.

*References pp. 60–61*

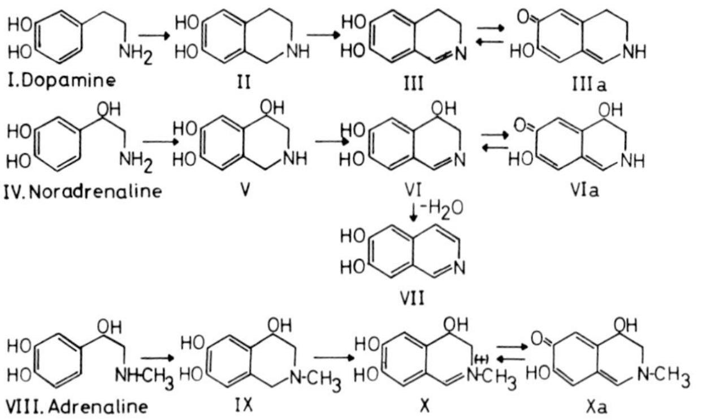

Fig. 2. The histochemical reaction between CA and formaldehyde. In the first step the CA (I, IV, VIII) condenses with formaldehyde to yield a 6,7-dihydroxy-1,2,3,4-tetrahydroisoquinoline (II, V, IX), which in a protein-promoted reaction is dehydrogenated by formaldehyde to the corresponding 3,4-dihydroisoquinoline (III, VI, X). The latter compound is in a pH-dependent equilibrium with the tautomeric quinone structure (IIIa, VIa, Xa), exhibiting strong fluorescence at 480 nm.

1962). The primary reaction involves a condensation of a $\beta$-arylethylamine with formaldehyde to yield a tetrahydro-derivative which in organic chemistry is known as the *Pictet–Spengler* reaction (see Whaley and Govindachari, 1951). In the next step the tetrahydro-compound is in a protein-promoted reaction dehydrogenated by formal-dehyde to its corresponding 3,4-dihydrocompound (see Fig. 1). The products formed in this way from CA are 6,7-dihydroxy-3,4-dihydroisoquinolines whereas inter-mediates in this reaction are the non-fluorescent 6,7-dihydroxy-1,2,3,4-tetrahydroiso-quinolines (see Fig. 2). The 6,7-dihydroxy-3,4-dihydroisoquinolines are in a pH-dependent equilibrium (maximum between pH 6 and 10) with their tautomeric quinone structures, which are responsible for the strong fluorescence; maximal excita-tion at 410 nm and maximal emission at 480 nm. This fluorescence is in fact bluish in nature, but appears as green to yellow-green when using a cut-off filter strongly absorbing below 490 nm.

The fluorescent product formed from NA, 4,6,7-trihydroxy-3,4-dihydroisoquino-line, has a labile hydroxyl group in position 4 which can easily be split off by *e.g.* HCl to form the fully aromatic 6,7-dihydroxyisoquinoline (Fig. 2). The structure of the different compounds formed during the formaldehyde treatment has been established by using synthetic compounds enclosed in model protein layers followed by spectral and chromatographic analyses (Corrodi and Hillarp, 1963, 1964; Corrodi *et al.*, 1964; Corrodi and Jonsson, 1965a, 1965b, 1966; Jonsson, 1966, 1967a, 1967b, 1967c, 1967d, see also Corrodi and Jonsson, 1967).

The first step, the so-called Pictet–Spengler reaction, proceeds as readily in solution as in the solid state and in the case of primary CA both quantitatively and with a high velocity at temperatures down to $+20°$. The second step, the protein-promoted de-hydrogenation reaction, also proceeds easily, but under the conditions used for histo-chemistry ($+50$–$80°$C, 1 hour) it is necessary for the reaction to take place in the presence of a protein with a high catalyzing power. Most proteins possess this property which in some way seems to be linked to certain amino acids, since only glycine and alanine and also dipeptides containing them have been found to be excellent catalyzers. The dehydrogenation reaction has previously been unknown in chemistry and its exact nature has so far escaped elucidation. Both the ring-closure reaction and the dehydrogenation step can occur in solution but the problems of diffusion of the amine and/or the fluorophors are great, especially as regards neuronal structures compared to the situation when the reaction is carried out in the solid state using dry formaldehyde vapour (see Eränkö and Räisänen, 1966; Eneström and Svalander, 1967; Sakharova and Sakharov, 1968).

The secondary CA, e.g. A, also reacts with formaldehyde to yield N-methyl-4,6,7-trihydroxy-3,4-dihydroisoquinoline (see Fig. 2). In this case the dehydrogenation step involves the formation of a quaternary nitrogen and therefore more energetic reaction conditions (e.g. longer incubation time) are needed to obtain good yields.

The amino acid DOPA gives a formaldehyde-induced fluorescence with spectral characteristics almost identical with those of primary CA. The structure of the fluorophor is 3-carboxy-6,7-dihydroxy-3,4-dihydroisoquinoline.

CA can under certain conditions undergo a side reaction resulting in a bathochromic shift in the emission maximum from 480 nm to 500–550 nm (Caspersson et al., 1966, Jonsson, 1967c). This side reaction has been found to occur when high concentrations of CA are present, e.g. in adrenal medullary cells and in model protein layers when the CA/protein ratio is very high. Primary CA more easily given this side reaction and spectral shift, but it is possible to prevent it by using a less energetic formaldehyde reaction (less humid gas, shorter incubation time and/or lower temperature). The exact molecular structure of the fluorophor(s) formed is not known, but the reaction in all probability proceeds via the tetrahydro- and dihydroisoquinoline compound to the final fluorescent product(s). The end product(s) may be the result of a polymerization and/or oxidation (Jonsson, 1967c).

The tryptamines, such as T, 5-HT, 5-HTP, 5,6-diHT and 6-HT, readily react with formaldehyde in the presence of proteins yielding fluorescent 3,4-dihydro-$\beta$-carbolines. Intermediates in this reaction are the non-fluorescent 1,2,3,4-tetrahydro-$\beta$-carbolines (see Fig. 3; Corrodi and Jonsson, 1965b, Jonsson and Sandler, 1969). The formaldehyde-induced fluorescence of 5-HT has its peak of excitation in the same wavelength region as that of CA (410 nm), while the emission maximum differs, being around 525 nm (see Fig. 6). This fluorescence appears as yellow in the fluorescence microscope The reaction between tryptamines and formaldehyde is thus in principle similar to that between CA and formaldehyde, but the former compounds require more energetic reaction conditions for obtaining optimal yields of the fluorophor compared with primary CA.

I. 5-Hydroxytryptamine    II    III

Fig. 3. The histochemical reaction between 5-HT and formaldehyde. 5-HT condenses with formaldehyde forming 6-hydroxy-1,2,3,4-tetrahydro-$\beta$-carboline (II) which is dehydrogenated to 6-hydroxy-3,4-dihydro-$\beta$-carboline (III).

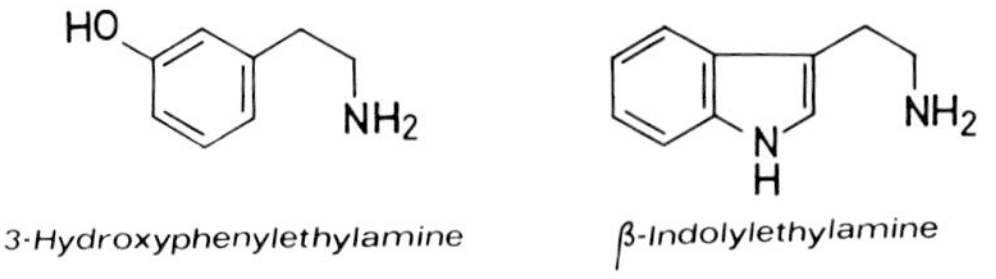

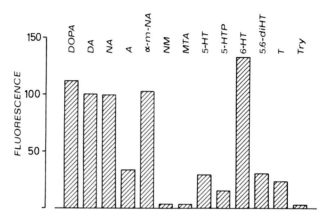

3-Hydroxyphenylethylamine              β-Indolylethylamine

Fig. 4.

Fig. 5. Relative fluorescence intensities obtained from biogenic monoamines and related compounds in dried protein spots at a concentration of 0.3 × 10⁻³ M in the protein solutions (2% w/v bovine serum albumin) used for preparing the spots, after exposure to formaldehyde vapour at +80° for 1 hour. Fluorescence expressed in arbitrary units.

The primary ring-closure reaction has been shown to be produced by an electrophilic attack on the benzene or indole nucleus and it is facilitated by an increased electron density of the carbon atom where the ring-closure takes place. This condition is amply fulfilled by *3-hydroxylated β-phenylethylamines*, *e.g.* NA, DA and *m*-tyramines, and also by *β-indolylethylamines* such as 5-HT and 5-HTP (see Fig. 4). These are the structural requirements for a compound to react with formaldehyde and to enter the primary condensation reaction during the histochemical procedure. In the β-phenylethylamine molecule it is the hydroxy group in position 3 and in the indole nucleus it is the heterocyclic nitrogen which facilitate the ring-closure due to their great activation. The protein-promoted dehydrogenation step is a general reaction for 1,2,3,4-tetrahydro-isoquinolines and β-carbolines. The amine must be either primary or secondary, since tertiary amines and amides do not give rise to any fluorescence. In complete agreement with these theoretical aspects it has been found that only 3-hydroxy- or 3,4-dihydroxy-phenylethylamines and their β-hydroxylated and α-methylated analogues (and their corresponding amino acids) react with formaldehyde during the conditions used in the histochemical procedure to form fluorescent 3,4-dihydroisoquinolines. The biogenic compounds structurally related to CA and 5-HT, *e.g.* phenylalanine, tyrosine, tyramine, octopamine, tryptophan, 5-hydroxyindole acetic acid and the deaminated and 3-*O*-methylated CA metabolites, do not give any formaldehyde-induced fluorescence or too little to be of any significance for the histochemical localization of biogenic monoamines (see Fig. 5). It is likely, however,

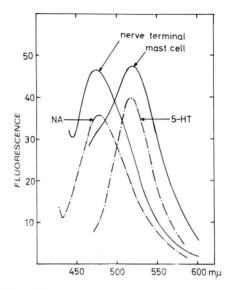

Fig. 6. Emission spectra of formaldehyde-treated model protein layers containing NA or 5-HT and NA-containing nerve terminals and a 5-HT-containing mast cell.

that the aromatic amino acids contribute at least to some of the background fluorescence exhibited by the tissue proteins.

The primary CA (NA and DA), DOPA and α-m-NA exhibit practically the same relative fluorescence yield on identical formaldehyde gas treatment, while the intensity of A is considerably less (see Fig. 5). The fluorescence intensity of A can be increased upon prolonged formaldehyde gas treatment, but never reaches the same strong intensity as that of primary CA. The 3-O-methylated CA, NM and MTA give only very weak fluorescence intensity. As regards the tryptamines, they all exhibit a relatively weak fluorescence compared to the primary CA and are in addition very sensitive to irradiation with ultraviolet light (see Fig. 6). An exception to this is, however, 6-HT which gives a very strong and fairly ultraviolet light resistant fluorescence.

SPECIFICITY

Considering the molecular requirements for a compound to give rise to formaldehyde-induced fluorescence, the chemical specificity must be regarded as very high for CA and 5-HT and their immediate precursors DOPA and 5-HTP. It must be pointed out, however, that it is of greatest importance to test whether the fluorescence observed is specific, *i.e.* due to the presence of one of the reactive monoamines. On the basis of the chemical–physical properties of the various fluorophors of monoamines, a number of histochemical criteria must be fulfilled if an observed fluorescence is to be regarded as specific. These criteria are discussed in a previous paper (Jonsson, 1967d) to which the reader is referred. The criteria are:
 1. The fluorescence must be formaldehyde-induced.
 2. Spectral characteristics (see below).

*References pp. 60–61*

3. Reduction of the fluorescence by NaBH$_4$.
4. Sensitivity of the fluorescence to ultraviolet light.
5. Quenching of the fluorescence by water.

## DIFFERENTIATION

The main differentiation problems in monoamine fluorescence histochemistry arise between the various CA and between CA and 5-HT.

### A. Differentiation of the various CA

Due to the almost identical spectral characteristics of the fluorescent compounds of CA and DOPA, they cannot be directly distinguished from one another in the fluorescence microscope.

*Primary CA* (*e.g.* NA and DA) can be differentiated from *secondary CA* (*e.g.* A) on the basis of the difference in reaction kinetics with formaldehyde: *e.g.* by incubation with formaldehyde for 1 or 3 h, respectively (Corrodi and Hillarp, 1963). Although this method can be employed with only subjective estimation of the fluorescence intensity, it is much safer to perform microfluorimetric measurements. Even then the results must be interpreted very carefully. *Differentiation between the primary CA*, NA and DA can be effected by spectral analyses after treatment with HCl. This is based on the finding that the fluorescent compound from NA can on HCl treatment form the fully aromatic 6,7-dihydroxyisoquinoline whose spectral characteristics are different from the 6,7-dihydroxy-3,4-dihydroisoquinolines formed from NA and DA (Corrodi and Jonsson, 1965; Björklund *et al.*, 1968).

### B. Differentiation of CA and 5-HT

(1) The differentiation of CA and 5-HT can be made directly in the fluorescence microscope, since CA will appear as green to yellow-green and 5-HT as yellow due to *differences in the peak of emission* (using a Hg lamp with a Schott BG12 filter and a cut-off filter absorbing strongly below 490 nm, see also Fig. 6). It must be remembered however, that a yellowish fluorescence cannot always be taken as evidence for the presence of 5-HT or 5-HTP. This is due to the fact that CA and especially primary CA when present in high concentrations can give rise to a fluorescent colour similar to that of 5-HT, maximal emission about 500–550 nm. This side reaction can be prevented by using milder reaction conditions. Another pitfall in this context are structures containing relatively high concentrations of CA which can give a yellowish fluorescence while objective measurements show typical CA-fluorescence, peak of emission at 480 nm. This is due to the fact that the maximum sensitivity of the human eye is shifted towards higher wavelengths with increasing intensity of the light. The differentiation between CA and 5-HT is facilitated by using narrow-band excitation (Ploem, 1969). The safest differentiation is of course done by use of microspectrophotofluorimetry.

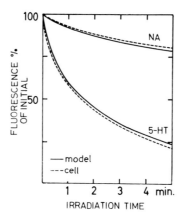

Fig. 7. Effect of irradiation of the maximal activation wavelength (410 nm) on the fluorescence intensity of formaldehyde-treated model protein layers (– –) containing NA or 5-HT and of NA-containing ganglion cells (– – –, upper curve) and 5-HT-containing mast cells (– – –, lower curve) exposed to formaldehyde gas.

(2) Another possibility for differentiation between 5-HT and CA employs studying the rate of decrease in fluorescence intensity upon irradiation with UV-light, since the rate of photodecomposition of 5-HT fluorescence is faster than that of CA (Fig. 7).

### QUANTITATION OF FLUORESCENCE

As regards primary CA, combined chemical assay and histochemical analysis have so far generally shown good correlation, especially in the case of distribution of CA neurones, although the general experience has been that relatively large changes in CA levels must have occurred to enable detection of differences in fluorescence intensity in the adrenergic neurone. Furthermore, an increase above normal fluorescence intensities cannot usually be detected, but if the increase is very high or if a redistribution of amine within the neurone has occurred, it can be observed. A more striking discrepancy, however, has been shown to exist between the levels of 5-HT in the brain as recorded by chemical assay and the number of 5-HT-containing nerve terminals as seen in the fluorescence microscope (see Fuxe, 1965a, 1965b; Fuxe and Jonsson, 1967). The difficulties involved in the demonstration of 5-HT are that 5-HT gives a fairly low fluorescence yield compared to primary CA (see Fig. 5) and that the fluorescence is extremely sensitive to ultraviolet light (see Fig. 7). The method for demonstration of 5-HT must therefore be considered as relatively unsensitive. An interesting observation is, however, that the isomer of 5-HT, namely 6-HT, has been found to give a formaldehyde-induced fluorescence which is in the same order of magnitude as that of primary CA (Jonsson and Sandler, 1969). 6-HT has furthermore been found to be taken up and accumulated in monoamine-neurones and preferentially in 5-HT-neurones. Incubation of brain slices from various parts of the brain *in vitro* in a medium containing 6-HT made it possible to discover new 5-HT nerve terminal systems in *e.g.* rhinencephalon, hypothalamus, cortex cerebri and cortex cerebelli (Jonsson *et al.,*

1969). These studies indicate that 6-HT will be a useful tool for detailed mapping out of 5-HT terminals in the central nervous system.

By use of model protein microdroplets and microfluorimetric techniques Ritzén investigated the fluorescence-concentration relationship of formaldehyde-treated primary CA and 5-HT (Ritzén 1966, 1967). He found that the fluorescence intensity is proportional up to a concentration corresponding to about 8000 $\mu$g/g wet weight of a cell. Above this value a considerable deviation from linearity occurred. The corresponding value for 5-HT is 16 000 $\mu$g/g. The average concentration of NA in the adrenergic nerve terminals has been estimated to be about 1000–3000 $\mu$g/g (see Dahlström, 1966). This value is thus lower than the quenching value, but since the transmitter is stored mainly in submicroscopic granules within the neurone, the local concentration of NA must be considerably higher than 1000–3000 $\mu$g/g, indicating that quenching of the fluorescence occurs. This seems in fact to be the case. In a combined microfluorimetric and [$^3$H]NA uptake study it was found that the fluorescence intensity of the adrenergic nerve terminals in rat iris is proportional to the NA concentration up to about 30–40% of the endogenous NA level. Above this value there is a deviation from linearity (Jonsson, 1969). It was observed, however, that this figure is somewhat lower for NA stored in the granules, but the relative fluorescence yield is higher when the amine is localized in the extragranular space. The subcellular localization of the transmitter will thus affect the fluorescence yield. In the linear part of the fluorescence–concentration relation it was possible to make a fairly reliable semiquantitative estimation of the fluorescence intensity directly in the fluorescence microscope (Olson et al., 1968; Jonsson, 1969). It may be concluded that if changes in fluorescence intensity as compared with the control are observed by eye, this certainly reflects true changes in amine concentration. On the other hand, changes in amine concentration may escape detection when the transmitter concentration is so high that quenching occurs. It has to be pointed out that adequate controls must always be used. Furthermore, it is not possible to extrapolate quenching values from one tissue to another. Taking all this together, it is of great importance in doubtful cases to correlate fluorescence estimations, both those obtained by microfluorimetry or those obtained by subjective estimation, with chemical analytical assays of the amine content.

## ACKNOWLEDGEMENTS

Parts of the work reviewed have been supported by grants from the Swedish Medical Research Council (B71-14X-2295-01, 02, 03, 04), Therese and Johan Andersson Memorial Foundation, "Magnus Bergvalls Stiftelse" and "Ollie och Elof Ericssons Stiftelse".

## REFERENCES

BJÖRKLUND, A., EHINGER, B. AND FALCK, B. (1968) J. Histochem. Cytochem., 16, 262–270.
CASPERSSON, T., HILLARP, N.-Å. AND RITZÉN, M. (1966) Exp. Cell Res., 42, 415–428.
CORRODI, H. AND HILLARP, N.-Å. (1963) Helv. Chim. Acta, 46, 2425–2430.

CORRODI, H. AND HILLARP, N.-Å. (1964) *Helv. Chim. Acta*, **47**, 911–918.

CORRODI, H., HILLARP, N.-Å. AND JONSSON, G. (1964) *J. Histochem. Cytochem.*, **12**, 582–586.

CORRODI, H. AND JONSSON, G., (1965a) *J. Histochem. Cytochem.*, **13**, 484–487.

CORRODI, H. AND JONSSON, G. (1965b) *Acta Histochem.*, **22**, 247–258.

CORRODI, H. AND JONSSON, G. (1966) *Helv. Chim. Acta*, **49**, 798–806.

CORRODI, H. AND JONSSON, G. (1967) *J. Histochem. Cytochem.*, **15**, 65–78.

DAHLSTRÖM, A. (1966) M.D. Thesis, Stockholm.

ENESTRÖM, S. AND SVALANDER, C. (1967) *Histochemie*, **8**, 155–163.

ERÄNKÖ, O. AND RÄISÄNEN, L. (1966) *J. Histochem. Cytochem.*, **14**, 690–691.

FALCK, B., HILLARP, N.-Å., THIEME, G. AND TORP, A. (1962) *J. Histochem. Cytochem.*, **10**, 348–354.

FUXE, K. (1965a) *Z. Zellforsch.*, **65**, 573–596.

FUXE, K. (1965b) *Acta Physiol. Scand.*, **64**, Suppl. 247.

FUXE, K. AND JONSSON, G. (1967) *Histochemie*, **11**, 161–166.

JONSSON, G. (1966) *Acta Chem. Scand.*, **20**, 2755–2762.

JONSSON, G. (1967a) *Histochemie*, **8**, 288–296.

JONSSON, G. (1967b) *Histochemie*, **8**, 122–130.

JONSSON, G. (1967c) *Acta Histochem.*, **26**, 379–390.

JONSSON, G. (1967d) The formaldehyde fluorescence method for the histochemical demonstration of biogenic monoamines. — A methodological study. *M.D. Thesis*, Stockholm.

JONSSON, G. (1969) *J. Histochem. Cytochem.*, **17**, 714–723.

JONSSON, G., FUXE, K., HAMBERGER, B. AND HÖKFELT, T. (1969) *Brain Res.*, **13**, 190–195.

JONSSON, G. AND SANDLER, M. (1969) *Histochemie*, **17**, 207–212.

OLSON, L., HAMBERGER, B., JONSSON, G. AND MALMFORS, T. (1968) *Histochemie*, **15**, 38–45.

PLOEM, J. S. (1969) *Arch. Intern. Pharmacodyn.*, **182**, 421–424.

RITZÉN, M. (1966) *Exp. Cell Res.*, **44**, 505–529.

RITZÉN, M. (1967) *Exp. Cell Res.*, **45**, 178–194.

SAKHAROVA, A. V. AND SAKHAROV, D. A. (1968) *Abstracts. The Third Congress of Histochemistry and Cytochemistry New York*, Springer-Verlag, New York, p. 231–232.

WHALEY, W. M. AND GOVINDACHARI, T. R. (1951) *Organic Reactions*, Coll. **6**, John Wiley and Sons, Inc., New York.

# Microspectrofluorimetric Characterization of Monoamines in the Central Nervous System: Evidence for a New Neuronal Monoamine-like Compound

ANDERS BJÖRKLUND, BENGT FALCK AND ULF STENEVI

*Institute of Anatomy and Histology, University of Lund, Lund (Sweden)*

## INTRODUCTION

The fluorescence histochemistry of biogenic monoamines, according to the formaldehyde condensation method devised almost ten years ago by Falck, Hillarp, and co-workers (Corrodi and Hillarp, 1963, 1964; Falck, 1962; Falck *et al.*, 1962), is now widely used. It is a very sensitive, precise, and versatile method, which has proven extremely useful, not only for morphological studies, but also in pharmacological and physiological research. A critical point in all such studies is the actual identification of the studied fluorogenic compound, *i.e.* the compound that yields fluorescence after formaldehyde gas treatment. Although a correct identification of the fluorogenic monoamine, especially the primary catecholamines, can often be achieved in the fluorescence microscope by means of the available specificity tests in combination with chemical analyses, this has frequently led to misinterpretations. For this reason, a final identification of a fluorogenic compound also requires a direct characterization of its fluorophore. The technique of analysing the formaldehyde-induced monoamine fluorophores by means of microspectrofluorimetry was introduced by van Orden *et al.* (1965), by Ritzén and co-workers (Caspersson *et al.*, 1966), and by Jonsson (1967). They demonstrated that the fluorophores formed from a number of phenylethyl-amine and indolylethylamine derivatives, particularly the catecholamines and 5-hydroxytryptamine, displayed characteristic and reproducible excitation and emission spectra. The spectral recordings thus provide not only a characterization of the fluorophore, but also permit a differentiation between various fluorogenic monoamines at their cellular storage sites. Although this analytical technique is still in its developmental stage, the necessary basis for the analysis is now so well known that microspectrofluorimetry must be considered indispensable for the basic identification in monoamine histochemistry. Because no basic microspectrofluorimetric characterization had previously been performed on the intraneuronal fluorogenic monoamines in the mammalian central nervous system, a study was initiated in our laboratory (Björklund *et al.*, 1970a, 1970c, 1971b). This led to the discovery of a hitherto unidentified intraneuronal fluorogenic compound in extensive neuron systems in the CNS of the rat. This study is reviewed and discussed in the present paper.

*References pp. 72–73*

TABLE 1

CHARACTERISTICS OF THE FORMALDEHYDE-INDUCED FLUOROPHORES OF A NUMBER OF PROPOSED BIOGENIC PHENYLETHYLAMINE AND INDOLYLETHYLAMINE DERIVATIVES ENCLOSED IN DRIED PROTEIN FILMS

| Substance group | Substance | Site of occurrence[a] | References | Relative fluorescence yield[b] | Exc. max. (nm) | Em. max. (nm) |
|---|---|---|---|---|---|---|
| Group A | 3,4,β-trihydroxyphenyl-ethylamine (noradrenaline) | Common, incl. brain | | 100 | 320 and 410 | 475 |
| | 3,4-dihydroxyphenylethyl-amine (dopamine) | Common, incl. brain | | 100 | 320 and 410 | 475 |
| | N-methyl-3,4,β-trihydro-xyphenylethylamine (adrenaline) | Adrenal medulla; Amphibian symp. nerv. syst; brain | Von Euler, 1963; Falck et al., 1963, 1969; Juorio and Vogt, 1967; Vogt, 1954 | 40 | 320 and 410 | 475 |
| | 3,4-dihydroxyphenylalanine (dopa) | Mammalian skin; brain | Cegrell et al., 1970; McGreer and McGreer, 1962; Montagu, 1957 | 120 | 320 and 410 | 475 |
| Group B1 | tryptamine (β3-indolyl)-ethylamine | Blood; liver after MAO-inhibition; nerve cords of Mollusc; skin of Salamandra | Cardot, 1963; Eccleston et al., 1966, 1963; Erspamer, 1966; Hess et al., 1959 | 20 | 370 | 495[c] |
| | tryptophan | Common, incl. brain | | 10 | 375 | 435 or 500[d] |
| Group B2 | 6-hydroxytryptamine | Heart of Crustacea | Kerkut and Price, 1964 | 130 | 385 (420)* | 505 |
| | 5,6-dihydroxytryptamine | Pericardial organ of Crustacea | Carlisle, 1964 | 30 | 310 and (380)*405 | (<340) 500 |
| | N-methyl-5-hydroxytrypt-amine | Amphibian skin | Erspamer, 1966 | 30 | 315 and (390)* 415 | 505 |
| | 5-methoxytryptamine | Pineal gland; blood | Gross and Franzen, 1965; Maickel and Miller, 1968 | 20 (410)* | (330)* and 380 (470)* | 505[e] |
| Group C | 5-hydroxytryptamine | Common, incl. brain | | 30 | (315)* 385 and 415[d] | 520–530 |
| | 5-hydroxytryptophan | Precursor of 5-hydroxy-tryptamine, detectable stores in invertebrate tissues | Erspamer, 1966 | 10 | 310, 385 and 415 | 520–530 |
| Other Compounds[f] | N-acetyl-5-hydroxy-tryptamine | Pineal gland | Maickel and Miller, 1968 | 0 | <310 and 420** | 420** (490)* |
| | N-acetyl-5-methoxy-tryptamine (melatonin) | Pineal gland; mammalian peripheral nerves; Amphibian brain | Maickel and Miller, 1968; Veerdonk 1967; Wurtman et al., 1968 | 0 | | |
| | N,N-dimethyltryptamine | Blood | Gross and Franzen, 1965; Heller et al., 1970 | – | | |
| | N,N-dimethyl-5-methoxy-tryptamine | Amphibian skin; blood | Erspamer, 1966; Heller et al., 1970 | – | | |

| Compound | Occurrence | References | | | |
|---|---|---|---|---|---|
| N,N-dimethyl-5-hydroxytryptamine (Bufotenine) | Amphibian skin; invertebrate tissue | Erspamer, 1966 | — | | |
| N,N-dimethyl-5-hydroxytryptamine-o-sulphate (Bufoviridine) | Amphibian skin | Erspamer, 1966 | — | | |
| N,N,N-trimethyl-5-hydroxytryptamine (Bufotenidine) | Amphibian skin | Erspamer, 1966 | — | | |
| Phenylethylamine | Blood; liver and kidney after MAO-inhibition | Asatoor and Dalgliesh, 1959, Nakajima et al., 1964 | 0 | | |
| 3-methoxy-4,β-dihydroxyphenylethylamine (normetanephrine) | Brain | Häggendal, 1963 | 0 | 310 and 370** | 470** |
| 3-methoxy-4-hydroxyphenylethylamine | Brain | Carlsson and Waldeck, 1964 | 0 | 310 and 370** | 470** |
| N-methyl-3,4-dihydroxyphenylethylamine (N-methyldopamine, epinine) | Amphibian tissue | Märki et al., 1962 | ? | | |
| N-acetyl-3,4-dihydroxyphenylethylamine (N-acetyldopamine) | Insect tissue | Sekeris and Karlsson, 1966 | ? | | |
| N-isopropyl-3,4,β-trihydroxyphenylethylamine (N-isopropylnoradrenaline, isoprenaline) | Adrenal gland (?) | Lockett, 1954 | ? | | |
| N,N-dimethyl-3,4,β-trihydroxyphenylethylamine (N-methyl-adrenaline) | Adrenal medulla | Axelrod, 1960 | — | | |
| 4-hydroxyphenylethylamine (p-tyramine) | Brain | Boulton and Majer, 1970 | 0 | | |
| 4,β-dihydroxyphenylethylamine (octopamine) | Sympathetic nerves; extra-cerebral tissues after MAO-inhibition | Kakimoto and Armstrong, 1962 Molinoff and Axelrod, 1969; Osumi and Fujiwara, 1969 | 0 | | |
| phenylalanine | Common, incl. brain | | 0 | | |
| p-tyrosine | Common, incl. brain | | 0 | | |

a.  The proposed identity of the isolated compounds has in many cases not been fully proved.
b.  Formaldehyde treatment for 1 h at +80°C according to the standard Falck–Hillarp procedure. The values are approximated from refs. Björklund et al., 1968b; Björklund and Stenevi, 1970; Falck et al., 1962; Jonsson, 1967; Jonsson and Sandler, 1969; Norberg et al., 1966. Values expressed with the intensities obtained from noradrenaline and dopamine as 100.
c.  The emission maximum of the tryptamine fluorophore exhibits a concentration-dependent variation from 450–520 nm (cf. Björklund et al., 1968b).
d.  The different peaks are observed under different conditions (cf. Björklund et al., 1968b).
e.  The emission maximum of the 5-methoxytryptamine fluorophore is higher (520–550 nm) under more intense reaction conditions, and at higher amine concentrations.
f.  This group includes compounds which give no or only very weak visible fluorescence after condensation with formaldehyde gas according to the Falck–Hillarp procedure. Three compounds with as yet unknown fluorescence characteristics are also included.
*  Position of shoulder given within brackets.
** Very weak visible fluorescence.

MICROSPECTROFLUORIMETRIC CLASSIFICATION OF THE FLUOROPHORES OF
SOME BIOGENIC MONOAMINES

In fluorescence histochemistry, we should bear in mind that there is actually a wide
variety of biogenic phenylethylamines and indolylethylamines, *i.e.* compounds known
to occur in animal tissues. Table 1 lists a number of these monoamines together with
their reported sites of occurrence. It should be noted that the chemical identification
of the different compounds has not always been conclusive and the suggested identity
of the isolated compounds may be only provisional.

As Table 1 shows, a number of phenylethylamines have been found in mammalian
nervous tissues, not only the well-known and widely distributed primary catecholamines, noradrenaline and dopamine, and their 3-*O*-methylated derivatives, but also
*p*-tyramine, octopamine, and possibly also adrenaline and DOPA. 5-Hydroxytrypt-
amine is the most studied biogenic indolylethylamine, having a distribution in nervous
and non-nervous tissues throughout the animal kingdom (for an extensive review of
this subject see Erspamer (1966)). However, a large number of closely related indolylethylamines are also probably biogenic (Table 1). Of these only melatonin has been
found in nervous tissues (van de Veerdonk, 1967; Wurtman *et al.*, 1968).

To what extent can these biogenic monoamines be visualized with the formaldehyde condensation procedure according to the Falck–Hillarp method? The studies
performed by Corrodi, Hillarp and Jonsson (for review and references, see Corrodi
and Jonsson, 1969) have demonstrated that in the cyclization reaction between monoamines and formaldehyde, only those primary and secondary amines with a high
electron density at the point of ring closure will cyclize under the conditions of the
Falck–Hillarp method; tertiary amines like bufotenine cannot cyclize. This means that
in this reaction the catecholamines and to a varying degree the indolylethylamines give
a high yield of fluorophores with strong visible fluorescence. Table 1 gives the approximate fluorescence yields of the proposed biogenic monoamines in the Falck–Hillarp
method. From this it can be seen that quite a few presumably biogenic indolylethylamines could be visualized histochemically, and that some of these amines give a
fluorescence as strong as, or stronger than, 5-hydroxytryptamine.

Microspectrofluorimetry makes possible the basic characterization and differentiation of the formaldehyde-induced fluorophores of these compounds necessary for their
actual identification. It is convenient to divide the fluorophores of these compounds
into three different groups on the basis of their emission peak maxima (see Table 1):
Group A has an emission peak maximum at about 475 nm and comprises the
fluorophores of the catecholamines. The substances in Group B have emission
peak maxima ranging from 495 to 510 nm. This group includes tryptamine, 6-
hydroxytryptamine, 5,6-dihydroxytryptamine, *N*-methyl-5-hydroxytryptamine, and
also 5-methoxytryptamine and tryptophan under certain conditions. Group C
comprises the fluorophores with emission peak maxima from 520 to 540 nm. 5-Hydro-
xytryptamine and 5-hydroxytryptophan belong to this group, as well as 5-methoxy-
tryptamine under certain conditions.

The classification of the monoamine fluorophores by their emission maxima means that the fluorophores within each group will have similar fluorescence colour. Thus, the catecholamine fluorophores of Group A have a clearly blue fluorescence, which, however, will appear green when viewed through the commonly used absorption filters with high absorption below 490 nm. The fluorophores of Groups B and C all have a colour in the yellow range, and it should be emphasized that a positive distinction between Group B and Group C fluorophores cannot usually be achieved subjectively in the fluorescence microscope.

Within each group of fluorophores, certain possibilities exist for the differentiation between individual compounds, mainly by means of their excitation spectra. Thus the two primary catecholamines, noradrenaline and dopamine, which are both widely distributed neuronal monoamines in the mammalian brain, can be differentiated on the basis of their different excitation spectra at acid pH (Björklund *et al.*, 1968, 1971a). In this differentiation procedure, adrenaline behaves like noradrenaline and DOPA like dopamine. On the basis of their excitation spectra, the indolylethylamine fluorophores in Group B can also be distinguished into two subgroups (Table 1). One is characterized by a single excitation peak with the maximum at about 370 nm. This group comprises the unsubstituted indolylethylamine, tryptamine (as well as tryptophan). In the other subgroup, the excitation spectrum is characterized by a double peak, one at 380–390 nm and the other at 405–420 nm. The relative predominance of these two peaks varies and depends on a number of factors such as concentration, reaction conditions, and pH. In addition to the double peak, many of these fluorophores have a peak or shoulder in the excitation spectrum at about 310–320 nm. The excitation spectra of the 5-hydroxytryptamine and 5-hydroxytryptophan fluorophores in Group C also have the characteristics of this second subgroup of Group B. Additional possibilities for further histochemical and microspectrofluorimetric characterization of monoamine fluorophores are outside the scope of this paper; they can be found in the papers by Björklund *et al.* (1968b, 1971b) and Björklund and Stenevi (1970).

CHARACTERIZATION OF NEURONAL MONOAMINES IN THE CNS OF THE RAT

Microspectrofluorimetry of specific, formaldehyde-induced fluorophores has been carried out on the rat spinal cord, brain stem, and hypothalamus by Björklund *et al.* (1970a, 1970c, 1971b). In the fluorescence microscope, *two types* of fluorophores can readily be distinguished: One has a blue fluorescence colour (or green under the most commonly used filter settings) and there is much evidence that this type of fluorophore is derived from the catecholamines, predominantly from the primary catecholamines (*cf.* Carlsson *et al.*, 1962; Fuxe *et al.*, 1969). The other is yellow and has generally been ascribed to 5-hydroxytryptamine (*cf.* Fuxe *et al.*, 1968). In the microspectrofluorimeter, spectra can readily be obtained from the blue fluorescence localized in cell bodies and nerve terminals in many localizations. The yellow fluorescence is generally weaker and, in non-pretreated animals, spectra can be recorded from cell bodies in the upper brain stem and from nerve terminals in the gray matter of the spinal cord and the subcommissural organ. To improve the conditionsf or the analysis, especially of the

TABLE 2

CHARACTERISTICS OF FOUR TYPES OF NEURONAL FLUOROPHORES IN THE RAT CENTRAL NERVOUS SYSTEM[†]

| Type of fluorophore | Identified monoamine | Exc. max. (nm) | Em. max. (nm) | Photodecomposition rate | Drugs** | | | | | |
|---|---|---|---|---|---|---|---|---|---|---|
| | | | | | — | p-Chlorophenylalanine[a] | Nialamide[b] | p-Chlorophenylalanine[a] + nialamide[b] | p-Chlorophenylalanine[a] + α-methyl-m-tyrosine[c] | Reserpine[d] |
| A-Type 1 | Noradrenaline | (320)*410[e] | 475 | Slow | Visible | Unchanged | Unchanged | Unchanged | Depleted | Depleted |
| A-Type 2 | Dopamine | (320)*410[f] | 475 | Slow | Visible | Unchanged | Unchanged | Unchanged | Depleted | Depleted |
| B-Type | ? | (315)* 370–380 (420) | 495–510 | Rather slow | Visible | Unchanged | Unchanged | Unchanged | Unchanged | Depleted |
| C-Type | 5-hydroxytryptamine | (315)* 380–390 | 520–535 | Rapid | Visible | Depleted | Increased | Depleted | Depleted | Depleted |

[†] Data compiled from Björklund *et al.*, 1970a and c, 1971b.

\* Low peak or shoulder.

\*\* The table reflects subjective evaluations in the fluorescence microscope after various drugs.

a. 350 mg/kg, i.p., 96 h + 100 mg/kg, i.p., 24 h.

b. 200–500 mg/kg, i.p., 3–5 h.

c. 400 mg/kg, i.p., 6 h.

d. 5 mg/kg, i.p., 24 h.

e. At acid pH, the main excitation peak is at 320 nm (Björklund *et al.*, 1968a).

f. At acid pH, the main excitation peak is at 365 nm (Björklund *et al.*, 1968a).

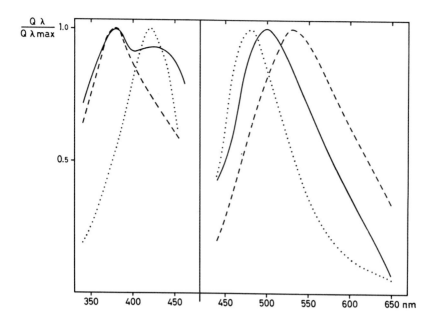

Fig. 1. Excitation (left) and emission (right) spectra of three types of fluorophores obtained after formaldehyde gas treatment in the rat spinal cord. . . . . . . = A-type (catecholamine) fluorophore; ———— = B-type fluorophore; —————— = C-type (5-hydroxytryptamine) fluorophore. The spectra are expressed as relative quanta *versus* wavelength. From Björklund *et al.* (1970c).

yellow type of fluorescence, spectra were also recorded in specimens from rats treated with a MAO-inhibitor, nialamide (*cf.* Table 2), and from animals with lesions in the spinal cord, brain stem, or hypothalamus. After such lesions, which were placed to transect axon bundles of monoamine neurons, a rapid piling up of the intraneuronal monoamines occurs in the axons just proximal to the transection. This accumulation gives rise to a strong intra-axonal monoamine fluorescence which is most convenient for reliable spectral recordings.

In the microspectrofluorimetric analysis of these different types of specimens, *four types* of formaldehyde-induced fluorophores can be demonstrated (Table 2). The blue fluorescence always displayed the spectra common for the different catecholamine fluorophores (exc. max./em. max. at 320 and 410/475 nm, Fig. 1). Upon acidification according to the procedure of Björklund and Ehinger (1971a) and Björklund *et al.* (1968a), one type of fluorophore showed the transformations in the excitation spectra characteristic of the noradrenaline and adrenaline fluorophores (A-type 1 fluorophore in Table 2); the other showed the transformation characteristic of the dopamine fluorophore (A-type 2 fluorophore in Table 2) (Björklund *et al.*, 1970a). These types of fluorophore also showed the relatively slow photodecomposition rate upon irradiation with ultraviolet or blue-violet light characteristic of the catecholamine fluorophores (Fig. 2; *cf.* Ritzén, 1966a), and they were not observed after pretreatment of the animals with reserpine or α-methyl-*m*-tyrosine (Table 2). The appearance of these fluorophores was not notably affected by pretreatment with nialamide or the tryptophan-5-hydro-

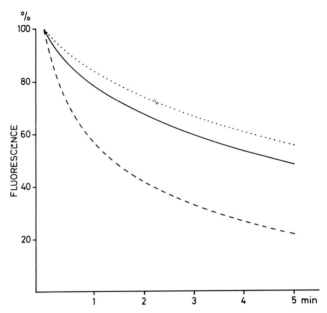

Fig. 2. Fluorescence fading of the three types of formaldehyde-induced fluorophores, recorded in the microspectrofluorimeter from the rat spinal cord. Time of irradiation (405 nm) is given on the x-axis. ...... = A-type (catecholamine) fluorophore; ——— = B-type fluorophore; —————— = C-type (5-hydroxytryptamine) fluorophore. From Björklund *et al.* (1970c).

xylase inhibitor, *p*-chlorophenylalanine (Table 2; Björklund *et al.*, 1970c). In all probability, these two blue-fluorescent types of fluorophores can be ascribed to noradrenaline and dopamine. It is not yet known to what extent adrenaline or DOPA fluorescence can be observed in the rat brain, for in this connection adrenaline fluorescence would be misinterpreted as noradrenaline, and DOPA fluorescence as dopamine.

The yellow fluorescence was found to be of two distinctly different types. One, the C-type fluorophore in Table 2, had the spectral characteristics of the fluorophores in Group C in Table 1 (comprising 5-hydroxytryptamine and 5-hydroxytryptophan). The exc./em. maxima were 315 and 385/520–535 nm (Fig. 1). This type of fluorophore showed a rapid photodecomposition rate (Fig. 2) similar to the 5-hydroxytryptamine and 5-hydroxytryptophan fluorophores (*cf.* Ritzén, 1966b). This fluorescence was markedly stronger in animals pretreated with the MAO-inhibitor (nialamide), but could not be observed in animals pretreated with reserpine or with the tryptophan-5-hydroxylase inhibitor, *p*-chlorophenylalanine. On the other hand, the catecholamine depletor, α-methyl-*m*-tyrosine, had no notable effect (Table 2; Björklund *et al.*, 1970c). From these data it can be concluded that this fluorophore is most probably derived from 5-hydroxytryptamine. From a purely histochemical standpoint, 5-hydroxytryptophan could also give rise to this type of fluorescence, but thus far no significant amounts of this compound have been found in the rat brain (Garattini and Valzelli, 1965). The 5-hydroxytryptamine fluorescence was observed in widespread cell bodies in the raphe regions of the brain stem, and in terminals in the gray matter of the spinal cord and the subcommissural organ. After the transecting lesions, 5-hydroxytryptamine accumulations were found in prominent pathways descending from the brain stem to the spinal cord, and ascending through the mesencephalon and hypothalamus (Björklund et al., 1970c, 1971b; cf. Fuxe et al., 1968).

The second type of yellow fluorescence (B-type fluorophore in Table 2) had the excitation maxima at 315 and 375 nm, with a shoulder at 420 nm, and the emission maximum at 495–510 nm (Fig. 1) characteristic of the Group B2 of monoamine fluorophores listed in Table 1. This fluorescence showed a photodecomposition rate that was notably slower than the 5-hydroxytryptamine type of fluorescence (Fig. 2). It could not be observed after pretreatment with reserpine, but was unaffected by the pretreatments with the tryptophan-5-hydroxylase inhibitor, p-chlorophenylalanine, by the catecholamine depletor, α-methyl-m-tyrosine, and by the MAO-inhibitor, nialamide (Table 2). This type of fluorophore was found in a large number of cell bodies with a distribution in the raphe region of the pons and mesencephalon rather similar to the 5-hydroxytryptamine type of cell bodies in this region, and these two types of cell bodies were to a varying extent intermingled. As observed in the lesioned animals, the B-type of yellow fluorophore occurred in a minor portion of the monoamine fibres descending to the spinal cord but, after combined treatment with p-chlorophenylalanine and α-methyl-m-tyrosine, this type of fluorophore was predominant. The B-type fluorophore was found in nerve terminals in the gray matter of the spinal cord in non-lesioned animals (Björklund et al., 1970c), and in a prominent system of neurons ascending from the upper brain stem through the mesencephalon and hypothalamus (Björklund et al., 1971b). The terminal distribution of these fibres is unknown, although fibres of this type have been observed to enter the median eminence–pituitary region (Björklund et al., 1970a).

## DISCUSSION

The intraneuronal, formaldehyde-induced fluorophores of noradrenaline, dopamine, and 5-hydroxytryptamine could be identified microspectrofluorimetrically in agreement with a bulk of chiefly pharmacological but also histochemical evidence (for discussion, see refs. Carlsson et al., 1962 and Dahlström and Fuxe, 1965). However, the microspectrofluorimetric analysis disclosed a fourth type of intraneuronal fluorophore with a yellow fluorescence that cannot be positively distinguished from the 5-hydoxytryptamine fluorescence in the fluorescence microscope. In the previous literature, this type of fluorophore has been ascribed to 5-hydroxytryptamine because it had not been subjected to microspectrofluorimetric analysis. The fluorogenic compound that gives rise to this new fluorophore has an intraneuronal localization, with a major storage in cell bodies and terminals. It is accumulated intra-axonally after axonal transection in a way suggesting that the compound is transported from cell bodies to terminals along axons. Further, its depletion by reserpine is compatible with a granular storage mechanism for the compound in the neuron. In all these properties, the fluorogenic substance that gives rise to the B-type of yellow fluorophore is similar to the known intraneuronal monamines. It is of particular interest that the spectral and histochemical properties of this new fluorophore are those of the indolylethylamines in Group B2 (Table 1). As Table 1 shows, this group comprises 6-hydroxytryptamine, 5,6-dihydroxytryptamine, *N*-methyl-5-hydroxytryptamine, and possibly also 5-methoxytryptamine. All these compounds are probably biogenic and, thus, the ability to synthesize and metabolize them can be expected in animal tissues. However, the intraneuronal fluorogenic compound has not yet been chemically isolated or identified. Such information is necessary to be able to state that the new fluorophore is derived from a hitherto unknown monoamine. Meanwhile, we are aware of other possible explanations for the observations of this new fluorophore in the rat brain.

### ACKNOWLEDGEMENTS

This study was supported by grants from the Magnus Bergwall Foundation, from the Åke Wiberg Foundation, and from the United States Public Health Service (NB 06701-04), and was carried out within a research organization sponsored by the Swedish Medical Research Council (Projects No. B70-14X-56-06 and B70-14X-712-05).

*N*-Methyl-5-hydroxytryptamine, *N*-acetyl-5-hydroxytryptamine, 5,6-dihydroxytryptamine and 6-hydroxytryptamine were gifts from Dr. John Daly, National Institutes of Health, Bethesda, Md. Bufotenine was a gift from Prof. Bo Holmstedt, Karolinska Institute, Stockholm, Sweden. 5-Hydroxytryptamine creatinine sulphate, noradrenaline-HCl, dopamine-HCl, 3-methoxytyramine-HCl, and L-DOPA were obtained from Sigma; tryptamine-HCl, 5-methoxytryptamine-HCl and *N*,*N*-dimethyl-tryptamine from Aldrich; 5-hydroxytryptophan and normetanephrine from Hoffmann–La Roche; and melatonin was obtained from Regis.

### REFERENCES

ASATOOR, A. M. AND DALGLIESH, C. E. (1959) *Biochem. J.*, **73**, 26 P.
AXELROD, J. (1960) *Biochim. Biophys. Acta*, **45**, 614.
BJÖRKLUND, A. AND EHINGER, B. (1971a) to be published.
BJÖRKLUND, A., EHINGER, B. AND FALCK, B. (1968a) *J. Histochem. Cytochem.*, **16**, 262.
BJÖRKLUND, A., FALCK, B., HROMEK, F., OWMAN, CH. AND WEST, K. A. (1970a) *Brain Res.*, **17**, 1.
BJÖRKLUND, A., FALCK, B. AND HÅKANSON, R. (1968b) *Acta Physiol. Scand.*, Suppl. 318.
BJÖRKLUND, A., FALCK, B. AND OWMAN, CH. (1971b) In I. KOPIN (Ed.), *Methods in Investigative and Diagnostic Endocrinology*, North Holland Publ. Comp., Amsterdam, to be published.
BJÖRKLUND, A. FALCK, B. AND STENEVI, U. (1970c) *J. Pharmacol. Exp. Therap.*, **175**, 525.
BJÖRKLUND, A., FALCK, B. AND STENEVI, U. (1971b) to be published.
BJÖRKLUND, A. AND STENEVI, U. (1970) *J. Histochem. Cytochem.*, **18**, 794.
BOULTON, A. A. AND MAJER, J. R. (1970) *J. Chromatogr.*, **48**, 322.
CARDOT, J. (1963) *C.R. Soc. Biol. (Paris)*, **157**, 853.
CARLISLE, D. B. (1964) The neurohumoral control of heart rate in crustaceans. In D. RICHTER (Ed.), *Comparative Neurochemistry*, Pergamon Press, Oxford, p. 323.
CARLSSON, A., FALCK, B. AND HILLARP, N.-Å. (1962) *Acta Physiol. Scand.*, **56**, Suppl. 196.
CARLSSON, A. AND WALDECK, B. (1964) *Scand. J. Clin. Lab. Invest.*, **16**, 133.
CASPARSSON, T., HILLARP, N.-Å. AND RITZÉN, M. (1966) *Exp. Cell. Res.*, **42**, 415.
CEGRELL, L., FALCK, B. AND ROSENGREN, A.-M. (1970) *Acta Physiol. Scand.*, **78**, 65.

CORRODI, H. AND HILLARP, N.-Å. (1963) *Helv. Chim. Acta*, **46**, 2425.
CORRODI, H. AND HILLARP, N.-Å. (1964) *Helv. Chim. Acta*, **47**, 911.
CORRODI, H. AND JONSSON, G. (1967) *J. Histochem. Cytochem.*, **15**, 65.
DAHLSTRÖM, A. AND FUXE, K. (1965) *Acta Physiol. Scand.*, **62**, Suppl. 232.
ECCLESTON, D., ASCHCROFT, G. W., CRAWFORD, T. B. B. AND LOOSE, R. (1966) *J. Neurochem.*, **13**, 93.
ECCLESTON, D., CRAWFORD, T. B. B. AND ASCHCROFT, G. W. (1963) *Nature*, **197**, 502.
ERSPAMER, V. (1966) Occurrence of indolealkylamines in nature. In *Handbuch der experimentellen Pharmacologie*, Springer, Berlin–Heidelberg–New York, p. 132.
EULER, U. VON (1963) Chromaffin cell hormones. In V. EULER AND HELLER (Eds.), *Comparative Endocrinology*, Academic Press, New York, p. 258.
FALCK, B. (1962) *Acta Physiol. Scand.*, **56**, Suppl. 197.
FALCK, B., HILLARP, N.-Å., THIEME, G. AND TORP, A. (1962) *J. Histochem. Cytochem.*, **10**, 348.
FALCK, B., HÄGGENDAL, J. AND OWMAN, CH. (1963) *Quart. J. Exp. Physiol.*, **48**, 253.
FALCK, B., JACOBSSON, S., OLIVECRONA, H. AND RORSMAN, H. (1966) *Arch. Dermatol.*, **94**, 363.
FALCK, B., LJUNGGREN, L. AND NORDGREN, L. (1969) *Life Sci.*, **8**, 889.
FUXE, K., HÖKFELT, T. AND UNGERSTEDT, U. (1968) *Adv. in Pharmacol.* 6A, 235.
FUXE, K., HÖKFELT, T. AND UNGERSTEDT, U. (1969) In: HOOPER, M. G. (Ed.), *Metabolism of Amines in the Brain*, Macmillan, London, p. 10.
GARATTINI, S. AND VALZELLI, L. (1965) *Serotonin*, Elsevier Publ. Comp., Amsterdam–London–New York, p. 202.
GROSS, H. AND FRANZEN, FR. (1965) *Nature*, **206**, 1052.
HÄGGENDAL, J. (1963) *Acta Physiol. Scand.*, **59**, 370.
HESS, S. M., REDFIELD, B. G. AND UDENFRIEND, S., (1959) *J. Pharmacol. Exp. Therap.*, **127**, 175.
HELLER, B., NARASIMHACHARI, N., SPAIDE, J., HASKOVEC, L. AND HIMWICH, H. E. (1970), *Experientia*, **26**, 503.
JONSSON, G. (1967) *Histochemie*, **8**, 288.
JONSSON, G. AND SANDLER, M. (1969) *Histochemie*, **17**, 207.
JUORIO, A. V. AND VOGT, M. (1967) *J. Physiol.*, **189**, 489.
KAKIMOTO, Y. AND ARMSTRONG, M. D. (1962) *J. Biol. Chem.*, **237**, 422.
KERKUT, G. A. AND PRICE, M. A. (1964) *Comp. Biochem. Physiol.*, **11**, 45.
LOCKETT, M. F. (1954) *Brit. J. Pharmacol.*, **9**, 498.
MAICKEL, R. P. AND MILLER, F. P. (1968) *Adv. Pharmacol.*, **6A**, 71.
McGREER, E. G. AND McGREER, P. L. (1962) *Can. J. Biochem. Physiol.*, **40**, 1141.
MOLINOFF, P. AND AXELROD, J. (1969) *Science*, **164**, 428.
MONTAGU, K. A. (1957) *Nature*, **180**, 244.
MÄRKI, F., AXELROD, J. AND WITKOP, B. (1962) *Biochim. Biophys. Acta*, **58**, 367.
NAKAJIMA, T., KAKIMOTO, Y. AND SANO, I. (1964) *J. Pharmacol. Exp. Therap.*, **143**, 319.
NORBERG, K.-A., RITZÉN, M. AND UNGERSTEDT, U. (1966) *Acta Physiol. Scand.*, **67**, 260.
ORDEN, L. S. VAN, VUGMAN, I. AND GIARMAN, N. J. (1965) *Science*, **148**, 642.
OSUMI, S. AND FUJIWARA, M. (1969) *Jap. J. Pharmac.*, **19**, 185.
RITZÉN, M. (1966a) *Exp. Cell. Res.*, **44**, 505.
RITZÉN, M. (1966b) *Exp. Cell. Res.*, **45**, 178.
SEKERIS, C. E. AND KARLSSON, P. (1966) In G. M. ACHESON (Ed.), *Second Symposium on Catecholamines, Pharmacol. Rev.*, **18**, 89.
VEERDONK, F. C. G. VAN DE (1967) *Currents in Modern Biology I*, North Holland Publ. Comp., Amsterdam, p. 175.
VOGT, M. (1954) *J. Physiol. (Lond.)*, **123**, 451.
WURTMAN, R. J., AXELROD, J. AND KELLY, D. E. (1968) *The Pineal*, Academic Press, New York–London, p. 47.

# II. AUTORADIOGRAPHY AND IMMUNOHISTOCHEMISTRY

# Histochemical Fluorescence Microscopy and Micro-autoradiography Techniques Combined for Localization Studies

DAVID T. MASUOKA, GIAN-FRANCO PLACIDI AND JOHN A. GOSLING

*Neuropharmacology Research Laboratory, Veterans Administration Hospital, Sepulveda, Calif., and Medical Pharmacology and Therapeutics, University of California–Irvine, 92664 Calif. (U.S.A.)*

The availability of [14]C- and [3]H-labeled compounds has permitted study of the distribution and localization at a whole-body, organ, cellular and subcellular level using the technique of autoradiography. With the development of a specific formaldehyde-induced histochemical fluorescence method for aromatic monoamines, the interesting possibility of combining this technique with that of autoradiography presents itself. Such studies might be of value in the localization of binding and storage of putative transmitters. Furthermore, the tissue distribution of a variety of drugs (*e.g.* sympathomimetics, adrenergic blockers, enzyme inhibitors and monoamine releasers) may be correlated with monoamine structures.

The present communication deals with procedures in which the histochemical fluorescence technique is combined with autoradiography in the complete absence of aqueous solutions. This criterion must be met in order to eliminate possible artifacts due to diffusion and dislocation of labeled water-soluble drugs and endogenous amines. Thus, liquid tissue fixation and dehydration through aqueous alcohol solutions before exposure to photographic emulsion, and the use of liquid or wet photographic emulsions over the tissue sections are steps which must be avoided when water-soluble compounds are employed.

## HISTOCHEMICAL FLUORESCENCE TECHNIQUE

The development of the formaldehyde-induced histochemical fluorescence method for the demonstration of aromatic monoamines (Barter and Pearse, 1953, 1955; Eränkö, 1955; Lagunoff *et al.*, 1961; Falck *et al.*, 1962) and its successful application to nervous tissue (Carlsson *et al.*, 1962) have led to significant advances in our knowledge of the distribution and function of monoaminergic nerves in the peripheral and central nervous systems. This method, which is presently the most specific and sensitive method for the localization of catecholamines and serotonin at a cellular level, is dependent upon the fact that these amines can be converted into highly fluorescent compounds when reacted with formaldehyde vapor (Corrodi and Jonsson, 1967).

As was pointed out by Eränkö (1967), the procedure is relatively simple but to obtain good, reproducible fluorescence all of the steps are quite critical. With respect to the present procedures, quick freezing of tissues is necessary to minimize ice crystal artifacts, and exposure of the dry tissue pieces to water or high atmospheric humidity can cause diffusion of fluorescence. The fluorophore in adrenergic nerve terminals appears to be most labile and that from serotonin in mast cells is least affected by water (Corrodi *et al.*, 1964). However, hydrocarbons such as xylene and liquid paraffin do not appear to affect fluorescence (Eränkö, 1967; Falck and Owman, 1965).

Details of the fluorescence microscope are covered adequately in papers by Dahlström and Fuxe (1964) and Falck and Owman (1965).

## AUTORADIOGRAPHY

Although many excellent studies have been done with whole-body and electron microscopic autoradiography, the present procedures deal specifically with auto-radiography only at the light microscope level. This technique consists of locating radioactivity at the cellular level by placing a tissue section containing a radioactive element against a photographic emulsion. The various micro-autoradiographic techniques which are available include: (1) covering a fixed, dehydrated, deparaffinized tissue section with liquid photographic emulsion (Belanger and Leblond, 1946); (2) covering a similarly treated tissue section with wet stripping film (Pelc, 1947); and (3) placing a freeze-dried cryostat section (Stumpf and Roth, 1966) or frozen section (Appleton, 1964) or freeze-dried, paraffin-embedded section (Hammarström *et al.*, 1965) over a microscope slide previously coated with emulsion. For autoradio-graphy of water-soluble substances, it is essential that steps involving an aqueous environment be eliminated completely; Stumpf and Roth (1966) have demonstrated that diffusion occurs in deparaffinized tissue sections dipped in liquid emulsion.

Consequently in developing a technique which combines fluorescence microscopy with micro-autoradiography the major factors for consideration are:

1. Water, aqueous alcohol and fixative solutions must be avoided to prevent diffusion of fluorophores and displacement of water-soluble radioactive drugs.

2. The tissue section (a) must be placed in direct contact with a dry, not liquid or wet, emulsion and (b) must remain attached to the emulsion during exposure, development, staining and final microscopy.

3. The distribution of monoamines and labeled compounds should be examined on the same section when the target site is relatively small (*e.g.* nerve terminals). If the target site is relatively large (*e.g.* neurons), thin adjacent sections may also be employed.

With these criteria in mind, two procedures are available, both of which are presently being used in this laboratory. These consist of a freeze-dried paraffin-embedding method and a cryostat method.

## FREEZE-DRIED PARAFFIN-EMBEDDING METHOD (F-D PARAFFIN) FOR HISTOCHEMICAL FLUORESCENCE AND AUTORADIOGRAPHY

The localization of radioactively labeled water-soluble substances studied in relation to monoaminergic structures has been described previously (Masuoka and Placidi, 1968). However, the method presented here incorporates certain improvements and modifications.

After treatment with radioactive material *in vivo* or *in vitro*, small tissue pieces are quenched in propane cooled by liquid nitrogen, freeze-dried at —40° for 3 to 7 days, heated with paraformaldehyde for 1 h at 80°, and embedded *in vacuo* in paraffin (Falck and Owman, 1965; Dahlström and Fuxe, 1964). Sections are cut at 6–8 $\mu$ and placed on Entellan-coated slides (Fig. 1A). These are clean, non-fluorescing, glass microscope slides which have been coated by dipping slightly more than one-half the length in a 1:1 (v/v) mixture of Entellan (E. Merck, Darmstadt, Germany) and xylene. The excess liquid is allowed to drain for 5–7 sec (a longer period of time may result in a coating which is too thin). The slides are then placed horizontally on a rack and dried in an oven at 80° for 10–15 min. Tissue sections placed on these Entellan-coated slides are allowed to flatten and adhere by warming at 60° for about 15 min. Just before fluorescence microscopy, one drop of mineral oil is placed over the section and pictures of the fluorescent structures are recorded on Kodak Tri-X Pan film and/or Polaroid 3000 film.

For micro-autoradiography, the mineral oil is removed from the section by washing carefully dropwise with *n*-heptane from a medicine dropper or pipette. (The section can shift or be lost at this step.) It must be determined in advance that the radioactive compound which is being investigated is not soluble in *n*-heptane. As far as norepinephrine in nerve terminals is concerned, the condensation product after reaction with formaldehyde is quite resistant to extraction with *n*-heptane (Masuoka and Placidi, 1970), hot paraffin and certain organic solvents (Falck *et al.*, 1962; Corrodi *et al.*, 1964). Since the catecholamine fluorophores are not affected by several solvents, it may be possible to find a suitable solvent compatible with fluorescence microscopy and one in which the radioactive compound being investigated is not soluble.

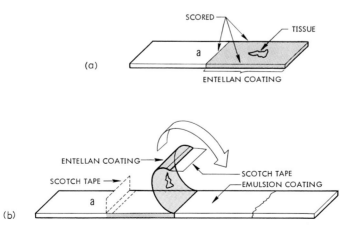

Fig. 1. A, Tissue section attached to Entellan-coated slide. B, tissue transferred to emulsion-coated slide.

In order to transfer the tissue to a dry emulsion-coated slide the Entellan coating is scored with a razor blade as illustrated in Fig. 1A, and a piece of 3-M Scotch transparent tape is attached to the coating at *a* (Fig. 1B). In the darkroom, this slide and another slide previously coated with emulsion are placed end-to-end, and by pulling the Scotch tape in the direction of the arrow, the thin Entellan film together with the adhering tissue are placed in contact with the dry emulsion. In this laboratory, emulsion-coated slides are prepared by dipping clean, glass microscope slides into G-5 or L-4 Nuclear Research Gel (Ilford, Ltd., Ilford, England) at 35°–40° and diluted with an equal volume of a 0.05 % aqueous solution of dioctyl sodium sulfosuccinate (Eastman Organic Chem., Rochester, N.Y.). The coated slides are allowed to dry in a vertical position with coated end up for several hours before tissue mounting. During autoradiographic exposure, the slide is placed with the Entellan side against a piece of polyethylene film and sandwiched between two blotters and two aluminum plates (all measuring approximately 5 cm × 10 cm) which are fastened together with a thin rubber band at each end. The slides are stored during exposure at —10° in a light-tight metal can containing dry silica gel.

After a suitable exposure period, the exposed slide with tissue and Entellan film still adhering to it are placed carefully into absolute alcohol for 1 min and dried 4–5 min. This step allows the tissue and emulsion to be moistened sufficiently to cause good adherence. The slide is placed in xylene for 6 min to dissolve the Entellan film covering the section and then passed through absolute, 95 % and 70 % ethanol before processing the emulsion. The period of time in developer and fixer should follow the recommendations of the manufacturer of the emulsion. After fixing, the slide is washed in water for 10–30 min, stained with H and E and mounted in Permount. This mounting medium gives good preservation of silver grains for a period of at least 2 years following development of the autoradiogram (N.B. some other media may cause loss of grains in a relatively short time). The autoradiogram is scanned now for areas previously photographed in the fluorescence microscope.

CRYOSTAT THIN-SECTION METHOD FOR HISTOCHEMICAL FLUORESCENCE AND AUTORADIOGRAPHY

Histochemical fluorescence (Placidi and Masuoka, 1968; Roth and Stumpf, 1969) and autoradiography (Stumpf and Roth, 1966) have been performed independently in freeze-dried, thin cryostat sections. Therefore, it is theoretically possible to correlate monoaminergic structures with the distribution of radioactivity in the same cryostat section. However, if one wishes to avoid a liquid medium of any sort for fear of dislocating radioactivity within the tissue, adjacent sections may be used, especially if the structures are sufficiently large as to be included in both sections. For example, since the diameters of autonomic ganglion cells are 15–55 $\mu$ (Hillarp, 1960) and fluorescent cell bodies of the brain are 15–30 $\mu$ (Fuxe *et al.*, 1970), if thin histological sections are prepared, it would be possible to observe the same cell in several consecutive sections. Therefore, it is possible to perform a variety of techniques on the same neuron, *e.g.* the histochemical fluorescence method on one section, micro-autoradiography on another section, and perhaps acetylcholinesterase "staining" on another. The low-temperature, frozen-sectioning method of Stumpf and Roth (1966) has been adapted and modified for the present purpose. They determined that it was possible to prepare thin and ultra-thin sections at temperatures down to —105° and dry-mount the freeze-dried sections onto photographic emulsion-coated slides.

Small tissue pieces (1–2 mm²) are placed on the tip of tapered 1/8″ (3 mm) diameter wooden rods (Placidi and Masuoka, 1968) and rapidly quenched in propane cooled by liquid nitrogen. The stick is placed in the chuck of an International Minot Custom Microtome with an ultra-thin sectioning attachment, and sections 1–2 $\mu$ are cut for micro-autoradiography and an adjacent section 1–2.5 $\mu$ for fluorescence microscopy. The temperature at the level of the knife is —50°. The sections for fluorescence microscopy are placed directly on clean microscope slides and the corresponding sections for micro autoradiography are placed on Entellan-coated slides (described above). Usually a non-radioactive control tissue section was placed on the same slide. All sections are covered with a 3-mm-diameter, 300-mesh specimen grid as used for electron microscopy. Otherwise bothersome curling invariably occurs, perhaps due to more rapid drying from the upper surface of the tissue. After many frustrating trials, it was found that these grids were the ideal material for maintaining the thin tissue sections flat during the drying process.

Without allowing the temperature to rise, the two sets of tissue sections are placed into separate vacuum desiccators containing phosphorus pentoxide and freeze-dried at —50° *in vacuo* for 24–48 h. The tissues are allowed to reach room temperature before the vacuum is broken in a dry atmosphere. The dried sections for fluorescence microscopy are then heated for 1 h at 80° together with paraformaldehyde (Matheson Coleman and Bell, N.J.) which has been previously equilibrated in an atmosphere of 30%–50% relative humidity. The importance of proper humidity and temperature conditions for optimum formaldehyde-induced fluorescence has been well documented (Eränkö, 1967; Hamberger *et al.*, 1965). After reaction, the slides are returned to a dry atmosphere, the sections are covered with a drop of mineral oil and a cover glass, and examined for fluorescence.

The dried sections for micro-autoradiography, mounted on Entellan-coated slides, are transferred in the darkroom to emulsion-coated slides as described above. Exposure, development, and tissue staining are conducted as described.

### DISCUSSION AND APPLICATIONS

There are, of course, advantages and disadvantages in the use of either method. Thus:

1. Paraffin-embedded tissue blocks can be stored until required for sectioning or resectioning, and the whole block can be reoriented to provide a different plane of section. With the cryostat method fresh tissues section more easily and should be prepared before dehydration of the block occurs, and attempts to reorient the block are hazardous.

2. The small size (1–2 mm²) of tissue blocks may be a disadvantage in the cryostat thin-section method.

*References p. 86*

3. Paraffin embedding could be a source of drug translocation, while the cryostat method requires no embedding.

4. Combining histochemical fluorescence and autoradiography in the same section is possible with either method. Removing the mineral oil from the section with *n*-heptane after fluorescence microscopy might cause redistribution of radioactivity within the tissue. This possibility can be reduced by employing the combined method only a) for radioactive substances which are water soluble but insoluble in non-polar liquids, and b) for radioactive substances which may be rendered immobile by treatment of the tissue with formaldehyde gas or other vapor.

5. Both the F–D Paraffin and cryostat methods can provide consecutive sections. Although individual nerve terminals cannot be compared, the cryostat thin-section

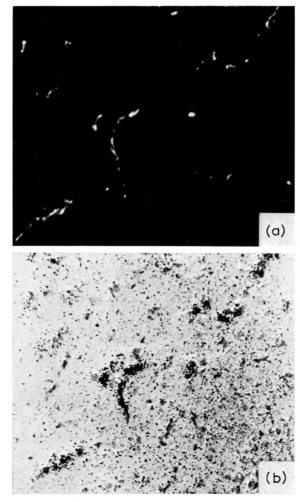

Fig. 2. Rat heart ventricle 5 min after intravenous injection of [³H]norepinephrine. a, fluorescence microphotograph and b, autoradiograph of the same section. (H and E stain). × 225.

technique has the capability of cutting several thin sections of the same nerve cell body for comparative fluorescence microscopy, micro-autoradiography, and other histochemical procedures (*e.g.* acetylcholinesterase activity). Each section can be processed separately, and thus one can be assured that maximum fluorescence can be obtained in one section, without altering enzyme activity by excess heat and formaldehyde treatment in the other sections. In addition, sections for micro-autoradiography are not in contact with any potential solvent.

The use of Entellan-coated slides has facilitated and resolved several difficult and annoying steps  in both procedures: 1) It forms a thin layer which does not fluoresce when exposed to UV light; 2) It peels readily, thus allowing the same section from fluorescence microscopy to be transferred to an emulsion-coated slide; 3) Since transferring is easy, tissue pieces can be freeze-dried directly on microscope slides. This aids not only the production of relatively flat sections, but also facilitates iden-

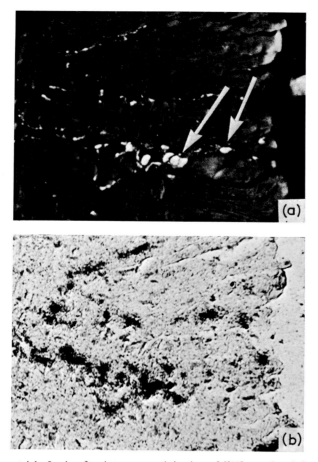

Fig. 3. Rat heart ventricle 5 min after intravenous injection of [³H]norepinephrine. a, fluorescence microphotograph with arrows pointing to probable mast cells (yellow fluorescence); b, autoradiograph of the same section. Note cells not radioactively labeled. (Hematoxylin). × 240.

tification and maintenance of tissue sections in proper sequence; 4) It reduces time expended in the darkroom.

The combined procedures in the same section have been used to demonstrate the localization of intravenously injected radioactively labeled NE in relation to fluorescent adrenergic nerves. Certain problems inherent in previous studies have been resolved by this technique since it is possible a) to delineate visually the uptake of a low concentration of NE into fluorescent nerve terminals in the absence of drug pretreatment (reserpine, nialamid, etc.) and b) to avoid the possibility that the special conditions of the experiment, such as drug pretreatment or a high concentration of NE, did not cause other nonadrenergic nerve structures to fluoresce. Fig. 2 shows a fluorescence photomicrograph (A) and a micro-autoradiograph (B) of a rat heart ventricle 5 min after intravenous injection of [³H]-NE. The deposition of silver grains

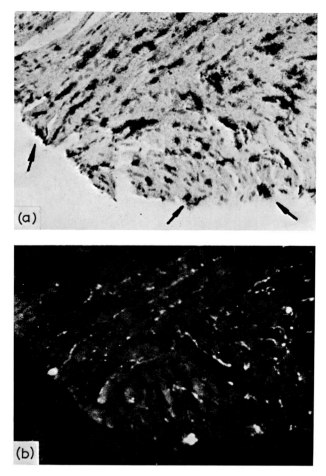

Fig. 4. Rat heart ventricle 1 h after intravenous injection of [³H]norepinephrine. a, autoradiograph of the same section; b, fluorescence microphotograph with probable mast cells (yellow fluorescence). Note cells and adrenergic nerves are radioactively labeled. (Hematoxylin). × 190.

indicating an accumulation of radioactivity forms a pattern corresponding exactly to the fluorescent nerves. Therefore uptake of [³H]-NE within 5 min was observed only in those structures which show a specific fluorescence reaction with formaldehyde (Masuoka and Placidi, 1970).

Studies are presently under way in this laboratory on the specificity of the uptake mechanism (data to be published). Fig. 3 shows a similar fluorescence photomicrograph (A) and micro-autoradiograph (B) of a rat heart ventricle. The arrows in Fig. 3A point to intensely yellow fluorescing mast cells, which upon careful comparison reveals that these cells 5 min after [³H]-NE injection have not accumulated significant amounts of radioactivity, whereas the fluorescent nerves are highly labeled. However, one hour after [³H]-NE injection, it is seen in Fig. 4 that both mast cells (arrows) and adrenergic nerves are highly labeled. These studies are being continued in other organs with other labeled monoamines.

In addition to histochemical fluorescence and autoradiography, it is possible to demonstrate acetylcholinesterase activity in adjacent thin cryostat sections. Fig. 5A is a fluorescence photomicrograph of a 2 μ thick section of a cat superior cervical

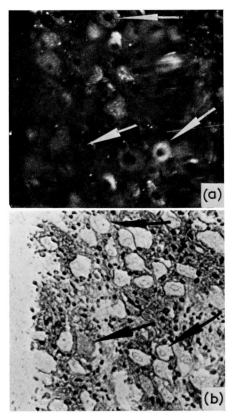

Fig. 5. Cryostat sections 2 μ thick of a cat superior cervical ganglion. a, fluorescence photomicrograph and b, adjacent section showing acetylcholinesterase activity. × 225.

*References p. 86*

ganglion and Fig. 5B is an adjacent 2 $\mu$ thick section which was developed for acetyl-cholinesterase activity (Karnovsky and Roots, 1964).

ACKNOWLEDGMENT

This study was aided by a grant from the American Medical Association Education and Research Foundation and by Veterans Administration institutional support. We thank Mr. Alcaraz for skilful technical assistance.

REFERENCES

APPLETON, T. C. (1964) *J. Roy. Microscop. Soc.*, **83**, 277.
BARTER, R. AND PEARSE, A. G. E. (1953) *Nature*, **172**, 810.
BARTER, R. AND PEARSE, A. G. E. (1955) *J. Pathol. Bacteriol.*, **69**, 25.
BELANGER, L. F. AND LEBLOND, C. P. (1946) *Endocrinology*, **39**, 8.
CARLSSON, A., FALCK, B. AND HILLARP, N.-Å. (1962) *Acta Physiol. Scand.*, **56**, Suppl. 196.
CORRODI, H., HILLARP, N.-Å. AND JONSSON, G. (1964) *J. Histochem. Cytochen.*, **12**, 582.
CORRODI, H. AND JONSSON, G. (1967) *J. Histochem. Cytochem.*, **15**, 65.
DAHLSTRÖM, A. AND FUXE, K. (1964) *Acta Physiol. Scand.*, **62**, Suppl. 232.
ERÄNKO, O. (1955) *Acta Endocrinol.*, **18**, 174.
ERÄNKÖ, O. (1967) *J. Roy. Microscop. Soc.*, **87**, 259.
FALCK, B., HILLARP, N.-Å., THIEME, G. AND TORP, A. (1962) *J. Histochem. Cytochem.*, **10**, 348.
FALCK, B. AND OWMAN, C. (1965) *Acta Univ. Lund.*, **2**, No. 7.
FUXE, K., HÖKFELT, T. AND UNGERSTEDT, U. (1970) In W. G. CLARK AND J. DEL GIUDICE (Eds.), *Principles of Psychopharmacology*, Academic Press, New York, p. 87.
HAMBERGER, B., MALMFORS, T. AND SACHS, C. (1965) *J. Histochem. Cytochem.*, **13**, 147.
HAMMARSTRÖM, L., APPELGREN, L.-E. AND ULLBERG, S. (1965) *Exptl. Cell Res.*, **37**, 608.
HILLARP, N.-Å. (1960) In J. FIELD (Ed.), *Handbook of Physiology*, Am. Physiol. Soc., Washington, D.C., Sect. 1, Vol. II, p. 979.
KARNOVSKY, M. J. AND ROOTS, L. (1964) *J. Histochem. Cytochem.*, **12**, 219.
LAGUNOFF, D., PHILLIPS, M. AND BENDITT, E. V. (1961) *J. Histochem. Cytochem.*, **9**, 534.
MASUOKA, D. T. AND PLACIDI, G. F. (1968) *J. Histochem. Cytochem.*, **16**, 659.
MASUOKA, D. T. AND PLACIDI, G. F. (1970) *J. Histochem. Cytochem.*, **18**, 660.
PELC, S. (1947) *Nature*, **160**, 749.
PLACIDI, G. F. AND MASUOKA, D. T. (1968) *J. Histochem. Cytochem.*, **16**, 491.
ROTH, L. J. AND STUMPF, W. E. (1969) In P. G. WASER AND B. GLASSON (Eds.), *International Conference on Radioactive Isotopes in Pharmacology*, Wiley–Interscience, London, p. 135.
STUMPF, W. E. AND ROTH, L. J. (1966) *J. Histochem. Cytochem.*, **14**, 274.

# Uptake of [³H]noradrenaline and γ-[³H]Aminobutyric Acid in Isolated Tissues of Rat: An Autoradiographic and Fluorescence Microscopic Study

TOMAS HÖKFELT AND ÅKE LJUNGDAHL

*Department of Histology, Karolinska Institutet, S-104 01 Stockholm 60 (Sweden)*

## INTRODUCTION

It is now well established that monoamine neurons possess an efficient mechanism for uptake of exogenous amines. This uptake is in all probability of great physiological significance, since it may inactivate circulating amines and especially since it may terminate the action of released monoamines at peripheral and central synapses (for references see monography by Iversen, 1967).

The existence of an efficient uptake mechanism has made it possible to use autoradiography (*e.g.* Wolfe *et al.*, 1962) and fluorescence histochemistry (*e.g.* Hamberger, 1967; Sachs, 1970) to study the localization and various properties of monoamine neurons, and the results obtained with these techniques have been of fundamental importance for the elucidation of the role of monoamines as possible transmitter substances.

In the search for other putative transmitter substances in the central nervous system much interest has been paid to a group of amino acids including γ-aminobutyric acid (GABA). Both biochemical and neurophysiological studies seem to indicate that at least one role of GABA may be to act as an inhibitory transmitter in certain brain regions (for references see, *e.g.*, recent reviews by Baxter, 1970; Curtis and Johnston, 1970; and Hebb, 1970). Recently attention has been focused on studies demonstrating that GABA, as well as many other amino acids, is taken up into isolated brain slices from the medium against a concentration gradient (Elliott and van Gelder, 1958). It has been suggested that this uptake could serve as an inactivation mechanism similar to that operating in monoamine neurons (Iversen and Neal, 1968). However, since no specific histochemical methods exist for GABA, there is, in contrast to monoamines, so far only little known concerning the exact cellular localization of both endogenous GABA and GABA taken up in isolated tissues. If hypothetical "GABA neurons" work in a similar way as monoamine neurons, *i.e.* GABA released at a synapse is inactivated by reuptake into the presynaptic nerve ending, then autoradiographic studies on the cellular localization of exogenous radioactive GABA may provide information on the localization of "GABA neurons" in the brain.

In the present paper the localization of exogenous and endogenous noradrenaline (NA) will be compared by means of autoradiography and fluorescence histochemistry according to the method of Falck and Hillarp (Falck *et al.*, 1962; Falck, 1962). Against this background results on the cellular localization of [³H]GABA as revealed by autoradiography will be presented and discussed.

## MATERIALS AND METHODS

Isolated irides (Malmfors, 1965) and thin slices (McIlwain and Rodnight, 1962) from different brain regions of rat were incubated either in a modified Krebs–Ringer bicarbonate buffer (Axelrod *et al.*, 1962) with added glucose (2 mg/ml) or in a Tyrode buffer (see Hökfelt *et al.*, 1970). Mostly Dextran (Pharmacia, Uppsala, Sweden) was present in various concentrations (1–10%) in the incubation medium. D,L-[³H]NA (5–10 C/mM; $10^{-8}$–$10^{-6}$ M) or [³H]GABA (2 C/mM; $4 \times 10^{-6}$ M) (both isotopes from New England Nucl. Corp., Boston, Mass.) was added and incubation performed for 30 and 45 min, respectively. In some cases of incubation with [³H]GABA, amino-oxyacetic acid (AOAA) ($10^{-5}$ M), which prevents breakdown of GABA by inhibiting GABA transaminase (Wallach, 1961), was added to the incubation medium. These brain slices were taken from rats previously injected with the same drug (25 mg/kg, i.p., 1 hour). After rinsing the irides were stretched on an object slide, dried and reacted with paraformaldehyde (Malmfors, 1965). The brain slices, after rinsing, were either freeze-dried, reacted with paraformaldehyde and embedded in Araldite (Hökfelt, 1965) or fixed in 5% glutaraldehyde (Sabatini *et al.*, 1963), dehydrated and embedded in Epon (Luft, 1961). 1–5 $\mu$ thick sections were cut on an LKB ultratome.

For autoradiography the stretch preparations or the sections were covered with Ilford L4 emulsion (Ilford Ltd., Essex, England) with the help of a loop technique (Miller *et al.*, 1964; Nagata and Nawa, 1966) and exposed for 2–10 weeks. For combined fluorescence histochemistry and autoradiography the stretch preparations and the sections were examined in a Zeiss fluorescence microscope, photographed and processed for autoradiography. The autoradiograms were examined in a Leitz Orthoplan light microscope equipped with an Ultropak system (E. Leitz, GmbH, Wetzlar, W. Germany).

### Comments on techniques used

The present results are in part based upon either freeze-dried tissues or stretch preparations. These procedures have been chosen to avoid translocation of diffusible substances which may occur when using chemically fixed tissues. Similarly, the autoradiographic procedure was chosen to obtain a comparatively "dry" technique in order to be able to study diffusible substances and to perform combined autoradiography and fluorescence histochemistry on the same section. A "dry" procedure is necessary when working with stretch preparations, since the isotopes in this case are completely unprotected and even the humidity of the air may cause profound diffusion within a short period. This problem is less crucial when working with freeze-dried tissue embedded in epoxy resins.

Combined autoradiography and fluorescence histochemistry has previously been

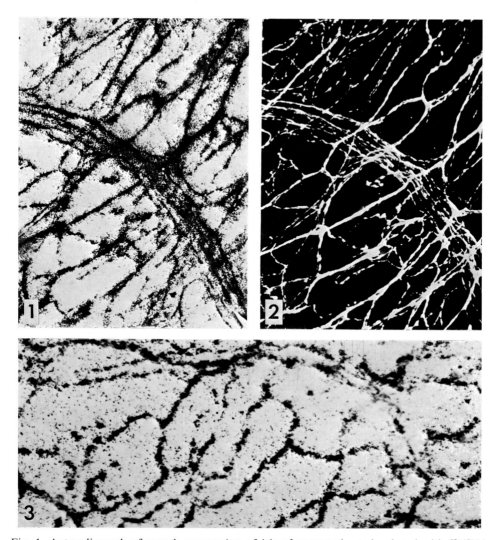

Fig. 1. Autoradiograph of stretch preparation of iris of untreated rat, incubated with [³H]NA (5 × 10⁻⁷ M) and reacted with paraformaldehyde vapours. Grains are concentrated in fiber-like strands running in various directions. From Ljungdahl, Farnebo and Hökfelt, to be published. Magnification 400 ×.

Fig. 2. Fluorescence micrograph of the same iris stretch preparation as in Fig. 1. Before performing autoradiography this stretch preparation was examined in a fluorescence microscope and photographed. Note the close correlation between NA-containing nerves and the distribution of grains as seen in Fig. 1. Magnification 400 ×.

Fig. 3. Autoradiograph of stretch preparation of mouse iris, incubated with 6-[³H]hydroxydopamine (10⁻⁵ M; supplied by Dr. H. Thoenen, Hoffmann–La Roche). The grains are concentrated in small dots with a similar distribution as the varicosities of the NA nerve terminals as revealed with fluorescence microscopy. This demonstrates directly an uptake and accumulation of 6-[³H]hydroxydopamine in the adrenergic neurons. From Ljungdahl, Hökfelt, Jonsson and Sachs, to be published. Magnification 640 ×.

performed by Hammarström *et al.* (1966), Ritzén (1967) and Fuxe *et al.* (1968). A "dry" method for combined autoradiography and fluorescence histochemistry has recently also been devised by Masuoka and Placidi (1968). Furthermore, for an extensive discussion of autoradiography of diffusible substances, see the book edited by Roth and Stumpf (1969).

RESULTS AND DISCUSSION

*Uptake of noradrenaline*

*Peripheral nervous system*

The localization of grains over an iris from an untreated rat, incubated with [³H]NA, stretched on an object glass and covered with an autoradiographic emulsion revealed a characteristic pattern (Fig. 1). Strong accumulations of grains were found running in fiber-like tracts all over the iris. Often these tracts were enlarged at more or less regular intervals. Thus, this pattern was very similar to the distribution of NA nerve terminals as revealed with the method of Falck and Hillarp (Malmfors, 1965). In fact, by performing combined fluorescence histochemistry and autoradiography on the same stretch preparation the almost identical localization of endogenous and exogenous NA was demonstrated (Figs. 1, 2) (Ljungdahl, Farnebo and Hökfelt, to be published), which is in good agreement with many earlier autoradiographic studies demonstrating at the ultrastructural level accumulation of grains over certain peripheral nerve endings (Wolfe *et al.*, 1962; Taxi and Droz, 1966a, b; Devine, 1967; Devine and Simpson, 1968; Esterhuizen *et al.*, 1968a, b; Graham *et al.*, 1968a; Lever *et al.*, 1968; Budd and Salpeter, 1969). Preliminary results indicate that pharmacological treatment and electric stimulation *in vitro* may influence both the number and distribution of grains over the nerve terminals (Ljungdahl, Farnebo and Hökfelt, to be published).

The use of iris stretch preparations for combined fluorescence histochemistry and autoradiography offers a valuable tool to study directly in the microscope the uptake and distribution pattern also of other labelled, water-soluble substances in relation to the NA nerve terminal plexus. Thus, it has been possible to demonstrate that 6-hydroxydopamine, a drug which causes degeneration of catecholamine neurons (Tranzer and Thoenen, 1968), is taken up and retained in the nerve terminals (Ljungdahl, Hökfelt, Jonsson and Sachs, to be published) (Fig. 3).

*Central nervous system*

Over thin hypothalamic slices incubated with [³H]NA, either glutaraldehyde fixed or freeze-dried and embedded in an epoxy resin, a characteristic distribution of grains was seen. Small accumulations (diameter about 1 $\mu$) of grains were seen *e.g.* in the periventricular zone, in the lateral basal hypothalamus, around the large blood vessels of the circle of Willis and especially in the external layer of the median eminence (Figs. 4–6). Accumulations of grains were also seen overlying a number of cell bodies in the arcuate nucleus (Figs. 4, 5). This distribution is in good agreement with the

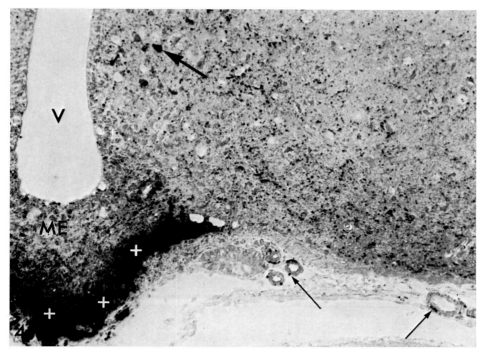

Fig. 4. Autoradiograph from a rat hypothalamic slice incubated with [³H]NA (10⁻⁶M) and fixed in glutaraldehyde. Small, strong accumulations of grains are localized in the periventricular zone, in the basal part of hypothalamus and in the median eminence (ME), especially in the external layer (+). Note accumulations also around blood vessels (thin arrows) and over cell bodies in the arcuate nucleus (thick arrow). V = third ventricle. Magnification 170 ×.

localization of monoamine neurons in the hypothalamus as described by Dahlström and Fuxe (1964) and Fuxe (1965). Combined autoradiography and fluorescence histochemistry in the same sections reveal that the grain accumulations overlie the fluorescent varicosities (Figs. 7, 8). In agreement with this, previous extensive auto-radiographic studies at the ultrastructural level on glutaraldehyde-fixed central nervous tissue have revealed that both [³H]NA and [5-³H]hydroxytryptamine mainly are taken up and accumulated within neurons, principally in the terminal parts (nerve endings, boutons) (Aghajanian and Bloom, 1966a, b, 1967; Lenn, 1967; Descarries and Droz, 1968, 1970).

## Uptake of γ-aminobutyric acid

### Radiometric assays

For many years it has been known that GABA is taken up and accumulated in brain slices (Elliott and van Gelder, 1958; Tsukada *et al.*, 1963; Blasberg and Lajtha, 1966; Weinstein *et al.*, 1965; Nakamura and Nagayama, 1966). Recently Iversen and Neal (1968) have studied the characteristics of this uptake from the viewpoint of GABA being a possible central transmitter substance and proposed that this up-

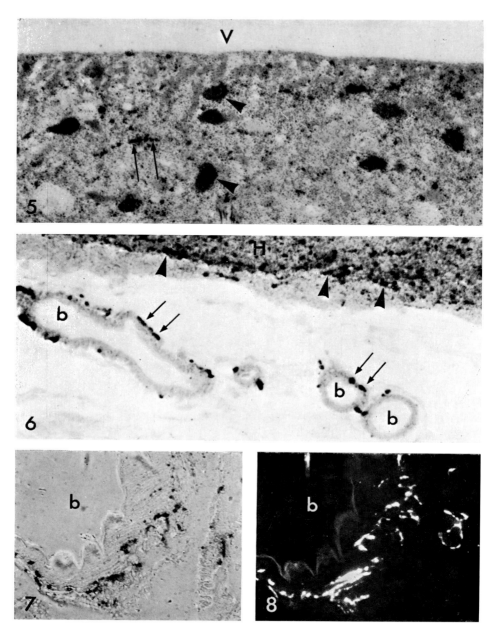

Fig. 5. The same tissue and treatment as Fig. 4. Periventricular zone. Note large, strong accumulations over cell bodies (arrow heads) and smaller accumulations (thin arrows) probably overlying nerve endings (boutons). Magnification 460 ×.

Fig. 6. The same tissue and treatment as Fig. 4. Note small accumulations around blood vessels (b) and in the basal part of hypothalamus (arrow heads). These small, strong accumulations are in all probability overlying nerve endings (boutons). Magnification 380 ×.

Figs. 7, 8. Autoradiograph (Fig. 7) and fluorescence micrograph (Fig. 8) from the same section. Hypothalamic slice incubated with [$^3$H]NA ($10^{-6}$M), freeze-dried, reacted with paraformaldehyde vapours and embedded in Araldite. Around blood vessel (b) belonging to the circle of Willis accumulations of grains are seen, which are well correlated to the distribution of NA nerve terminals as revealed by fluorescence microscopy. Magnification 300 ×.

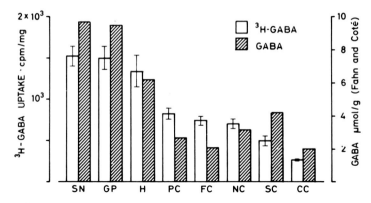

Fig. 9. Comparison between uptake and accumulation of [³H]GABA in various brain regions of ra and endogenous GABA levels in corresponding brain regions of monkey after Fahn and Coté (1968) Correlation coefficient = 0.92. CC = Cerebellar cortex; FC = frontal cortex; GP = globus pallidus; H = hypothalamus; NC = nucleus caudatus putamen; PC = parietal cortex; SC = superior colliculus; SN = substantia nigra. (From Hökfelt *et al.*, 1970).

take may serve as an inactivation mechanism similar to that operating in monoamine neurons (see Iversen, 1967). Subcellular fractionation studies furthermore indicate that at least a large part of the exogenous GABA is taken up into neuronal elements and seems to mix with endogenous pools, possibly localized to neurons (Iversen and Neal, 1968; Iversen and Snyder, 1968; Neal and Iversen, 1969; Hökfelt *et al.*, 1970). In agreement with this, regional uptake studies have revealed that GABA is taken up to a different degree in different brain regions (Hökfelt *et al.*, 1970) and that this uptake closely parallels endogenous GABA levels (Fahn and Coté, 1968) (Fig. 9). It may be added that other amino acids such as alanine (Hökfelt *et al.*, 1970) or glutamic acid (Hökfelt, Jonsson and Ljungdahl, unpublished) under the same experimental conditions also show specific regional uptake patterns which, however, differ from that of GABA. These results are in agreement with previous extensive studies by Lajtha and colleagues (*e.g.* Kandera *et al.*, 1968; Lajtha, 1968; Battistin *et al.*, 1969; Battistin and Lajtha, 1970).

*Autoradiographic studies*

To obtain a more exact knowledge on the cellular localization of exogenous GABA we have performed autoradiographic studies on freeze-dried or glutaraldehyde-fixed tissue (Hökfelt and Ljungdahl, 1970). So far our studies have mainly been concerned with the cerebellar cortex, but some preliminary results from other brain regions will also be presented.

Compared to background activity an increased number of grains were found diffused over the *cerebellar cortex*. Furthermore, numerous strong and well-defined accumulations of grains were found as described below. Principally both diffuse and well-defined activities were highest in sections from the superficial layer of the slices.

In the *molecular layer* strong accumulations of grains were found over cell bodies, mainly in its outer zone (Fig. 10). Sometimes also a few cell bodies near the Purkinje

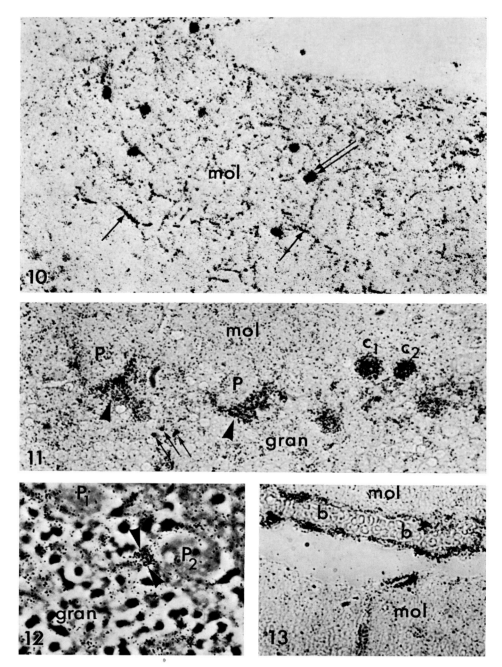

Figs. 10–13. Autoradiographs from slices of rat cerebellar cortex incubated with [³H]GABA. Fig. 10 from an AOAA-treated rat and slice incubated with AOAA (see text). In Fig. 10 large accumulations of grains over cell bodies (double arrow) and fiber-like accumulations (arrows) running in various directions are seen. In Fig. 11 large accumulations (arrow heads) are seen near Purkinje cell bodies (P). Two dense accumulations (C₁ and C₂) over cell bodies are lying deep in the molecular layer (mol). Small accumulations in the granular layer (gran) overlie the neuropile (thin arrows). In Fig. 12 (phase contrast) an accumulation of grains is seen in the immediate neighbourhood of a Purkinje cell (arrow heads). In this area the axon of the Purkinje cell leaves the cell body. In Fig. 13 accumulations of grains are found over the walls of a small blood vessel (b) in the fissure between the molecular layers of two laminae. (Fig. 11 from Hökfelt and Ljungdahl, 1970). Magnifications 400 ×, 620 ×, 800 ×, and 540 ×, respectively.

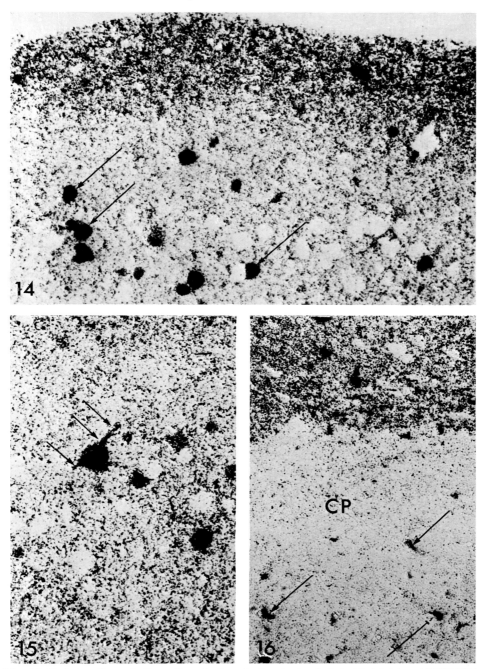

Figs. 14–16. Autoradiographs from slices of rat cerebral cortex incubated with AOAA and [³H]GABA. Rat pretreated with AOAA. In Fig. 14 a strong diffuse activity is observed in the outer layer of the cerebral cortex. Many cell bodies (arrows) are covered by high numbers of grains. In Fig. 15 the grains seem to cover processes of a cell body (arrows). In Fig. 16 the border between the grey (upper third) and white matter of corpus callosum (CP) is seen. Note accumulation of grains over small cell bodies in the white matter. Magnifications 380 ×, 640 × and 320 ×, respectively.

cell layer were covered with grains (Fig. 11). Mainly in the outer zone of the molecular layer smaller accumulations (1–3 $\mu$ in diameter) of grains were seen (Fig. 10). In the *Purkinje cell layer* large, comparatively weak accumulations were observed lying in the immediate vicinity of the Purkinje cell bodies, sometimes almost investing its basal part (towards the granular layer) (Figs. 11, 12). Sometimes these accumulations *seemed* to have processes "extending towards" (or "coming from") the molecular layer. Generally, these accumulations were not covering cell bodies. In the *granular layer* small, strong accumulations were found over the neuropile and occasionally accumulations were found over large cell bodies. In addition accumulations of grains were found over the walls of blood vessels and cell bodies associated with them (Fig. 13). Also the brain meninges and associated cell bodies were covered with grains. It may be pointed out that the Purkinje cells and most of the granular cells showed only a low activity.

In general the same results were obtained from slices taken from rats pretreated with AOAA and incubated with [³H]GABA and AOAA, a drug which inhibits GABA transaminase and thus the breakdown of GABA (Wallach, 1961). However, a higher diffuse activity was observed, especially over the molecular layer. Furthermore, in the molecular layer thin fiber-like accumulations of grains were seen running both parallel and perpendicular to the surface (Fig. 10). In the white matter increased numbers of grains were also found over several small cell bodies, over which we, so far, have not seen any accumulations of grains in sections from untreated rats.

Also in slices from other brain regions specific patterns for the uptake and accumulation of [³H]GABA have been found. Thus, in the *cerebral parietal cortex* a high diffuse activity was found in layer I (*cf.* Hirsch and Robins, 1962) (Fig. 14). Strong accumulations of grains were found over several cell bodies, mainly in layers II and III (Figs. 14, 15), sometimes also in deeper layers. The grains sometimes seemed to cover a process emanating from the cell body (Fig. 15). Over the underlying white matter of corpus callosum a comparatively low number of grains were observed. However, after AOAA treatment accumulations could be observed over small cell bodies (Fig. 16). In the *hippocampal region* (Fig. 17) a high diffuse activity was found, mainly in the stratum pyramidale, in the region surrounding the obliterated hippocampal fissure and in the molecular layer of area dentata. The number of grains was considerably lower over stratum radiatum and stratum oriens. Sometimes the grains seemed to be concentrated in small clusters in the stratum pyramidale (Fig. 18). Single cell bodies covered by high numbers of grains were found mainly in the stratum pyramidale (Figs. 18, 19), in the neighbourhood of the granular layer, and scattered in the stratum locunosum–moleculare (Fig. 19). It should, however, be emphasized that the vast majority of cell bodies, *e.g.* in the stratum pyramidale, showed only a low activity. In the *globus pallidus* the grains were sometimes seen forming a patchy pattern, but mostly a high diffuse activity was observed over the marginal zone of the section of the sliced tissue which decreased rapidly towards the middle. Also over sections from the *hypothalamus* a strong gradient of diffuse activity decreasing from the border was observed. Most cell bodies were only covered by few grains and so far we have not observed true accumulations of grains over cell bodies in this area.

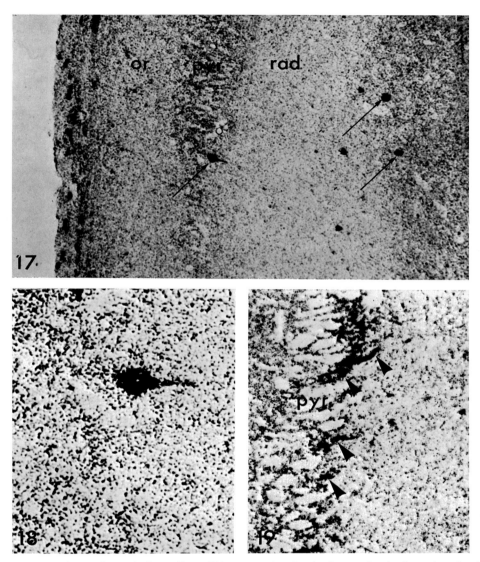

Figs. 17–19. Autoradiographs from slices of hippocampal region (regio superior, horizontal sections) incubated with AOAA and [³H]GABA. Rats pretreated with AOAA. In Fig. 17 stratum oriens (or,) stratum pyramidale (pyr) and stratum radiatum (rad) are seen with a medium, high and low activity, respectively. Note higher activity towards hippocampal fissure (to the right). Accumulations of grain are seen over some cell bodies (arrows). Fig. 18 shows accumulation over a cell body. In Fig. 19 small, dense accumulations of grain are seen between the cell bodies of the pyramidal layer. Magnifications 160 ×, 600 × and 300 ×, respectively.

*Aspects of interpretation*

The interpretation of the present results is complicated by insufficiencies in various steps of the experimental procedure used. Firstly, it is well known that the slicing and/or incubation procedure cause profound biochemical and morphological changes mainly in the superficial zone of the slices (Gerschenfeld *et al.*, 1959; Pappius *et al.*, 1962; Cohen and Hartmann, 1964; Thorack *et al.*, 1965; Hökfelt, 1968), which *inter alia* makes the identification of the structures difficult. Furthermore, the damage caused may prevent uptake and/or accumulation of the very substance leading to a "false" negative autoradiographic result. For these and other problems related to incubation of tissues we refer to articles by Elliott (1970), Harvey and McIlwain (1970), Pappius (1970) and Levin *et al.* (1970). Secondly, during fixation, embedding and/or application of the emulsion, isotopes may be extracted or translocated leading to erroneous results. Thirdly, the low resolution power of the light microscope adds to difficulties in the identification of the structures accumulating the labelled substance. In conclusion, the results should be interpreted with caution.

The various accumulations of grains observed in the present study in all probability correspond to sites, where [³H]GABA has been taken up and retained in unchanged form, since GABA metabolites formed during the incubation procedure do not seem to be retained in the slices (Iversen and Neal, 1968). Furthermore, accumulations of grains are found over the same structures in sections from AOAA-treated rats as in those of untreated rats. Thus metabolites mainly do not seem to be responsible for the autoradiographic patterns obtained. However, it is of interest that accumulations occur over small cell bodies in the white matter both in cerebrum and cerebellum after GABA transaminase inhibition. Since these accumulations so far have not been observed over untreated tissues, these cell bodies may normally have a high GABA turnover preventing an accumulation of this substance.

In the present study cell bodies accumulating [³H]GABA have been identified in various brain regions. However, it cannot be stated with certainty whether they are neurons or glial cells or both (see above). For example as to the cerebellum the cell bodies found in the outer zone of the molecular layer may be stellate cells; those deeper in this layer may represent basket cells. Also cell bodies identified in layers II and III in cerebral cortex and in various places in the hippocampal region may be neurons. However, the small cell bodies found in the white matter in cerebellum and cerebrum may instead represent glial elements. Furthermore, the accumulations surrounding the basal part of the Purkinje cell body could correspond to axons of basket cells or to collaterals of the Purkinje cell axon. On the other hand, it cannot be excluded that uptake of [³H]GABA into Bergmann glia is responsible for these accumulations. Similarly, the small dot-like or fiber-like accumulations of grains in the cerebellar molecular and granular layer could represent either axon terminals or glial processes.

Previous knowledge of the localization of GABA based on autoradiographic studies is poor. Whole-body autoradiography has shown the distribution of exogenous GABA outside the central nervous system (Hespe *et al.*, 1969) and intraventricular injections of [¹⁴C]GABA have demonstrated a strong diffuse activity in the periventricular zones (Clark *et al.*, 1968). Recently, Ehinger (1970) has obtained data that [³H]GABA is accumulated within retinal neurons, probably in amacrine cells, which is in good agreement with biochemical results (Graham *et al.*, 1968b; Roberts and Kuriyama, 1968).

However, information on the possible localization of GABA in the central nervous system has been obtained with other techniques such as biochemistry and neurophysiology and has been summarized in several review articles (Curtis, 1968; Krnjević and Schwartz, 1968; Roberts, 1968; Baxter, 1970; Curtis and Johnston, 1970; Hebb, 1970). As to cerebellum, GABA has been associated with the inhibitory neuron systems, especially the Purkinje neurons (Hirsch and Robins, 1962; Van Gelder, 1965; Kuriyama et al., 1966; Obata et al., 1967).

This has recently been further underlined by Obata (1969) demonstrating four times higher GABA concentration in isolated Purkinje neurons as compared to spinal motoneurons and by Fonnum et al. (1970), demonstrating a 50–70% decrease of glutamate decarboxylase activity in the dorsal part of the lateral vestibular nucleus after lesions in the vermis of the anterior cerebellar lobe.

Against this background the low activity over Purkinje cells observed in this study is remarkable. It may, however, be added that Csillik and Knyihár (1970) have failed to demonstrate accumulation in Purkinje cells of $[^{14}C]$thiosemicarbazide which is thought to indicate localization of glutamate decarboxylase, the GABA synthesizing enzyme.

It should, however, be strongly emphasized once more that failure to demonstrate activity over certain structures may have numerous explanations. The uptake mechanism of these cells might have been damaged during slicing and/or incubation procedure, or GABA taken up in Purkinje cells may diffuse during fixation and/or embedding procedure. This is especially crucial in glutaraldehyde-fixed material, where about 40% of the isotope is lost during the fixation and dehydration procedure (unpublished results).

Finally it should be remembered that GABA may have a number of important functions in brain not directly related to neurotransmission (see review by Baxter, 1970). Furthermore, various pools of GABA seem to exist (Varon et al., 1965a, b; see also review by Baxter, 1970) and we have so far only poor knowledge concerning possible connections between the distribution of endogenous and exogenous GABA in these various pools and the autoradiographic pattern obtained in the present study.

## CONCLUSIONS

Isolated tissues incubated in physiological buffer solutions take up and accumulate NA. This uptake is mainly localized to NA neurons as can be *directly* shown by performing combined autoradiography (demonstrating the localization of exogenous NA) and fluorescence histochemistry (demonstrating the localization of endogenous NA in NA neurons) on the same section or stretch preparation. The procedure used for this purpose includes stretch preparations or sections of freeze-dried and plastic-embedded tissues. Furthermore, the emulsion is applied in a dry state by the so-called loop technique of Miller et al. (1964). The results obtained demonstrate that for NA autoradiography is a useful tool both for studying the localization of NA neurons and also for studying, *e.g.* the effect of drugs on the uptake mechanism.

Also GABA, which has been proposed to act as an inhibitory transmitter substance in certain brain regions, is taken up and accumulated in brain slices. Regional uptake studies show that the amount of GABA retained is different in different regions of the brain. Using a similar autoradiographic technique as described for NA, an attempt has been made to determine the cellular localization of exogenous GABA in various brain regions. Diffuse accumulations of grains over neuropile as well as well-defined accumulations of grains have been found over certain cell bodies in the cerebellar and cerebral cortex and in the hippocampal formation. After inhibition of the breakdown of GABA by AOAA, accumulations of grains were also observed over small cell bodies in the white matter. Furthermore, small well-defined dot-like or fibre-like accumulations over neuropile have been found in the molecular and granular layer of the cerebellar cortex. These results should, however, be interpreted with great caution. Thus, due to the low resolution power of the light microscope and to the inferior morphology of the brain slices caused by the slicing and incubation procedure, it has so far not been possible to identify with certainty the structures which accumulate [$^3$H]GABA. Thus, it is premature to decide whether the cell bodies accumulating GABA are "GABA-neurons" or glial cells or maybe both. If the first turns out to be right, we now have the possibility of mapping "GABA-neurons" in the brain and of studying their uptake mechanism. If, on the other hand, the second alternative is correct, then a possible inactivating mechanism for GABA may be localized to glial components, revealing a quite different principle as compared to monoamine neurons. Autoradiographic studies at the ultrastructural level are in progress and they will hopefully help to solve this problem.

## ACKNOWLEDGEMENTS

This work has been supported by grants from the Swedish Medical Research Council (B70-14X-2887-01 and B71-14X-2887-02A) and by grants from Therese och Johan Anderssons Minne, Ollie och Elof Ericssons Stiftelse and Magnus Bergvalls Stiftelse.

## REFERENCES

AGHAJANIAN, G. K. AND BLOOM, F. E. (1966a) *Science*, **153**, 308–310.

AGHAJANIAN, G. K. AND BLOOM, F. E. (1966b) *J. Pharmacol. Exp. Therap.*, **156**, 23–30.

AGHAJANIAN, G. K. AND BLOOM, F. E. (1967) *J. Pharmacol. Exp. Therap.*, **156**, 407–416.

AXELROD, J., GORDON, E., HERTTING, G., KOPIN, I. J., AND POTTER, L. T. (1962) *Brit. J. Pharmacol.*, **19**, 56–63.

BATTISTIN, L., GRYNBAUM, A. AND LAJTHA, A. (1970) *J. Neurochem.*, **16**, 1459–1468.

BATTISTIN, L. AND LAJTHA, A. (1970) *J. Neurol. Sci.*, **10**, 313–322.

BAXTER, C. F. (1970) In A. LAJTHA (Ed.), *Handbook of Neurochemistry*, Plenum Press, New York, London, Vol. 3, pp. 289–353.

BLASBERG, R. AND LAJTHA, A. (1966) *Brain Res.*, **1**, 86–104.

BUDD, G. C. AND SALPETER, M. M. (1969) *J. Cell Biol.*, **41**, 21–32.

CLARK, W. G., VIVONIA, C. A. AND BAXTER, C. F. (1968) *J. Appl. Physiol.*, **25**, 319–321.

COHEN, M. M. AND HARTMAN, J. F. (1964) In M. M. COHEN AND R. S. SNYDER (Eds.), *Morphological and Biochemical Correlates of Neural Activity*, Harper & Row, New York, pp. 57–74.

CSILLÍK, B. AND KNYIHÁR, E. (1970) *Nature*, **225**, 562–563.

CURTIS, D. R. (1968) In C. V. EULER, S. SKOGLUND AND U. SÖDERBERG (Eds.), *Structure and Function of Inhibitory Neuronal Mechanisms*, Pergamon Press, Oxford, London, Edinburgh, New York, Toronto, Sydney, Paris, Braunschweig, Vol. 10, pp. 429–455.

CURTIS, D. R. AND JOHNSTON, G. A. R. (1970) In A. LAJTHA (Ed.), *Handbook of Neurochemistry*, Plenum Press, New York, London, pp. 115–134.

DAHLSTRÖM, A. AND FUXE, K. (1964) *Acta Physiol. Scand.*, **62**, Suppl. 232, 1–55.

DESCARRIES, L. AND DROZ, B. (1968) *Compt. Rend.*, **266**, 2480–2482.

DESCARRIES, L. AND DROZ, B. (1970) *J. Cell Biol.*, **44**, 385–399.

DEVINE, C. E. (1967) *Proc. Univ. Otago Med. Sch.*, **45**, 7–8.

DEVINE, C. E. AND SIMPSON, F. O. (1968) *J. Cell Biol.*, **38**, 184–192.

EHINGER, B. (1970) *Experientia*, in the press.

ELLIOTT, K. A. C. (1970) In A. LAJTHA (Ed.), *Handbook of Neurochemistry*, Plenum Press, New York, London, Vol. 2, pp. 103–114.

ELLIOTT, K. A. C. AND VAN GELDER, N. M. (1958) *J. Neurochem.*, **3**, 28–40.

ESTERHUIZEN, A. C., SPRIGGS, T. L. B. AND LEVER, J. D. (1968a) *Diabetes*, **17**, 33–36.

ESTERHUIZEN, A. C., GRAHAM, J. D. P., LEVER, J. D. AND SPRIGGS, T. L. B. (1968b) *Brit. J. Pharmacol. Chemotherap.*, **32**, 45–56.

FAHN, S. AND COTÉ, L. J. (1968) *J. Neurochem.*, **15**, 209–213.

FALCK, B. (1962) *Acta Physiol. Scand.*, **56**, Suppl. 197, 1–25.

FALCK, B., HILLARP, N.-Å., THIEME, G. AND TORP, A. (1962) *J. Histochem. Cytochem.*, **10**, 348–354.

FONNUM, F., STORM-MATHISEN, J. AND WALBERG, F. (1970) *Brain Res.*, **20**, 259–276.

FUXE, K. (1965) *Acta physiol. scand.*, **64**, Suppl. 247, 39–85.

FUXE, K., HÖKFELT, T., RITZÉN, M. AND UNGERSTEDT, U. (1968) *Histochemie*, **16**, 186–194.

GERSCHENFELD, H. M., WALD, F., ZADUNAISKY, J. A. AND DE ROBERTIS, E. (1959) *Neurology*, **9**, 421–425.

GRAHAM, J. D. P., LEVER, J. D. AND SPRIGGS, T. L. B. (1968a) *Brit. J. Pharmacol. Chemotherap.*, **33**, 15–20.

GRAHAM, JR., L. T., LOLLEY, R. N. AND BAXTER, C. F. (1968b) *Federation Proc.*, **27**, 463.

HAMBERGER, B. (1967) *Acta physiol. scand.*, **295**, 1–59.

HAMMERSTRÖM, L., RITZÉN, M. AND ULLBERG, S. (1966) *Experientia (Basel)*, **22**, 213.

HARVEY, J. A. AND MCILWAIN, H. (1970) In A. LAJTHA (Ed.), *Handbook of Neurochemistry*, Plenum Press, New York, London, Vol. 2, pp. 115–136.

HEBB, C. (1970) *Ann. Rev. Physiol.*, **32**, 165–192.

HESPE, W., ROBERTS, E. AND PRINS, H. (1969) *Brain Res.*, **14**, 663–671.

HIRSCH, H. E. AND ROBINS, E. (1962) *J. Neurochem.*, **9**, 63–70.

HÖKFELT, T. (1965) *Histochem. Cytochem.*, **13**, 518–519.

HÖKFELT, T. (1968) *Z. Zellforsch.*, **91**, 1–74.

HÖKFELT, T., JONSSON, G. AND LJUNGDAHL, Å. (1970) *Life Sci.*, **9**, 203–212.

HÖKFELT, T. AND LJUNGDAHL, Å. (1970) *Brain Res.*, **22**, 391–396.

IVERSEN, L. L. (1967) *The Uptake and Storage of Noradrenaline in Sympathetic Nerves*, Cambridge University Press, Cambridge.

IVERSEN, L. L. AND NEAL, M. J. (1968) *J. Neurochem.*, **15**, 1141–1149.

IVERSEN, L. L. AND SNYDER, S. (1968) *Nature*, **220**, 796–798.

KANDERA, J., LEVI, G. AND LAJTHA, A. (1968) *Arch. Biochem. Biophys.*, **126**, 249–260.

KRNJEVIĆ, K. AND SCHWARTZ, S. (1968) In C. V. EULER, S. SKOGLUND AND U. SÖDERBERG (Eds.), *Structure and Function of Inhibitory Neuronal Mechanisms*, Pergamon Press, Oxford, London, Edinburgh, New York, Toronto, Sydney, Paris, Braunschweig, Vol. 10, pp. 419–427.

KURIYAMA, K., HABER, B., SISKEN, B. AND ROBERTS, E. (1966) *Proc. Natl. Acad. Sci. U.S.*, **55**, 856–852.

LAJTHA, A. (1968) In A. LAJTHA AND D. H. FORD (Eds.), *Brain Barrier Systems*, *Progr. Brain Res.*, Elsevier, Amsterdam, Vol. 29, pp. 201–218

LENN, N. J. (1967) *Amer. J. Anat.*, **120**, 377–390.

LEVER, J. D., SPRIGGS, T. L. B. AND GRAHAM, J. D. P. (1968) *J. Anat.*, **103**, 15–34.

LEVIN, E., WOLOSIUK, R., SCIDI, G. AND GLANCSZPIGEL, R. (1970) *Neurology*, **20**, 584–593.

LUFT, J. H. (1956) *J. Biophys. Biochem. Cytol.*, **2**, 799–802.

MALMFORS, T. (1965) *Acta Physiol. Scand.*, **64**, Suppl. 248, 1–93.

MASUOKA, D. AND PLACIDI, G.-F. (1968) *J. Histochem. Cytochem.*, **16**, 659–662.

MCILWAIN, H. AND RODNIGHT, R. (1962) *Practical Neurochemistry*, J. A. Churchill, London.

MILLER, JR., O. L., STONE, G. E. AND PRESCOTT, D. M. (1964) *J. Cell Biol.*, **23**, 654–658.

NAGATA, T. AND NAWA, T. (1966) *Histochemie*, **7**, 370–371.

NAKAMURA, R. AND NAGAYAMA, M. (1966) *J. Neurochem.*, **13**, 305–313.

NEAL, M. J. AND IVERSEN, L. L. (1969) *J. Neurochem.*, **16**, 1245–1252.

OBATA, K. (1969) *Experientia*, **25**, 1283.

OBATA, K., ITO, M., OCHI, R. AND SATO, N. (1967) *Exptl. Brain Res.*, **4**, 43–57.

PAPPIUS, H. M. (1970) In A. LAJTHA (Ed.), *Handbook of Neurochemistry*, Plenum Press, New York, London, pp. 1–10.

PAPPIUS, H. M., KLATZO, I. AND ELLIOTT, K. A. C. (1962) *Can. J. Biochem. Physiol.*, **40**, 885–898.

RITZÉN, M. (1967) *Acta Physiol. Scand.*, **70**, 42–53.

ROBERTS, E. (1968) In C. V. EULER, S. SKOGLUND AND U. SÖDERBERG (Eds.), *Structure and Function of Inhibitory Neuronal Mechanisms*, Pergamon Press, Oxford, London, Edinburgh, New York, Toronto, Sydney, Paris, Braunschweig, Vol. 10, pp. 401–418.

ROBERTS, E. AND KURIYAMA, K. (1968) *Brain Res.*, **8**, 1–35.

ROTH, L. J. AND STUMPF, W. E. (Eds.) (1969) *Autoradiography of diffusible substances*, Academic Press, New York, London.

SABATINI, D. D., BENSCH, K. AND BARRNETT, R. J. (1963) *J. Cell Biol.*, **17**, 19–58.

SACHS, CH. (1970) *Acta Physiol. Scand.*, Suppl. 341, 1–67.

TAXI, J. AND DROZ, B. (1966a) *Compt. Rend.*, **263**, 1237–1240.

TAXI, J. AND DROZ, B. (1966b) *Compt. Rend.*, **263**, 1326–1329.

THORACK, R. M., DUFTY, M. L. AND HAYNES, J. M. (1965) *Z. Zellforsch.*, **66**, 690–700.

TRANZER, J. P. AND THOENEN, H. (1968) *Experientia*, **24**, 155–156.

TSUKADA, Y., NAGATA, Y., HIRANO, S. AND MATSUTANI, T. (1963) *J. Neurochem.*, **10**, 241–256.

VAN GELDER, N. M. (1965) *J. Neurochem.*, **12**, 231–237.

VARON, S., WEINSTEIN, H., BAXTER, C. F. AND ROBERTS, E. (1965a) *Biochem. Pharmacol.*, **14**, 1755–1764.

VARON, S., WEINSTEIN, H., KAKEFUDA, T. AND ROBERTS, E. (1965b) *Biochem. Pharmacol.*, **14**, 1213–1224.

WALLACH, D. P. (1961) *Biochem. Pharmacol.*, **5**, 323–331.

WEINSTEIN, H., VARON, S., MUHLEMAN, D. R. AND ROBERTS, E. (1965) *Biochem. Pharmacol.*, **14**, 273–288.

WOLFE, D. E., AXELROD, J., POTTER, L. T., AND RICHARDSON, K. C. (1962) *Science*, **138**, 440–442.

# The Role of Sheath Cells in Glutamate Uptake by Insect Nerve Muscle Preparations

MIRIAM M. SALPETER AND ISABELLE R. FAEDER*

*Section of Neurobiology and Behavior and Department of Applied Physics, Cornell University, Ithaca, N.Y. 14850 (U.S.A.)*

Nervous tissue is rich in amino acids, among which glutamic acid appears to be one of the most prominent. A facilitated transport mechanism specific for glutamic acid has been demonstrated in peripheral vertebrate nerve by Wheeler and Boyarsky (1968) and a similar mechanism has been demonstrated in crustaceans by Iverson and Kravitz (1968).

Although the role of glutamic acid in vertebrate peripheral nerves is still completely obscure, its importance in the arthropod nervous system has recently promised to become more tangible. It is now generally accepted that the excitatory neuromuscular synapses in both crustaceans and insects are non-cholinergic. Neither acetylcholine nor cholinesterase inhibitors are able to affect the neuromuscular response (see Faeder et al., 1970, for review). Although some workers believe that a very effective barrier or other special factors may have prevented investigators from detecting a cholinergic effect, the search for some other transmitter has gained momentum.

An attractive candidate for this role is glutamic acid. Perfusion or iontophoretic application of glutamate mimics transmitter action both in crustacean (Van Harreveld and Mendelson, 1959; Takeuchi and Takeuchi, 1964) and in insects (Usherwood and Machili, 1966; Beranek and Miller, 1968; Usherwood and Machili, 1968a; Faeder and O'Brien, 1970). Glutamic acid has also been recovered from perfusates of stimulated insect neuromuscular preparations (Kerkut et al., 1965; Usherwood and Machili, 1968b). Furthermore, glutamate appears to be acting on the postjunctional membrane since its effectiveness in producing muscle contraction persists after denervation eliminates all neurally evoked action (Beranek and Miller, 1968; Usherwood, 1969; Faeder et al., 1970).

Several considerations have cast doubt that glutamate could be the excitatory neurotransmitter at the insect endplates. One is the high concentration of free glutamic acid in the haemolymph ($10^{-3}$ to $10^{-2}$ M) (Frontalis, 1961; Florkin and Jeuniaux, 1964; Benassi et al., 1959, 1961; Stevens, 1961; Corrigan and Kearns, 1963), although this has recently been disputed (Usherwood and Machili, 1968a). Another is the

---

* Dr. Faeder's current address is: Department of Anatomy, Duke University Medical College, Durham, North Carolina.

*References pp. 113–114*

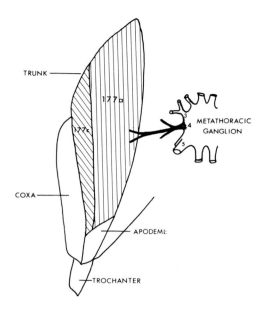

Fig. 1. Ventral view of the metathoracic coxal adductors 177a and c of *Gromphadorhina portentosa*. Overlying coxal muscles and their apodemes have been removed to expose the whole length of the muscle. In dissecting the nerve muscle preparation, muscles 177a and c are removed from the body by cutting the apodeme close to its insertion into the trochanter as well as the portion of the trunk muscle containing the muscle origins. Nerve 4 is cut close to the ganglion, and those branches which do not innervate muscles 177a and c are also cut to allow removal of the nerve trunk with the muscle.

fact that no enzymes for inactivating glutamate have been found at the insect endplate (see also discussion by Beranek and Miller, 1968). Finally, a concentration of glutamate considerably higher than expected of a neural transmitter ($\sim 10^{-4}$ M) is usually necessary to produce an optimum neuromuscular response in perfused insect preparations, although the concentration is considerably lower ($\sim 10^{-4} - 10^{-8}$) for iontophoretic application (Beranek and Miller, 1968).

We have studied the response to glutamate of isolated insect nerve muscle preparations by combined pharmacological, fine structural and autoradiographic techniques in an attempt to clarify some of the contradictions. The preparation used was the metathoracic coxal adductor muscle from the large Madagascar cockroach, *Gromphadorhina portentosa* (Fig. 1). This muscle is *homo*logous to 135 in *Periplaneta* (Dresden and Nijenhuis, 1958) and has only a fast excitatory motor innervation. The preparation is much sturdier than the one from *Periplaneta* and is ideal for experiments involving lengthy manipulations.

The fine structure of this preparation has been described (Faeder and Salpeter, (1970b). A characteristic endplate is illustrated in Fig. 2. The insect muscle is striated and the endplate resembles chemical synapses elsewhere. The nerve contains characteristic vesicles and mitochondria, and there is a synaptic cleft of about 200 Å, with an elaborate sub-synaptic specialization. The insect does not have junctional

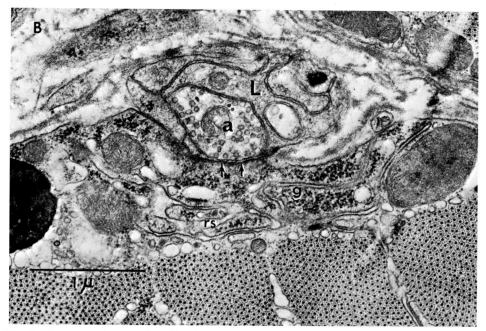

Fig. 2. Neuromuscular junction. Sheath processes are absent from axon surface only at zone of synaptic contact (arrows); aposynaptic granules (g); rete synapticum (rs); axon (a); and lemnoblast sheath (L). × 30600.

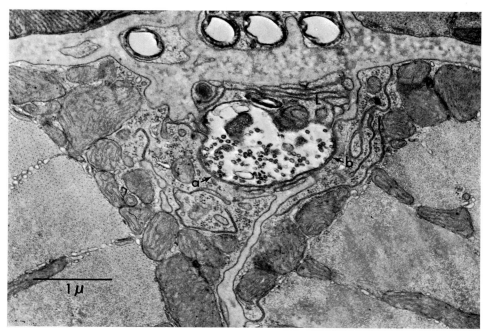

Fig. 3. Axon terminal making synaptic contacts with two muscle fibers (a, b); lemnoblast sheath (L). × 23700.

folds as seen in the vertebrate but has a loose membranous infolding called rete synapticum (Edwards *et al.*, 1958). Lemnoblast or sheath cells envelop the axon along its full length and are absent only at the region of synaptic contact. Tracheoles follow with the sheath, and the tracheolar cytoplasm is hard to distinguish from that of the lemnoblast. It is important to remember that the insect has a multiterminal muscle innervation (*i.e.* many neuromuscular junctions along one fiber, $\sim 100$ $\mu$ apart) and that synapses usually occur on the inner surface of a fiber, tightly surrounded by several other fibers. One axon innervates the same fiber many times, as well as several adjacent fibers. Synapses made by one axon terminal on several adjacent muscle fibers are frequently seen (Fig. 3).

The pharmacology of an isolated leg preparation of Gromphadorhina has been described (Faeder *et al.*, 1970; Faeder and O'Brien, 1970). Glutamate ($10^{-5}$ to $10^{-4}$M) causes contractures and enhances neurally evoked contractions. Higher concentrations produced effects to be expected from desensitization. Glutamate application also produced contractures in the isolated coxal adductor preparation.

The coxal adductor preparation also shows preferential uptake of glutamate (Faeder and Salpeter, 1970a). Matched nerve–muscle preparations (two bilateral muscles per animal) were used in this study. In one preparation of each set, the nerve was stimulated electrically at 0.5/sec for 1 hour (pre-stimulated preparation) while the matched preparation was merely incubated for the same period in insect saline (non-stimulated or passive preparation). Both preparations were then placed either in L-[$^3$H]glutamate or L-[$^3$H]leucine ($10^{-5}$ M) in a metabolic shaker for 1 hour at room temperature.

TABLE 1

A. NONPROTEIN AMINO ACID (AND SMALL MOLECULE METABOLITES)

| Pretreatment | Uptake[1] ( $\times$ 10$^{-5}$ mmoles/g) | |
|---|---|---|
| | Glutamate[2] | Leucine |
| Non-stimulated | 1.25 $\pm$ 0.43 | 0.21 $\pm$ 0.07 |
| Stimulated | 2.78 $\pm$ 0.84 | 0.16 $\pm$ 0.07 |

B. PROTEIN-BOUND AMINO ACID

| Pretreatment | Uptake[1] ( $\times$ 10$^{-5}$ mmoles/g) | |
|---|---|---|
| | Glutamate[3] | Leucine[3] |
| Non-stimulated | 0.004 $\pm$ 0.001 | 0.005 $\pm$ 0.003 |
| Stimulated | 0.011 $\pm$ 0.003 | 0.011 $\pm$ 0.003 |

[1] Based on average of five animals. An extracellular space of 20% of tissue wet weight has been estimated on the basis of results obtained by Iverson and Kravitz (1968). Uptake values have been corrected for extracellular space, assuming equilibration with the incubating medium.
[2] Difference between glutamate uptake by stimulated and non-stimulated preparations significant (by *t* test) at 1% level.
[3] Difference in incorporation into protein of both glutamate and leucine between stimulated and non-stimulated preparations significant (by *t* test) at 1% level.

After incubation with the radioactive amino acids, the tissues were either:

(1) weighed and homogenized in 0.4 M perchloric acid and the radioactivity determined both in the supernatant and in the pellet; or

(2) fixed and embedded for electron microscope (EM) autoradiography. For a detailed description of these procedures see Faeder and Salpeter (1970a).

*The chemical results* are summarized in Table 1. These results are based on an average of 5 animals. In the non-protein fraction, glutamate is taken up preferentially over leucine, and this glutamate uptake is enhanced by prior nerve stimulation. The protein fraction on the other hand contains about the same amounts of both amino acids (which constitutes less than 1% of the total glutamate taken up and about 2 to 7% of the leucine). Nerve stimulation increases subsequent protein synthesis significantly.

*Autoradiographic results*: Control studies indicate that about 50–60% of the radioactivity due to glutamate uptake is retained in the non-stimulated tissue after processing for electron microscopy (fixing in glutaraldehyde followed by osmium tetroxide and embedding in Epon 812). Light microscope autoradiography from 0.5 $\mu$ sections coated with Ilford L4 indicated that there is a considerable label in the muscle fibers both in the passive and pre-stimulated glutamate preparations. In the pre-

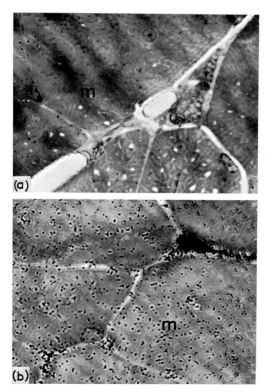

Fig. 4. Light microscope autoradiogram of muscle (m): (a) of passive preparation; (b) of pre-stimulated preparation. Note "hot spots" between muscle fibres. × 1000.

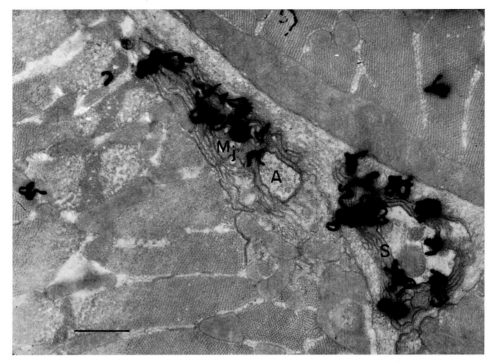

Fig. 5. Over-exposed radioautograph of nerve branch and neuromuscular junction in tissue exposed to
[³H]glutamate after nerve stimulation. High grain density over sheath cells (s) and post-synaptic
region of muscle fiber (Mj) is demonstrated. × 15000.

stimulated preparation this label was much less homogeneous, however, and varied
considerably from fiber to fiber. Another difference was that only in the pre-stimulated preparations did we see intensely labeled "hot spots" in the intercellular space
between muscle fibers (Fig. 4). These small "hot spots" corresponded with the location
of nerve fibres and tracheoles. The detailed localization of this intense label was
determined by EM autoradiography.

Autoradiograms were prepared by the "flat substrate" method of Salpeter and
Bachmann (1964). Pale gold sections (∼1000 Å) were coated with monolayers of
Ilford L4 (purple interference color) and developed with Microdol X. An over-
exposed autoradiogram to illustrate what an endplate of a pre-stimulated glutamate
preparation looks like is given in Fig. 5. The label is primarily in the sheath and in the
post-synaptic rete synapticum.

Autoradiograms of 2 pre-stimulated and 2 control preparations, were analyzed
quantitatively and the results are summarized in Tables 2 and 3. To accomplish this
quantitation, autoradiograms were scanned in the electron microscope and all areas
containing nerve or endplates were photographed at constant magnification. Sufficient
areas of muscle near the nerve branches were included for a balanced analysis. Grain
densities were obtained (*i.e.* grains per unit area) for different cellular components.

TABLE 2

RADIOAUTOGRAPHIC LOCALIZATION OF GLUTAMATE UPTAKE ($\times 10^{-5}$ M)[1]

| Pretreatment | Axon (average) | Axon at junction | Sheath (average) | Sheath at junction | Muscle[2] (interior) | Muscle[2] (surface) | Muscle[3] Post-synaptic region | Tracheae |
|---|---|---|---|---|---|---|---|---|
| Non-stimulated | 0.23 ± 0.05 | 0.24 ± 0.01 | 0.25 ± 0.02 | 0.34 ± 0.09 | 0.18 ± 0.01 | 0.20 ± 0.02 | 0.26 ± 0.05 | 0.21 ± 0.04 |
| Stimulated | 2.0 ± 0.4 | 6.85 ± 2.99 | 4.8 ± 0.5 | 12.4 ± 2.5 | 0.83 ± 0.04 | 1.01 ± 0.11 | 3.8 ± 0.8 | 5.6 ± 0.8 |

[1] In obtaining the tissue concentrations given above, it should be recalled that grain densities were converted to molar concentrations using the specific activity of administered glutamate. Therefore, the concentrations given describe the total amount of exogenously obtained glutamate (both labeled and carrier molecules) retained by the tissue after processing for electron microscopy.
[2] Muscle surface represents a zone of 1 $\mu$ inside the sarcolemma. The remaining muscle fiber volume is called muscle interior.
[3] The post-synaptic region was delineated by its fine structural specialization (see text).

TABLE 3

RATIO OF GLUTAMATE UPTAKE AT JUNCTIONAL ($j$) VS NON-JUNCTIONAL ($n$-$j$) REGIONS

| Pretreatment | $Sheath_j/Sheath_{n-j}$ | $Axon_j/Axon_{n-j}$ | Post-synaptic muscle region/ non-synaptic muscle surface |
|---|---|---|---|
| Non-stimulated | $1.60 \pm 0.40$ | $1.01 \pm 0.48$ | $1.32 \pm 0.26$ |
| Stimulated | $3.67 \pm 0.91$ | $7.51 \pm 3.84$ | $5.86 \pm 1.10$ |

(The center of the smallest circle which would just circumscribe a developed grain defined its location. The areas occupied by the various cellular components were obtained by placing a calibrated grid of points, 1 point to $\sim 3\ \mu^2$, over the autoradiogram and then tabulating the number of points which fell over each component.) Since the autoradiographic technique that we use has been calibrated for sensitivity (*i.e.*, it has been determined how many radioactive decays are necessary to give on the average one developed grain, Bachmann and Salpeter (1967), we could easily convert the grain densities to decays per $\mu^3$ (or $cm^3$) per exposure day. (Control studies confirm that no latent image fading or chemography affects the sensitivity over the exposure periods used in this study.) Since the specific activity of the bathing solution tells us the number of decays to be expected per mole of glutamate per day, a simple division gives us the molar concentration ($mM/cm^3$) of glutamate retained in the different cellular components.

From Tables 2 and 3 we see that in the passive preparation tissue radioactivity was more or less uniformly distributed over all tissue components with a slightly higher concentration in the sheath at the endplate (junction). In the pre-stimulated preparation on the other hand, in addition to an overall higher concentration of radioactivity, there was distinct differentiation between tissue components. The nerve and tracheae were labeled significantly higher than muscle, and a distinct gradient between junctional (endplate) and non-junctional regions was established. The sheath cell at the endplate was the most heavily labeled tissue component.

From independent random sampling we determined that the muscle volume is more than 80 times greater than that of sheath and tracheole combined. The chemical results (Table 1) are thus predominantly determined by the muscle uptake and only from quantitative E.M. autoradiography can we hope to determine the role of the nerve in this process.

Before speculating on the significance of these results and discussing future experimental prospects it is important to assess the reliability of the quantitation obtained from our autoradiograms. We have to deal with two major classes of error. The first stems from random statistical factors due to variations in section thickness and in the sensitivity of the autoradiograms, as well as in the Poisson distribution of the grain density sampling. The limits here are well defined. The color judgements of our sections were checked interferometrically and found to be accurate to $\pm\ 10\%$. The sensitivity calibration was determined by Bachmann and Salpeter (1967) to be accurate

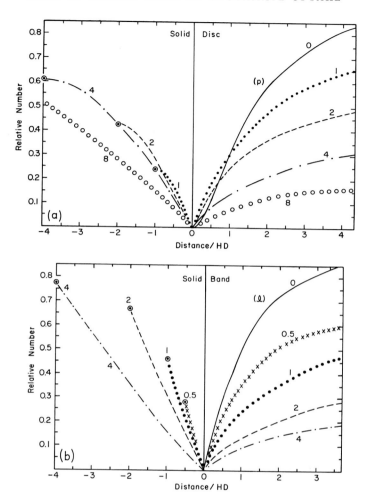

Fig. 6a and b. The relative number of total grains (integrated curve) with distance inside and outside a uniformly labeled circular (a) or band (b) source. The radius (half-thickness) of the source is marked on the individual curves. The positive $x$-axis represents successive distances outside the source; the negative $x$-axis represents successive distances inside the source approaching the center; and the origin represents the circumference (a) or edge (b) of the source. The curves are all normalized to unity ($y$ axis) for the sum of all grains (inside plus outside). The relative number of grains found outside the source obviously increases as the source size decreases; — the limit is reached at o which is a point (p) for the circle (a) and a line for the band (b) where all the grains are outside.

to $\pm 20\%$. Since that study, we have tested every batch of new emulsion before using it in our laboratory and found them all to fall within these limits. The sampling errors depend on the number of grains and points tabulated (the SE of a Poisson distribution of sample size $N$ is $\sqrt{N}$.) and is represented as the standard error in Tables 2 and 3.

The second class of error is a systematic one and stems from the fact that we tabulated only the grains immediately over a given cellular structure. We, thus, did not correct for those grains that lie at a distance from the radioactive structure due to radiation spread. The extent of radiation spread depends on the resolution of the specimen and on the size of the radioactive structure. Recently we have determined this spread experimentally and obtained a measure of resolution (which we called HD) for different autoradiographic specimens (Salpeter *et al.*, 1969). We then generated families of curves which give the expected spread of developed grains from radioactive structures differing in size and shape. These curves can be universally applied in analyzing autoradiograms of any specimen provided the resolution (or HD) value of that particular specimen is used as the unit of measure both for distance and size. In the present study (1000 Å sections, monolayer Ilford L4, Microdol X development) the HD value is 1600 Å.

Characteristic families of curves most relevant to the present analysis are given in Fig. 6a and b (Figs. 13 a and 15 of Salpeter *et al.*, 1969). These curves tell us what fraction (relative number) of the total grains due to a uniformly labeled circular or band structure will lie over the structure and what fraction will scatter outside it. It is clear that this depends on the size of the structure (radius or half-thickness of the structures in units of HD are marked on the individual curves). For instance 60% of the grains due to a circular source of 4 HD radius (*i.e.*, 6400 Å with our specimen) will lie over the structure or 80% of those due to a band source of 4 HD half-thickness (8 HD or 12,800 Å total thickness) will do so. Thus, if a structure is just over 1 $\mu$ in diameter or thickness, values obtained by merely tabulating grains over the structure are systematically 20–40% too low depending on the shape of the structure. With structures half that size, these values become 35–55% too low. In the present study the sheath cell was the smallest structure tabulated, especially at the endplate where its average diameter (thickness) approached 0.5 $\mu$. The values for sheath concentrations given in Tables 2 and 3 were therefore a lower limit, estimated to be accurate to within a factor of 2. The problem is further complicated with two adjacent radioactive structures, as is the case in the present study. It should be remembered that in such an instance the final net grain density favors the less radioactive neighbor. Thus, the value for the axon is systematically too high. Because of the more complicated geometry, however, (the axon is like the hole in a radioactive doughnut), an assessment of the extent of the true label must await completion of further studies using higher resolution specimens and more detailed analysis.

We can now return to a discussion of the biological results. There appears to be a selective uptake of glutamate by an insect nerve muscle preparation and this uptake is enhanced by nerve stimulation. The highest concentration of exogenously derived glutamate was bound in the sheath cells, especially at the endplate. Here it was concentrated by more than 12 fold over the bathing solution. The existence of such a glutamate sink may eliminate some of the stumbling blocks to accepting glutamate as a transmitter in this system. The sheath fully surrounds the axon and thus, could provide a barrier and protection against the haemolymph glutamate (as well as against the externally applied glutamate of pharmacological studies). Most important, it could provide an inactivating mechanism by reuptake, analogous to that for norepinephrine in the vertebrate nervous system (see Iverson, 1967 for review). Finally one could speculate that the sheath cells may contain a reserve pool of glutamate to be transferred to the axon as needed for transmission. The last hypothesis needs extensive study to verify, but is not outside the realm of possibility. A metabolic relationship between satellite cells and neurons has been discussed in the central nervous system of vertebrates by Hyden (1967), in the peripheral nerves of vertebrates by Singer and Salpeter (1966) and Singer (1968) and in the central ganglia of insects by Smith and Treherne (1963). The possible transport of transmitter material from sheath to axon provides a highly attractive mechanism for an expanded role of sheath cells in nervous function. Yet, whether glutamate is the actual transmitter or not, there is no doubt that it plays an important role in excitatory neuromuscular transmission in the insect. The location of the large glutamate sink in the sheath indicates an active partnership between axon and sheath in this function. These considerations must force us to reassess the current view of the limited metabolic capabilities of peripheral nerves and the dependence of peripheral axons on the nerve cell body for their every need. It is, for instance, interesting to speculate what the maintenance role of the sheath cell may be in crustaceans where severed distal nerve segments do not degenerate for months and are capable of regenerating by fusing with their proximal stump (Hoy *et al.*, 1967).

Finally, we would like to touch upon the evolutionary implications of the facilitated transport mechanism for glutamate in vertebrate nerve (Wheeler and Boyarski, 1968). The excitatory neuromuscular transmitter in annelid worms appears to be acetylcholine as it is in vertebrates (see Sakharov, 1970; and Florey, 1962 for review). Yet, the arthropods have taken on another transmitter at these sites, suggesting a transmitter switch. An efficient and successful transmitter switch may be expected to utilize a mechanism already in existence in the animal. Glutamate transport may have been such a mechanism. Its persistence in the vertebrate nervous system possibly represents the remains of an old and universal neural process, may be as a general excitant (see for instance Curtis and Watkins, 1963). More extensive studies on the role of glutamate and other amino acids in neural function of lower forms may contribute to our understanding of its role in the vertebrate nervous system.

ACKNOWLEDGEMENTS

This study was supported by United States Public Health Service, grants GM10422, NS09315, by postdoctoral fellowship IF2NB39010 and by Career Development Award K3-NB-3738.

REFERENCES

BACHMANN, L. AND SALPETER, M. M. (1967) *J. Cell Biol.*, **33**, 299.
BENASSI, C. A., COLOMBO, G. AND ALLEGRI, G. (1961) *Biochem. J.*, **80**, 332.
BENASSI, C. A., COLOMBO, G. AND PERETTI, G. (1959) *Experientia*, **15**, 457.
BERANEK, R. AND MILLER, P. L. (1968) *J. Exp. Biol.*, **49**, 83.
CORRIGAN, J. J. AND KEARNS, C. W. (1963) *J. Insect Physiol.*, **9**, 1.
CURTIS, D. R. AND WATKINS, J. C. (1963) *J. Physiol.*, **166**, 1.
DRESDEN, D. AND NIJENHUIS, E. D. (1958) *Kon. Nederl. Akad. Wetensch. Proc. Ser. C.*, **61**, 213.

EDWARDS, G. A., RUSKO, H. AND DE HARVEN, E. (1958), *J. Biophys. Biochem. Cytol.*, **4**, 251.

FAEDER, I. R., O'BRIEN, R. D. AND SALPETER, M. M. (1970) *J. Exp. Zool.*, **173**, 187.

FAEDER, I. R. AND O'BRIEN, R. D. (1970) *J. Exp. Zool.*, **173**, 203.

FAEDER, I. R. AND SALPETER, M. M. (1970a), *J. Cell Biol.* **46**, 300.

FAEDER, I. R. AND SALPETER, M. M. (1970b) *J. Morph.*, **132**, 225.

FLOREY, E. (1962) *Neurochemistry, Chap. XXVIII*, Chas. Thomas, Springfield, Ill., p. 673.

FLORKIN, M. AND JEUNIAUX, CH. (1964) *Physiology of Insecta, III*, 110.

FRONTALIS, N. (1961) *Nature*, **191**, 178.

HOY, R. R., BITTNER, G. D. AND KENNEDY, D. (1967) *Science*, **156**, 251.

HYDEN, H. (1967) *The Neurosciences*, The Rockefeller Univ. Press, New York, p. 248.

IVERSON, L. L. (1967) *The Uptake and Storage of Noradrenaline in Sympathetic Nerves*, Cambridge Univ. Press, Cambridge.

IVERSON, L. L. AND KRAVITZ, E. A. (1968) *J. Neurochem.*, **15**, 609.

KERKUT, G. A., LEAKE, L. D., SHAPIRO, A., COWAN, S., AND WALKER R. J. (1965) *Comp. Biochem. Physiol.*, **15**, 485.

SALPETER, M. M. AND BACHMANN, L. (1964) *J. Cell Biol.*, **22**, 469.

SALPETER, M. M., BACHMANN, L. AND SALPETER, E. E. (1969) *J. Cell Biol.*, **41**, 1.

SAKHAROV, D. A. (1970) *Ann. Rev. Pharmacol.*, **10**, 335.

SINGER, M. AND SALPETER, M. M. (1966) *J. Morphol.*, **120**, 280.

SINGER, M. (1968) *Ciba Found. Symp. on Growth of Nervous System*, Churchill, London, p. 200.

SMITH, D. S. AND TREHERNE, J. E. (1963) *Advan. Insect Physiol.*, **1**, 401.

STEVENS, T. M. (1961) *Comp. Biochem. Physiol.*, **3**, 304.

TAKEUCHI, A. AND TAKEUCHI, N. (1964) *J. Physiol.*, **170**, 296.

USHERWOOD, P. N. R. (1969) *Nature*, **223**, 411.

USHERWOOD, P. N. R. AND MACHILI, P. (1968b) *Nature*, **219**, 1169.

USHERWOOD, P. N. R. AND MACHILI, P. (1966) *Nature*, **210**, 634.

USHERWOOD, P. N. R. AND MACHILI, P. (1968a) *J. Exp. Biol.*, **49**, 341.

VAN HARREVELD, A. AND MENDELSON, M. (1959) *J. Cellular Comp. Physiol.*, **54**, 85.

WHEELER, D. D. AND BOYARSKY, L. L. (1968) *J. Neurochem.*, **15**, 1019.

# On the Kinetics of $^{35}$S-labelled L-Cysteine in the Hypothalamic-Hypophyseal Neurosecretory System of the Rat

## An Experimental Study by Autoradiography*

SEPPO TALANTI, ULJAS ATTILA AND MATTI KEKKI

*Department of Anatomy and Embryology, Veterinary College, Helsinki (Finland)*

In numerous previous studies accumulation of labelled cysteine in the region of the hypothalamic–hypophyseal system has been demonstrated at distinctly greater intensity than in surrounding brain tissues (for references, see Sloper, 1966). It is suggested that the uptake of labelled cysteine reflects the synthesis and storage of proteins or polypeptides in this system (Sloper *et al.*, 1960). These substances probably include the posterior pituitary principles which are known to be rich in cystine. The idea is supported by the observation that the neurosecretory material (NSM) has a rather high cystine content (Adams and Sloper, 1956).

The incorporation of cysteine in the neurosecretory system has been employed as an indicator of the dynamics governing the neurosecretory processes (Rinne, 1966). This is valid if indeed the NSM is labelled by the incorporation mentioned, and on this basis we then possess a method by which the secretory activity of the hypothalamic–hypophyseal neurosecretory system and the flow rate of NSM can be assessed. Experimental studies have in fact been undertaken on this basis. Dehydration was noted to cause increased and accelerated incorporation (Wells, 1963), which has been ascribed to activated neurosecretion. For the same reason, administration of thyroxine has been thought to trigger neurosecretory activation, and at the same time the release of NSM has also presumably increased, as evidenced by rapid disappearance of the incorporated isotope (Talanti and Pasanen, 1968). Thiouracil had an opposite effect on incorporation.

It has become a widely used approach in various disciplines of physiological research, and one which may yield very valuable information on the system studied by its aid, to evaluate experimental data from tests performed with a tracer-labelled substance by means of kinetic model analysis. Such analysis is based on stipulation of a model comprising a number of discrete pools of the compounds under consideration and which obeys simple mathematics in respect of the flow of substance by the paths connecting the pools, or compartments. The compartments represent

* This study was supported by a grant from the Sigrid Jusélius Foundation, Helsinki.

certain anatomical structures, metabolic steps or the like which are involved in the phenomenon under investigation. Kinetic compartment analysis can be undertaken if one has a set of data stating, as a function of time, the amount of label present in at least one of the compartments after a dose of labelled substance has been administered. Methods and calculating formulae by which various models can be treated have been presented in a great number of publications (for references, see Kekki, 1964).

The present study was undertaken because it seemed evident from the reports cited above that detailed study of cysteine incorporation may throw significant light upon the problems associated with neurosecretion. Its aim was to carry out in suitably extensive material systematic measurements of the incorporation of $^{35}$S-labelled cysteine in various parts of the neurosecretory system after intraperitoneal injection of labelled cysteine. While kinetic analysis of the findings was not included in the original plans, part of the observations was found to contain such a wealth of detail and of such apparent accuracy that it could be subjected to analysis by the mathematical tools mentioned. This analysis is looked upon as a first tentative application of a mode of study which, to our knowledge, has not previously been employed in the domain of neurosecretion research. The results are tendered merely as a first, orientative approximation, and it is realized that a great deal of further research along these lines will be needed. However, it is thought that such research may prove highly rewarding, since the present preliminary results are very promising.

## MATERIAL AND METHODS

### *Material*

The material of the present study consisted of 64 adult male albino rats weighing 229–247 g. These animals were used in two series, comprising 31 and 33 rats, respectively. Similar experiments were carried out with both series. The results obtained in the first series were not completely satisfactory from the point of view of the aims set for the study; they could not by themselves be evaluated unequivocally. The series was consequently mainly useful as a preliminary study, pointing out necessary refinements of technique. When these points were taken into careful consideration, the second series produced results which could be treated by the principles of kinetic analysis. Observing those points in which the findings of the first series were analogous to those of the second, the first series too could be similarly evaluated so that it confirmed the inferences drawn from the other set of experiments.

### *Methods of experimentation*

The rats received a basic pellet diet of constant composition *ad libitum*. Tap water was available in an unrestricted amount. All rats were kept in the same room throughout the test period.

All rats received by intraperitoneal injection $^{35}$S-labelled L-cysteine ("L-Cysteine-S 35 Hydrochloride", The Radiochemical Centre, Amersham, Bucks., England). The specific activity was 35.4 mC/mmole in the first and 40.0 mC/mmole in the second series. The dose was 150 $\mu$C per animal. The injections were given in the morning between 9:00 and 9:20 a.m. Each group (I to XI) comprised three rats, with the exception of groups X and XI in the first series, which had two members each. The animals were sacrificed at the following times after injection of labelled cysteine:

| Group | Series I | Series II |
|-------|----------|-----------|
| I | 10 min | 30 min |
| II | 30 | 45 |
| III | 45 | 1.5 h |
| IV | 1 h | 3 |
| V | 1.5 h | 4.5 |
| VI | 2 | 6 |
| VII | 4 | 12 |
| VIII | 6 | 24 h 45 min |
| IX | 24 | 25 h 30 min |
| X | 48 | 27 h |
| XI | 72 | 30 |

The rats were killed by rapid decapitation without anaesthesia. The brains and hypophysis were removed *en bloc* and embedded in paraffin after fixing in Bouin's fluid. Serial sections were made sagittally at 7 $\mu$, mounted on glass slides and coated with Kodak NTB 2 emulsion. The slides were placed in light-proof boxes with calcium chloride as dehydrating agent and stored for 28 days at 4°C. They were developed in Kodak D 11 developer and fixed with Kodak Rapid Fixer. The sections were then stained with haematoxylin–eosin.

Grain counts were made with a $\times$ 10 eye-piece and a $\times$ 100 objective using the eye-piece micrometer. The area counted was 75 $\mu$ $\times$ 75 $\mu$ (150 $\mu$ $\times$ 37.5 $\mu$ for the median eminence). All counts were made by one examiner. The counting error varied between 1 and 3% when the same area was counted several times. The objects counted were: the supraoptic nucleus (SON), the paraventricular nucleus (PVN), the median eminence (ME), and the neurohypophysis (NH). Ten areas of each object were counted in each rat. Only one area of each object was counted in each section. From the counts thus obtained the means and standard deviations were calculated. The calculations were made by the Computer Centre of the University of Helsinki.

### Method of kinetic analysis — Mathematical theory

In the kinetic compartment analysis employed in this study, the substance to which the label attaches is assumed to travel by steady-state flow from one compartment or pool to another in accordance with a first-order law (Fig. 1). Any label arriving in a given compartment is immediately mixed with the previous contents. From these assumptions it follows that the amount (or concentration) of label in any compartment as a function of time, must be a sum of exponential terms

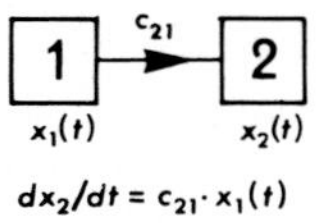

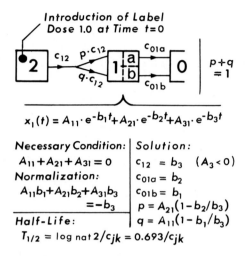

$$dx_2/dt = c_{21} \cdot x_1(t)$$

Fig. 1. Illustrating the principle of steady-state, first-order transfer of the substance being investigated from one discrete pool to another.

Introduction of Label
Dose 1.0 at Time $t=0$

$$x_1(t) = A_{11} \cdot e^{-b_1 t} + A_{21} \cdot e^{-b_2 t} + A_{31} \cdot e^{-b_3 t}$$

| Necessary Condition: | Solution: |
|---|---|
| $A_{11} + A_{21} + A_{31} = 0$ | $c_{12} = b_3 \quad (A_3 < 0)$ |
| Normalization: | $c_{01a} = b_2$ |
| $A_{11}b_1 + A_{21}b_2 + A_{31}b_3$ | $c_{01b} = b_1$ |
| $\quad = -b_3$ | $p = A_{21}(1 - b_2/b_3)$ |
| Half-Life: | $q = A_{11}(1 - b_1/b_3)$ |
| $T_{1/2} = \log$ nat $2/c_{jk} = 0.693/c_{jk}$ | |

Fig. 2. Kinetic compartment model employed in analysis of cysteine kinetics in the SON and PVN, and formulae valid for this model.

$$x_i = A\hat{I}_i\, e^{-b_1 t} + \ldots + A_{ni}\, e^{-b_n t}.$$

If these components are known from observation in terms of their 'amplitudes' $A$ and exponents $b$ for one compartment, 'No. 1', then the kinetic parameters $c$ of the flow model can be calculated.

For analysis of events in the SON as well as PVN the model reproduced in Fig. 2 was chosen from among several possible alternatives. The respective nucleus under consideration — pool 1 — is assumed to receive 'carrier' of the label by first-order kinetics from a body pool 2. This input is immediately split into two fractions, a and b, in the proportion $p/q$. Both partial pools have their own respective first-order output. This system is solved by the formulae shown in Fig. 2. Instead of the various rate constants $c_{jk}$, it is more illustrative to state the biological half-life time, $T_{1/2}$, of the respective pool of departure.

With regard to the rate constant $c_{12}$ and the corresponding half-life it should be noted that they refer not to the total body pool of cysteine, but to a constant fraction of it, which is accessible for supply to the SON or to the PVN, as the case may be. Taking biological considerations into account, it is also virtually certain that $c_{12}$ does not represent the true fractional turnover rate of the body pool; it must be a combination of at least two functions, most probably exponential, resulting from the

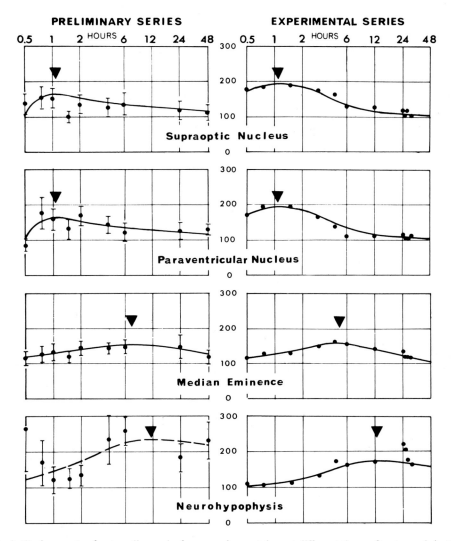

Fig. 3. Grain counts of autoradiographs from specimens taken at different times after tracer injection from the objects studied in the preliminary and experimental series.

absorption of cysteine from the peritoneal space into the blood stream and the turn-over of this pool. The former function in particular would seem to occur too rapidly to be revealed separately by the present experimental data.

RESULTS

The means of the grain counts found for the different objects studied at different times after the introduction of label have been plotted over the logarithm of time (in hours) in Fig. 3. In the graphs referring to the preliminary series the $\pm$ S.D.

*References p. 125*

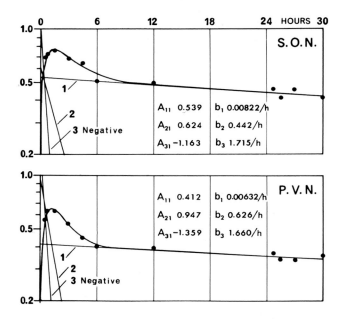

Fig. 4. Normalized grain counts observed at different times (means of three animals, ten microscopic fields of vision each) in the experimental series with reference to SON and PVN, plotted semilogarithmically over time. Both curves could be approximated by a sum of three exponential components (1, 2, 3). The parameters of these components (entered in the graphs) constitute the basis of kinetic analysis.

ranges have been entered; in the experimental series all standard deviations were considerably less than 10 grain counts units.

It is noted that the grain counts of the SON and PVN as functions of time were virtually identical in both series. There is a distinct maximum about 1 h after label introduction. The final decline of activity is rather slow: after two days the value was still one-half of the maximum or higher.

The range in which the activity recorded in the ME varied is narrower than that for the nuclei, and the persistence of activity is even more notable here. The activity can be said to have its maximum about 6 h after injection.

The results referring to the NH are not easy to fit with a smooth curve. If there is a maximum in the time interval from 0 to 48 h, it would be in the neighbourhood of 12 h. It is possible, however, that in actual truth the activity of the NH ascends throughout the period of observation, and its maximum has not been bracketed by the present times of sampling.

It is particularly worth noticing that all activities seem to lie between 100 and about 200 grain counts units, *i.e.*, the label concentrations are very much of the same order in all the objects studied.

The data concerning the SON and PVN, with reference to the experimental series, could be very successfully approximated by a function composed of three exponential terms, as Fig. 4 illustrates. In this semilogarithmic presentation, the straight lines

TABLE 1

VALUES OF KINETIC PARAMETERS FOUND BY ANALYSIS OF THE SON AND PVN DATA OF THE EXPERIMENTAL AND PRELIMINARY SERIES ACCORDING TO THE MODEL OF FIG. 2

| . Kinetic parameter | Experimental series | | Preliminary series |
| | SON | PVN | SON & PVN |
| --- | --- | --- | --- |
| $p$ | 0.46 | 0.59 | 0.22 |
| $q$ | 0.54 | 0.41 | 0.78 |
| $c_{12}$ | 1.72 | 1.66 | 2.16 |
| $T_{1/2}$ | 24 min | 25 min | 19 min |
| $c_{01a}$ | 0.442 | 0.626 | 0.530 |
| $T_{1/2}$ | 1.57 h | 1.11 h | 1.31 h |
| $c_{01b}$ | 0.00822 | 0.00632 | 0.00378 |
| $T_{1/2}$ | 84 h | 109 h | 183 h |

1, 2 and 3 represent these components, while the heavy line is their sum, showing a good fit with the observed values. The $A_{v1}$ and $b$ values consistent with the plots have been entered in the figure.

By means of the formulae given above, the kinetic parameter values compiled in Table 1 were found for the SON and PVN in the experimental series. The values are strikingly close for both nuclei.

In view of this evidence suggesting nearly equal function of the SON and PVN and considering the fairly wide scatter of the observations in the preliminary series, these two nuclei were considered as one entity in an attempt to analyse the preliminary observations kinetically. This was done by subjecting to kinetic analysis the curve determined by the means (on a logarithmic level) of the SON and PVN findings. Biologically, this is equivalent to the concept that both nuclei operate in parallel and with identical functions. The resulting kinetic parameters are seen in the last column of Table 1.

On the basis of the factor which had to be used for normalizing the $A_{v1}$ values of the SON and PVN functions, the grain count of 254 and 306, respectively, in the sample volume would be equivalent to the total label throughout. The sample volume was $7 \mu \times 75 \mu \times 75 \mu = 39.375 \mu^3$. In the literature, the number of ganglion cells in the right and left SON has been given as $6955 \pm 476$ and $6891 \pm 470$, respectively, and in the PVN, as $1339 \pm 77$ and $1310 \pm 65$, respectively (Olivecrona, 1957). The volume of one cell body is $2.742 \mu^3$ (Edström and Eichner, 1960). From these data the approximate cellular volumes of 38 mill. $\mu^3$ for both SON and 7.3 mill. $\mu^3$ for both PVN can be calculated, and these in turn lead to total label throughput figures of 245000 for both SON and 58000 for both PVN. From this, the uptake rates and cysteine processing rates are in the ratio 4.2:1.

The information to be found in the literature concerning the ME states that this structure consists of about 12000 axons from the nuclei running, parallel and each about 1 $\mu$ in diameter (Green and Maxwell, 1959). Since the ME has a length on the order of 2.5 mm, its volume would be something like 15 mill. $\mu^3$. As this is roughly

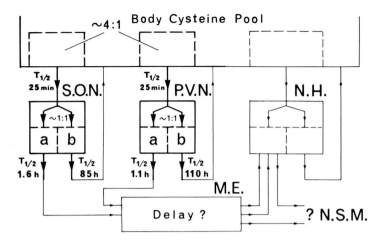

Fig. 5. Tentative model of cysteine kinetics in the hypothalamic–hypophyseal system. Thin lines indicate parts which are hypothetical so far.

one-third of the combined SON and PVN volumes, and on the other hand, the activities in the ME were on the same order as those in the nuclei, it is concluded that the label found in the ME may all have come from the SON and PVN. It would seem that no external source for its supply to the ME need be assumed.

Kinetic analysis of the passage of label through the ME was not considered justified on the basis of existing observations. One should particularly bear in mind the lineal configuration of this structure, which suggests the idea that any substance travelling through it from the nuclei to the NH probably moves by laminar flow. The assumption of instant mixing would therefore be inadmissible; instead, the ME would in all likelihood act as a delaying element between the nuclei and NH. This is compatible with the position of the peaks in the different curves.

The total volume of the NH has been given as 570 mill. $\mu^3$ (Olivecrona, 1957). This is more than ten times the combined cellular volumes of SON and PVN, and since the activity level in the NH was on the same order as the level in the nuclei, it seems evident that the NH must obtain something like nine-tenths of its cysteine supply by a path not involving these nuclei. For this structure, too, kinetic analysis was not thought to be feasible as yet on the basis of our data. Indications could be derived from the curve which would not be contradictory to the scheme tentatively suggested for the NH in Fig. 5. In this diagram all the results given above have been combined, and thin lines indicate the parts of the scheme which are as yet entirely hypothetical.

DISCUSSION

The narrow ranges of the standard deviations found in the experimental series proper of this study can be taken to indicate that the experimental technique has been satisfactorily mastered. This observation, and the ultimate criterion of smoothly running label-uptake curves, which upon kinetic analysis yield reasonable results, also serves to show that no grave errors are likely to have resulted from the unavoidable necessity of combining data from different experimental subjects to describe the activities in the different objects as functions of time. Thus, the impossibility in autoradiographic studies of brain tissues of taking several consecutive samples from one and the same animal, which is standard practice in many other fields employing the kinetic approach, is not an insurmountable obstacle; it merely involves a very great amount of work coupled with extremely careful experimentation. The same criteria also support the practice of pooling the observations relating to several animals to give a picture of their mean behaviour; this has also previously been successfully applied (*e.g.* Kekki, 1964).

As regards the counting procedure applied in this study, it is reliable when the grains occur uniformly in the autoradiograms, that is in the case of homogeneous incorporation of the isotope in the tissues. This requirement is best fulfilled in the NH, where the grains are usually quite uniformly distributed. However, in the neurohypophysis the present results do not seem quite satisfactory for some reason which is not yet understood. Rather uniform distribution is also noted in the areas of the neurosecretory nuclei studied with the magnification used in this study. The ME shows more uneven distribution; endeavours were accordingly made to perform the counts in equivalent parts of this structure in every instance. In view of the suggested function of the ME as a delay element, it seems appropriate to make a closer study of its isotope uptake in relation to various topological sites along the structure. Such studies are in progress.

The administration of label was different from the procedures used in previous studies on the neurosecretory system: in earlier works different amino acid preparations have been used, or there has been no count of autoradiographically produced silver grains, which may have been replaced by mere visual, 'semi-quantitative' assessment, for example, or by densitometry. No results directly comparable to those obtained in the present study can therefore be found in the literature, other than those from an experimental work by Talanti and Pasanen (1968). The latter agree on the whole with the present results.

The previously reported tendency of subarachnoidally applied cysteine to be maximally incorporated first in the ganglia of the nuclei and comparatively late in the NH (Sloper *et al.*, 1960) is visible, though not as marked, in the present findings. This has been considered to indicate flow of the NSM in the hypothalamic–hypophyseal system in a distal direction toward the NH. Sloper thinks that cysteine is included by synthesis in the NSM, which it thus labels. Although evidence in support of the transport theory can be seen in the present results, it is difficult to explain the rapid incorporation of cysteine in the distal parts of the system on this basis alone. Another theory put forward previously, namely, that of progressive synthesis of the NSM (see for references Bargmann, 1967), would of course account for the discrepancy. The theory claims that neurosecretory synthesis takes place in the entire region of the neurosecretory neuron. The possibility occurs that, at least in part, cysteine is also incorporated in the cells of the neurosecretory system in association with some process other than attachment to the NSM. This would mean bonding of cysteine to proteins other than those constituting the neurosecretion.

Astonishingly prolonged retention of the isotope in the neurosecretory system was noted: there was remarkable activity in all parts of the system as late as two or three days after injection. Two explanations have been tendered for this observation: either the process of neurosecretion is not very fast after all, or part of the $^{35}S$ might be recirculated in the organism. As the present findings reveal no 'humps' in the curves, typical of such recirculation, one further possibility has to be considered, namely, that part of the label attaches to non-neurosecretory proteins, possibly involved in the production of NSM, which are only slowly replaced from the body pool.

The kinetic model which emerged from the present analysis of the neurosecretory nuclei would seem to be consistent with the last idea. If one assumes that the fast output of the SON and PVN represents their respective neurosecretory principles, the slow output might consist of cysteine-containing protein which has participated in the mechanism by which the NSM is produced, and which is being replaced in a steady-state fashion by virgin protein. The cysteine taken up from the body pool would be distributed in about a 1:1 ratio between the two uses.

Both nuclei were found to behave in a very similar manner as regards rates of uptake and output and cysteine distribution between both outputs. It remains to be shown by further studies whether the slight differences between the kinetic parameters are real or not. What seems to be real is that the slow output of the SON and PVN present a quantitative ratio of about 4:1. The present approach cannot furnish any answer to the question of whether the outputs of both nuclei consist of identical material or whether both produce different neurosecretory principles.

Hardly any definite conclusions as to the function of the ME are possible from the present results. It is hoped that studies in progress may disclose evidence either in favour of or against the idea that the fast outputs of the nuclei would be delivered into the ME and thence to the NH, in which connection the ME would probably act as a delaying element.

Concerning the NH, too, little can be said so far with any degree of confidence. The level of activity observed in the NH, together with the tissue volume of this organ, seems to support the idea that the NH has its own input of cysteine, possibly used to form the hypothetical protein which is involved in NSM synthesis or handling. The fast output of the NH might be the NSM proper, which may consist of the outputs from the nuclei, via the ME, alone or augmented by principles synthesized in the NH.

As regards our future plans, we have already outlined the work now in progress concerning the special behaviour of the ME. The kinetics of the NH require special study, and we have thought of the possibility of excluding other components of the hypothalamic–hypophyseal system by surgical interference. A fairly obvious extension of our preliminary experiments will be their repetition under different experimental conditions, particularly under stress or with other stimuli. Substitution of other proteins or amino acids for the labelled cysteine in experiments of the kind described may be worthwhile.

From the preliminary results reported it seems to us that the approach of kinetic analysis is applicable to studies of neurosecretory phenomena, provided that observations of a high technical standard are available. We believe it can be a powerful tool for the clarification of a wealth of problems in this field which remain to be answered.

## REFERENCES

ADAMS, C. W. M. AND SLOPER, J. C. (1956) *J. Endocrinol.*, **13**, 221.
BARGMANN, W. (1967) *Intern. Rev. Cytol.*, **19**, 183.
EDSTRÖM, J. E. AND EICHNER, D. (1960) *Anat. Anz.*, **108**, 312.
GREEN, J. D. AND MAXWELL, D. S. (1959) *Comparative Endocrinology*, Wiley, New York, p. 368.
KEKKI, M. (1964) *Acta Endocrinol.*, 46, Suppl. **91**, 1.
OLIVECRONA, H. (1957) *Acta Physiol. Scand.*, 40, Suppl. **136**, 1.
RINNE, U. K. (1966) *Methods and Achievements in Experimental Pathology*, Vol. I, S. Karger, Basel, p. 169.
SLOPER, J. C. (1966) *Brit. Med. Bull.*, **22**, 209.
SLOPER, J. C., ARNOTT, D. J. AND KING, B. C. (1960) *J. Endocrinol.*, **20**, 9.
TALANTI, S. AND PASANEN, V. (1968) *Z. Zellforsch.*, **88**, 220.
WELLS, J. (1963) *Exp. Neurol.*, **8**, 470.

# Cellular Localization of Dopamine-β-hydroxylase and Phenylethanolamine-N-methyl Transferase as Revealed by Immunohistochemistry

KJELL FUXE, MENEK GOLDSTEIN, TOMAS HÖKFELT AND TONG HYUB JOH

*Department of Histology, Karolinska Institutet, 104 01 Stockholm 60 (Sweden) and Department of Psychiatry, New York University Medical Center, New York, N.Y. 10016 (U.S.A.)*

The studies with the histochemical fluorescence method for the demonstration of catecholamines (CA) and 5-hydroxytryptamine (5-HT) on the central nervous system have clearly indicated that the mapping out of new specific neuron systems in the brain will result in markedly increased knowledge of the function of the brain. This progress was made on the basis of the localization of the transmitters themselves, dopamine (DA), noradrenaline (NA) and 5-hydroxytryptamine (5-HT) respectively. Another approach to map out specific neuron systems is to purify the enzymes specifically involved in transmitter synthesis and to produce antibodies towards these enzymes with subsequent demonstration of their cellular localization using fluorescent antibodies. We have started out by studying the enzymes involved in CA synthesis. In the present paper the results from our immunohistochemical studies on dopamine-β-hydroxylase (DBH) and phenylethanolamine-N-methyl transferase (PNMT) will be reported. Studies on the cellular localization of DBH in tissues have previously been made by Geffen *et al.* (1969) and Hartman and Udenfriend (1970). Our own results on the localization of DBH in the peripheral and central nervous system have previously been summarized in a short paper (Fuxe *et al.*, 1970).

## MATERIAL AND METHODS

Bovine DBH and PNMT were purified as described in previous papers (Fuxe *et al.*, 1970; Goldstein *et al.*, 1970) and after purification DBH appears as a single band and PNMT shows several enzymatically active bands on disc gel electrophoresis.

Immunization was performed in rabbits. The purified DBH and PNMT, in 0.9% NaCl, were emulsified with complete Freund's adjuvant before being injected into the rabbits (for details see Fuxe *et al.*, 1970; Goldstein *et al.*, 1971). The antibodies were tested against the antigens by micro-immunodiffusion and electrophoresis in agarose. The active sera were stored at —20°C.

Since cross-reactivity exists between DBH or PNMT of various species and between adrenal and nervous DBH or PNMT, tissues of rats have been used in these studies. A few rabbits have also been studied.

The immunohistofluorescent procedure used has already been described in part (Fuxe *et al.*, 1970). The tissues were rapidly frozen with $CO_2$ gas or with the help of propane cooled by liquid nitrogen. Cryostat sections (10–15 $\mu$ in thickness) were made from the unfixed frozen tissue. The sections were fixed for 10 min in pure acetone of room temperature, after which they were stained in the following procedure. The staining was made with the indirect (multiple layer) technique (for technical details, see reviews by Nairn, 1969 and Kawamura, 1969; see also Jonsson and Knutsson, 1968). The sections were incubated at room temperature with the undiluted active antibodies for 30 min, after which the sections were carefully rinsed with the help of phosphate buffer at pH 7.1 during a period of 15 min. After rinsing the sections were incubated in fluoresceine–isothiocyanate (FITC) labelled sheep anti-rabbit immuno-globulin which is commercially available at the National Bacteriological Laboratory in Stockholm. The $\gamma_1$-globulin fraction of sheep is purified in a two-step procedure involving precipitation with polyethylene glycol and ion-exchange chromatography on DEAE-Sephadex A-50 before the conjugation procedure (Bergquist and Schilling, 1970). The protein concentration was 10 mg per ml and the fluoresceine–isothiocya-nate:protein ratio was 0.45 mg per 100 mg of protein. After 30 min incubation the sections were rinsed as above and then mounted in a mixture of glycerine and phos-phate buffer (pH 7.1) in proportion 9:1. As a specificity test the specific antibody serum against DBH and PNMT respectively was replaced by pre-immune serum taken from the rabbit before immunization. Non-specific staining of the tissues mainly occurred in brain tissue.

A Zeiss fluorescence microscope was used with a dark-field condensor. As activation filter was used BG12 (3 mm) or UG1 (1 mm) and as secondary filter Zeiss 47 with BG12 and Zeiss —65 with UG1.

The indirect method has the advantage as compared with the direct method that it possesses a higher degree of sensitivity, since the specific antibodies contain more reactive sites than the antigen itself. On the other hand the specificity of the reaction is decreased due to the fact that the FITC-labelled immunoglobulin consists of a large number of different fluorescent antibodies which can react with the tissue proteins of the section either due to an antigen–antibody interaction or to electrostatic binding of the cationic antibodies to the anionic proteins of the section. The latter cause of unspecific staining may be avoided by increasing the pH which also increases fluores-cence efficacy of the fluorophor. In view of the above, specificity was further ensured in the present experiments by checking whether disappearance of immunofluorescence occurred in the section after preincubation of the antiserum with its antigen before staining (see Nairn, 1969).

RESULTS AND DISCUSSION

*Dopamine-β-hydroxylase (DBH)*

*Rat adrenal gland*

Most of the adrenal medullary cells showed a relatively weak green fluorescence

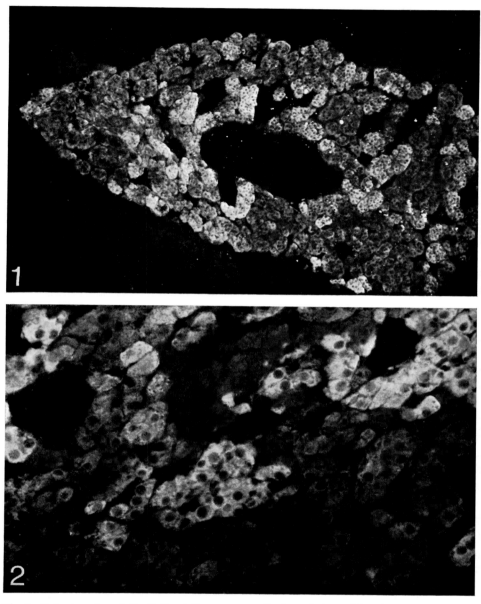

Fig. 1. Rat adrenal medulla. Indirect fluorescent antibody technique. DBH immunofluorescence revealed with FITC-conjugated immunoglobulin. Several cell islands are observed with a strong specific fluorescence in the cytoplasm. Most gland cells exhibit a weak to moderate specific immuno-fluorescence. No fluorescence is observed in the surrounding adrenal cortex. × 100.

Fig. 2. Same tissue and species as in Fig. 1. DBH immunofluorescence. Same techniques used as described in text to Fig. 1. Strongly fluorescent cell islands are illustrated. × 200.

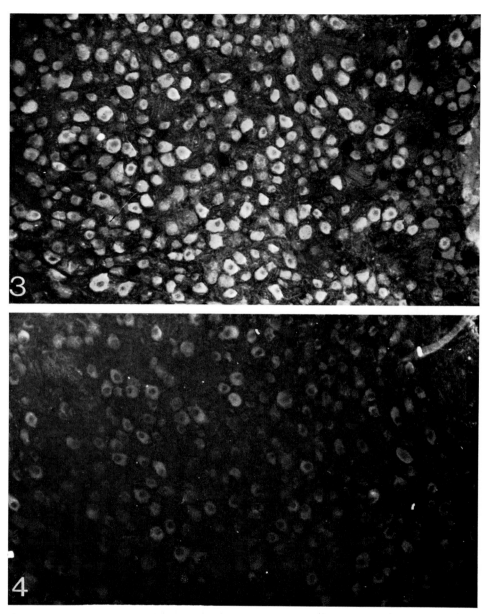

Fig. 3. Rat superior cervical ganglion. DBH immunofluorescence. For technique see text to Fig. 1. Weakly to strongly fluorescent CA ganglion cells are observed with fluorescence evenly distributed in the cytoplasm. × 160.

Fig. 4. Rat superior cervical ganglion. Pre-immune serum used instead of specific antiserum against DBH. Only very weakly fluorescent CA ganglion cells are observed. × 160.

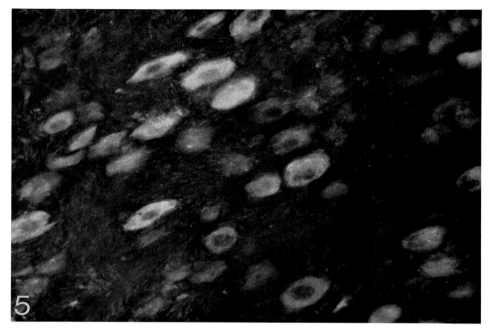

Fig. 5. Rat superior cervical ganglion. DBH immunofluorescence. Same rat as in Fig. 3. Weakly to strongly green-fluorescent ganglion cell bodies are observed. × 400.

and a few exhibited no specific fluorescence at all. Several islands of adrenal medullary cells (10–20 % of total population) exhibited a strong specific green fluorescence (Figs. 1, 2). In view of these results the adrenal medullary cells are probably heterogeneous with regard to their content of DBH. It may be that the strongly fluorescent cells represent the NA cells which are present in similar numbers and also are found in islands of similar morphology (Hillarp and Hökfelt, 1953, 1955; Eränkö, 1951, 1955a; Coupland *et al.*, 1964). No specific fluorescence was found in the cells of the adrenal cortex.

### Rabbit adrenal gland

All rabbit medullary cells exhibited a strong specific green immunofluorescence which was not the case in the rat adrenal glands. No specific staining occurred in the adrenal cortex. These results indicate that the population of adrenal medullary cells in the rabbit is homogeneous with regard to contents of DBH. This is in line with the fact that practically all gland cells in the rabbit store adrenaline (A) (Hökfelt, 1951; Hillarp and Hökfelt, 1955; Eränkö, 1955b).

### Rat superior cervical ganglion

The cytoplasm of the vast majority of the NA ganglion cells contained specific green immunofluorescence (Figs. 3–5). The brightness of fluorescence varied from weak to strong, and the fluorescence was localized diffusely throughout the cytoplasm. No specific fluorescence was found in axon terminals or non-terminal axons, nor in the primitive CA-storing system of these ganglia which consists of small CA-containing cells containing large concentrations of CA (Norberg *et al.*, 1966).

These results indicate that the DBH contents of NA ganglion cells varies considerably, which is true also for their contents of NA (Norberg and Hamberger, 1964). However, the NA is mainly localized in the periphery of the NA cells whereas the DBH is evenly distributed throughout the cytoplasm. This may indicate that some NA storage granules do not contain DBH, which has been shown to be localized in amine storage particles (Levin *et al.*, 1960; Potter, 1967). The distribution of DBH in the cell bodies mainly coincides with that of the large amine granular vesicles (Grillo and Palay, 1962). The small amine granular vesicles are mainly found in the periphery (Hökfelt, 1969).

In view of the probable lack of DBH in the primitive CA cells, these cells probably store DA and not NA.

### *Rat iris*

The adrenergic ground plexus has not been found to contain any specific immunofluorescence. This may be due to the poor penetration of the antibodies into the nerve terminals since the nerve terminals are not cut in stretch preparations. Experiments will therefore be performed with, *e.g.*, histamine and phospholipase C to open up the nerve membranes before incubation with the antibodies. Preliminary results with various concentrations (0.05–0.2%) of Tritone, a detergent, suggest that non-terminal axons contain a weak specific immunofluorescence. However, the terminals still lacked fluorescence. This may be an artefact, but it cannot be excluded that the present observations are due to the fact that the DBH is mainly bound to the large granular amine vesicles (Grillo and Palay, 1962) which are scarce in the terminals and mainly found in the non-terminal axons and cell bodies (see, *e.g.*, Hökfelt, 1969, and above).

### *Rat sciatic nerve*

Nerve fibres containing specific immunofluorescence could only be identified following ligation of the nerve. Twenty-four hours following operation, a strong immunofluorescence was observed immediately cranial to the ligation in nerve fibres with the same distribution and appearance as NA fibers have following such ligations (Figs. 6, 7) (Dahlström and Fuxe, 1964a; Dahlström, 1965). Increased reaction to antisera against DBH has also been found by Geffen *et al.* (1969) cranial to a ligation and increased DBH activity has been measured biochemically above a ligation by Laduron and Belpaire (1968). All these results are in accordance with the view that DBH may mainly be localized in the large granular vesicles, since high amounts of such vesicles are found in transected adrenergic fibres (Kapeller and Mayor, 1967; Geffen and Ostberg, 1969; Hökfelt and Dahlström, 1971) The accumulation of NA and DBH above a transection is therefore probably the result of interruption of the axonal flow of large granular amine vesicles which are synthesized in the cell bodies and transported down to the terminals.

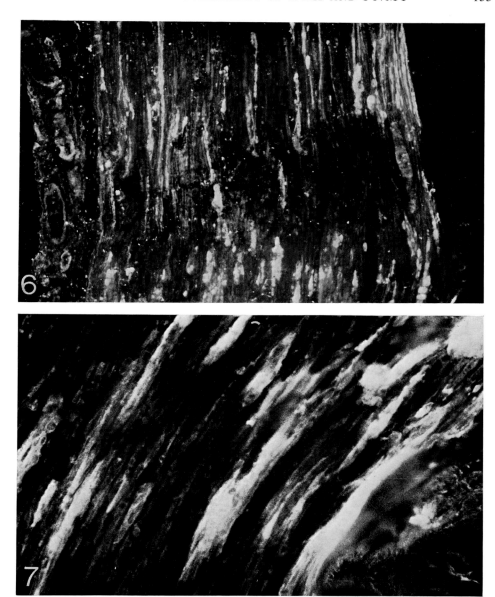

Fig. 6. Rat sciatic nerve 24 h after ligation. Cranial is up in the picture. DBH immunofluorescence. For technique see text to Fig. 1. Strongly fluorescent fibres are observed both cranial and caudal to the ligation. These fibres seem to be identical in number, distribution and appearance to the NA fibres. × 100.

Fig. 7. Same rat as in Fig. 6. DBH immunofluorescence. The strongly fluorescent fibres lie cranial to the transection. × 400.

*Rat central nervous system*

Specific immunofluorescence was only found in the CA-containing cell bodies of the pons and medulla oblongata (Figs. 8–10). These CA cell bodies constitute the CA cell

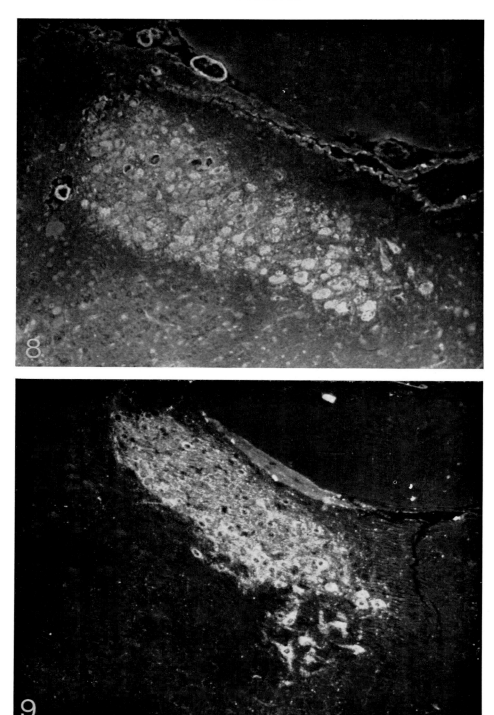

Fig. 8. Rat locus coeruleus. DBH immunofluorescence. For technique see text to Fig. 1. Moderately to strongly green-fluorescent cell bodies are observed. The immunofluorescence is found diffusely all over the cytoplasm. × 160.

Fig. 9. Same area as in Fig. 8. The histochemical fluorescence method for demonstration of CA has been used. A strong specific CA fluorescence is observed in the nerve cells of locus coeruleus. × 160.

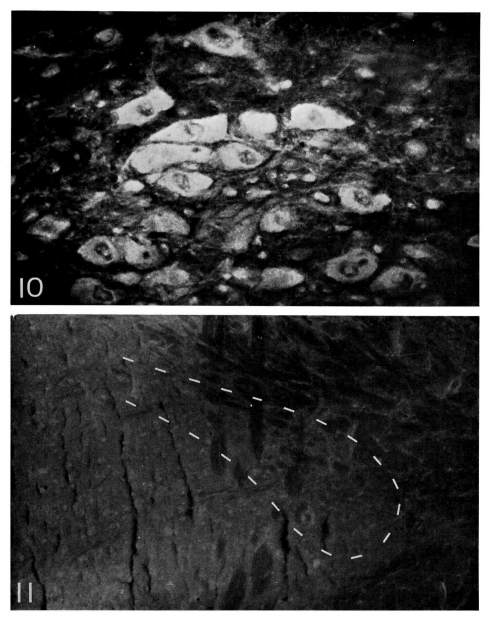

Fig. 10. Rat locus coeruleus. DBH immunofluorescence. For technique see text to Fig. 1. Moderately to strongly fluorescent nerve cells are observed. The fluorescence is evenly distributed throughout the cytoplasm. × 400.

Fig. 11. Rat substantia nigra. DBH immunofluorescence. For technique see text to Fig. 1. No specific immunofluorescence is observed in the CA cell bodies of this area (within marked area). × 160.

groups A1–A2 and A4–A7 of Dahlström and Fuxe (1964b). They are localized mainly in the reticular formation and group A6 is practically identical with locus coeruleus. These results show that the NA cell bodies are exclusively located in the pons and the medulla oblongata.

No specific fluorescence was observed in the DA cell bodies of the mesencephalon (Fig. 11) and hypothalamus and in the 5-HT cell bodies.

No specific immunofluorescence was observed in the NA pathways unless stereotaxic lesions had been made. When the lesion was placed in the ascending CA bundles from the pons and the medulla oblongata on the border between pons and mesencephalon, strong specific immunofluorescence was observed in the CA fibers close to the lesion on the cell body side. These results demonstrate that the ascending CA bundles from the pons and the medulla oblongata are NA bundles. After a corresponding lesion of the nigro-neostriatal DA pathway no specific immunofluorescence was observed in the DA fibers on the cell body side of the lesion. However, it is known that DA does accumulate in these fibers (Andén *et al.*, 1964, 1965). Thus the negative results indicate the absence of DBH in these fibers.

The failure of demonstrating the DBH in the central NA nerve terminal network may be due to the same reasons as discussed already under peripheral NA neurons.

The results with DBH definitely indicate that studies of this type will be of great value for mapping out specific neuron systems in the brain and in the spinal cord as underlined in the introduction.

### Pharmacological studies

Reserpine, a monoamine-depleting agent (see Carlsson, 1966) and a new potent DBH inhibitor, (4-methyl-1-homopiperazinylthiocarbonyl) disulphide (FLA63) have not been found to decrease the brightness of the specific immunofluorescence observed. This indicates that DBH contents in the adrenal gland cells and the NA nerve cells is not markedly influenced by depletion of amine stores. However, further studies are now in progress to determine the sensitivity of this procedure. The finding that FLA63, a DBH copper-chelating type inhibitor, does not decrease the DBH content may suggest that the copper moiety of the enzyme is not required for the antigenic activity.

### *Phenylethanolamine-N-methyl transferase (PNMT)*

### Rat adrenal gland

Most of the adrenal medullary cells exhibited a diffuse strong green immunofluorescence in their cytoplasm (Figs. 12, 13). The rest of the cells showed no specific immunofluorescence. In contrast to the case with the DBH reaction in which the fluorescent islands were sharply defined, the immunofluorescence developed in the cells in the PNMT reaction showed indistinct borders and the cell islands appeared indistinct. This difference towards DBH may be related to the fact that PNMT is a cytoplasmic enzyme which is localized in the supernatant fraction (Axelrod, 1962; Laduron and Belpaire, 1968) while DBH is a particulate enzyme (see Potter, 1967).

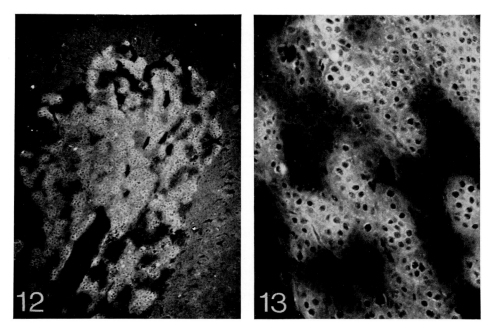

Fig. 12. Rat adrenal gland. PNMT immunofluorescence. For technique see text to Fig. 1. A strong green-fluorescence is observed in most of the gland cells. Several islands of non-fluorescent cells are present. × 100.

Fig. 13. Rat adrenal gland. PNMT immunofluorescence. For technique see text to Fig. 1. Strongly fluorescent bands of gland cells are observed. The cell borders are not distinctly outlined probably due to diffusion of PNMT which is a cytoplasmic enzyme. The dark islands are built up of non-fluorescent cells not containing PNMT. These cells probably represent the NA gland cells. × 200.

The morphology and number of the PNMT-positive gland cells correspond well with the number of A-containing gland cells present in rat (Eränkö, 1955a).

*Rat superior cervical ganglion, rat sciatic nerve*

No specific immunofluorescence was found in the CA ganglion cells or in the CA fibers, not even after ligation of the nerve. These results are in agreement with the view that the rat autonomic nervous system is practically entirely built up of NA neurons.

CONCLUSIONS

Our immunohistochemical work with DBH is principally in agreement with that of Geffen *et al.* (1969) and that of Hartmann and Udenfriend (1970). Our findings show that antibodies towards adrenal bovine DBH can react with rat DBH of both adrenal and nervous origin. In view of this it was possible to localize DBH at the cellular level in both the peripheral and central nervous system. The findings in the central nervous system have greatly contributed to the mapping out of central NA neurons.

Our immunohistochemical work on rats with bovine PNMT represents the first paper in which this enzyme has been localized at the cellular level. PNMT-positive cells have been found in most of the gland cells of rat adrenal medulla. They are in all probability identical with the A gland cells.

## ACKNOWLEDGEMENTS

We are grateful to Dr. G. Biberfeld for valuable advice as to the immunohistochemical procedure. This work has been supported by grants (B71-14X-715-06C, B71-14X-2887-02A) from the Swedish Medical Research Council and by grants from Ollie och Elof Ericssons Stiftelse and Magnus Bergvalls Stiftelse.

## REFERENCES

ANDÉN, N.-E., CARLSSON, A., DAHLSTRÖM, A., FUXE, K., HILLARP, N.-Å. AND LARSSON, K. (1964) *Life Sci.*, **3**, 523–530.

ANDÉN, N.-E., DAHLSTRÖM, A., FUXE, K. AND LARSSON, K. (1965) *Amer. J. Anat.*, **116**, 329–333.

AXELROD, J. (1962) *J. Biol. Chem.*, **237**, 1657–1660.

BERGQUIST, N. R. AND SCHILLING, W. G. E. E. (1970) in E. J. HOLBOROW (Ed.), *Standardization of Immunofluorescence*, Blackwell Sci. Publ., Oxford-Edinburgh, 171–176.

CARLSSON, A. (1966) In V. ERSPAMER (Ed.), *Handbuch der Experimentellen Pharmakologie, Vol. XIX*, Springer, Berlin, Heidelberg, New York, pp. 529–592.

COUPLAND, R. E., PYPER, A. S. AND HOPWOOD, D. (1964) *Nature*, **201**, 1240–1242.

DAHLSTRÖM, A. (1965) *J. Anat.*, **99**, 677–689.

DAHLSTRÖM, A. AND FUXE, K. (1964a) *Z. Zellforsch.*, **62**, 602–607.

DAHLSTRÖM, A. AND FUXE, K. (1964b) *Acta Physiol. Scand.*, **62**, Suppl. 232, 1–55.

ERÄNKÖ, O. (1951) *Acta Physiol. Scand.*, **25**, Suppl. 89, 22–23.

ERÄNKÖ, O. (1955a) *Endocrinology*, **57**, 363–368.

ERÄNKÖ, O., (1955b) *Nature*, **175**, 88–89.

FUXE, K., GOLDSTEIN, M., HÖKFELT, T. AND TONG HYUB JOH (1970) *Res. Commun. Chem. Pathol. Pharmacol.*, in press.

GEFFEN, L. B., LIVETT, B. G. AND RUSH, R. A. (1969) *J. Physiol.*, **204**, 593–605.

GEFFEN, L. B. AND OSTBERG, A. (1969) *J. Physiol.*, **204**, 583–592.

GOLDSTEIN, M., HÖKFELT, T., FUXE, K. AND TONG HYUB JOH (1971) *Experientia*, in press.

GRILLO, M. AND PALAY, S. L. (1962) In S. S. BREESE, JR. (Ed.), *Electron Microscopy, Vol. 2*, Academic Press, New York, p. u–1.

HARTMANN, B. K. AND UDENFRIEND, S. (1970) *Mol. Pharmacol.*, **6**, 85–94.

HILLARP, N.-Å. AND HÖKFELT, B. (1953) *Acta Physiol. Scand.*, **30**, 55–68.

HILLARP, N.-Å. AND HÖKFELT, B. (1955) *J. Histochem. Cytochem.*, **3**, 1–5.

HÖKFELT, B. (1951) *Acta Physiol. Scand.*, **25**, Suppl. 92, 5–130.

HÖKFELT, T. (1969) *Acta Physiol. Scand.*, **76**, 427–440.

HÖKFELT, T. AND DAHLSTRÖM, A. (1971) *Z. Zellforsch.*, in press.

JONSSON, J. AND KNUTSSON, K. (1968) *Tidskriften Laboratoriet*, **5**, 1–10.

KAPELLER, K. AND MAYOR, D. (1967) *Proc. Roy. Soc. B*, **167**, 282–292.

KAWAMURA, JR., A. (1969) *Fluorescent Antibody Techniques and their Applications*, University of Tokyo Press, Tokyo and University Park Press, Baltimore and Manchester.

LADURON, P. AND BELPAIRE, F. (1968) *Biochem. Pharmacol.*, **17**, 1127–1140.

LEVIN, E. Y., LEVENBERG, B. AND KAUFMAN, S. J. (1960) *J. Biol. Chem.*, **235**, 2080–2086.

NAIRN, R. C. (1969) *Fluorescent Protein Tracing*, E. & S. Livingstone Ltd., Edinburgh and London.

NORBERG, K.-A. AND HAMBERGER, B. (1964) *Acta Physiol. Scand.*, **63**, Suppl. 238, **1**–42.

NORBERG, K.-A., RITZÉN, M. AND UNGERSTEDT, U. (1966) *Acta Physiol. Scand.*, **67**, 260–270.

POTTER, L. T. (1967) *Circulation Res.*, **21**, Suppl. 3, 13–24.

# Effect of Thyrotropin-Releasing Factor on Thyrotropic Cells *in vitro* *

PAUL K. NAKANE

*University of Colorado, School of Medicine, Denver, Colorado, 80220 (U.S.A.)*

## INTRODUCTION

The case for neurohumoral control of the pituitary was built using data from experiments in which the anatomical connection between the hypothalamus and the pituitary had been observed and from studies in which specific areas of the hypothalamus had been destroyed or stimulated electrically. The existence of the postulated regulators of anterior pituitary function was demonstrated experimentally by Saffran and Schally (1955) in an experiment utilizing hypothalamic and neurohypophyseal extract. Since then, a number of hypothalamic extracts and materials with high potency have been prepared which selectively stimulate release of corticotropic, gonadotropic, thyrotropic and somatotropic hormones from the pituitary and inhibit release of prolactin and melanocyte-stimulating hormones. The work of various investigators clearly established the existence of thyrotropic hormone-releasing factor (TRF) capable of stimulating the release of thyrotropic hormone (TSH) in hypothalamic extracts of several animal species. The purification of ovine TRF was reported by Guillemin *et al.* (1962, 1965), while Schally *et al.* (1966) described the purification of porcine and bovine materials.

Recently Burgus *et al.* (1970a, 1970b) isolated 1.0 mg of a preparation of highly purified TRF from a total of 300 000 sheep hypothalamic fragments. From this preparation they were able to determine the molecular structure of TRF as 2-pyrrolidone-5-carboxylyl-histidyl-proline amide. Synthetic TRF was produced by Burgus *et al.* (1970a, 1970b) consisting of L-2-pyrrolidone-5-carboxylyl-L-histidyl-L-proline amide ($PCA-His-Pro-NH_2$). They found that the synthetic TRF behaves in an identical manner to the isolated TRF of ovine origin. Using the synthetic TRF, Burgus *et al.* (1970a, 1970b) were also successful in inducing the release of TSH from the pituitary gland *in vitro*.

In this study the effect of TRF on the thyrotropic cells (TSH cells) was investigated *in vitro* and it was found that the TSH cells undergo degranulation rapidly following exposure to the TRF *in vitro*.

* This investigation was supported in part by research grants E105 from the American Cancer Society, Inc., and United States Public Health Service AI09109 and AM13112 and a United States Public Health Service Research Career Development Award GM46228.

*References pp. 144–145*

## MATERIALS AND METHODS

Anterior pituitary glands of adult male albino Swiss rats were used for these studies. The rats were maintained in a temperature-controlled room on Purina laboratory chow and water *ad libitum* for one month before sacrifice. The animals were sacrificed by decapitation between 9:00 a.m. and 10:00 a.m. and the anterior pituitary gland was removed immediately. The posterior lobe was removed from the gland and the anterior pituitary gland was cut into two halves. The left half was used as experimental and the right half was used as a control.

Pituitaries were incubated according to the procedure described by Meites (Mittler and Meites, 1966). Synthetic media 199 (Colorado Serum, Denver, Colorado) was adjusted to pH 7.2 to 7.4 with 5.6 % sodium carbonate and was used as the incubation medium. As a preliminary experiment, synthetic TRF with the polypeptide sequence of L-2-pyrrolidone-5-carboxylyl-L-histidyl-L-proline amide (PCA-His-Pro-NH$_2$), synthesized by Dr. John M. Stewart of the University of Colorado School of Medicine, was added to the incubation medium in concentrations of 10 ng/ml. The pituitary glands were incubated in 1.5 ml of the incubation medium in 10-ml Erlenmeyer flasks. The flask was shaken gently (60 cycles/min) at 37°C under a 95 % oxygen and 5 % carbon dioxide atmosphere. Some tissues were placed in the incubation medium with TRF immediately after they were removed from the animals. Others were incubated for 60 min without TRF, then placed in a medium with TRF. The tissues were exposed to TRF for 5, 10, 15, 20, 30 and 60 min. At the end of the incubation, pituitary glands were removed and fixed in 4 % p-formaldehyde–picric acid solution (Zamboni and DeMartino, 1967) for 6 h. The fixed tissues were washed overnight with 0.01 M phosphate-buffered saline (PBS), dehydrated in increasing concentrations of alcohol, cleared in xylene and embedded in paraffin. Thyrotropic hormone (TSH) was localized on the tissue sections using peroxidase-labeled antibody method (Nakane and Pierce, 1966, 1967; Nakane, 1968; and Nakane, 1970). For this, the sections were hydrated and reacted with rabbit antisera against human TSH and washed. The washed sections were then reacted with sheep anti-rabbit IgG labeled with horseradish peroxidase (Sigma type VI) and washed. The sites of peroxidase, hence the sites of TSH, were revealed histochemically using hydrogen peroxide and 3,3-diaminobenzedine as substrates.

Some of the pituitary glands were incubated with tritium-labeled thymidine in addition to the TRF to determine if DNA synthesis would be elevated by the presence of TRF. For this, an incubation medium containing 2 $\mu$C/ml of [$^3$H]thymidine and TRF (10 ng/ml) was used. Two pituitary halves were placed as before and were incubated in the oxygen–carbon dioxide atmosphere for two days. Immediately after incubation, the flask was placed on ice, the medium discarded, and the glands rinsed twice with cold PBS and stored at —30° for later analysis. DNA was extracted with 0.5 M perchloric acid by the Schneider technique (1945) as modified by Kuff and Hymer (1966). The acid-precipitable material was collected by centrifugation, washed extensively with 0.5 M perchloric acid, and hydrolyzed in 0.5 M perchloric acid at 70°C. The concentration of DNA in hydrolysate was determined by the Burton procedure (1956) as modified by Giles and Meyers (1965). Highly polymerized salmon sperm DNA was used as a standard. Radioactivity in the hydrolysate was measured in a Nuclear-Chicago liquid scintillation counter.

RESULTS

*Distribution of TSH cells in the anterior pituitary gland*: TSH cells were more frequently found in clusters in the center of the gland (Fig. 1). The cells were polygonal to stellate in shape and were usually located in the center of the cord (Fig. 2). In a

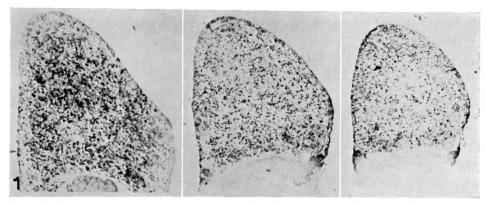

Fig. 1. Horizontal sections of an anterior pituitary gland from ventral (left) to dorsal (right). Sections were stained for TSH. TSH cells were not found at the peripheries of the gland. ( × 30).

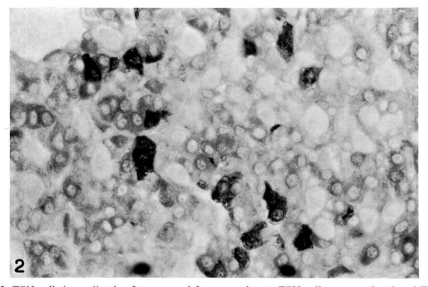

Fig. 2. TSH cells immediately after removal from a male rat. TSH cells are angulated and TSH is distributed in the cytoplasm in a granular form. Immunohistochemically stained for TSH. ( × 800).

*References pp. 144–145*

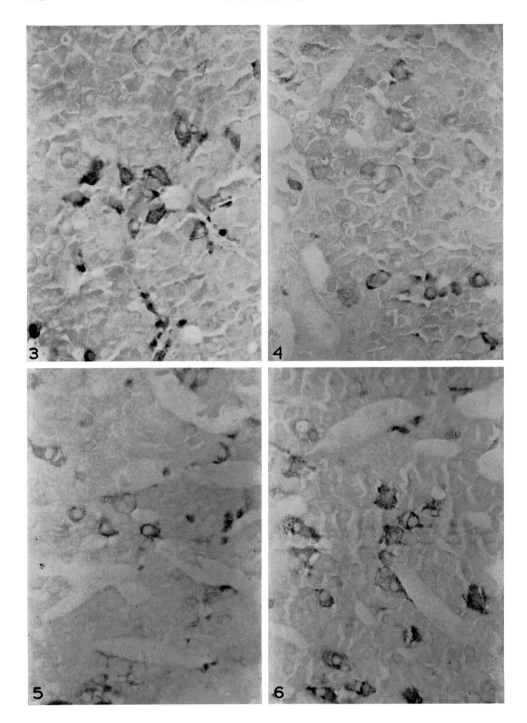

previous ultrastructural study, it was found that secretion granules with TSH were more frequently situated near the plasma membrane and large vacuoles containing little or no hormone were dispersed throughout the cytoplasm. Round oval mitochondria were found among the vacuoles (Nakane, 1970).

*Effect of TRF on TSH cells*: Signs of TSH release were noticed in those pituitary glands which were placed in the incubation medium immediately after removal from the animals. After 5 min exposure of the gland to TRF, some TSH cells were degranulated, their cytoplasm filled with hydropic vacuoles, and anti-TSH positive granules found among the vacuoles. Some of the cells contained a normal amount of TSH but with small vacuoles near the nucleus. Some TSH cells appeared normal (Fig. 3). In the gland exposed to TRF for 10 min, the majority of the TSH cells were degranulated and their cytoplasm was filled with hydropic vacuoles (Fig. 4). In those tissues with 30-min and 60-min exposure to the TRF, small TSH cells with condensed clumps with TSH were found among the dilated TSH cells (Fig.5).

Some signs of the effect of the incubation of the TSH cells were observed in those tissues which were incubated without TRF. Ten min after the start of the incubation, some TSH cells began to dilate and lost some of their TSH. At 30-min and 60-min incubation, the cytoplasm of the TSH cells lost their granular appearance and became diffused (Fig. 6).

TSH cells in the pituitaries which were preincubated for 60 min without TRF underwent changes similar to those in the pituitaries which were exposed to the TRF immediately after removal from the animals except that the pattern of release started with a diffused cytoplasm.

In the control specimens with 2 h of incubation, TSH cells lost the majority of the TSH and became very much like that of TSH cells 10 min with TRF.

*Effect of TRF on tritium-labeled thymidine uptake*: Tissues incubated with TRF and tritium-labeled thymidine and those tissues incubated with tritium-labeled thymidine without TRF took up a similar amount of tritium-labeled thymidine. (Tissues with TRF $= 296 \pm 50$ counts/min/mg DNA, tissues without TRF $= 364 \pm 76$ counts/min/mg DNA).

## DISCUSSION

The central distribution of TSH cells in the anterior pituitary gland suggests that TSH cells may be totally regulated by TRF since the portal blood supply of this area

---

Fig. 3. TSH cells exposed to TRF for 5 min. Vacuoles begin to appear in the cytoplasm and near nuclei. Immunohistochemically stained for TSH. ($\times$ 600).

Fig. 4. TSH cells exposed to TRF for 10 min. The majority of TSH cells are vacuolated and appear hydropic. Immunohistochemically stained for TSH. ($\times$ 600).

Fig. 5. TSH cells exposed to TRF for 60 min. Small TSH cells with a little cytoplasm begin to appear among the dilated TSH cells. Immunohistochemically stained for TSH. ($\times$ 600).

Fig. 6. TSH cells incubated for 60 min without TRF. Some TSH cells become hydropic, and the TSH stains are rather diffuse. Compared to Fig. 2, the intensity of TSH staining is reduced. Immunohistochemically stained for TSH. ($\times$ 600).

*References pp. 144–145*

is solely by the so-called "long portal vessels" whose primary bed lies in the median eminence and pituitary stalk (Porter *et al.*, 1967).

The formation of vacuoles near the nuclei of TSH cells and eventual vacuolation of the cytoplasm appears to be a common process of secretion of hormone from the pituitary cells. A similar process has been observed in luteotropic cells during the post-partum hormone release (Nakane *et al.*, 1968) and ACTH cells also undergo a similar vacuolation during their hormone release (Mazurkiewicz and Nakane, 1970). The reappearance of the small clumps of TSH-positive granules within small TSH cells shortly after the completion of the first wave of release of TSH appears to be a sign of the synthesis of the new TSH.

It may be speculated that the TRF may also stimulate the synthesis of TSH as well as that of the release, since those cells in the control specimens underwent gradual release, but did not begin to accumulate TSH. Whether these small TSH cells originated from cells which did not produce TSH prior to TRF stimulation, or resulted by shrinkage of the larger vacuolated cells remains to be seen.

The gradual loss of TSH from the control specimens was expected since Guillemin *et al.* (1963), in an earlier study conducted on the effect of TRF on pituitary glands *in vitro*, observed the release of TSH into the incubation medium from their control tissues although at a slow rate.

The lack of initiation of the mitotic activity with the TRF suggests that TRF will not initiate the new synthesis of DNA in order to increase the population of the TSH cells.

The primary sites of the activity of TRF on TSH cells is not yet known, however eventual development of antisera against TRF and its localization on TSH cells may answer the question.

In conclusion, the synthetic TRF is capable of releasing the TSH cells *in vitro*. The morphological changes associated with the release of TSH are similar to those observed in other cell types and it may be concluded that the phase of the release of the pituitary hormones from the pituitary glands are very similar.

## ACKNOWLEDGEMENTS

I wish to express my sincere thanks to Miss Mildred Van Der Schouw and Mrs. Leoner Wenger for their technical assistance.

## REFERENCES

BURGUS, R., DUNN, T. F., DESIDERIO, D. M., WARD, D. N., VALE, W. AND GUILLEMIN, R. (1970a) *Endocrinology*, **866**, 573.
BURGUS, R., DUNN, T. F., DESIDERIO, D., WARD, D. N., VALE, W. AND GUILLEMIN, R. (1970b) *Nature*, **226**, 321.
BURTON, K. (1956) *Biochem. J.*, **62**, 315.
GILES, K. W. AND MEYERS, A. (1965) *Nature*, **206**, 93.
GUILLEMIN, R., SAKIZ, E. AND WARD, D. N. (1965) *Proc. Soc. Exp. Biol. Med.*, **118**, 1132.
GUILLEMIN, R., YAMAZAKI, E., GARD, D. A., JUTISZ, M. AND SAKIZ, E. (1963) *Endocrinology*, **73**, 564.
GUILLEMIN, R., YAMAZAKI, E., JUTISZ, M. AND SAKIZ, E. (1962) *Compt. Rend.*, **255**, 1018.

KUFF, E. AND HYMER, W. C. (1966) *Biochemistry*, **5**, 959.

MATTLER, J. C. AND MEITES, J. (1966) *Endocrinology*, **78**, 500.

MAZURKIEWICZ, J. AND NAKANE, P. K. (1970) In preparation.

NAKANE, P. K. (1968) *J. Histochem. Cytochem.*, **16**, 557.

NAKANE, P. K. (1970) *J. Histochem. Cytochem.*, **18**, 9.

NAKANE, P. K. AND PIERCE, G. B. (1966) *J. Histochem. Cytochem.*, **14**, 929.

NAKANE, P. K. AND PIERCE, G. B. (1967) *J. Cell Biol.*, **33**, 307.

NAKANE, P. K., REBAR, W. AND MIDGLEY, A. R. (1968) *Excerpta Medica*, No. **157**, 103.

PORTER, J. C., HINES, M. F. M., SMITH, K. R., REPASS, R. L. AND SMITH, J. K. (1967) *Endocrinology*, **80**, 583.

SCHALLY, A. V., BOWERS, C. Y., KUROSHIMA, S., ISHIDA, Y. AND REDDING, T. W. (1966) *Endocrinology*, **78**, 726.

SCHALLY, A. V., BOWERS, C. Y. AND REDDING, T. W. (1966) *Proc. Soc. Exp. Biol. Med.*, **121**, 718.

SCHNEIDER, W. C. (1945) *J. Biol. Chem.*, **161**, 293.

ZAMBONI, L. AND DE MARTINO, C. (1967) *J. Cell Biol.*, **35**, 148A.

# III. ELECTRON-MICROSCOPIC HISTOCHEMISTRY OF MONOAMINE TRANSMITTERS

# The Fine Structural Characterization of Different Types of Synapse

E. G. GRAY

*Department of Anatomy, University College, London (U.K.)*

In this account an attempt has been made to summarize recent observations on synaptic morphology and relate them to the more well-known structural variations already reviewed (see Gray and Guillery, 1966; Gray, 1969a). More detailed accounts on specific topics can be found in symposia edited by Barondes (1969) and Akert and Waser (1969). A book by Peters, Palay and Webster (1970) gives a well-illustrated account of mammalian synaptology. Diagrams have been used here, because of the strict limit on half-tone illustrations.

## SYNAPSES WITH OPEN CLEFTS

The criteria of the presence in nerve tissue of vesicles of rather uniform size related to surface membranes with attached material that makes them look thickened have withstood intense investigation over two decades, and the morphologist now uses these criteria to recognise a synapse with justifiable confidence. Where there is physiological evidence for chemical transmission at neuro-neuronal and neuro-muscular contacts, the electron microscope reveals a presynaptic bag containing synaptic vesicles thought to contain the transmitter, and the synaptic cleft is open along its entire length with a gap of 120 to 300 Å and 600 Å or more at the vertebrate endplate.

The introduction of heavy metal staining techniques, phosphotungstic acid (PTA), uranium and lead salts, for example, which clearly reveal differences in the synaptic thickenings, has permitted classification of synapses into different categories. Gray (1959), using PTA on the rat cerebral cortex, showed that Type 1 synapses with well-defined synaptic thickenings are located specifically on pyramidal cell dendritic spines (Fig. 1 A), whereas Type 2 synapses on the cell bodies have a poorly defined thickening. Similar arrangements were later described in the cerebellar cortex (Gray, 1961). However, subsequent observations of other regions of the brain and spinal cord with PTA often failed to reveal two clear-cut categories. The situation became confused when other workers using different staining methods applied the Type 1 — Type 2 classification uncritically to their observations.

No functional implications were originally intended (Gray, 1959a). However, Eccles (1964, 1969) noted that in the hippocampus and cerebellar cortex known excitatory synapses had a Type 1 morphology, whereas inhibitory synapses were Type 2. The plot thickened when Uchizono (1965), working on the cerebellar cortex, showed that,

E. G. GRAY

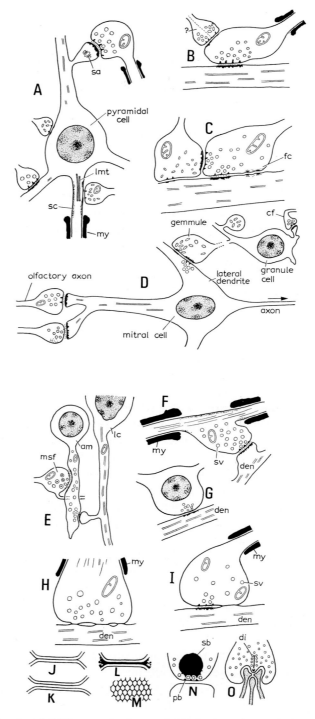

Figs. 1 and 2. Diagrams to show variation in synaptic morphology.

ABBREVIATIONS USED IN THE FIGURES

| | | | | |
|---|---|---|---|---|
| am | = amacrine cell | | my | = myelin sheath |
| cf | = ending of centrifugal fibres | | pb | = one of parallel bars |
| cv | = complex vesicle | | sa | = spine apparatus |
| den | = dendrite | | sb | = spheroid body |
| di | = synaptic disc (ribbon) | | sc | = sub-surface dense material (under-coating) |
| dp | = dense projection | | | |
| fc | = filamentous contact | | sh | = shell of complex vesicle |
| lc | = large cell | | shf | = shell fragments |
| lmt | = linked microtubules | | sp | = spinous body on synaptic vesicle |
| msf | = axons from median superior frontal lobe of octopus brain | | sv | = synaptic vesicle |

after initial aldehyde fixation, excitatory endings (with Type 1 thickening) showed spherical synaptic vesicles while inhibitory ones (Type 2) contained flattened (ellipsoid, polymorphic) synaptic vesicles.

Since then numerous investigations with aldehyde initial fixation on a number of sites where the physiology is known have supported Uchizono's observations (see Gray, 1969a, b). Three main problems emerge and are at present under investigation: why does aldehyde pre-fixation result in the flattening of the vesicles only in certain types of synapse?; are endings with flattened vesicles always (chemically) inhibitory?; are Type 1 and Type 2 contacts always related to round and flat vesicles, respectively?

Although it is often assumed that 'all' the synaptic vesicles are spherical *in vivo* so that initial osmium fixation in this respect gives a truer representation than aldehyde initial fixation, this is very difficult to prove. Indeed, some workers (*e.g.* Robertson, 1970) still question whether vesicles exist *in vivo* and argue that they could be arti-factually derived from tubular systems. The flattening effect could result from some sort of reaction between aldehyde and the inhibitory substance within the vesicle. It is not easy to understand how different types of transmitter in different categories of synapse could produce this flattening effect, however. Certainly the tonicity of the fixing solutions plays an important part. Valdivia (1971) has shown that it is the os-molarity of the buffer, either contributing to the aldehyde fixative or used for the post-aldehyde rinse, which is responsible for the degree of flattening of the vesicles. The highest osmolarities were seen to produce flattening even in vesicles which usually remained spherical. Bodian (1970) has shown that passage through cacodylate buffer can flatten certain categories of vesicle that are otherwise resistant to the effect of aldehyde. From both these observations we come to understand why some workers have not been able to find clear-cut round- and flat-vesicle categories in spite of the fact that they have used initial aldehyde fixation. Why osmotic effects on the synaptic vesicle should differ between excitatory and inhibitory synapses is not understood at present.

The problem is complicated in that Dennison (1970), using a goniometer stage on the EM, finds that the 'flat' vesicles in mammalian synapses are in fact discoidal, while in the fishes and amphibia some endings have 'flat' vesicles which are in fact discoidal and others are cylindrical. Fukami (1969) has shown round- and flat-vesicled endings in snake and frog spinal cord, using initial osmium fixation, to complicate the problem even further.

In answer to the second question there is good correlation between the presence of round and flat-vesicled endings and physiological evidence for excitation and inhibition, respectively, in a number of situations where aldehyde initial fixation has been used. Examples are the various cerebellar contacts (see Gray, 1969a, b) in the different classes of vertebrates. The Purkinje cell, for example, is an inhibitory neuron. Its extrinsic endings in Deiters' nucleus have flat vesicles (Mugnaini and Walberg, 1967) and so have the terminals of their recurrent collaterals (Mugnaini, 1970) — a morphological correlation with Dale's principle. The connections in the olfactory bulb (see below) fit the pattern remarkably well (Price and Powell, 1970); also in the hippocampus (Gottlieb, 1970). Vertebrate motor endplates, which are, of course, excitatory, have spherical vesicles. The Mauthner cell collateral synapses are excitatory (Diamond and Ysargil, 1969) and these have spherical vesicles (Gray, 1969a, b). The synaptic vesicles in the hair cells of the fish lateral line canal organ are round, while the efferent inhibitory synapses on them have flat vesicles (Flock, 1965). Endings on axonal initial segments (Fig. 1A), the majority of which are probably inhibitory, also usually have flat vesicles. There is also a clear correlation in the excitatory and inhibitory synapses of the crustacean stretch receptors and neuromuscular contacts (Uchizono, 1967; Atwood, 1968). Strangely enough, aldehyde fixation has not yet been shown to reveal two clear-cut categories of round-vesicled and flat-vesicled endings in the other invertebrate groups.

In answer to the third question, in regions where, with the appropriate stain, Type 1 and Type 2 synaptic thickenings can be differentiated, there is usually a clear correlation with the presence (after aldehyde initial fixation) of round or flat vesicles respectively (see Gray, 1969a). Recently, however, Mugnaini (1970) has described exceptions to this rule in the cerebellar cortex where, although endings with round vesicles always showed Type 1 contacts, certain endings with flat vesicles also showed Type 1 contacts. Mugnaini has elaborated an interesting theory, based on the time sequence of the establishment of the different connections, to explain this apparent anomaly. Mugnaini gave no figures to indicate the frequency of occurrence of these anomalous types, however. It could be that these are incorrect connections made during ontogeny, which are non-functional. Indeed, it is usually assumed that when a profile of a synapse looks apparently normal then it is functional. We have no means of knowing this, however. Westrum and Black (1971) have shown that when a Type 1 (round-vesicled) synaptic knob has undergone degeneration a neighbouring Type 2 (flat-vesicled) synapse may extend and overlie the remaining postsynaptic type 1 thickening. Thus, when anomalous synapses are seen, the possibility of previous 'natural' degenerative changes having taken place in the animal's brain must be seriously considered. Keeping in mind the various interpretive problems mentioned above a variety of synaptic configurations (Figs. 1 and 2), at present under investigation by various workers, will be considered briefly.

*Pyramidal and stellate cell contacts — cerebral cortex*

Fig. 1 A shows a diagram of a pyramidal cell. Most of the dendritic spines have Type 1 synapses with round vesicles (Colonnier's, 1968, asymmetrical type), while the cell bodies have Type 2 (Colonnier's symmetrical type) contacts. The initial axon segment, which incidentally contains linked microtubules (lmt) and has a subsurface web of dense material (sc) similar to that found at nodes of Ranvier, has synaptic contacts most of which are of the flat vesicle Type 2 (see Westrum, 1966; Conradi, 1969; Jones and Powell, 1970). Thus the evidence suggests that dendritic spines receive excitatory contacts while cell bodies and initial segments receive inhibitory contacts. This scheme also holds for certain cell types in the cerebellar cortex, hippocampus, lateral geniculate nucleus, olfactory bulb and spinal cord (see Gray 1959, 1969a; Colonnier, 1968; Guillery, 1969; Westrum, 1969; Jones and Powell, 1970; Price and Powell, 1970). In the cerebral cortex the stellate cells have both types of synapse on the cell bodies (see Jones and Powell, 1970; Peters, 1970).

*Presynaptic (axo–axonal) contacts*

In certain regions of the vertebrate CNS (spinal cord and cuneate nucleus) and crustacean muscle synaptic knobs can be seen contacted by other synaptic knobs (Fig. 1 B). Briefly, there is evidence to indicate that where presynaptic inhibition can be recorded physiologically then such serial synapses (axo–axo-dendritic or axo–axo-somatic) can be detected with the electron microscope. There is also important negative evidence in that in the cerebral and cerebellar cortices no serial synapses have been described, nor is there physiological evidence for presynaptic inhibition. The evidence remains controversial and incomplete, however.

In the spinal cord the first knob (Fig. 1 B) is thought to liberate an excitatory transmitter and the inhibition is effected by depolarisation of the second knob, resulting in a diminution of its output of excitatory transmitter (see Eccles, 1964). After aldehyde initial fixation, then, one would expect to see spherical vesicles in both knobs. Khattab (1968) in fact described such a situation. Conradi (1969), however, describes 'small synaptic vesicles of an irregular shape' in the first knob, so the situation needs further investigation, with particular attention paid to the tonicities of the fixing and rinsing media (see above). (See Gray, 1969a, for a consideration of the crustacean muscle serial synapse.)

*Lateral geniculate synapses*

A complex situation, for example, exists in the encapsulated synaptic zones of the mammalian lateral geniculate nucleus (Fig. 1C). Here (in aldehyde fixed material) an axo-dendritic knob with spherical vesicles and Type 1 contact synapses with a dendrite (filamentous contacts, fc, are also made, but will not be considered here — see Colonnier and Guillery, 1964). These are the terminals of the optic tract axons. They are probably excitatory and so the spherical shape of the vesicle agrees. However, these knobs are also presynaptic to knobs with flat vesicles, which in turn are presynaptic to dendrites. Thus, if our vesicle morphology is correct, then, as Saavedra and Vaccarezza (1968) point out, excitation of the second knob by the optic axon should result in a diminution of the output of the former's presumed (because of flat vesicles) inhibitory transmitter, resulting in the inhibition of an inhibitory pathway. Since the optic axon knobs are not themselves contacted by other knobs, *i.e.*, the optic knobs are not postsynaptic to other knobs, the morphology suggests that the optic fibres are not subject to presynaptic inhibition. This is contrary to early physiological observations, but these are now apparently open to alternative interpretations (see Guillery, 1969).

### Olfactory bulb connections

As in the cerebellar cortex, many of the connections in the olfactory bulb are now well understood (Price and Powell, 1970) and, similarly, there is a remarkable correlation between morphological type of synapse and its excitatory or inhibitory physiology. Briefly, the excitatory olfactory axons (Fig. 1 D) make Type 1 round-vesicle contacts with the tips of the apical dendrites of the mitral cells. The mitral cell lateral dendrite connects with gemmules from the granule cells, and here we find a reciprocal synapse (Andres, 1965; Rall *et al.*, 1966). After aldehyde fixation it can be seen that the mitral-to-granule cell synapse has spherical presynaptic vesicles, while the adjacent granule-to-mitral synapse has flat presynaptic vesicles. There is good physiological evidence that the mitral cells are excitatory and the granule cells are inhibitory (see Nicoll, 1969). Thus this could represent a negative feed-back system, excitation leading to reciprocal inhibition from the granule cell. The granule cells have excitatory endings on them (Fig. 1 D, cf) with round vesicles and Type 1 thickenings, the centrifugal fibres from the basal forebrain (Price, 1969; Price and Powell, 1970) and these also activate the granule cells to inhibit the mitral cells.

The granule cells have no axons (see Price and Powell, 1970) and so they could be termed amacrine cells. The amacrine cells of the retina (see Dowling and Boycott, 1966) participate in similar types of connections. However, in the retina, aldehyde initial fixation does not seem to produce two categories of round and flat vesicles.

Interneurons without axons occur in the autonomic ganglia (see Matthews and Raisman, 1969; Williams and Palay, 1969), also in the vertical lobe of the octopus brain (Young, 1964; Gray and Young, 1964; Gray, 1970) several millions of amacrine cells occur (Fig. 2 E). They are contacted by axons (msf) from the median superior frontal lobe and in turn are presynaptic to dendritic collaterals of the large cells. Thus it can be seen that the neuronal surface membrane, whether it be perikaryon (Fig. 2 G), dendrite (see Famiglietti, 1970), terminal axon knob or undifferentiated process of amacrine cell, can possess isolated patches capable either of ejecting transmitter substance or of receiving and transducing transmitter substance. Two interesting exceptions to this general rule are the vertebrate initial segments (see above) and axonal regions of the nodes of Ranvier. The IS can be postsynaptic but so far morphological observations indicate that it is never presynaptic to another neurite. The converse occurs at CNS nodes of Ranvier. The modal axon bare area can often be found to be presynaptic to another neurite but never postsynaptic, *i.e.*, the bare area is never seen to have synaptic knobs contacting it. Nodal synapses are further described in the next section.

### Synapses at nodes of Ranvier

Dilatations of the nodal axoplasm in the form of the presynaptic bags are commonly seen throughout the vertebrate central nervous system (Fig. 2 F). The synaptic vesicles can be either round or flat suggesting that nodal synapses might be either excitatory or inhibitory. The undercoating of dense material that lines the cytoplasmic surface of the axon membrane at the node is absent from the surface of the membrane that actually forms the wall of the bag. As mentioned in the previous section, the nodal regions of axons are apparently never postsynaptic to other synaptic knobs.

#### SYNAPSES WITH CLOSED CLEFTS

Where electrical coupling has been demonstrated between neural and other types of cell, specialised contacts, where the surface membranes come into very close opposition, have in most cases been demonstrated by electron microscopy. Examples are vertebrate and invertebrate electrical synapses, vertebrate cardiac muscle cells (at the intercalated discs), smooth muscle cells and vertebrate neuroglia (astrocytes and oligodendroglia).

Fig. 2 H is a diagram of a club ending on the Mauthner cell lateral dendrite (Robertson *et al.*, 1963). The membranes appear closely applied together in three places along the region of axo-dendritic apposition. Fig. 2 I shows a type of synapse seen frequently in the fish spinal cord and much less frequently in the frog spinal cord (Charlton and Gray, 1966). One region of close membrane apposition can usually be seen in the plane of section and frequently membrane specialisations (described above at chemical synapses) can be seen. Only certain aspects of these synapses will be described here (see Gray, 1969a for detailed references to the literature).

Now, at higher magnification and with the appropriate preparative technique, the unit membranes can be seen to come together (Fig. 2 J) to form a three-lined (in micrographs) junction. This has become known as a tight junction (external compound membrane, nexus, closed contact, quintilaminate contact) and it would seem that the outer leaflets of the synaptic membranes are fused together to make a low resistance pathway for current flow. However, when certain categories of tight junctions are examined after aldehyde fixation and staining with *aqueous* uranyl acetate a small gap —20Å across is revealed between the apposed unit membranes (Fig. 2 K) (Revel and Karnovsky, 1967). This gap is permeable to lanthanum and in some cases horse-radish peroxidase (Fig. 2 L), and when tilted in the electron beam the lanthanum in the gap can be seen to form a hexagonal array (Fig. 2 M). Freeze-etching indicates that there are regularly arranged particles spanning the cleft and the lanthanum penetrates between and around them (Goodenough and Revel, 1970). These junctions are now referred to as 'gap' junctions rather than tight junctions and they are found at electrical synapses, between glia and at epithelial contacts in the ependyma (except near the choroid plexus, area postrema and median eminence, where the blood–brain barrier is absent). True 'tight' junctions are those that appear always as in Fig. 2 J, whatever the preparative technique. They are equivalent to the *zonula occludens* type described in epithelia (Farquhar and Palade, 1963), (including that of the choroid plexus, area postrema and median eminence) and are also found at the endothelia of blood vessels. Incidentally, in the latter the tight junctions occur as isolated patches ('spot welded'), so that there are diffusion pathways out from the capillary lumina between the endothelia, the tight junctions being small patches and easily circum-vented. In the brain, however, the tight junctions between the endothelia are suffi-ciently extensive to block diffusion between the endothelial cells so that the only pathway available is intra-cytoplasmic across the endothelial cells, micro-pinocytosis playing a role. This arrangement probably constitutes the blood–brain barrier (see Brightman and Reese, 1969).

Returning to the gap junctions, these have also been demonstrated with the hexa-gonal array in the cleft, at the electrical septate synapse of the crayfish giant fibres by Payton *et al.* (1969). Most intriguing is their experiment showing that the fluorescent dye Procion Yellow will pass intracellularly from one side of the synapse to the other.

The presence of synaptic vesicles at synapses with gap junctions (Fig. 2, H and I) presents a problem in that electrical but not chemical transmission can be demonstra-ted, although the vesicles are thought to contain transmitter substance (Bennett *et al.*, 1967). In the fish and frog CNS, vesicles aggregated against specialised contacts indistinguishable from those found at known chemically transmitting synapses are commonly seen (Fig. 2 I) (see Charlton and Gray, 1966). Does this mean that our morphological criteria for recognising a chemical synapse may not be entirely reliable? Curiously enough, the vesicles at electrical synapses always appear spherical and never flat after aldehyde fixation (Gray, 1969a, b; Dennison, 1971), correlating with the fact that such synapses are excitatory, but not apparently chemically so! Dennison (1971) has shown that these spherical vesicles are zinc iodide positive (see Akert, Kawana and Sandri in this volume). We need to know whether this technique reflects the presence or absence of transmitter in the vesicles.

Synapses with gap junctions occur in the CNS of some invertebrate groups; are very common in the brain stem and spinal cord of fishes and much less common in amphibia (see Charlton and Gray, 1966; Gray, 1969a). In the mammals they have long been thought absent, until recently when they have been described in the lateral vestibular nucleus of the rat (but not the cat!) (Sotelo and Palay, 1970). They are also said to occur at synapses in the primate retina (Dowling and Boycott, 1966) and at inter-receptor contacts in the guinea pig retina (personal observations).

*Receptor cell synapses*

Many types of receptor cell have the basal region specialized to form a presynaptic zone with synaptic vesicles and membrane thickenings at the region of apposition with the second order neurite. Thus these contacts are just like those found at known chemical synapses. Certain receptor cells have an elaborate presynaptic morphology, the functional implications of which are not understood at present, nor for that matter is much known about the transmission mechanism at such junctions. The presence of synaptic vesicles and open synaptic clefts and not tight junctions suggests a chemical mode of transmission at receptor cell synapses.

Two examples illustrate the complexity mentioned above. Mullinger (1964) has described a large spheroidal body (sb) in the electric receptor cells of a fish (Fig. 2 N). They have spikes which project opposite dense parallel bars (pb) that lie on the synaptic membrane. In this way a number of tunnels are formed with synaptic vesicles in them. Mullinger suggests that the tunnels guide the vesicles to and along the surface of the presynaptic membrane (see also Flock, 1965). In the rod and cone synapse of the vertebrate retina a disc or ribbon (di) occurs with a dense v-shaped structure between it and the surface membrane. The disc is lined by rows of synaptic vesicles, and the vesicles of the outermost file come into close relationship with the presynaptic membrane (personal observations).

### THE ORIGIN OF SYNAPTIC VESICLES

The way synaptic vesicles form, their life span, the point in time at which they become charged or recharged with transmitter, the relationship of the formative enzymes (*e.g.*, choline acetyltransferase) to the vesicle membrane, the mode of release of transmitter, *e.g.*, exocytosis or discharge, through the intact vesicle wall, are under intensive investigation at present, but there is still much to be learnt. In adrenergic neurons (see other papers in this symposium) there is evidence that at least some of the synaptic vesicles (recognised by their dense cores) form in the cell body (probably from the Golgi apparatus) and move down the axon. Whether some of the synaptic vesicles form at the endings remains uncertain. Recent observations on non-adrenergic endings with plane synaptic vesicles suggest that they do.

Gray (1961) described vesicles with shells of subunits around them in the mossy fibre endings of the cerebellar cortex using phosphotungstic acid staining. They could often be seen apparently forming by invagination from the surface membrane. Subsequently he observed that complex vesicles are common in presynaptic knobs of the CNS of all the gnathostome vertebrate groups. Later Westrum (1965) obtained further evidence and suggested that the vesicles inside the shells were in fact synaptic vesicles, which formed by invagination from the surface membrane with a shell around them. Gray in his early observations was puzzled by the fact that shells or parts of shells could often be seen in the presynaptic knob without vesicles inside. This observation was clarified by Kanaseki and Kadota (1969) who, using a novel method of fixation on fractionated material, showed that the shells (baskets) were made up of pentagonal and hexagonal subunits and inside the shells vesicles could be seen with their unit membranes clearly delineated. Other shells or fragments were empty and they pointed out that after formation the vesicles were extruded from the shells. Gray and Willis (1970) used the fixation method of Kanaseki and Kadota on whole brain tissues. Their observations confirm those of Kanaseki and Kadota and lead to

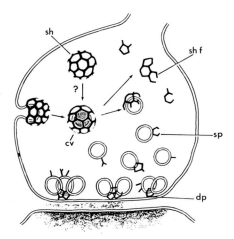

Fig. 3. Diagram to show the way synaptic vesicles are thought to originate from complex vesicles, and how the shells of complex vesicles may be related to dense projections (from Gray and Willis, 1970).

further suggestions summarised in Fig. 3. The vesicle forms by invagination with the shell around it. (Vesicles could form *de novo* inside empty shells (sh), the latter acting as a template — arrow marked with question mark, but this seems less likely.) This is the complex vesicle (cv). The vesicle then leaves the shell, which fragments (shf) and some of the fragments adhere to the vesicle. These could be seen as spiky projections (sp) with the appropriate stain. The vesicles then move to the presynaptic membrane and the spiky attachments become inserted into specific points on the presynaptic membrane. The spiky attachments are, or contribute to, the dense projections (dp) that can be seen in regular hexagonal arrays on the presynaptic membrane (Gray, 1963). Staining techniques which reveal the shells clearly also reveal the shell fragments, spiky attachments to the vesicles and the dense projections. Staining techniques which do not show the shells also do not show these other structures (see Gray and Willis, 1970 for detailed discussion).

### SYNAPSES AND LEARNING

The normal fine structure of synapses still presents so many problems of interpretation that looking for subtle changes that might be related to learning is, to say the least, hazardous at present. The changes might take place in the molecular organisation of the synaptic membranes, intra-neuronal fibrous proteins, the enzyme systems or the nucleic acids that control the turnover of these structures. We cannot say whether the physico-chemical changes involved in learning will ever be *morphologically* detectable even with the highest resolution techniques available to the electron microscopist. Much is known about localisation in the brain related to different forms of learning and something is known about fine structural changes correlated with learning in given brain centres. These two approaches present no insuperable difficulties, but they do not in themselves reveal the engram. The real problem is to detect structural changes which can be shown to contain in some form or other a representation of certain past environmental events.

My own observations on most invertebrate and vertebrate groups reveal that there is nothing obviously different about the general structure of a synapse in the most primitive groups compared with the most advanced. In the platyhelminth, annelid or mollusc, the CNS synapse with its synaptic vesicles and pre- and postsynaptic thickenings and cleft material looks very much the same as a synapse in the human cerebral cortex. Also synapses in the mammalian cerebral cortex, where learning changes probably occur, look no different from those in the spinal cord, where such changes probably do not occur. One striking difference, however, is that most synapses in the cerebrum contact dendritic spines whereas in the cord the synapses are mostly directly on dendritic trunks and cell bodies. A structure termed a spine apparatus unique to mammals (Gray, 1959) occurs in the majority of spines of the cerebrum (Fig. 1 A). In other vertebrate and invertebrate groups synapses on dendritic spines are common, but the spines never contain a spine apparatus, which, of course, means the spine apparatus is not an essential component of a learning circuitry. Recent work (Diamond et al., 1970) indicates that the dendritic spines may serve to isolate the synaptic membranes from synaptic noise in the parent dendrite (the spine apparatus may play a part in this) so that subtle changes related to learning taking place at the synapse would not be interfered with. Changes in spine numbers have been shown to be related to changes in activity in their input connections, but such changes have not yet been detected by electron microscopy. Whether these are plastic changes related to the learning mechanism remains to be seen.

## REFERENCES

AKERT, K. AND WASER, P. G. (1969) Mechanisms of synaptic transmission. In: *Progr. Brain Res.*, **31**, Elsevier, Amsterdam.

ANDRES, K. H. (1965) *Z. Zellforsch.*, **65**, 530–561.

ATWOOD, H. L. (1968) *Experientia*, **24**, 753–763.

BARONDES, S. H. (1969) *Cellular dynamics of the neuron. J.S.C.B. Symposium, Paris*, Academic Press, New York.

BENNETT, M. V. L., PAPPAS, G. D., GIMENEZ, M. AND NAKAJIMA, Y. (1967) *J. Neurophysiol.*, **30**, 161–300.

BODIAN, D. (1970) *J. Cell Biol.*, **44**, 115–124.

BRIGHTMAN, M. W. AND REESE, T. S. (1969) *J. Cell Biol.*, **40**, 448–677.

CHARLTON, B. T. AND GRAY, E. G. (1966) *J. Cell Sci.*, **1**, 67–80.

COLONNIER, M. (1968) *Brain Res.*, **9**, 268–287.

COLONNIER, M. AND GUILLERY, R. W. (1964) *Z. Zellforsch.*, **62**, 333–355.

CONRADI, S. (1969) *Acta Physiol. Scand.*, Suppl. **332**, 1–115.

DENNISON, M. (1971) *Brain Res.* and *J. Cell. Sci.*, In press.

DIAMOND, J., GRAY, E. G. AND YSARGIL, G. M. (1970) The function of the dendritic spine — an hypothesis. In: P. ANDERSEN AND J. K. S. JANSEN (Eds.), Excitatory synaptic mechanisms, 213–222, Scand. Univ. Books, Oslo.

DIAMOND, J. AND YSARGIL, G. M. (1969) *Progr. Brain Res.*, **31**, 201–209.

DOWLING, J. E. AND BOYCOTT, B. B. (1966) *Proc. Roy. Soc. B.*, **166**, 80–111.

ECCLES, J. C. (1969) *The inhibitory pathways of the CNS*, Thomas, Springfield, Ill.

FAMIGLIETTI, E. V. (1970) *Brain Res.*, **20**, 181–192.

FARQUHAR, M. G. AND PALADE, G. E. (1963) *J. Cell Biol.*, **17**, 375–412.

FLOCK, A. (1965) *Acta Otolaryngol.*, Suppl. **199**, 1–90.

FUKAMI, Y. (1969) *Brain Res.*, **14**, 127–145.

GOODENOUGH, D. A. AND REVEL, J. P. (1970) *J. Cell Biol.*, **45**, 272–290.

GOTTLIEB, D. I. (1970) *Anat. Rec.*, **166**, 309.

GRAY, E. G. (1959) *J. Anat. Lond.*, **93**, 420–433.

GRAY, E. G. (1961) *J. Anat. Lond.*, **95**, 345–356.

GRAY, E. G. (1963) *J. Anat. Lond.*, **97**, 101–106.

GRAY, E. G. (1969a) *Progr. Brain Res.*, **31**, 141–155.

GRAY, E. G. (1969b) *Symp. Intern. Soc. Cell Biol.*, **8**, 211–227.

GRAY, E. G. (1970) *Phil. Trans. Roy. Soc. London, B.*, in press.

GRAY, E. G. AND GUILLERY, R. W. (1966) *Intern. Rev. Cytol.*, **19**, 111–182.

GRAY, E. G. AND WILLIS, R. A. (1970) *Brain Res.*, **24**, 149–168.

GRAY, E. G. AND YOUNG, J. Z. (1964) *J. Cell Biol.*, **21**, 87–103.

GUILLERY, R. W. (1969) *Z. Zellforsch.*, **96**, 1–38.

JONES, E. G. AND POWELL, T. P. S. (1970) *Phil. Trans. Roy. Soc. London, B.*, **257**, 1–62.

KANASEKI, T. AND KADOTA, K. (1969) *J. Cell Biol.*, **42**, 202–220.

KHATTAB, F. I. (1968) *Experientia*, **24**, 690–691.

MATTHEWS, M. R. AND RAISMAN, G. (1969) *J. Anat. Lond.*, **105**, 255–282.

MUGNAINI, E. (1970) *Brain Res.*, **17**, 169–180.

MUGNAINI, E. AND WALBERG, F. (1967) *Exp. Brain Res.*, **4**, 212–236.

MULLINGER, A. M. (1964) *Proc. Roy. Soc. London, B*, **160**, 345–359.

NICOLL, R. A. (1969) *Brain Res.*, **14**, 157–172.

PAYTON, B. W., BENNETT, M. V. L. AND PAPPAS, G. D. (1969) *Science*, **166**, 1641–1643.

PETERS, A. (1970) *Anat. Rec.*, **166**, 362.

PETERS, A., PALAY, S. L. AND WEBSTER, H. DE F. (1970) *The fine structure of the nervous system*, Harper & Row, New York.

PRICE, J. L. (1969) *J. Physiol.*, **204**, 77–78P.

PRICE, J. L. AND POWELL, T. P. S. (1970) *J. Cell Sci.*, **7**, 91–187.

RALL, W., SHEPHERD, G. M., REESE, T. S. AND BRIGHTMAN, M. W. (1966) *Exp. Neurol.*, **14**, 44–56.

REVEL, J. P. AND KARNOVSKY, M. J. (1967) *J. Cell Biol.*, **33**, C7–C12.

ROBERTSON, J. D. (1970) *Neurosciences Res. Prog. Bull.*, **8**, 350–352.

ROBERTSON, J. D., BODENHEIMER, T. S. AND STAGE, D. E. (1963) *J. Cell Biol.*, **19**, 159–199.

SAAVEDRA, J. P. AND VACCAREZZA, O. C. (1968) *Brain Res.*, **8**, 389–393.

SOTELO, C. AND PALAY, S. L. (1970) *Brain Res.*, **18**, 93–116.

UCHIZONO, K. (1965) *Nature*, **207**, 642–643.

UCHIZONO, K. (1967) *Nature*, **214**, 833–834.

VALDIVIA, O. (1971) *Anat. Rec.*, **166**, p. 392.

WESTRUM, L. E. (1965) *J. Physiol.*, **179**, 4–6P.

WESTRUM, L. E. (1966) *Nature*, **210**, 1289–1290.

WESTRUM, L. E. (1969) *Z. Zellforsch.*, **98**, 157–187.

WESTRUM, L. E. AND BLACK, R. G. (1971) *Brain Res.*, in press.

WILLIAMS, T. H. AND PALAY, S. L. (1969) *Brain Res.*, **15**, 17–34.

YOUNG, J. Z. (1964) *A model of the Brain*, University Press, Oxford.

# Differentiation between 5-Hydroxytryptamine and Catecholamines in Synaptic Vesicles

AMANDA PELLEGRINO DE IRALDI, ROBERTO GUEUDET AND ANGELA MARÍA SUBURO

*Instituto de Anatomía General y Embriología, Facultad de Medicina Buenos Aires (Argentina)*

Knowledge of the subcellular localization of monoamines is indispensable in establishing the biochemical organization of the synaptic region and in determining the physiological role of monoamines in neurotransmission.

After the demonstration that noradrenaline (v. Euler, 1946), serotonin (Twarog and Page, 1953) and dopamine (Carlsson, 1959) are present in nervous tissue, many different methods have been used to establish their precise localization. At the ultrastructural level these led to the conclusion that monoamines are mainly stored in some of the different granulated vesicles described in peripheral (De Robertis and Pellegrino de Iraldi, 1961a, b; Bondareff, 1965) and central (Pellegrino de Iraldi *et al.*, 1963; Höckfelt, 1968) nerve endings and varicosities. These granulated vesicles correspond to the morphological entity postulated in different models based upon the available information on uptake, synthesis, storage, release and inactivation of monoamines.

All these vesicles are morphologically characterized by an electron-dense core and a clear space between the core and the surrounding membrane. However, it is now evident that a great deal of heterogeneity must be considered in the granulated vesicles of different nerve endings, even in the granulated vesicles of the same nerve.

Taking into account their size, at least two types of granulated vesicles may be distinguished in nervous tissue. These have been classified as the "small" and "intermediate" types by Pellegrino de Iraldi and De Robertis (1964). The first group is formed by vesicles with a diameter of 400–600 Å, similar to that of the synaptic vesicles first described by De Robertis and Bennett (1954). The second group includes vesicles ranging from 700 Å to 1500 Å and different populations may be distinguished among them (Pellegrino de Iraldi and Jaim Etcheverry, 1967; Suburo and Pellegrino de Iraldi, 1969).

The heterogeneity of granulated vesicles is not limited to their variance in size. The dense core can be visualized in different ways in the various populations of granulated vesicles. While in some of the small ones it can be revealed with osmium

\* The original work contained in this paper was supported by grants from the Consejo Nacional de Investigaciones Científicas y Técnicas, Argentina and the National Institutes of Health. (5 R01 NS 06953-05 NEUA)

*References pp. 169–170*

tetroxide (De Robertis and Pellegrino de Iraldi, 1961a, b), glutaradehyde 10llowed by osmium tetroxide (Pellegrino de Iraldi and Gueudet, 1969) or permanganate (Richardson, 1966), in others a core can only be revealed with permanganate fixation (Höckfelt, 1968). Although the dense core of intermediate granulated vesicles is revealed by all the previously mentioned fixatives, its electron density differs from that of the small vesicle cores as revealed by the same fixatives. Furthermore heterogeneity is also present in the so-called clear space as this reacts in a different way with the osmium tetroxide–zinc iodide mixture of Champy–Maillet (Pellegrino de Iraldi and Gueudet, 1969; Pellegrino de Iraldi and Suburo, 1970) depending on the particular population under study. However this morphological heterogeneity is not enough to characterize the different types of granulated vesicles because similar vesicles may be found in tissues storing different monoamines. This situation is complicated by the fact that similar vesicles may be found in nerves storing more than one amine. This fact pointed to the necessity of differentiating catechol- and indolamines at the electron microscopic level to determine whether these amines are located in the same or in different synaptic vesicles. This problem will be considered in the nerves of the pineal gland of the rat which are peculiar in that they contain both noradrenaline (NA) and serotonin (5-HT).

The axons and nerve endings of the pineal gland of the rat contain the plurivesicular component which is now considered to be characteristic of adrenergic nerves (De Robertis and Pellegrino de Iraldi, 1961, a,b). This component is formed by clear and granulated vesicles of about 400–600 Å and a few granulated vesicles of about 800–900 Å (Bondareff, 1965).

Several pharmacological and biochemical studies supported the hypothesis formulated by De Robertis and Pellegrino de Iraldi (1961a) that the granulated vesicles of the pineal nerves contain NA (Pellegrino de Iraldi and De Robertis, 1963, 1964; Pellegrino de Iraldi and Zieher, 1966). This line of evidence was also supported by the uptake of [³H]noradrenaline in relation to granulated vesicles radioautographically observed at the electron microscopic level (Wolfe *et al.*, 1962).

The finding of Bertler *et al.* (1963) and Pellegrino de Iraldi *et al.* (1963) that denervation reduces the 5-HT content of the rat pineal body by 50% was interpreted as a demonstration of the existence of a large pool of 5-HT in the pineal nerves.

The presence of 5-HT in the pineal nerves of different mammals was reported using fluorescence microscopy (Bertler *et al.*, 1963) and interpreted as due to the fixation of 5-HT synthesized in the parenchymal cells (Owman, 1964). Taxi and Droz (1966) using radioautography at the electron microscopic level found that 35 min after injection of [5-³H]hydroxytryptophan there is a selective labeling of the preterminal and terminal axons, while the parenchymal cells show less incorporation. These findings tend to indicate that the axons could synthesize serotonin themselves.

More recently Bloom and Giarman (1967) using *p*-chorophenylalanine (*p*-CPA), a drug which selectively inhibits the synthesis of 5-HT (Koe and Weissman, 1966), found that nerve endings and axons in the pineal gland of the rat were greatly depleted of granulated vesicles. To obtain more information about the localization of 5-HT in the pineal nerves the action of *p*-CPA on the pineal gland of the rat was

TABLE 1

EFFECT OF DL-*p*-CHLOROPHENYLALANINE ON SEROTONIN AND CATECHOLAMINE CONTENT
OF THE PINEAL GLAND

|  | Control | DL-*p*-Chlorophenyl-alanine | % Control | t | P |
|---|---|---|---|---|---|
| Serotonin | (8) 30.66 ± 2.6 | (7)  3.9 ± 2.7 | —87 | 7.101 | <0.001 |
| Noradrenaline | (11)  5.8 ± 1.1 | (3)  9.4 ± 2.2 | +62 | 1.468 | >0.1* |
| Dopamine | (9) 20.3  ± 2.5 | (3) 18.3 ± 4.3 | —10 | 0.390 | >0.7* |

Data are expressed as $\mu$g/g wet weight (mean standard error) of serotonin, noradrenaline and dopamine. In parentheses number of determinations. Animals injected with saline were used as controls.
*t* Student's "*t*" value.
* Non-significant value.

studied in our laboratory (Pellegrino de Iraldi and Gueudet, 1969) using a combined biochemical, histochemical and ultrastructural approach. In this work we confirmed the observation of Bloom and Giarman (1967) that this drug depletes serotonin in the pineal gland of the rat while NA and dopamine (DA) levels do not decrease (Table 1). 5-HT was determined according to Anden and Magnusson (1967), NA according to Häggendal (1963) and DA with the method of Carlsson and Waldeck (1958). Treated and control glands were studied under the electron microscope after two fixation schedules: 1) 1% osmium tetroxide in "Periston" (Bayer), pH 6.7, for 2 h, followed by immersion in uranyl acetate 2% in distilled water for 2 h; 2) 3% glutaraldehyde in phosphate buffer 0.1 M, pH 7.2, overnight, washing in 4% sucrose in the same phosphate buffer for 1 h, postfixation in 1% osmium tetroxide in phosphate buffer for 2 h, brief washing and immersion in 2% uranyl acetate in distilled water for 2 h.

After both fixation methods the typical population of clear and granulated vesicles could be observed with minor differences, such as a greater density of the intermediate type of vesicles after glutaraldehyde–osmium tetroxide, and darker and better defined cores of the small vesicles after osmium tetroxide alone. We found that the dense core of granulated vesicles disappeared in *p*-CPA-treated glands fixed in glutaraldehyde–osmium tetroxide (compare Figs. 1 and 2) but remained in those fixed in osmium tetroxide alone (compare Figs. 3 and 4). Table 2 shows the proportions of granulated vesicles in control and treated glands after the two fixatives used. After *p*-CPA there is an increase in the number of granulated vesicles of the osmium tetroxide-treated glands but this is not significant. On the contrary, they are considerably reduced after glutaraldehyde fixation. The correlation between morphological and biochemical data indicates that the granulated vesicles of the pineal nerves store both catechol- and indolamines. It also shows that both fixation methods, done as described, preserve different components in the pineal nerves, although they give a similar picture in control glands. This behavior of the dense core of the granulated vesicles, correlated with the decrease in 5-HT content without reduction in NA and DA levels seems to indicate that NA is preserved in osmium tetroxide-fixed nerves while

TABLE 2

GRANULATED VESICLES IN NERVE ENDINGS OF THE PINEAL GLAND

| | ( *% of total vesicles* ) | | *% Control* | *t* | *P* |
|---|---|---|---|---|---|
| | *Control* | DL-*p-Chlorophenyl alamine* | | | |
| Osmium tetroxide 1% Periston Bayer | (7) 37 ± 3 | (7) 47 ± 3 | +25 | 1.893 | >0.05* |
| Glutaraldehyde 3% phosphate buffer | (7) 33 ± 1 | (7) 5 ± 1 | —85 | 14.860 | <0.001 |

Data are expressed as mean percent of total number of vesicles ± S.E.
*t* Student's "*t*" value.
In parentheses number of pineals studied; 1000 vesicles were counted in each gland. Animals injected with saline were used as controls.
* Non-significant value.

in glutaraldehyde–osmium tetroxide-fixed material the dense core represents a 5-HT store (Histogram 1).

The importance of the fixative used in the preservation of biogenic amines in granulated vesicles has been stressed by many authors (Coupland *et al.*, 1964; Tranzer and Thoenen, 1967a, b; Duncan and Yates, 1967; Machado, 1967). The influence of the fixation procedure has been further investigated in our laboratory (Pellegrino de Iraldi and Suburo, to be published). We arrived at the conclusion that not only is the fixative used of crucial importance in revealing the different biogenic amines, but all the details of the procedure are of paramount importance. Tranzer and Thoenen (1967b) have offered strong evidence that 5-hydroxydopamine (5-OH-DA) accumulates in vesicles of sympathetic nerve terminals filling them completely. We found that this was a useful basis for the evaluation of the influence of fixation on the preservation of the amines. Figs. 5 and 6 show nerve endings of a vas deferens from the same rat after the treatment with 5-OH-DA. In both cases the tissue was fixed in 3% glutaraldehyde in phosphate buffer 0.1 M, pH 7.4, washed in 4% sucrose in the same buffer and postfixed in 1% osmium tetroxide in the same buffer. The only difference between the procedures was that in the first case the tissue was fixed in glutaraldehyde overnight, while in the second it was immersed in the fixative for 1 hour only. It is observed that with the short fixation method an electron-opaque deposit fills both kinds of granulated vesicles, as reported by Tranzer and Thoenen (1967b), while they appeared almost emptied with the long fixation method.

In 5-OH-DA-treated pineal glands the short fixation method produces an electron-opaque deposit which fills both kinds of vesicles, while with the long fixation method only a small dense core, similar to that present in nontreated glands, can be observed. It is interesting to correlate these results with the fact that according to the Wood (1967) histochemical technique, granulated vesicles of the rat vas deferens store NA

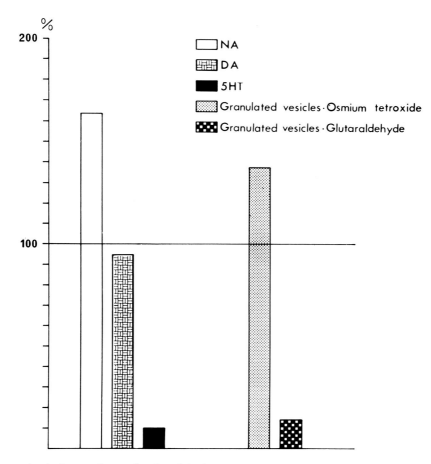

Histogram 1: Amines and granulated vesicles in *p*-chlorophenylalanine-treated glands. Data are expressed as percentage of control values: There is a significant decrease in serotonin (5-HT) level which can be correlated with the significant decrease in the number of granulated vesicles in glands fixed with glutaraldehyde–osmium tetroxide. The persistence of noradrenaline (NA) and dopamine (DA) can be correlated with the preservation of granulated vesicles in osmium tetroxide-fixed glands. Changes in catecholamines and granulated vesicles revealed by osmium tetroxide are non-significant.

only, while those of the pineal nerves contain both NA and 5-HT (Jaim Etcheverry and Zieher, 1968a, b).

The results obtained after 5-OH-DA treatment suggest that catecholamines are more loosely bound than 5-HT and that they may be washed out when the glutaraldehyde fixation is too long. The results can also be correlated with our previous experiments with *p*-CPA, where NA is not preserved in the pineal nerves of the rat after an overnight glutaraldehyde fixation. Other authors (Coupland *et al.*, 1964; Elfvin, 1965; Wood and Callas, 1966; Tramezzani *et al.*, 1964) have reported a good preservation of NA stores in the adrenal gland with glutaraldehyde. However, they used

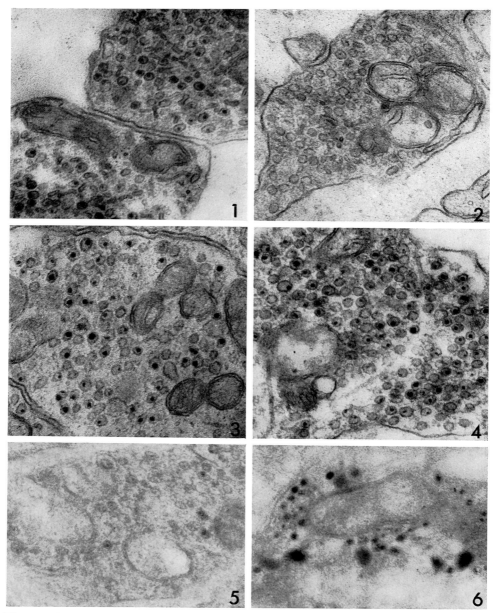

Figs. 1 and 2. Nerve endings of the pineal gland of the rat fixed with glutaraldehyde–osmium tetroxide. Fig. 1 from a control gland and Fig. 2 after *p*-chlorophenylalanine treatment. Observe the
disappearance of the dense core in the treated gland. × 60 000.

Figs. 3 and 4. Pineal nerve endings fixed with osmium tetroxide. Fig. 3 from a control gland and
Fig. 4 after *p*-chlorophenylalanine treatment. There is no disappearance of the dense cores in the
treated gland. × 60 000.

Figs. 5 and 6. Nerve endings of the vas deferens of a rat treated with 5-hydroxydopamine fixed in
glutaraldehyde–osmium tetroxide. When the fixation in glutaraldehyde was done overnight the
vesicles appeared almost empty (Fig. 5). After one-hour fixation in glutaraldehyde small and intermediate vesicles appeared completely filled by an electron-opaque material (Fig. 6). × 60 000.

shorter fixation times. Furthermore, it may be postulated that the NA binding is not the same in the adrenal gland and the adrenergic nerves.

Different histochemical techniques have been developed to reveal the localization of biogenic amines. Most of them are based on a primary glutaraldehyde fixation to obtain an insoluble product with monoamines, and the subsequent exposure of the tissue to one of the metal-containing oxidizing agents such as dichromate (Wood and Barnett, 1964), ammoniacal silver (Tramezzani *et al.*, 1964) or osmium tetroxide (Coupland *et al.*, 1964). It has also been demonstrated that permanganate fixation is a useful tool in investigating monoamines (Richardson, 1966; Hökfelt, 1968). All of these techniques may reveal more than one amine depending on the schedule used. In 1967, Wood published a new method based on the use of dichromate, which made possible the differentiation between catechol- and indolamines. Experiments made *in vivo* and *in vitro* demonstrated that with a glutaraldehyde fixation dichromate reveals NA, DA and 5-HT (Wood, 1965 and 1966). If formaldehyde is used prior to glutaraldehyde, the reaction between catecholamines and dichromate becomes negative while that of indolic sites remains unaffected (Wood, 1967).

This technique has been applied in our laboratory (Pellegrino de Iraldi and Gueudet, 1969) after *p*-CPA treatment. The results obtained are shown in Figs. 7–10. In normal glands fixed with glutaraldehyde (Fig. 7) or formaldehyde–glutaraldehyde (Fig. 8) followed by oxidation with potassium dichromate, electron-dense granules were observed in the pineal nerves. Most of them were 200–300 Å in diameter and a few 500–700 Å. These two types of reactive granules can be matched by their diameter and relative frequency with the dense cores of the two types of granulated vesicles described in adrenergic nerves (De Robertis and Pellegrino de Iraldi, 1961a, b; Bondareff 1965). As this technique shows, both of them can store biogenic amines. This does not mean that both kinds of vesicles play the same role in the adrenergic nerve terminal.

In *p*-CPA-treated glands similar dense granules were observed only when the tissue was fixed in glutaraldehyde (Fig. 9). The reaction was negative in treated glands previously fixed in formaldehyde (Fig. 10). The disappearance of reactive granules after formaldehyde–glutaraldehyde fixation can be correlated with the decrease of serotonin content, and the persistence of reactive granules after glutaraldehyde with the preservation of noradrenaline stores (Table 2). This correlation indicates that this histochemical technique is able to differentiate between catechol- and indolamines. The fact that *p*-CPA specifically inhibits the enzyme tryptophan hydroxylase (Koe and Weissman, 1967) shows that the histochemical assay has a great degree of specificity for revealing 5-HT. The specificity of the histochemical technique of Wood has also been tested in blood platelets with a different experimental approach by Jaim Etcheverry and Zieher (1968b).

CONCLUDING REMARKS

The results presented here show that it is possible to differentiate between catechol- and indolamines in synaptic vesicles. Two methods have been successfully assayed in the pineal nerves of the rat, one of them based on the use of current fixation methods

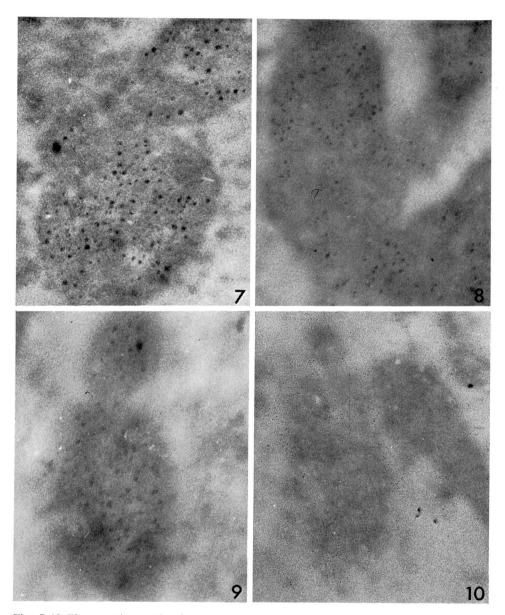

Figs. 7–10. Electron micrographs of nerve endings of the pineal gland studied with the histochemical technique of Wood to differentiate catechol- and indolamines.

Fig. 7. Normal nerve endings after glutaraldehyde–potassium dichromate treatment. Numerous reactive granules of 200–300 Å and one of 600 Å diameter may be observed. × 55 000.

Fig. 8. Normal nerve endings after formaldehyde–glutaraldehyde–potassium dichromate treatment. A similar aspect to Fig. 9 may be observed with paler reactive granules. × 55 000.

Fig. 9. Nerve endings treated with *p*-chlorophenylalanine processed with glutaraldehyde–potassium dichromate. Similar aspect to Fig. 9 with reactive granules of lesser density. × 55 000.

Fig. 10. Nerve endings after treatment with *p*-chlorophenylalanine processed with formaldehyde–glutaraldehyde–potassium dichromate. Observe the disappearance of reactive granules. × 55 000.

combined with pharmacological treatment and the other using a histochemical technique. However, the heterogeneity of monoamine-containing vesicles as revealed by current and special fixation methods indicates that these results cannot be extrapolated to other granulated vesicles without demonstration.

It has also been shown that different fixatives may preserve different components in synaptic vesicles even if they give a similar picture at the electron microscopic level. Furthermore, not only the fixative employed but also the precise schedule used may involve substantial differences in the preservation of monoamines. Differences in binding may be an important parameter in the localization of monoamines in synaptic vesicles.

## REFERENCES

ANDEN, N. AND MAGNUSSON, T. (1967) *Acta Physiol. Scand.*, **69**, 87.
BERTLER, Å., FALCK, B. AND OWMAN, CH. (1963) *Kl. fisiogr. Sällsk. hund Forh.*, **33**, 13.
BLOOM, F. E. AND GIARMAN, N. J. (1967) *Anat. Rec.*, **157**, 351.
BONDAREFF, W. (1965) *Z. Zellforsch.*, **67**, 211.
CARLSSON, A. (1959) *Pharmacol. Rev.*, **11**, 300.
CARLSSON, A. AND WALDECK, B. (1958) *Acta Physiol. Scand.*, **44**, 293.
COUPLAND, R. E., PYPER, A. S. AND HOPWOOD, D. (1964) *Nature*, **201**, 1240.
DE ROBERTIS, E., AND BENNETT, H. S. (1954) *Federation Proc.*, **13**, 35.
DE ROBERTIS, E. AND PELLEGRINO DE IRALDI, A. (1961a), *Anat. Rec.*, **139**, 299.
DE ROBERTIS, E. AND PELLEGRINO DE IRALDI, A. (1961b) *J. Biophys. Biochem. Cytol.*, **10**, 361.
DUNCAN, D. AND YATES R. (1967) *Anat. Rec.*, **157**, 667.
ELFVIN, L. G. (1965) *J. Ultrastruct. Res.*, **12**,263.
EULER, V. S. VON (1946) *Acta Physiol. Scand.*, **12**, 73.
HÄGGENDAL, J. (1963) *Acta Physiol. Scand.*, **59**, 242.
HÖKFELT, T. (1968) *Z. Zellforsch.*, **91**, 1.
JAIM ETCHEVERRY, G. AND ZIEHER, L. M. (1968a) *Z. Zellforsch.*, **86**, 393.
JAIM ETCHEVERRY, G. AND ZIEHER, L. M. (1968b) *J. Histochem. Cytochem.*, **16**, 162.
KOE, B. K. AND WEISSMAN, A. (1966) *J. Pharmacol. Exp. Therap.*, **154**, 499.
MACHADO, A. B. M. (1967) *Stain. Technol.*, **42**, 293.
OWMAN, CH. (1964) *Intern. J. Neuropharmacol.*, **2**, 105.
PELLEGRINO DE IRALDI, A. AND DE ROBERTIS, E. (1963) *Intern. J. Neuropharmacol.*, **2**, 231.
PELLEGRINO DE IRALDI, A. AND DE ROBERTIS, E. (1964) *Excerpta Med. Intern. Congr. Series*, **83**, 355.
PELLEGRINO DE IRALDI, A. AND GUEUDET, R. (1968) *Z. Zellforsch.*, **91**, 178.
PELLEGRINO DE IRALDI, A. AND GUEUDET, R. (1969) *Intern. J. Neuropharmacol.*, **8**, 9.
PELLEGRINO DE IRALDI, A. AND JAIM ETCHEVERRY, G. (1967) *Z. Zellforsch.*, **81**, 283.
PELLEGRINO DE IRALDI, A. AND SUBURO, A. M. (1970) *The Pineal Gland*, Ciba Symposium, London, in press.
PELLEGRINO DE IRALDI, A. AND ZIEHER, L. M., (1966) *Life Sci.*, **5**, 149.
PELLEGRINO DE IRALDI, A., FARINI DUGGAN, H. AND DE ROBERTIS, E. (1963) *Anat. Rec.*, **145**, 521.
PELLEGRINO DE IRALDI, A., ZIEHER, L. M. AND JAIM ETCHEVERRY, G. (1968) *Advan. Pharmacol.*, **6**, 257.
RICHARDSON, K. C. (1966) *Nature*, **210**, 756.
SUBURO, A. M. AND PELLEGRINO DE IRALDI, A. (1969) *J. Anat.*, **105**, 439.
TAXI, J. AND DROZ, B. (1966) *Compt. Rend.*, **263**, 1326.
TRAMEZZANI, J., CHIOCCHIO, S. AND WASSERMANN, G. (1964) *J. Histochem. Cytochem.*, **12**, 890.
TRANZER, J. P. AND THOENEN, H. (1967a) *Experientia*, **15**, 123.
TRANZER, J. P. AND THOENEN, H., (1967b) *Experientia*, **15**. 743.
TWAROG, B. AND PAGE, I. A. (1953) *Amer. J. Physiol.*, **175**, 157.
WOLFE, D. E., POTTER, L. T., RICHARDSON, K. C. AND AXELROD, J. (1962) *Science*, **138**, 440.

WOOD, J. (1965) *Texas Rep. Biol. Med.*, **23**, 828.
WOOD, J. (1966) *Nature*, **209**, 1131.
WOOD, J. (1967) *Anat. Rec.*, **157**, 343.
WOOD, J. AND BARNETT, R. J. (1964) *J. Histochem. Cytochem.*, **12**, 197.
WOOD, J. AND CALLAS, G. (1966) *Z. Zellforsch.*, **71**, 261.

# Electron Microscopy of Developing Sympathetic Fibres in the Rat Pineal Body
## The Formation of Granular Vesicles

ANGELO B. M. MACHADO

*Institute of Biological Sciences, University of Minas Gerais (Brazil)*

## INTRODUCTION

The pineal body of the rat is innervated exclusively by post-ganglionic sympathetic fibres from the superior cervical ganglion (Kappers, 1960) that are very important for its metabolic activity (Axelrod and Wurtman, 1968). There is evidence that these fibres are adrenergic, taking up serotonin from the parenchyma (Owman, 1964), but cholinergic sympathetic fibres were also recently demonstrated (Machado and Lemos, 1971; Eränkö *et al.*, 1970). The development of the adrenergic component of pineal innervation has been studied in the rat by Håkanson *et al.* (1967) and Machado *et al.* (1968b) using fluorescence histochemistry. The understanding of the pattern of development of pineal adrenergic innervation provided by this research offered an interesting opportunity for a study at the ultrastructural level. Except for our own preliminary studies (Machado, 1967a; Machado *et al.*, 1968a) it seems that only Yamauchi and Burnstock (1969) have dealt with the ultrastructure of post-ganglionic sympathetic fibres during development. In the present paper the development of the sympathetic innervation of the rat pineal body was studied at the ultrastructural level. Special attention was paid to the so-called granular vesicles, in the hope of obtaining some further insight into their mechanism of formation. There is now considerable evidence that these vesicles play an important role in the synthesis, uptake, storage and release of catecholamines (see Potter, 1967; Hökfelt, 1968a, b). Studies on the formation of granular vesicles may contribute to the understanding of adrenergic transmission and the origin of the other types of synaptic vesicles.

## MATERIAL AND METHODS

Holtzman rats of the following ages were used: 2–24 h, 18; 2–3 days, 9; 5–8 days, 9; 15 days, 3; 21 days, 3. Most pineal bodies were fixed by immersion in (or perfusion with) 3% glutaraldehyde in 0.1 M phosphate buffer adjusted to pH 7.3, followed by $OsO_4$ (Machado, 1967b). Three pineals of 1-day-old rats were fixed in 3% $KMnO_4$ in 0.1 M phosphate buffer, pH 7 (Richardson, 1966). The specimens were embedded in epoxy resin, sectioned, double-stained and studied with a Hitachi HU 11 A or

Zeiss EM-9A electron microscope. Most pictures were taken at an original magnification of 15 000 and enlarged 3 or more times.

## RESULTS

### *General features of pineal innervation in the immature rat*

Immediately after birth coarse nerve bundles were seen in the pineal capsule (Fig. 1), especially under the vein of Gallen, and they probably represent the nervi conarii and their main branches. At this age an exhaustive search for nerve fibres inside the gland demonstrated at least one nerve terminal already in contact with a pinealocyte (Fig. 5). The number of nerve fibres inside the gland increased considerably by day 2–3, and at day 7 most vessels had sympathetic fibres in their perivascular spaces. It seems that between days 15 and 21 the adult nerve density is attained. Some of the presumably neuroeffector contacts observed in the immature animal were very intimate, the axon being completely enveloped by the pineal cell (Fig. 2). The cytoplasm of the pineal cell adjacent to the point of contact had no consistent specialization, but the axoplasm contained agranular and granular vesicles, the number of the latter increasing with age of the animal.

During the first days after birth nerve bundles were wrapped by Schwann cells and a basement lamina (Fig. 1). The Schwann cell cytoplasm did not invest individual axons which were naked and in close contact with one another (Fig. 1). At days 7–15, processes of Schwann cells were seen separating large groups of axons. At day 21 (Fig. 3) they wrapped around individual axons or small groups of axons thus establishing the relationship observed in the adult. A few growth cones were found during the first week after birth. Typical microfilaments and neurotubules were also observed. The neurotubules were frequently seen dilating to form saccular or tubular profiles which were interpreted as smooth endoplasmic reticulum (Fig. 14). Usually the mitochondria had a very dense matrix. Glycogen particles were observed in the

---

Fig. 1. Sympathetic nerve in the pineal capsule of 1-day-old rat. The whole bundle of axons is enveloped by a Schwann cell (SC). Outside the Schwann cell and the basement lamina is a leptomeningeal cell (LC) from the pineal capsule. $\times$ 18 000.

Fig. 2. A supposed neuroeffector contact formed by an axon terminal containing many SGV completely enveloped by a pineal chief cell. 7-day-old-rat $\times$ 37 700.

Fig. 3. Sympathetic nerves from the pineal body of a 21-day-old rat. Virtually every axon is enveloped by the Schwann cell. $\times$ 33 000.

Fig. 4. Axons of a 5-hour-old rat pineal body fixed in $KMnO_4$ containing many LGV and a few SGV with small granules (arrows). $\times$ 73 000.

Fig. 5. Neuroeffector contact in a 5-hour-old rat. The dilated axon is in close contact with pineal chief (CC) and interstitial cells (IC) and contains many agranular vesicles, three typical LGV, possibly three SGV (arrows). At this age no cholinergic nerve was detected inside the gland (Machado and Lemos, 1971) while a few adrenergic terminals could be detected by fluorescence microscopy after injection of exogenous norepinephrine. Supported by this fact and by the presence of two doubtful SGV, this axon is tentatively classified as adrenergic. Glutaraldehyde–$OsO_4$ fixation. $\times$ 55 000.

Fig. 6. Axon with a large number of SGV and one LGV (arrow). Glutaraldehyde–$OsO_4$ fixation. 15 day-old rat. $\times$ 73 000.

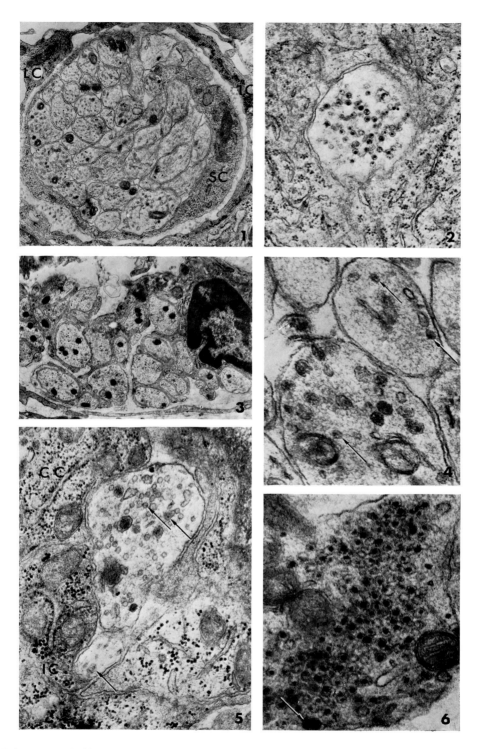

axons during the first month of life (Fig. 13), disappearing almost completely in the adult. Multivesicular bodies were frequent and the smooth endoplasmic reticulum was abundant (Figs. 10, 15). Coated, granular, and agranular vesicles were observed in the fibres from birth. The granular vesicles were large or small, according to the classification of Grillo and Palay (1962) modified by Bondareff (1965).

*The small granular vesicles*

In glutaraldehyde–$OsO_4$-fixed tissues unequivocal small granular vesicles (SGV) were virtually absent at day 1. However, after $KMnO_4$ fixation they could be observed at this age (Fig. 4). The number of these vesicles was considerably greater at day 7 (Fig. 2), and at 2 weeks, clusters of more than 100 SGV were seen (Fig. 6). Although the size (525 Å mean diameter) of the SGV observed in the first 3 days after birth corresponds to that observed in vesicles found in older or adult animals (516 Å; Machado, 1967b), the size and position of their granules were different. The majority of the SGV found in the first three days after birth had a small and eccentric granule attached to the vesicle membrane (Figs. 4, 7 , and 9). The inner lamina of the vesicle membrane was frequently encrusted with tiny specks similar to those described in glutaraldehyde-fixed vesicles of adult rats (Machado, 1967b). Many SGV observed at day 1 after $KMnO_4$ fixation had dense contents, though never as dense as their granules (Fig. 4). In order to evaluate the differences in the size of the granules of the SGV at different ages, their mean diameters were measured 1, 2–3, 7 and 15 days after birth. The values obtained are shown in the histograms (Fig. 11). It is evident that there is a shift toward larger granule sizes between days 1–3 and day 15. The difference between the sizes of the granules at day 1 (mean = 160 Å) and day 7 (mean = 223 Å) is highly significant ($t = 4.102$; $P < 0.001$). The same is true for those between day 7 and day 15 (mean = 272 Å; $t = 2.793$; $P < 0.01$). At day 7 a comparison was made between the sizes of the granules of SGV in the large branches of the nervi conarii of the pineal capsule (mean = 212 Å) and those found in nerve terminals and preterminals inside the gland (mean = 223 Å). No difference could be observed (Fig. 11). In pineal nerves of 1-day-old rats the SGV with small eccentric granules (immature SGV) were frequently associated with agranular vesicles (AV) of about the same size which usually outnumbered them (Figs. 7 and 9). Tubular or saccular profiles of smooth endoplasmic reticulum occurred frequently in these clusters of vesicles (Figs. 7–9). Some profiles suggested that the AV were forming from the endoplasmic reticulum (Figs. 8 and 9), but the evidence for this was not unequivocal. On the other hand, transitions were seen between SGV and AV, and in some cases classification of a vesicle as agranular or immature granular was rather difficult. In spite of this, vesicle countings were made in order to evaluate the changes with age in the proportions of SGV to LGV and AV. To exclude cholinergic fibres, only axons containing at least one typical SGV were counted. The results are shown in Table 1.

It is clear that there was an age-dependent increase in the percentage of SGV simultaneously with a decrease in the percentages of LGV and AV. At day 1 the percentage of SGV was slightly higher than at day 2–3, probably due to the use of

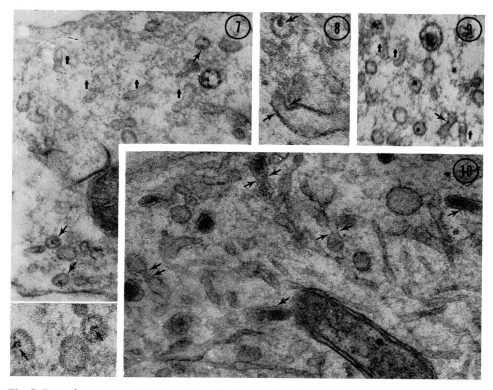

Fig. 7. Part of an axon containing tubules (t) of smooth endoplasmic reticulum, agranular vesicles, one LGV (upper right), and three immature SGV (arrows). Except for the larger size, the LGV in this picture is very similar to the SGV and appears to be formed by a similar mechanism. 3-day-old rat. × 80 000.

Fig. 7. (inset). Detail of the two SGV in the lower part of fig. 7. Note that they contain a small eccentric granule (arrows) which is regarded as the first step in the formation of these vesicles from agranular ones. The granules consist of a less dense globular component surrounded by another component of increased density, resembling the two subcellular elements variously distributed to form the granule of SGV in the adult (Bondareff, 1965). × 149.

Fig. 8. The LGV in this axon has a small eccentric granule (arrow) which is probably in a more advanced stage of maturation than the one in Fig. 7. A sac of smooth endoplasmic reticulum apparently is budding off an agranular vesicle (arrows). 3-day-old rat. × 45 000.

Fig. 9. Axon containing agranular vesicles, LGV and three immature SGV. Tubules (t) of smooth endoplasmic reticulum, one of which appears to be budding off an agranular vesicle (arrow). 3-day-old-rat. × 82 000.

Fig. 10. Dilated axon with many sacs and tubules of smooth endoplasmic reticulum some of which contain dense or semidense material (single arrows) apparently in the process of forming LGV (facing arrows). One granular vesicle seems to be pinching off from SER (double arrows). 5-hour-old rat. × 73 000.

$KMnO_4$ as fixative at this age. The ratio between the percentages of SGV and AV also increased with age, and the values were 0.4, 1.9, 3.4 and 4.2 for animals aged 1, 7, 15 days and adults, respectively. This ratio at day 7 was slightly lower in the extrapineal branches of the nervi conarii (1.4) than in their intrapineal terminals and preterminals (1.9). The apparent increase in the size of the granules of the SGV

TABLE 1

PROPORTION OF THE TWO TYPES OF GRANULAR VESICLES* AND AGRANULAR VESICLES AT
DIFFERENT AGES IN ADRENERGIC AXONS OF THE RAT PINEAL BODY

|      | 1 day** | 2–3 days | 7 days (EP)*** | 7 days (IP) | 15 days | Adult§ |
|------|---------|----------|----------------|-------------|---------|--------|
|      | %       | %        | %              | %           | %       | %      |
| LGV  | 13§§    | 15       | 15             | 9           | 4       | 2.3    |
| SGV  | 25      | 23       | 49             | 60          | 74      | 79     |
| AV   | 62      | 62       | 36             | 31          | 22      | 18.7   |

* The border line between large and small granular vesicle was considered to be 700 Å.
** Fixatives were: $KMnO_4$ (1 day) and glutaraldehyde–$OsO_4$ (other ages).
*** EP = extrapineal; IP = intrapineal; LGV = large granular vesicles; SGV = small granular vesicles; AV = agranular vesicles.
§ Data obtained from Machado (1967b).
§§ 500–700 vesicles were counted for each age using 15–30 random pictures per age.


and in the proportion of granular to agranular vesicles observed during development suggest that the SGV were forming from the agranular vesicles. Our theory of the steps of this formation is presented in Fig. 12.

### The large granular vesicle

Large granular vesicles (LGV) with a mean diameter of 820Å were frequently present in pineal sympathetic fibres of newborn rats. Occasionally axon dilatations with more than twenty LGV were observed (Fig. 13). The number of LGV per unit axon area was counted in pictures of sympathetic axons taken at random from pineal bodies of rats aged 1 day (20 pictures) and adults (30 pictures). This number in 1-day-old rats (1.1 vesicles/$\mu^2$) was slightly higher than in the adult (0.8 vesicles/$\mu^2$), but the difference was not significant ($t = 1.13$; $P > 0.5$).

It was possible particularly in the early postnatal period to trace the origin of the LGV from sacs of smooth endoplasmic reticulum (Figs. 10 and 13–21) as suggested before (Machado, 1967a). It seems that the fundamental process consists in the accumulation of dense or semidense material within sacs or tubules of the smooth endoplasmic reticulum (Figs. 10 and 13–21) from which the vesicles pinch off (Figs. 10, 17, and 21). A constriction observed in the middle portion of some of these elongated sacs probably results in the formation of two vesicles (Figs. 10, 14, 17, 18 and 20). A few LGV vesicles contained a small excentric granule (Figs. 7 and 8) with all transition stages to a larger granule (Figs. 7–9). The existence of these vesicles suggests

Fig. 11. Distribution of diameters of granules of small granular vesicles in adrenergic axons of the pineal body of rats of different ages. The granules were measured in intrapineal terminal and preterminal axons except at day 1 and day 7 when extrapineal (EP) branches of the nervi conarii were used. All the specimens were fixed in glutaraldehyde–$OsO_4$ except the 1-day-old material which was fixed in $KMnO_4$. 120–200 vesicles from 15–30 pictures were measured for each age.

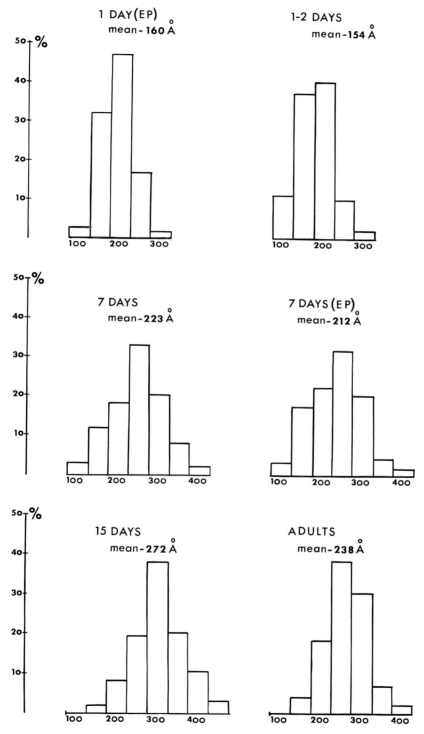

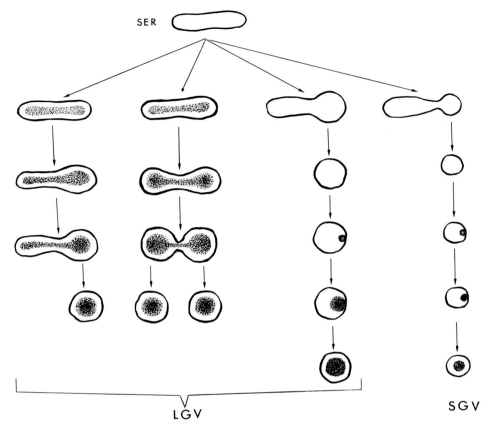

Fig. 12. Diagram showing the author's interpretation of the formation of granular synaptic vesicles based on morphological evidence discussed in the text. SER = smooth endoplasmic reticulum; LGV = large granular vesicle; SGV = small granular vesicle.

another mechanism of formation for the LGV in which dense material accumulates within an empty vesicle in a manner similar to that described for the formation of the SGV (Figs. 7–9, and diagram of Fig. 12). It seems that LGV formed by this mechanism resemble the SGV in core density as well as in the presence of tiny dense specks attached to the inner component of the vesicle membrane.

DISCUSSION

*Pattern of development of the sympathetic innervation and the granular vesicles in the rat pineal body*

The developmental pattern of the adrenergic innervation of the rat pineal body as studied by electron microscopy agrees with the results obtained by fluorescence microscopy except for the time of penetration of the first nerve terminals into the

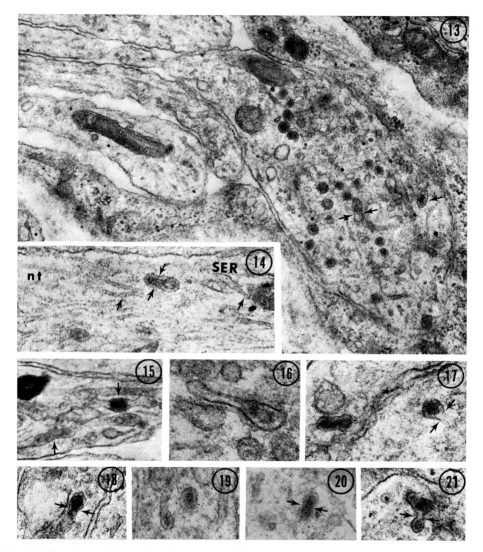

Fig. 13. Dilated axon from a pineal nerve containing many LGV and a few glycogen particles. The arrow points to an elongated LGV. A small sac of smooth endoplasmic reticulum appears to be forming a LGV in one of its extremities (facing arrows). 24-hour-old rat. × 44 000.

Fig. 14. Axon containing typical neurotubule (nt) and slightly dilated neurotubules (arrows) one of which is widening to form smooth endoplasmic reticulum (SER). A slightly constricted sac of SER containing dense material can be observed (facing arrows). 2-day-old rat. × 45 000.

Fig. 15. Axon with smooth endoplasmic reticulum containing material of different densities (arrows). 1-day-old rat. × 55 000.

Fig. 16. An elongated LGV is apparently budding off from a tubule of smooth endoplasmic reticulum. 2-day-old rat. × 100 000.

Fig. 17. On the right a LGV is continuous with smooth endoplasmic reticulum and appears to be pinching off from it (arrows). On the left a sac of smooth endoplasmic reticulum about twice as large as the LGV contains material of the same density as the vesicle. 5-hour-old rat. × 75 000.

Fig. 18. A LGV appears to be forming from smooth endoplasmic (facing arrows) reticulum containing dense material. 5-hour-old rat. × 60 000.

Fig. 19. A LGV is apparently budding off from a tubule of smooth endoplasmic reticulum. 2-day-old rat. × 75 000.

Fig. 20. Probably a sac of smooth endoplasmic reticulum containing dense material constricted in the middle to form two LGV. However, an artefact caused by overlapping of two LGV could not be completely ruled out in this picture. 3-day-old rat. × 60 000.

Fig. 21. A LGV is pinching off (arrows) from the smooth endoplasmic reticulum which contains dense material. A SGV is shown in the upper left. 15-day-old rat . × 50 000.

gland. Studies with fluorescence microscopy showed this to occur at day 5–6 (Håkanson *et al.*, 1967) or 2–3 (Machado *et al.*, 1968b), while electron microscopy showed a few nerve terminals to be inside the gland at day 1. Indeed varicose terminals could be detected inside the rat pineal gland a few hours after birth (Machado and Machado, unpublished data) by injecting norepinephrine (NE), a technique recently proposed by Read and Burnstock (1969). The progressive postnatal investment of the sympathetic nerves by the Schwann cells (Machado, 1967a) agrees with the observations of Yamauchi and Burnstock (1969) in nerves of the mouse vas deferens. The Schwann cell–axon relationship in sympathetic nerves during the first postnatal week corresponds to those observed in somatic nerves of 17-day-old intrauterine rat embryos (Peters and Armuir, 1959).

Earlier we studied the development of the sympathetic fibres of the rat pineal body using only glutaraldehyde–$OsO_4$ fixation (Machado *et al.*, 1968a). It was stated that the SGV were absent at day 1, appeared at day 2, and that their number considerably increased by day 7–15, while the LGV were already present at day 1. However, after $KMnO_4$ fixation SGV were observed at day 1. This fact indicates that although glutaraldehyde–$OsO_4$ is a good fixative for SGV in the rat pineal body (Machado, 1967b) it is not as sensitive as $KMnO_4$ for detecting the small amount of NE that presumably exists in the small granules of the SGV of the early postnatal adrenergic fibres. Nevertheless in the adult rat pineal body Bloom and Giarman (1970) observed no superiority of $KMnO_4$ over glutaraldehyde–$OsO_4$ in revealing intravesicular granules. The postnatal increase in the number of SGV within pineal adrenergic fibres agrees with the data obtained by Yamauchi and Burnstock (1969) in the mouse vas deferens. This increase parallels the increase in the number of intrapineal nerve terminals and neuroeffector contacts, a fact which further emphasizes the relationship of the SGV to adrenergic transmission. The same statement cannot be made regarding the LGV whose amount is the same in the adult and at birth, when very few terminals occurred inside the gland. The significance of the LGV is a matter of considerable controversy (see Hökfelt, 1968a, b). The fact that these vesicles were present in adult amounts around birth suggests that they might have some functional significance very early in the development of the adrenergic fibre.

There is now considerable evidence relating the SGV to the synthesis and binding of NE (Potter, 1967) which is stored in their granules (Bondareff and Gordon, 1966; Van Orden *et al.*, 1966). During the maturation of the adrenergic fibres there is an increase in the number of SGV as well as in the number of vesicles with large granules. It seems therefore that the maturation of the adrenergic fibres and not only the density is a factor in the increase in the amount of the endogenous NE observed in several tissues during development (Iversen *et al.*, 1967; Ignarro and Shideman, 1968; Friedman *et al.*, 1968).

### *Origin of the small granular vesicle*

The maturation of the adrenergic neuron during development offers a unique opportunity for studying the formation of granular vesicles under normal conditions.

The mechanism of formation of these vesicles should be considered in two steps which may be independent, namely, the formation of the granule or dense core and the formation of the vesicle membrane. These steps will now be considered for the SGV. Our results showed that the SGV/AV ratio and the proportion of SGV with large granules increased from days 1–3 to day 15. It is difficult to explain this increase simply by the arrival from the superior cervical ganglion of a new population of SGV containing predominantly large granules. In this case, assuming a uniform axonal flow of both SGV and AV, the SGV/AV ratio and the proportion of SGV with large granules on the 7th day should have been greater in the extrapineal trunks of the nervi conarii than in their smaller intrapineal branches. However, the opposite was seen. If we assume that no selective destruction of AV or AGV with small granules occurred at the periphery, we are led to conclude that there was an actual increase in the sizes of the granules of the SGV, as well as a formation of SGV from AV, both phenomena occurring at the periphery. This fact suggests the existence of a developmental continuum beginning at the AV and ending with a vesicle containing a large dense core or a mature SGV. This view is further supported by the finding of transition stages between these two extremes and especially between the AV and SGV with an eccentric tiny granule. It seems therefore legitimate to consider the SGV with a small eccentric granule observed in the newborn or even adult animals as an immature SGV. It has been suggested (Machado, 1967b) that the few AV remaining in the adrenergic fibres after an adequate fixation represent maturational or else functional stages of the norepinephrine-storing vesicles. The present results support the first assumption and there is evidence that agranular and granular vesicles represent a homogenous population differing only in the degree of amine filling (Tranzer and Thoenen, 1967), which may depend on functional situations at the nerve terminal.

The origin of the vesicle membrane is more difficult to trace. The frequent association of AV with tubular profiles of smooth endoplasmic reticulum suggest that they could originate from the latter. Indeed some profiles suggest that the vesicles are pinched off from the reticulum. The present results do not support the view of Geffen and Ostberg (1969) that the SGV is formed from the LGV and the two populations of vesicles represent different states of maturity.

### Origin of the large granular vesicle

In a preliminary study on developing sympathetic axons in the rat pineal body I suggested in 1967 that the LGV originate in the axons by accumulation of dense material within sacs of smooth endoplasmic reticulum (Machado, 1967a), a view that is supported by the present observations. However, Pellegrino de Iraldi and De Robertis (1968) studying regenerating axons proximal to a nerve constriction reported that these vesicles are formed by dilatation and pinching off of neurotubules. Indeed profiles very similar to those presented by Pellegrino de Iraldi and De Robertis showing "dilated neurotubules" forming LGV were observed in my material; and it seems to me that the disagreement is a matter of interpretation. I think that the dilatation of the neurotubules to form tubular or saccular structures with a unit membrane is a transformation of these neurotubules into smooth endoplasmic reticulum. The endoplasmic reticulum in turn, may accumulate dense material and give rise to the LGV, a phenomenon which is independent of the formation of the smooth endoplasmic reticulum from the neurotubule. It is not known whether all the axonal endoplasmic reticulum is formed from the neurotubules and if it is totally used for the formation of vesicles. Dilatations of axonal neurotubules to form smooth endoplasmic reticulum have been reported by Sandborn who proposed a model to explain the phenomenon (Sandborn, 1966). Continuities between typical neurotubules and vesicles were not observed in our material, and if the phenomenon really occurs it must be very rapid; on the other hand dilatation of neurotubules to form smooth endoplasmic reticulum was frequently seen, although apparently the phenomenon was not as pronounced as demonstrated by Pellegrino de Iraldi and De Robertis in constricted nerves. In these nerves Kapeller and Mayor (1969) observed an increase in the endoplasmic reticulum which was interpreted as an active reaction to the effect of axonal injury.

It seems that the dense material forming the granules of most of the LGV accumulates within the sacs of smooth endoplasmic reticulum before the vesicles are pinched off. This means that in the formation of most of the LGV there apparently is at no stage an empty or agranular vesicle as described for the SGV. However, some vesicles of the same size as the LGV probably form their granules by a mechanism similar to that described for the SGV, *i.e.*, by forming a tiny eccentric granule at the membrane, which then enlarges. It is tempting to suggest that these two mechanisms for LGV formation may be related to the two types of LGV that have been described by Bloom and Aghajanian (1968), namely the dense and semidense types.

### Site of formation of the granular vesicles

Pellegrino de Iraldi and De Robertis (1968) observed the local formation of LGV in peripheral regenerating axons. Our results indicate that during development, part of the LGV, the granules and probably the membrane of the SGV are also formed locally in peripheral axons and nerve terminals. However, it is usually accepted that these vesicles are manufactured in the cell body and transported down the axon by axoplasm flow. The main evidence in favor of this hypothesis is that NE accumulates above a nerve section or a ligature (Dahlström and Fuxe, 1964; Dahlström, 1965; Eränkö and Härkönen, 1965), and granular vesicles pile up above the lesion (Kapeller and Mayor, 1967). In addition, Hökfelt (1969) demonstrated granular vesicles in cell bodies of the rat superior cervical ganglion. They were also observed in the perikaryon of developing nerve cells in the sympathetic trunks of the chick embryo (Wechsler and Schmekel, 1966). It seems therefore that granular vesicles can be formed both in the perikaryon and in peripheral axons and nerve terminals, which is consistent with the fact that NE can be synthesized at these sites (Austin et al., 1967). It would be interesting to correlate the appearance of the granular vesicles in the cell body and in the corresponding axon terminals during development. Such a study, however, is likely to be difficult for there is evidence that in the same ganglion, the maturation of groups of neurons supplying different organs may be heterochronic (Machado and Machado, 1970). The formation of granular vesicles in both the axon and the perikaryon raises the problem of which of these two sites provides a larger amount of vesicles and whether this varies with age. In the newborn, part of the SGV are formed from AV at the periphery. It is possible that part of these AV forms locally and part comes from the perikaryon. In the adult the formation of the granule may be faster, for the enzymatic machinery for synthesis of granule components is presumably well developed. Under these conditions, in the adult more than in the newborn there would be more chance for an AV to complete the formation of its granule in the cell body or on the way down to the nerve terminal.

*Onset of functional activity in the sympathetic innervation of the rat pineal body*

A few contacts between sympathetic terminals and pineal cells were seen in rats immediately after birth. A this age the pinealocytes are undifferentiated as judged by histochemical (Håkanson *et al.*, 1967; Machado *et al.*, 1968b), biochemical (Håkanson *et al.*, 1967; Klein and Lines, 1969), and ultrastructural (Machado, 1966, and unpublished data) criteria. The nerve terminals have only a small population of "immature" SGV, and the fact that at day 1 they can be detected only by administration of exogenous NE indicates that their NE content is probably very small. It therefore seems unlikely that the neuroeffector contacts observed in the rat pineal in the early postnatal period are already functioning. However, at some moment during pineal differentiation the sympathetic nervous system begins the regularory control that it exerts over many aspects of pineal metabolism (Axelrod and Wurtman, 1968).

The serotonin content of the rat pineal body shows a circadian rhythm (Quay, 1963) which in the adult depends on the integrity of the sympathetic innervation (Fiske, 1964). The fact that in the immature rat this rhythm persists after immunosympathectomy (Machado *et al.*, 1969a) or superior cervical ganglionectomy (Machado *et al.*, 1969b) might suggest that this innervation is not functioning at this early age. However, it has been shown that extending the light period into the normal dark period prevents the nocturnal fall in serotonin in immature rats (Zweig *et al.*, 1966). This phenomenon can be blocked by immunosympathectomy in 8-day-old rats (Machado *et al.*, 1968a). This result indicates that at this age the sympathetic innervation is capable of functional transmission and conveys the effect of the exposure to an additional period of light. Although the innervation density at this age is smaller than in the adult animal, the proportion of granular vesicles and the sizes of their cores are very close to the adult pattern. It seems that the onset of the transmission at the neuroeffector adrenergic junction requires a period of maturation of both the effector cell and the nerve terminal. This is supported by the recent findings of Furness *et al.* (1970) who were unable to demonstrate neuromuscular transmission in the ductus deferens of the developing mouse until 18 days after fluorescent nerves were first detectable. The maturation of the adrenergic terminal involves the development of a certain number and possibly the attainment of a certain proportion of fully formed granular vesicles.

*References pp. 184–185*

ACKNOWLEDGEMENTS

This work was initiated at the Department of Anatomy, Northwestern University, Chicago, and finished at the University of Minas Gerais, Brazil (Centro de Microscopia Eletrônica da Faculdade de Medicina). I am deeply indebted to Dr. J. C. Hampton for his unfailing support and his guidance in electron microscopy, and to Dr. W. L. Tafuri for his attention. I am grateful to my wife, Dr. C. R. S. Machado, for performing the tedious work of measuring and counting hundreds of vesicles.

This work was supported by the National Research Council of Brazil (CNPq), C.A.P.E.S., and the Rockefeller Foundation.

SUMMARY

The development of the sympathetic innervation of the rat pineal was studied at the ultrastructural level with special attention to the morphology and distribution of the granular vesicles. Immediately after birth few nerve fibres were seen inside the gland although branches of the nervi conarii occur on the capsule. The quantity of intrapineal nerves increased and adult nerve density was attained between two and three weeks. Small granular vesicles could be observed in small amounts a few hours after birth. Their number increased enormously during the first two weeks, while the number of the large granular vesicles remained within the range observed in the adult from the day of birth. There was also an increase in the proportion of small granular to granular vesicles as well as in the size of their granules. This fact was taken as evidence that SGV were forming from AV with the appearance at the vesicle membrane of a small granule which progressively increased in size. Some of the LGV appeared to be formed by a similar mechanism. However most of the LGV originate by pinching off from sacs and tubules of smooth endoplasmic reticulum which had accumulated dense material. In developing adrenergic fibres part of the LGV, the granules, and probably the membranes of the SGV are formed locally in peripheral axons and nerve terminals. Evidence was presented that in 8-day-old rats the pineal sympathetic innervation is functional and able to convey the effect of light on the gland. The attainment of a certain quantity of fully formed granular vesicles may be an important factor for the onset of functional transmission at the neuroeffector adrenergic junction.

REFERENCES

AXELROD, J. AND WURTMAN, R. J. (1968) *Advan. Pharmacol.*, **6A**, 157.
AUSTIN, L., LIVETT, B. G. AND CHUBB, I. W. (1967) *Circulation Res.*, **21**, *Suppl.* **3**, 11.
BLOOM, F. E. AND AGHAJANIAN, G. K. (1968) *J. Pharmacol. Exp. Therap.*, **159**, 261.
BLOOM, F. E. AND GIARMAN, N. J. (1970) *Biochem. Pharmacol.*, **19**, 1213.
BONDAREFF, W. (1965) *Z. Zellforsch.*, **67**, 211.
BONDAREFF, W. AND GORDON, B. (1966) *J. Pharmacol. Exp. Therap.*, **153**, 42.
DAHLSTRÖM, A. (1965) *J. Anat.*, **99**, 677.
DAHLSTRÖM, A. AND FUXE, K. (1964) *Z. Zellforsch.*, **62**, 602.

DAHLSTRÖM, A. AND HAGGENDAL, J. (1966) *Acta Physiol. Scand.*, **67**, 278.
ERÄNKÖ, O. AND HÄRKÖNEN, M. (1965) *Acta Physiol. Scand.*, **63**, 411.
ERÄNKÖ, O., L. RECHARDT, ERÄNKÖ, L. AND CUNNINGHAM, A. (1970) *Histochem. J.*, **2**, 479.
FISKE, V. M. (1964) *Science*, **146**, 253.
FRIEDMAN, W. F., POOL, P. E., JACOBOWITZ, D. AND SEAGREN, S. C. (1968) *Circulation Res.*, **23**, 25.
FURNESS, J. B., MCLEAN, J. R. AND BURNSTOCK, G., (1970) *Develop. Biol.*, **21**, 491.
GEFFEN, L. B. AND OSTBERG, A., (1969) *J. Physiol.*, **204**, 583.
GRILLO, M. A. AND PALAY, S. L. (1962) in S. S. BREESE (Ed.), *Vth Intern. Congr. Electron Microscopy*, Philadelphia, 1962, Vol. 2, p. U-1, Academic Press, New York.
HÅKANSON, R., LOMBARD DES GOUTTES, M. N. AND OWMAN, C. (1967) *Life Sci.*, **6**, 2277.
HÖKFELT, T. (1968a) *Z. Zellforsch.*, **91**, 1.
HÖKFELT, T. (1968b) Electron microscopic studies on peripheral and central monoamine neurones. *Thesis*, Stockholm, pp. 30.
HÖKFELT, T. (1969) *Acta Physiol. Scand.*, **76**, 427.
IGNARRO, L. J. AND SHIDEMAN, F. E. (1968) *J. Pharmacol. Exp. Therap.*, **159**, 38.
IVERSEN, L. L., CHAMPLAIN, J., GLOWINSKI, J. AND AXELROD, J. (1967) *J. Pharmacol Exp. Therap.*, **157**, 509.
KAPELLER, K. AND MAYOR, D. (1967) *Proc. Roy. Soc. London*, **167**, 282.
KAPELLER, K. AND MAYOR, D. (1969) *Proc. Roy. Soc. London*, **172**, 39.
KAPPERS, J. A. (1960) *Z. Zellforsch.*, **52**, 163.
KLEIN, D. C. AND LINES, S. V. (1969) *Endocrinology*, **84**, 1523.
MACHADO, A. B. M. (1966) *Anat. Rec.*, **154**, 381.
MACHADO, A. B. M. (1967a) *Anat. Rec.*, **157**, 282.
MACHADO, A. B. M. (1967b) *Stain Technol.*, **42**, 293.
MACHADO, A. B. M. AND MACHADO, C. R. S. (1970) *Comm. IXth Intern. Congr. Anatomists*, Leningrad.
MACHADO, A. B. M., MACHADO, C. R. S. AND WRAGG, L. E. (1968a) *Experientia*, **24**, 464.
MACHADO, A. B. M. AND LEMOS, V. P. J. (1971) *J. Neuro-Visc. Relations*, **32**, 104.
MACHADO, C. R. S., MACHADO, A. B. M. AND WRAGG, L. E. (1969a) *Endocrinology*, **85**, 846.
MACHADO, C. R. S., WRAGG, L. E. AND MACHADO, A. B. M. (1968b) *Brain Res.*, **8**, 310.
MACHADO, C. R. S., WRAGG, L. E. AND MACHADO, A. B. M. (1969b) *Science*, **164**, 442 .
OWMAN, C. (1964) *Intern. J. Neuropharmacol.*, **2**, 105.
PELLEGRINO DE IRALDI, A. AND DE ROBERTIS, E. (1968) *Z. Zellforsch.*, **87**, 330.
PETERS, A. AND ARMUIR, A. R. (1959) *Quart. J. Exp. Physiol.*, **44**, 117.
POTTER, L. T. (1967) *Circulation Res.*, **21** and **22**, Suppl. 3, 13.
QUAY, W. B. (1963) *Gen. Comp. Endocrinol.*, **3**, 473.
READ, J. B. AND BURNSTOCK, G., (1969) *Histochemie*, **20**, 197.
RICHARDSON, K. C. (1966) *Nature*, **210**, 756.
SANDBORN, E. B. (1966) *Can. J. Physiol. Pharm.*, **44**, 329.
TRANZER, J. P. AND THOENEN, H. (1967) *Experientia*, 23, 123.
VAN ORDEN, L. S., BLOOM, F. E., BARRNETT, R. J. AND GIARMAN, N. J. (1966) *J. Pharmacol. Exp. Therap.*, **154**, 185.
WECHSLER, W. AND SCHMEKEL, L. (1966) *Experientia*, **22**, 296.
YAMAUCHI, A. AND BURNSTOCK, G. (1969) *J. Anat.*, **104**, 17.
ZWEIG, M., SNYDER, S. H. AND AXELROD, J. (1966) *Proc. Natl. Acad. Sci. U.S.*, **56**, 515.

# Morphological Studies on the Mechanism of Adrenergic Transmission in the Central Nervous System

## I. Granulated Vesicles

SEIJI ISHII

*Department of Neurology and Gynecology, Center for Adult Disease, Osaka (Japan)*

### INTRODUCTION

The functional significance of catecholamine in nervous tissue, especially the role it plays in nervous transmission, is a subject of great interest, but its significance in the central nervous system has not yet been ascertained.

Before a certain substance is definitely determined to be a nervous transmitter substance, it should satisfy the following conditions (McLennan, 1962). The substance is contained in the synaptic terminals in a moderate quantity and is liberated from its terminals when it is stimulated. The synthetic enzymes of this substance are contained in the terminal, and its metabolizing enzymes exist in the synaptic cleft. When this substance is applied to the posterior part of the synapse (for example, by way of microelectrophoresis), an effect similar to that of nerve stimulation should be produced.

To study the action of catecholamine in nervous transmission, its localization and distribution should first be clarified; then, the distribution of the enzyme system which takes part in the metabolism and synthesis of catecholamine should be made clear. By electron microscopy the vesicles containing cores with high density are found in large number in the axons and terminals of the hypothalamus and other parts of the brain, and these granulated vesicles are considered to have some relation to the storage of noradrenaline (De Iraldi *et al.*, 1963; Ishii *et al.*, 1965).

This paper is concerned with the fine structure and distribution of granulated vesicles in the brain, and also reports some properties of these vesicles correlated with microassay of amine, drug administration, and electron microscopic radioautography and cytochemistry.

### MATERIALS AND METHODS

Twenty adult male mice (20–25 g), 35 adult male rats (180–200 g), 6 adult male guinea pigs (290–310 g) and 155 adult male and 20 female rabbits (1800–2100 g) were used.

### 1. Method of study of normal distribution of the granulated vesicles

To obtain rapid fixation without anoxic changes of the brain, animals were treated by the perfusion method (Palay et al., 1962). Five per cent glutaraldehyde, adjusted to pH 7.2 with cacodylate buffer, was perfused for 20 min. Then the brain was quickly excised and cut into 0.2-mm-thick frontal sections with an automicrochopper. The sections were refixed in $OsO_4$ for 2.5 h after rinsing with cacodylate buffer, pH 7.2, containing 0.2 M sucrose. The required nuclei embedded in Epon 812 were cut into 1–2 $\mu$ thick sections and were identified by light microscopy. Ultra-thin sections were stained with uranyl acetate or lead hydroxide and observed under a HU-11B electron microscope.

### 2. Microassay of catecholamine in the brain

The medial and lateral hypothalamic areas and nucleus caudatus of rabbit brain were removed for microassay of catecholamine. The tissue from ten animals was pooled for a single analysis. Each sample was extracted with 0.4 $N$ perchloric acid and the extract was fractionated on a Duolite C-25 resin column (Ito et al., 1962). Noradrenaline was estimated by the trihydroxyindole method (Euler and Floding, 1955) and dopamine by the ethylenediamine condensation method (Weil-Malherbe and Bone, 1952) after absorption of each sample with aluminum hydroxide.

### 3. Administration of various drugs

Experimental animals were sacrificed 1.$\frac{1}{2}$, 3, 4, 24, and 48 h after intraperitoneal injection of Win 18501-2, and some reserpinized animals were treated with DOPA (500 mg/kg) 30 min before sacrifice. Reserpine (5–10 mg/kg) or Win 18501-2 (70 mg/kg) was injected into the abdominal cavity of the rabbit pretreated with Iproniazid (100 mg/kg). The distribution of the granulated vesicles and contents of catecholamine were studied as described in sections 1 and 2.

### 4. Demonstration of acetylcholinesterase (AchE) in the brain

Rats were fixed by the perfusion method described in section 1 using 2% glutaraldehyde or 4% formaldehyde adjusted to pH 7.4 with a cacodylate buffer. After perfusion fixation, frontal sections were cut and rinsed overnight in 0.1 M cacodylate buffer containing 0.2 M sucrose in a cold room. The incubation medium was prepared by the method of Karnovsky (1964). Incubation was carried out at room temperature for 30 min or 60 min. After incubation, sections were refixed in $OsO_4$ for 60 min and embedded in Epon 812 as usual.

### 5. Light and electron microscopic autoradiography using the precursor of noradrenaline ([³H]DOPA)

[³H]DOPA (5 $\mu$C/g) was intraperitoneally injected into mice. The brain was quickly excised, fixed in dichromate and embedded in paraffin. 10-$\mu$-thick paraffin sections were covered with NTB₂ (Kodak) by dipping method (Kopriwa and Leblond, 1962). Sections coated with film were exposed 1 or 2 months at 0°C in a dark box and developed with Fuji Rendol and stained with Giemsa solution. The average number of grains in 100 $\mu^2$ of the desired areas or nuclei were calculated by Wipflers micrometer under the light microscope.

In order to inhibit endogenous monoamine oxidase, Catron (0.01 mg/kg) was injected intraperitoneally into rats 24 h and 2 h before DL-[³H]DOPA administration. Rats were killed 30 min, 3 h and 24 h after [³H]DOPA (5 $\mu$C/g) injection by the method described in section 1. Ultra-thin sections were coated with a film of Sakura NR-H1 (diluted 10 times) by the wire-loop method (Caro, 1964; Montrose and Moses, 1964). Sections coated with film were exposed for 6 or 8 weeks at 0°C in a dark box and developed with Fuji Rendol for 3 min at 10°C. After fixation with Fuji fix for 2 min, sections were stained with a solution of lead hydroxide (Karnovsky, 1962) and observed under an electron microscope.

### OBSERVATIONS

Granulated vesicles in the hypothalamus are found in large number in the nuclei hypothalamicus anterior, paraventricularis and ventromedialis. The granulated vesicles are nearly identical in size (150–170 nm in diameter) with that of type 1 of the peripheral nervous system as classified by Grillo and Palay (1962). Granulated vesicles are mixed with synaptic vesicles, and a synaptic terminal that exclusively contains granulated vesicles is never found when specimens are prepared by double

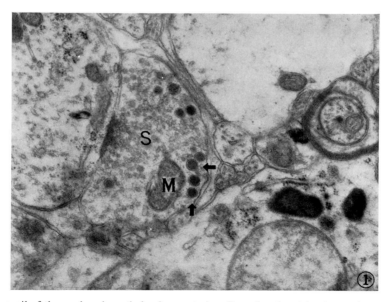

Fig. 1. Neuropil of the nucleus hypothalamicus anterior. Granulated vesicles (arrows) are observed within the synaptic terminal (S). M: mitochondria. Rabbit. × 25000.

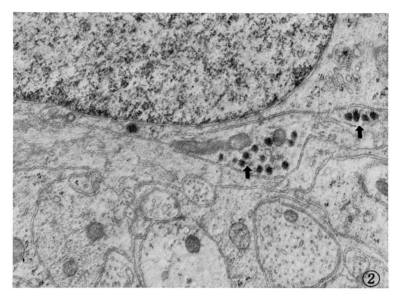

Fig. 2. Neuropil of the area postrema. The varicose axons are filled with granulated vesicles (arrow).
Rabbit. × 24000.

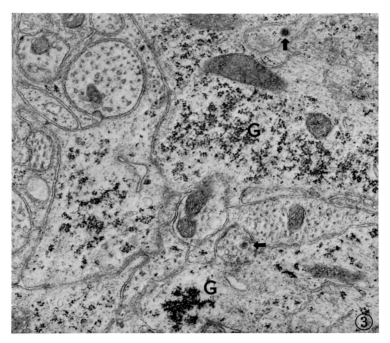

Fig. 3. Neuropil of the area postrema. Note the large amount of glycogen particles (G) in the astro-
cyte-like cells and their processes which surround the axon terminal and small axon containing
granulated vesicles (arrow). Rabbit. × 24000.

fixation with glutaraldehyde and OsO₄. Granulated vesicles always exist at a certain distance from the presynaptic membrane, while the synaptic vesicles are observed clustering together adjacent to the presynaptic membrane (Fig. 1). The synaptic terminals containing granulated vesicles and contacting dendritic processes are always covered with the processes of astrocytes in which fine particles believed to be glycogen are contained. A moderate amount of granulated vesicles is found in the subependymal layer of the third ventricle. In the nucleus hypothalamicus lateralis, they are found not only in the unmyelinated but also in the myelinated axons. In the nucleus hypothalamicus posterior an appreciable number of granulated vesicles were detected, not merely at the terminals of axons but also in the vicinity of the Golgi field within the cell bodies.

The area postrema and the supraoptic crest belong to the paraventricular structure where the blood–brain barrier is lacking. In the former site, the existence of a large amount of noradrenaline was biochemically proven by Vogt (1954). In the area

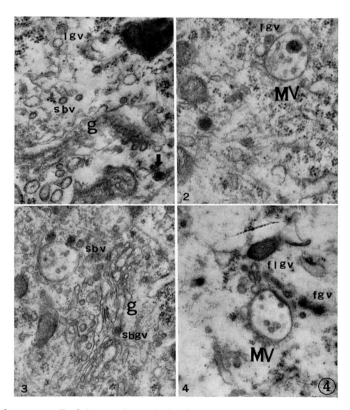

Fig. 4. Part of a nerve cell of the pontine reticular formation. Four kinds of vesicles are seen (sbv, sbgv, lgv, gv), mixed with ordinary Golgi vesicles within the Golgi apparatus (g) or near the multivesicular body (MV). The chain-like structure of the granulated vesicles (flgv, fgv) is seen in the neighborhood of the multivesicular body. sbv: spine border vesicle, sbgv: spine border granulated vesicle, lgv: less dense core granulated vesicle, flgv: chain-like less dense core granulated vesicle, fgv: chain-like granulated vesicle. Rabbit. 1: × 29000. 2: × 30000. 3: × 22000. 4: Guinea pig. × 25000.

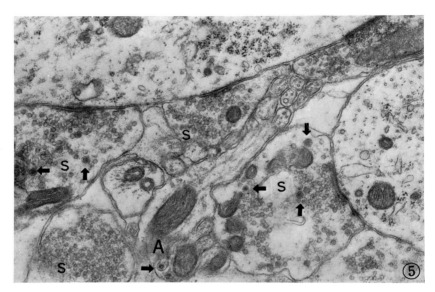

Fig. 5. Neuropil of the pontine tegmentum (nucleus reticularis pontis caudalis). The axonal bouton (S) which contains granulated vesicles (arrow) form the axosomatic synapse on the cytoplasmic membrane. Guinea pig. × 21000.

postrema, the varicose axons were often filled with granulated vesicles (Fig. 2). Moreover, granulated vesicles exist in the cytoplasm of the small nerve cell and a large number are found in the synaptic terminals surrounded by astrocytic processes, with disseminated glycogen particles (Fig. 3). In the neuropil of the supraoptic crest, the parenchymal cells overlap one another, forming a complicated structure by piling up these membranes on each other, and axons containing granulated vesicles are seen among them.

A fairly large number of granulated vesicles were seen within the cytoplasm, especially in the vicinity of the Golgi fields of large cells of the midbrain and the pontine reticular formation of rabbits and guinea pigs. The granules existing in the neighborhood of the Golgi field are classified into 5 types according to their morphological characteristics (Fig. 4). The nerve cells of the midbrain and pontine reticular formation were often surrounded by numerous axosomatic synapses with granulated vesicles in the presynaptic bags (Fig. 5). In the Golgi field of the locus coeruleus of guinea pig, a moderate number of granulated vesicles and vesicles that seem to be an immature stage were observed.

The fluctuation of granulated vesicles in the hypothalamus when 5–10 mg/kg of reserpine was administered was reported by us (Shimizu and Ishii, 1964). Win 18501-2 depleted only noradrenaline without loss of dopamine and serotonin content in the brain, suggesting that the sedative effect of the drug is closely related to loss of brain noradrenaline (Spector *et al.*, 1962; Matsuoka, 1964). The hypothalamus is divided into the medial and lateral part by the line passing the mamillothalamic tract and the fornix. Pooling the tissues of 10 rabbits, dopamine and noradrenaline were determined

TABLE 1

EFFECT OF WIN 18501-2 ON THE CONTENT OF CATECHOLAMINES AND THE NUMBER OF GRANULATED VESICLES IN RABBIT HYPOTHALAMUS

| Area | Treatment | No. of samples | Noradrenaline (µg/g) | | Dopamine (µg/g) | | Number of granulated vesicles per area (200 µ²) | | |
|------|-----------|----------------|----------|------|----------|------|--------------|--------|------|
| | | | Range | Mean | Range | Mean | No. of areas | Range | Mean |
| Medial part | Control | 5 | 1.27–2.12 | 1.61 | 0.69–1.03 | 0.86 | 10 | 53–116 | 77 |
| | Win 18501-2 | 3 | 0.33–0.82 | 0.50 | 1.12–1.41 | 1.26 | 10 | 6– 20 | 12 |
| Lateral part | Control | 5 | 0.24–1.26 | 0.56 | 0.54–1.18 | 0.64 | 10 | 7– 36 | 19 |
| | Win 18501-2 | 3 | 0.31–0.55 | 0.34 | 1.20–1.61 | 1.43 | 10 | 6– 16 | 9 |

Animals were killed by decapitation 3 h after intraperitoneal injection of Win 18501-2 (70 mg/kg), and tissues of the hypothalamus from 8–10 animals were pooled for each assay. The hypothalamus was divided into medial and lateral parts by a dorso-ventral section passing through the fornix and mammillothalamic tract, the medial part containing mainly anterior and ventromedial nuclei, and the lateral part the lateral nucleus of the same level. Ten areas (200 µ²) of the neuropil of both the medial and lateral parts of 5 control and 3 experimental animals were chosen at random and examined by electron microscopy.

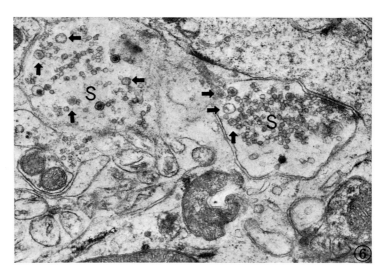

Fig. 6. Neuropil of the nucleus hypothalamicus anterior of the rabbit injected with Win 18501-2 (70 mg/kg) 3 h before sacrifice. Most granulated vesicles change in appearance, either the granulated vesicles disappearing to leave empty vesicles or the electron density of dense core of the remaining vesicles decreasing (arrow). A few vesicles are of a density similar to normal vesicles. S: synaptic terminal. Rabbit. × 26000.

biochemically, and were compared in amount with the number of granulated vesicles seen in the electron micrographs of the corresponding parts. Three hours after Win injection, the amount of noradrenaline decreased by less than 1/3 in the medial part, and by about 3/5 in the lateral part, whereas the amount of dopamine markedly increased both in the medial and lateral parts. Electron microscopic studies showed that the number of granulated vesicles decreased markedly in the medial hypothalamus. Similarly to the case of reserpine, some normal granulated vesicles and granulated vesicles with decreased electron density of their core and vacuoles were observed (Table 1) (Fig. 6).

Thirty min after DOPA (500 mg/kg) was administered to the reserpinized animals and the Win-pretreated animals, the empty vesicles almost disappeared in the medial hypothalamus, and typical granulated vesicles with dense cores reappeared (Fig. 7). The animals were excited then. From the results of a quantitative determination, there was scarcely any change in the noradrenaline content. On the other hand, the dopamine content, which decreased after reserpine administration, increased markedly after DOPA. In the caudate nucleus the noradrenaline content showed almost no change throughout the experiment. However, the dopamine content decreased markedly after reserpine administration and increased greatly after DOPA injection (Table 2). From this observation of a large rise in the content of dopamine, granulated vesicles may be considered capable of storing dopamine.

When pretreated with MAO inhibitor (Iproniazid), the vacuolization and decrease of granulated vesicles caused by reserpine and Win are appreciably suppressed (Fig. 8).

TABLE 4

ELECTRON MICROSCOPIC AUTORADIOGRAPHY

Grain distribution in nucleus hypothalamicus anterior and ventromedialis after intraperitoneal injection of [³H]DOPA into rats pretreated with Catron

| | 30 min | 3 h | 24 h |
|---|---|---|---|
| Cell body | 76.56% | 66.78% | 25.56% |
| Nucleus | 28.48 | 23.02 | 29.07 |
| (Nucleolus) | 15.76 | 11.45 | 24.50 |
| (Chromatin) | 12.60 | 11.76 | 5.59 |
| Golgi ap. | 7.62 | 6.49 | 8.40 |
| M.V.B. | 37.66 | 38.23 | 26.71 |
| E.R. | 3.81 | 6.48 | 4.44 |
| Mit. | 3.93 | 2.73 | 3.33 |
| Free | 57.08 | 43.83 | 38.89 |
| Neuropil | 23.23% | 33.20% | 74.43% |
| Synapse | 27.58% | 41.98% | 42.22% |
| pre | 0.39 | 1.35 | 3.14 |
| G.V. | | 0.11 | |
| S.V. | | | |
| post | 1.57 | 3.18 | 11.1 |
| Dend. | 0.79 | 0.34 | |
| Axon | 21.69 | 29.18 | 34.35 |
| Myelin | 10.62 | 3.11 | 1.51 |

G.V.: Presynaptic terminal containing synaptic vesicles and granulated vesicles.
S.V.: presynaptic terminal containing synaptic vesicles exclusively.
Golgi ap.: Golgi apparatus.
M.V.B.: Multivesicular body.
E.R.: Endoplasmic reticulum.
Dend.: Dendrite.
pre: presynaptic terminal.
post: postsynaptic terminal.

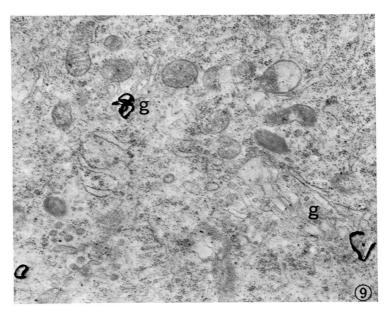

Fig. 9. Cytoplasm of nucleus hypothalamicus ventromedialis of an animal given [³H]DOPA 3 h previously. The silver grains are located within the Golgi apparatus (g). Rat. × 22000.

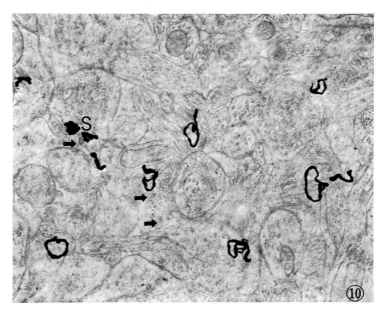

Fig. 10. Neuropil of nucleus hypothalamicus ventromedialis of an animal administered [³H]DOPA 24 h previously. The silver grains are in the synaptic endings (S) which contain granulated vesicles (arrow). Exposure 8 weeks. Rat. × 22000.

silver grains in the neuropil were in the axon and synaptic terminal, and an appreciable number (27 ~ 38 %) existed on the dendrite. To study the relationship between granulated vesicles and the presence of silver grains, the number of grains on synaptic terminals with and without granulated vesicles were compared. Thirty min and 3 h after the intraperitoneal injection, half the silver grains were located on the synaptic terminals containing granulated vesicles. After 24 h, 80 % of the silver grains were located on the synaptic terminals containing granulated vesicles (Fig. 10). Thus I observed that the silver grains tended to concentrate on the terminals containing granulated vesicles with a lapse of time after the injection.

The localization of AchE activity in the neuropil of the mossy fibre endings of the cerebellum was demonstrated by the electron microscope. In the cerebellum of the rat only the nodule and uvula exhibited AchE, as shown by a histochemical method. As shown in Fig. 11, the precipitate of the reaction was seen in the synaptic cleft between the mossy fiber endings and the granule cell dendrites. Their presynaptic boutons were filled with the synaptic vesicles and mitochondria, and granulated vesicles were not observed within them. The locus coeruleus and the nucleus dorsalis nervi vagi also showed AchE activity on the plasma membrane of the axon terminals which contained both granulated vesicles and synaptic vesicles. Dendritic tubules in the dendritic branches attached to the presynaptic terminals also showed activity (Fig. 12). In the hypothalamus a weak reaction occurred and was only seen after

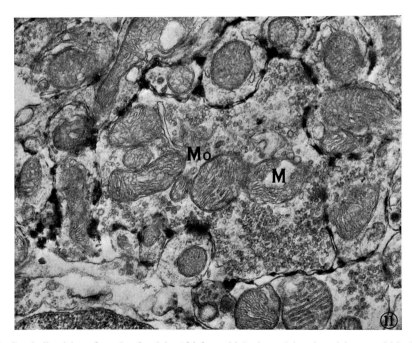

Fig. 11. Cerebellar islet of uvula, fixed in 4% formaldehyde and incubated in acetylthiocholine. Reaction deposits are demonstrated on the plasma membrane and synaptic clefts between mossy fiber endings (Mo) and granule cell dendrites. M: mitochondria. Rat. × 26000.

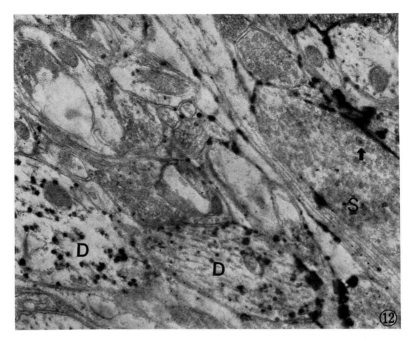

Fig. 12. Neuropil of locus coeruleus, fixed in 2% glutaraldehyde and incubated in acetylthiocholine. The reaction products are attached to the tubules of the dendrites (D) and are also seen on the plasma membrane of the synaptic terminal (S) containing granulated vesicles (arrow). Rat. × 25000.

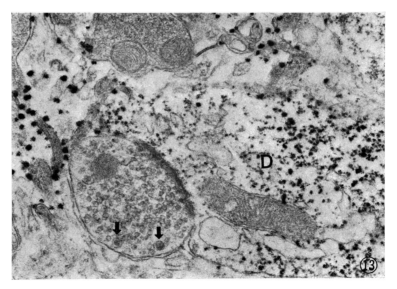

Fig. 13. Neuropil of medial hypothalamus, fixed in 4% formaldehyde and incubated in acetylthiocholine. Small amounts of the reaction product are seen on the dendritic tubules in the synaptic terminals which contain granulated vesicles (arrow) in the presynaptic bag. Rat. × 26000.

formaldehyde fixation. Sparse deposits were seen along the plasma membranes. Some synapses showed a positive reaction in both the plasma membranes of the presynaptic bags containing granulated vesicles and dendritic tubules of the attached dendritic branches, but other synapses showed a positive reaction only on the dendritic tubules (Fig. 13).

## DISCUSSION

In a part of brain such as the hypothalamus which is rich in noradrenaline, granulated vesicles are mainly observed on the synaptic terminals and preterminal axons, while in the nucleus caudatus, few granulated vesicles are found (Mori, 1966), and the relationship between dopamine and granulated vesicle is hardly recognizable (following the double fixation with glutaraldehyde and $OsO_4$). A large number of granulated vesicles are found in the nerve cells, especially in the vicinity of the Golgi field and in the neighborhood of the multivesicular body of nerve cells of the midbrain and pontine reticular formation, locus coeruleus, nucleus hypothalamicus posterior and area postrema. The investigation using fluorescence (Dahlström and Fuxe, 1964) indicated the presence of strong green fluorescence in the cytoplasm of the nerve cell in the above-described nuclei. In other words, there appears to be a correlation between the granulated vesicles and fluorescent substances. Fuxe (1966) and Lenn (1965) implied that in some parts of the brain, no parallel relation between the fluorescent materials and granulated vesicles could be observed, and they suggested that the amines might be contained in the synaptic vesicles. It cannot be said that the distribution of granulated vesicles in the brain as found in this experiment exactly agrees with the distribution of fluorescence. One reason for this is that both soluble and insoluble forms of amine have been shown to exist by the fluorescence method, whereas only the firmly bound form is demonstrable in the electron microscopic sample. This may be clearly understood from the fact that where the existence of granulated vesicles is proven, the nerve cells and nerve fibers are invariably positive for noradrenaline while the reverse is not always true. Wood (1966) supposed that granulated vesicles contain these amines, since dopamine, noradrenaline and serotonin yield precipitates with high electron densities when they react with glutaraldehyde–$OsO_4$ or potassium bichromate. As to the form in which amines exist in brain, the binding form contained in granulated vesicles, the form loosely bound to other objects (for example, the synaptic vesicle) and the free form must be considered. Hökfelt (1966) considered small granulated vesicles (500 Å) demonstrated by permanganate fixation to be the storage site of noradrenaline.

From the results of Andén et al. (1966) who applied the fluorescence method to fibre connections, it becomes clear that in the dorsal part of the midbrain and pontine reticular formation, many cells containing noradrenaline, the locus coeruleus being the main nucleus, send their axons mostly to the part of the forebrain belonging to the limbic system and the hypothalamus through the medial forebrain bundle. In the present work, electron microscopic studies demonstrated the existence of a large number of granulated vesicles and various immature types of granulated vesicles in the

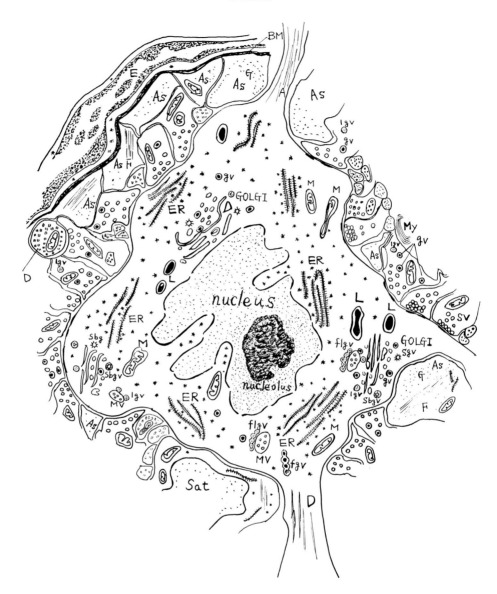

Schema 1. Diagram of a catecholamine-type cell of the reticular formation. This cytoplasmic membrane was surrounded by many axon terminals containing granulated vesicles (gv) and was in contact
with astrocytes containing glycogen particles. Free gv and gv with a less dense core were seen in the
cytoplasm. There are four types of vesicles (sgv, sbgv, lgv, gv) in the Golgi apparatus. A, axon;
As, astrocyte; BM, basement membrane; ER, endoplasmic reticulum; D, dendrite; F, filament;
MV, multivesicular body; G, glycogen; Sat, satellite cell; M, mitochondria; L, lysosome; E, endothelium; gv, granulated vesicle; sbv, spine border vesicle; sbgv, spine border gv; lgv, gv with less
       dense core; flgv, chain-like gv with less dense core; fgv, chain-like gv; sv, synaptic vesicle.

Golgi apparatus and in the neighborhood of the multivesicular body in the cytoplasm of the nerve cells of the midbrain and pontine reticular formation and locus coeruleus. The most reasonable explanation of these electron microscopic findings is that the granulated vesicles are formed in the Golgi apparatus or multivesicular body within the perikaryon, and are transferred along the varicose axon of the ascending fibre to the axon terminals of the hypothalamus and accumulated there. The nerve cells producing granulated vesicles seemed to be cell groups which have been identified as catecholamine-type cells by fluorescence light microscopy (Andén et al., 1966). These nerve cells are often surrounded by numerous axosomatic synapses which contain granulated vesicles in the presynaptic boutons, as shown in Fig. 5. A summary of these observations is shown in Schema 1. This transferred system of granulated vesicles closely resembles the neurosecretion system in the hypothalamic–hypophyseal system.

In the experiment of infusing [$^3$H]noradrenaline into the lateral ventricle, 80% of the incorporation in the hypothalamus was found in the synaptic terminals of the neuropil, most of which contain granulated vesicles (Aghajanian and Bloom, 1966; Lenn, 1967). Accordingly it seems that these results indicate far more clearly the relation between granulated vesicles and noradrenaline than our experiment using labeled precursor. However, careful consideration is necessary before deducing the localization of endogenous noradrenaline directly from the incorporation of the exogenous noradrenaline.

The decarboxylase which takes part in the formation of catecholamine and 5-hydroxytryptamine denotes a distribution similar to that of amine in the brain, being located in the soluble fraction (Kuntzman et al., 1961). According to De Robertis et al. (1964), 5-hydroxytryptophan decarboxylase exists in the nerve ending fraction, and when the fraction is disrupted under low osmotic pressure, it migrates to the soluble fraction. Monoamine oxidase exists in the mitochondria of the nerve terminals (De Robertis et al., 1964), and 50% of the total catechol-o-methyl-transferase is concentrated in the particulate fraction of nerve ending (Alberichi et al., 1965). In our experiment conducted with labeled DOPA, the grains are observed in mainly the neuropil and they are scarce in the cytoplasm. These results point to the possibility of the primary formation of the amines at the nerve terminals.

As TPNH has been recognized to be important in the hydroxylation of tyrosine and phenylalanine (Kaufman, 1966), the production of TPNH by glucose-6-phosphate dehydrogenase has been thought to have an intimate relationship with the formation of catecholamine. Abe (1963) had proven the enzyme to be strongly positive in the hypothalamus, paraventricular structures, nucleus dorsalis nervi vagi, etc. On the other hand, dopamine -$\beta$-hydroxylase which takes part in the synthesis of noradrenaline from dopamine is a copper protein. This enzyme requires ascorbic acid and dicarboxylic acid as co-enzymes. The fact that ascorbic acid is contained in the nerve cells in the hypothalamus, locus coeruleus, and nucleus dorsalis nervi vagi was shown by Shimizu et al. (1960), and an interrelationship with the formation of catecholamine in these nuclei was suggested.

Granulated vesicles were usually localized at some distance from the presynaptic membrane and never accumulated in contact with this membrane. The amine-in-activating enzyme (MAO) exists in the mitochondria, and is independent of the pre- and postsynaptic membranes. AchE activity has been demonstrated in the plasma membrane of the synaptic terminals containing granulated vesicles in the autonomic region of the brain, such as the locus coeruleus and nucleus dorsalis nervi vagi as well as in the hypothalamus, although the activity in the last of these is rather weak.

Koelle (1961) suggested that in non-cholinergic nerve ending, acetylcholine might be released first, and that this changes the permeability of the presynaptic membrane resulting in the secondary release of noradrenaline which acts as transmitter of nervous impulse. In view of the present results, the acetylcholine has a primary significance and it seems unreasonable to regard catecholamine as a nerve transmitter itself.

Noradrenaline activates adenyl cyclase and facilitates the formation of cyclic nucleotide from ATP. By the action of the cyclic nucleotide, the phosphorylase converts to its active form through phosphorylation, and it promotes glycolysis by decomposing glycogen (Sutherland and Rall, 1960). Catecholamine is believed to exert its effect on the nervous function indirectly through the glycolysis of glycogen. Those concepts seem to be justified from the histochemical observation that glycogen and phosphorylase exist in a large amount in the hypothalamus and paraventricular structure (Shimizu and Kubo, 1957). From the electron microscopic observation of the brains of mammals it appears that glycogen is not found at the nerve endings which contain granulated vesicles, but exists in the astrocyte which surrounds the terminal. On these observations is based a hypothesis that the noradrenaline liberated from the adrenergic synapse acts on the astrocyte, where it promotes the glycolysis within the glial cell, thereby affecting secondarily the nervous function of synapse. However, the relation between the granulated vesicles and glycolysis requires further study. Since the hypothalamus and the paraventricular structure are weakly active for succinic dehydrogenase and cytochrome oxidase (Shimizu et al., 1957), it may hardly be surmised that the glycolysis is connected to the TCA cycle, resulting in the production of a large amount of ATP.

Finally, I reported here on granulated vesicles nearly identical with those of type 1 as classified by Grillo et al. (1962). Furthermore, minute granulated vesicles are observed at the axon terminals in the autonomic region when a permanganate fixation is used. Dr. P. H. Hashimoto will discuss the correlation between these minute vesicles and catecholamine (this volume, p. 000).

## SUMMARY

The distribution and fine structure of the granulated vesicles in the central nervous system of rodents have been investigated by means of electron microscopy. Some properties of these vesicles were studied by the administration of certain drugs, radioautography and cytochemistry at the fine structural level.

Granulated vesicles were most numerous in the nuclei hypothalamicus anterior, paraventricularis and ventromedialis and less numerous in the subependymal layer of the third or fourth ventricle and the nuclei hypothalamicus lateralis and posterior. A moderate number of granulated vesicles were demonstrated in the formatio reticularis, locus coeruleus, nucleus dorsalis nervi vagi, area postrema and supraoptic crest.

The midbrain and pontine reticular formation showed many axosomatic synapses, and some presynaptic bags contained both granulated and synaptic vesicles. In the perikaryon of the nerve cell of the formatio reticularis, locus coeruleus, area postrema, and nucleus hypothalamicus posterior, mature and immature types of granulated vesicles were concentrated around the Golgi apparatus and in the neighborhood of the multivesicular bodies.

On the basis of the effects of various drugs upon the biochemical determination and electron microscopic image, granulated vesicles are believed to be related more to noradrenaline than to dopamine except under some special conditions.

The distribution of acetylcholinesterase activity was studied on electron microscopic levels. In the mossy fiber endings of the cerebellum, activity was demonstrated on the plasma membranes and synaptic cleft between the mossy fiber ending and the granule cell dendrite. The locus coeruleus, nucleus dorsalis nervi vagi and medial hypothalamus also showed activity on the plasma membrane of the axon terminals which contained both granulated and synaptic vesicles.

Electron microscopic autoradiography of the nuclei hypothalamicus anterior and ventromedialis showed that two-thirds and three-quarters of the total silver grains were located on the neuropils, where about 70% of the silver grains were localized on the synaptic endings and dendrites. There was a tendency for the number of silver grains on the presynaptic terminals containing granulated vesicles to increase with time after the administration of [$^3$H]DOPA.

## REFERENCES

ABE, T., YAMADA, Y., HASHIMOTO, P. H. AND SHIMIZU, N. (1963) *Med. J. Osaka Univ.*, **14**, 67.

AGHAJANIAN, G. K. AND BLOOM, F. E. (1966) *Science*, **153**, 308.

ANDÉN, N. E., DAHLSTRÖM, A., FUXE, K., LARSSON, K., OLSSON, L. AND UNGERSTEDT, U. (1966) *Acta Physiol. Scand.*, **67**, 317.

CARO, L. D. (1964) In D. M. PRESCOTT (Ed.), *Method in Cell Physiology, Vol. 1*, Academic Press, New York, p. 327.

DAHLSTRÖM, A. AND FUXE, K. (1964) *Acta Physiol. Scand.* **62**, Suppl. **232**, 1.

DE IRALDI, A. P., DUGGAN, H. F. AND DE ROBERTIS, E. (1963) *Anat. Rec.*, **145**, 521.

DE ROBERTIS, E. (1964) In H. E. HIMWICH AND W. A. HIMWICH (Eds.), *Progress in Brain Research, Vol. 8*, Elsevier, Amsterdam, p. 118.

EULER, U. S. AND FLODING, I. (1955) *Acta Physiol. Scand.*, **33**, Suppl. **118**, 57.

FUXE, K., HÖKFELT, T., NILSSON, O. AND REINIUS, S. (1966) *Anat. Rec.*, **155**, 33.

GRILLO, M. A. AND PALAY, S. L. (1962) *Electron microscopy, Vol. 2*, U-1, Academic Press, New York.

HÖKFELT, T. (1966) *Experientia*, **22**, 56.

ISHII, S., SHIMIZU, N., MATSUOKA, M. AND IMAIZUMI, R. (1965) *Biochem. Pharmacol.*, **14**, 183.

ITO, T., MATSUOKA, M., NAKAJIMA, K., KAWATA, K. AND IMAISUMI, R. (1962) *Jap. J. Pharmacol.*, **12**, 130.

KARNOVSKY, M. J. (1962) *J. Biophys. Biochem. Cytol.*, **11**, 729.

KARNOVSKY, M. J. AND ROOTS, L. (1964) *J. Histochem. Cytochem.*, **12**, 219.

KAUFMAN, S. (1966) *Pharmacol. Rev.*, **18**, 61.

KOELLE, G. G. (1961) *Nature*, **190**, 208.

KOPRIWA, B. M. AND LEBLOND, C. P. (1962) *J. Histochem. Cytochem.*, **10**, 269.

KUNTZMAN, R., SHORE, P. A., BOGDANSKI, D. F. AND BRODIE, B. B. (1961) *J. Neurochem.*, **6**, 226.

LENN, N. J. (1965) *Anat. Rec.*, **153**, 399.

LENN, N. J. (1967) *Amer. J. Anat.*, **120**, 377.

MATSUOKA, M. (1964) *Jap. J. Pharmacol.*, **14**, 151.

McLENNAN, H. (1962) *Synaptic Transmission*, Saunders, Philadelphia.

MONTROSE, J. AND MOSES, M. J. (1964) *J. Histochem. Cytochem.*, **12**, 115.

MORI, S. (1966) *Z. Zellforsch.*, **70**, 461.

PALAY, S. L., McGEE-RUSSELL, S. M., GORDON, S. AND GRILLO, M. A. (1962) *J. Cell Biol.*, **12**, 385.

SHIMIZU, N. AND ISHII, S. (1964) *Arch. Histol. Jap.*, **24**, 489.

SHIMIZU, N. AND KUBO, Z. (1957) *J. Neuropathol. Exp. Neurol.*, **16**, 40.

SHIMIZU, N., MATSUNAMI, T. AND ONISHI, S. (1960) *Nature*, **186**, 479.

SHIMIZU, N., MORIKAWA, T. AND ISHII, Y. (1957) *J. Comp. Neurol.*, **108**, 1.

SPECTOR, S., MELMON, K. AND SJOERDSMA, A. (1962) *Proc. Soc. Exp. Biol. Med.*, **111**, 79.

SUTHERLAND, E. W. AND RALL, T. W. (1960) In J. R. VANE (Ed.), *Ciba Foundation Symposium on Adrenergic Mechanisms*, Churchill, London, p. 295.

VOGT, M. (1954) *J. Physiol.*, **123**, 451.

WEIL-MALHERBE, H. AND BONE, A. D. (1952) *Biochem. J.*, **51**, 311.

WOOD, J. G. (1966) *Nature*, **209**, 1131.

MORTA ALBERICHI, G. B., DE LOVEZ ARNAIZ AND DE ROBERTIS, E. (1965) *Life Sci.*, **4**, 1951.

# Morphological Studies on the Mechanism of Adrenergic Transmission in the Central Nervous System

## II. Minute Vesicles

PAULO H. HASHIMOTO

*Department of Anatomy, Osaka University Medical School, Osaka 530 (Japan)*

Even in the early reports on the fine structure of synapses, the size of the synaptic vesicles seemed to vary according to the location (Palay, 1956), and probably the functional state (De Robertis, 1959) of the synaptic bulb. However, there is no general agreement as to the significance of the size of synaptic vesicles. In the ventral cochlear nucleus, Lenn and Reese (1966) observed synaptic boutons which contain smaller vesicles than those present in the calyciform endings. On the other hand, Grillo and Palay (1962) reported 3 types of granular vesicles in autonomic nerve endings outside the central nervous system. Ishii (this volume, p. 187) has mentioned mainly the first type or the large granular vesicles. I should like to present some suggestive evidence for a relationship between central monoaminergic transmission and the smaller synaptic vesicles.

### MATERIAL AND METHODS

Twenty-one male and female albino rats, ranging in body weight between 120 and 390 g, were used for this study. Tritiated Dopa* or 5-HTP* (5 to 10 $\mu$C/g body wt.) was injected intraperitoneally into animals which had been treated with iproniazid (60 $\mu$g/g body wt.), intraperitoneally, 16 to 18 h previously. Tritiated norepinephrine* was injected into the fourth ventricle stereotaxically by a method modified from that used for the rabbit (Kurotsu *et al.*, 1958).

Most animals were fixed by perfusion successively with 200 ml of 4% paraformaldehyde in 0.1 M phosphate buffer 7.3, 20 ml of the same buffer, and 50 ml of 1% osmium tetroxide in 0.1 M phosphate buffer pH 7.3, at room temperature. After being removed from the skulls, the brains were cut into serial frontal sections about 1 mm thick, and immersed in ice-cold 1% osmium tetroxide for another 2 h. The remaining specimens were fixed with permanganate as follows.

---

*DL-3(3,4-Dihydroxyphenyl)alanine-T (G) 200 mC/mmole, or L-3(3,4-Dihydroxyphenyl)alanine (*ring*-2,5,6-T) 134 mC/mg; DL-5-Hydroxytryptophan-T (G) 250 mC/mmole, or 12.6 mC/mg, The Radiochemical Centre, Amersham, England; DL-[7-³H]Noradrenalin 1100 mC/mmole, Radioisotope Dept., Mol, Belgium.

*References p. 212*

The dorsal surfaces of the brain and spinal cord were exposed under anesthesia. The animal was hung by its tail, and quickly lowered into a thermos containing a dry ice/acetone mixture. The entire CNS was then taken out of the skull and vertebrae, and placed on a wax plate in an ice box together with a lump of dry ice, in order to keep the environmental temperature at around –10°C, where it was cut, under the dissection microscope, into coronal slices of about 0.8 mm thick using an ice-cold fresh razor blade. The appropriate slices were found, and put into 6% KMnO₄ in deionized water (4°C) for 2 h.

During dehydration in ascending concentrations of ethanol, permanganate-fixed slices were block-stained with 2% uranyl acetate for 10 min, and all slices at the level of the obex were sketched under the dissection microscope. They were then immersed *in toto* in an Epon mixture after a propylene oxide bath. The slices were finally cut into small pieces according to the sketches, and embedded in gelatin capsules. Thin sections were made on a Porter–Blum MT-2 microtome with glass knives, and ex- amined in a Hitachi HU-11E electron microscope.

Electron microscope autoradiography was done with Ilford L4 or Sakura NR-H2 emulsion according to the method of Caro (1969), but special care had to be taken in the photographic processing of the permanganate-fixed samples: It is very important to limit the fixation time to 30 sec. Both the developer (Microdol-X, 20°C, 3 min) and fixer (20% simple hypo) should be dropped from a pipette onto the emulsion-coated grids which are supported on a glass slide. The stop bath should be omitted, and the developer washed out with excess of simple hypo.

OBSERVATIONS AND DISCUSSION

The visceral brain stem nuclei at the level of the obex are representative of central monoaminergic autonomic nuclei (Hashimoto, 1962; Fuxe, 1965), and highly ame- nable to electron microscopic examination. We have examined a type of synaptic terminal common in the medulla oblongata but most abundant in the nucleus tractus solitarii at the level of the obex, which contains small, near spherical or ellipsoidal vesicles, measuring 250 to 400 Å in diameter, and 350 to 600 Å in length. Most ter- minals with these minute vesicles lack typical postsynaptic membrane specialization (Gray, 1959), and also contain large granular vesicles (Grillo and Palay type I vesicles), tubular profiles of smooth endoplasmic reticulum, and glycogen particles. The large granulated vesicles have already been discussed by Ishii in Part I of the present paper.

In Fig. 1, a terminal containing minute vesicles (M) can be clearly distinguished from terminals containing flat vesicles (F), spherical vesicles of about 500 Å in diameter (S), and mixed large granulated vesicles and spherical vesicles (L). Following intraperi- toneal administration of [³H]Dopa (Fig. 2), or intraventricular administration of [³H]- norepinephrine (Hashimoto *et al.*, 1970), electron microscopic autoradiography on aldehyde and osmium tetroxide-fixed specimens showed developed silver grains localized on the synapses with minute vesicles. In the electron micrographs in Des- carries and Droz's recent paper (1970) using a similar method, the labeled endings can be seen to contain vesicles which are smaller and more irregular in size and

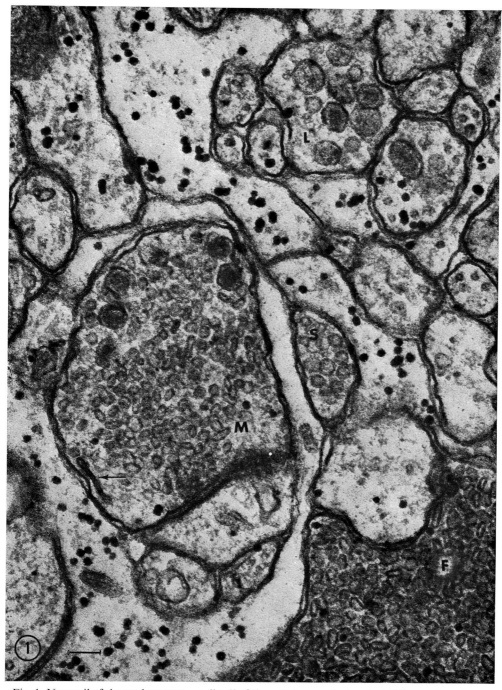

Fig. 1. Neuropil of the nucleus tractus solitarii of the rat. A synaptic terminal (M) contains minute, near spherical or ellipsoidal vesicles, together with large granular vesicles, glycogen particles, and a tubular profile of smooth endoplasmic reticulum (arrow). A bouton (F) is filled with flat vesicles. In profiles L and S, spherical vesicles about 500 Å in diameter accumulate with and without large granular vesicles. Fixed by successive perfusion with formaldehyde and osmium tetroxide. Scale, 0.1 $\mu$ $\times$ 85 000.

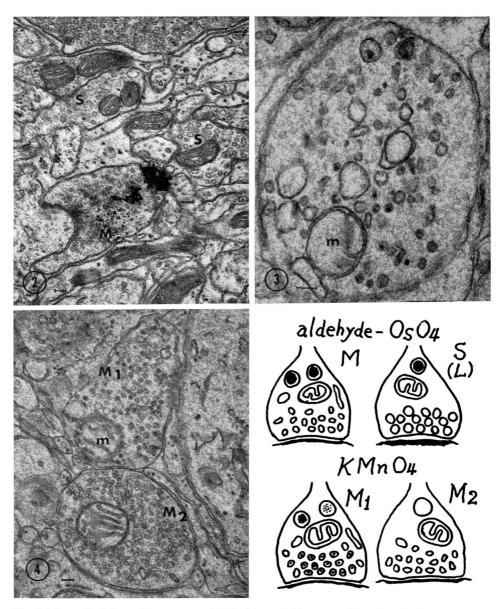

Fig. 2. Neuropil of the nucleus tractus solitarii of iproniazid-pretreated rat. 15 min after [³H]Dopa injection. Silver grains are found on a terminal with minute vesicles (M). Boutons containing 500 Å vesicles (S) are not labeled. EM autoradiography on aldehyde–osmium-fixed specimen. Scale, 0.1 μ. × 31 000.

Fig. 3. A bouton containing minute vesicles with core in the dorsal motor nucleus of vagus. m, mito chondrion. Permanganate fixation. Scale, 0.1 μ. × 55 000.

Fig. 4. Two boutons containing minute vesicles with (M₁), and without (M₂) core. Nucleus tractus solitarii. m, mitochondrion. Permanganate fixation. Scale, 0.1 μ. × 33 000.

distribution than those in the unlabeled endings, although the authors did not mention this point.

After permanganate fixation according to Richardson's scheme (1966), Hökfelt (1967) observed small granular vesicles of about 500 Å in diameter (Grillo and Palay type II vesicles) in boutons in the locus coeruleus of the rat. In permanganate-fixed material taken from he level of the obex, we found the minute vesicles in some boutons to contain a small core of 70 to 200 Å in diameter (Fig. 3 and Fig. 4 $M_1$). The core varies in density, and either lies centrally or more often, eccentrically as if it was stuck to the inner surface of the vesicle near its apex. The majority of the vesicles measure $250 \times 350$ Å to $300 \times 400$ Å. They are very similar to Grillo and Palay type III vesicles. Besides mitochondria, the boutons contain tubular profiles of endoplasmic reticulum, and large vesicles of 1000 Å or more in diameter, some of which show cores of various densities, but generally less dense than those in aldehyde and osmium-fixed samples. Postsynaptic membrane specializations are generally not remarkable.

There are also terminals with minute vesicles which never show cores after permanganate fixation (Fig. 4 $M_2$). By autoradiography after intraperitoneal administration of tritiated 5-HTP, developed silver grains were found to be localized on terminals containing minute vesicles without cores. Rude *et al.* (1969) examined 5-HT-containing colossal cells of the leech, and reported that formaldehyde or permanganate fixatives did not preserve the core.

At the present time, it seems reasonable to state that it is impossible to associate particular neurotransmitters with particular morphological features of vesicles or terminals. Further detailed observation of the fine structure of chemical synapses of the kind already attempted by various authors (Uchizono, 1967; Bodian, 1970), may allow us to identify other morphological characteristics of synapses, which can be correlated with their physiological and chemical specialization.

## SUMMARY

1. In the rat medulla oblongata at the level of the obex, a type of synaptic terminal which contains small, near spherical or ellipsoidal vesicles of 250 to 400 Å in diameter was distinguished from terminals containing flat vesicles, and spherical vesicles of about 500 Å in diameter with or without large granular vesicles.

2. Developed silver grains were localized on the terminal containing minute vesicles after intraperitoneal administration of [³H]Dopa, or intraventricular administration of [³H]norepinephrine.

3. Permanganate fixation visualized small cores of 70 to 200 Å in diameter within the minute vesicles in some boutons, but not all.

4. Boutons containing minute vesicles without core were labeled after intraperitoneal administration of [5-³H]hydroxytryptophane and permanganate fixation.

## REFERENCES

BODIAN, D. (1970) *J. Cell Biol.*, **44**, 115–124.

CARO, L. G. (1969) *J. Cell Biol.*, **41**, 918–919.

DE ROBERTIS, E. (1959) *Intern. Rev. Cytol.*, **8**, 61–96.

DESCARRIES, L. AND DROZ, B. (1970) *J. Cell Biol.*, **44**, 385–399.

FUXE, K. (1965) *Acta Physiol. Scand.*, **64**, *Suppl.* **247**, 37–85, Illus.

GRAY, E. G. (1959) *J. Anat.*, **93**, 420–433.

GRILLO, M. A. AND PALAY, S. L. (1962) *Electron Microscopy*, U-1, Academic Press, New York.

HASHIMOTO, P. H. (1970) *Microscopie Électronique*, III-711, Société Française de Microscopie Électronique, Paris.

HASHIMOTO, P. H., MAEDA, T., TORII, K. AND SHIMIZU, N. (1962) *Med. J. Osaka Univ.*, **12**, 425–465.

HÖKFELT, T. (1967) *Z. Zellforsch.*, **79**, 110–117.

ISHII, S. (1971) Morphological studies on the mechanism of adrenergic transmission in the central nervous system. I. Granulated vesicles. In: *Progr. Brain Res,*, **34**, Elsevier, Amsterdam.

KUROTSU, T., HASHIMOTO, P. H., MATSUSHIMA, C. I. AND BAN, T. (1958) *Med. J. Osaka Univ.*, **9**, 227–241.

LENN, N. J. AND REESE, T. S. (1966) *Amer. J. Anat.*, **118**, 375–389.

PALAY, S. L. (1956) *J. Biophys. Biochem.* Cytol., **2** (4, Suppl.), 193–202.

RICHARDSON, K. C. (1966) *Nature*, **210**, 756.

RUDE, S., COGGESHALL, R. E. AND VAN ORDEN, III, L. S. (1969) *J. Cell Biol.*, **41**, 832–854.

UCHIZONO, K. (1967) *Nature*, **214**, 833.

# Ultrastructural Localization of Intraneuronal Monoamines Some Aspects on Methodology

TOMAS HÖKFELT

*Department of Histology, Karolinska Institutet, S-104 01 Stockholm 60 (Sweden)*

## INTRODUCTION

Since several years a number of histochemical methods are available for the visualization of certain biogenic monoamines at the light microscopic level (see Pearse, 1960). The majority of these methods are, however, limited to non-nervous tissues like adrenal medulla, enterochromaffin cells or mast cells. Based on findings of Erös (1932) and Eränkö (1955), Falck, Hillarp and coworkers (Falck *et al.*, 1962; Falck, 1962) developed a histochemical fluorescence technique which permits the demonstration also of intraneuronal monoamines both in the peripheral and central nervous system.

At the ultrastructural level amine storage sites were early correlated to electron-dense granules found *e.g.*, in the adrenal medulla in a number of species (Lever, 1955; Sjöstrand and Wetzstein, 1956; De Robertis and Ferreira, 1957; De Robertis and Sabatini, 1960; Eränkö and Hänninen, 1960; Yates *et al.*, 1962). A more profound knowledge of the nature of these granules was obtained when using a fixation procedure including glutaraldehyde (Sabatini *et al.*, 1963) followed by various metallic oxidants (Coupland *et al.*, 1964; Tramezzani *et al.*, 1964; Wood and Barrnett, 1964). Using this and other improved fixation techniques it is now possible to visualize monoamines and monoamine storage sites also in nerves and in the present article some aspects on this topic will be summarized.

In recent years, various review articles have been published dealing with the ultrastructural localization of monoamines (Grillo, 1966, Bloom and Aghajanian, 1968; Bloom and Giarman, 1968; Hökfelt, 1968a, b, 1970; Tranzer *et al.*, 1969; Bloom, 1970; Jaim-Etcheverry and Zieher, 1970; Hökfelt and van Orden, 1971) and the methodological background has been thoroughly covered by Bloom (1970). Therefore this paper does not intend to cover the whole field but mainly present some aspects partly based on the work in our laboratory.

## TEST TUBE EXPERIMENTS

Almost all routine fixatives for electron microscopy can be shown to react and form a precipitate with various monoamines in test tube experiments. This approach offers possibilities, *e.g.*, to screen various fixatives and amines, to elucidate the chemical

TABLE 1

REACTION BETWEEN VARIOUS FIXATIVES AND AMINES IN TEST TUBE EXPERIMENTS

The formation of a precipitate is indicated by a plus.

| | $OsO_4$[1] | $KMnO_4$[2] | $PF$[3] | $Glut.$[4] | $Glut. + OsO_4$[4] or $K_2Cr_2O_7$ |
|---|---|---|---|---|---|
| Noradrenaline | + | + + | 0 | + | + |
| Dopamine | + | + + | 0 | + | + |
| Adrenaline | + | + + | 0 | 0 | |
| 5-Hydroxytryptamine | + | + + | 0 | + | + |
| L-DOPA | + | + + | | | |
| Metaraminol | 0 | + | | | |
| β-Phenylethylamine | | 0 | | | |

[1] Orden *et al.*, 1966; [2] Hökfelt and Jonsson, 1968; [3] Hopsu and Mäkinen, 1966; [4] Wood and Barrnett, 1964; Coupland *et al.*, 1964.

reaction occurring and to work out optimal reaction conditions, etc. Such experiments have been presented in many papers some of which are summarized in Table 1. The fixatives tested are either metallic oxidants or various aldehydes, partly in combination with metallic oxidants.

### Metallic oxidants

Both osmium tetroxide ($OsO_4$) and potassium permanganate ($KMnO_4$) react with most substances listed in Table 1 forming a precipitate. Although it has been assumed that a redox reaction occurs leading to a reduction of $OsO_4$ to $OsO_2$ or metallic osmium and of $KMnO_4$ to $MnO_2$ (brownstone) the process is not exactly known. However, in all probability the hydroxyl groups (mainly the phenolic ones) (Fig. 1) are responsible for the reducing capacity of the amines. This is indicated by the fact that no precipitate is found when mixing $KMnO_4$ and β-phenylethylamine, a monoamine analogue lacking hydroxyl groups (Fig. 1). It can directly be seen in the test tube that the reaction between amine and $KMnO_4$ is more vigorous than between amine and $OsO_4$. This is in good agreement with the higher redox potential of $KMnO_4$ (1.51) as compared to $OsO_4$ (0.85). Furthermore, this difference in reactivity is also demonstrated by the fact that $KMnO_4$ but not $OsO_4$ reacts with metaraminol, a monoamine analogue containing only *one* phenolic hydroxyl group (Fig. 1).

Noradrenaline          Metaraminol          β-Phenylethylamine

Fig. 1. Molecular structure of three monoamine analogues — noradrenaline, metaraminol and β-phenylethylamine. Noradrenaline (two phenolic hydroxyl groups) reacts *in vitro* with both $KMnO_4$ and $OsO_4$ forming a precipitate. Metaraminol (one phenolic hydroxyl group) reacts only with $KMnO_4$ and β-phenylethylamine (no hydroxyl group) reacts neither with $KMnO_4$ nor with $OsO_4$.

# Functional Importance of Subcellular Distribution of False Adrenergic Transmitters

H. THOENEN and J. P. TRANZER

*Department of Experimental Medicine, F. Hoffmann–La Roche & Co. Ltd.
Basle (Switzerland)*

Rapid progress has been made in the knowledge of the physiology, biochemistry and pharmacology of the sympathetic nervous system since the identification of norepinephrine as the neurohumoral transmitter of mammalian postganglionic adrenergic nerves. The single steps in the pathway of norepinephrine synthesis proposed by Blaschko more than 30 years ago have been verified, and the enzymes involved have been characterized and localized at the cellular and subcellular level. Remarkable advances have also been made in understanding the mechanism of storage, transport through neuronal membranes, enzymatic degradation and action on effector organs (for references see Iversen, 1967; and Thoenen, 1969).

Fig. 1 shows a schematic summary of the pathway of norepinephrine synthesis in the adrenergic neuron and the events taking place after arrival of a nerve impulse.

Concomitant with the elucidation of these basic physiological processes, a great number of drugs have been developed which interferere with these different mechanisms (for references see Iversen, 1967; Thoenen, 1969).

Since the enzymes involved in the synthesis of the adrenergic transmitter and the mechanisms of transport and storage reveal no strict chemical specificity (Iversen, 1966, 1967; Thoenen, 1969; Hagen, 1962; Fischer *et al.*, 1965; Goldstein and Anagnoste, 1965) a further possibility for the modification of the postganglionic sympathetic

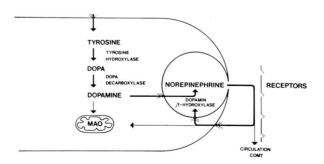

Fig. 1. Scheme of physiological processes taking place in the adrenergic nerve terminal: Pathway of synthesis of norepinephrine, liberation by nerve impulses, action on effector organs, inactivation by re-uptake and enzymatic degradation.

*References pp. 235–236*

transmission arose, namely the replacement of norepinephrine by false adrenergic transmitters. The replacement of norepinephrine by a transmitter substance which under physiological conditions is entirely absent or present only in very small, functionally insignificant quantities provides an opportunity for a more differentiated modification of the adrenergic transmission than could be achieved by the possibilities known so far, such as impairment of storage and re-uptake, inhibition of synthesis and enzymatic degradation or interference with the action on the effector organs (for references see Iversen, 1967; Thoenen, 1969). The replacement of the physiological transmitter by a false one implies not only quantitative but also qualitative functional consequences depending on the transmitter liberated and the receptors involved.

There are three possibilities for replacing norepinephrine by false transmitters:

(a) administration of the amines acting as false transmitters themselves,

(b) administration of false precursors,

(c) blockage of particular steps in the synthesis or enzymatic degradation of physiological amines.

(a) The administration of amines acting as false transmitters themselves results in a striking rise in blood pressure caused by the liberation of large amounts of norepinephrine (indirect sympathomimetic effect). This procedure is therefore unsuitable for therapeutic purposes such as the treatment of hypertension, although the desired hypotensive effect may occur after the initial (unwanted) blood pressure rise (Crout et al., 1965, 1966). However, for the investigation of the stereochemical requirements of amines necessary for their transport, storage, and liberation by nerve impulses, this procedure proved to be very useful, as will be shown later.

(b) The enzymes involved in the synthesis of norepinephrine reveal only a limited chemical specificity for the substrates to be transformed. Therefore it is possible to administer precursors which are absent under physiological conditions but which resemble the physiological precursors to such an extent that they are handled by the corresponding enzymes in a very similar way. The metabolic products formed are stored, transported, and liberated by nerve impulses very similar to the natural ones. Well known examples are α-methyl-dopa (Carlsson and Lindquist, 1962; Day and Rand, 1963; Muscholl and Maître, 1963; Haefely et al., 1967), α-methylmetatyrosine (Carlsson and Lindquist, 1962; Andén, 1964; Udenfriend and Zaltzman-Nirenberg, 1963; Crout et al., 1964) and 5-hydroxydopa (Thoenen, 1969; Thoenen et al., 1967; Tranzer and Thoenen, 1967a).

(c) If enzymes involved in the synthesis or degradation of physiological amines are blocked, an accumulation of substances occurs, which normally represent only short-lived transitory products which are barely detectable and have no functional importance. In the peripheral sympathetic nervous system, for instance, dopamine is only present in very small amounts which are generally below the sensitivity of the available assay methods (Seiden and Carlsson, 1964; Carlsson et al., 1966; Thoenen et al., 1967a). However, inhibition of dopamine-$\beta$-hydroxylase, the enzyme responsible for the conversion of dopamine to norepinephrine, results in an accumulation of dopamine which partially replaces the missing norepinephrine and which is liberated as a false transmitter (Thoenen et al., 1967a). Here, the term false transmitter is used in a more extensive way, merely indicating that an amine which normally plays no significant role takes over the function of norepinephrine. It does not, however, mean that the amine is entirely absent under physiological conditions.

The replacement of norepinephrine by dopamine is of particular interest, since dopamine has in both dog and man not only a weaker vasoconstrictive effect than norepinephrine in the muscle and skin vessels but even produces a dilatation of renal arteries (McNay and Goldberg, 1966; McDonald et al., 1964). The substitution of norepinephrine by dopamine as an adrenergic transmitter could be of particular interest in the treatment of hypertension.

Octopamine like dopamine is also present only in very small quantities under physiological conditions (Molinoff and Axelrod, 1969), since tyramine, the decarboxylation product of tyrosine, is a very good substrate for monoamine oxidase and only very small amounts are available for $\beta$-hydroxylation.

However, after inhibition of monoamine oxidase more tyramine is available for $\beta$-hydroxylation and there is a 5- to 10-fold increase in the amount of octopamine present in sympathetically innervated organs (Molinoff and Axelrod, 1969). Whether this accumulation of octopamine is responsible for the impaired postganglionic sympathetic transmission after treatment with monoamine oxidase inhibitors is not yet established: Octopamine does not displace norepinephrine under these experimental conditions but is stored in addition to it. Furthermore, Van Orden and co-workers (1966, 1967) have provided good evidence that any treatment (among others inhibition of monoamine oxidase) which leads to an increase in the concentration of free norepinephrine in the axoplasm of adrenergic nerves impairs the liberation of norepinephrine by nerve impulses. Although the mechanism of this inhibition is poorly understood it could at least provide just as good an explanation for the impaired postganglionic adrenergic transmission after treatment with monoamine oxidase inhibitors as does the liberation of octopamine.

To evaluate the functional consequences of the replacement of the physiological transmitter by false transmitters it is not sufficient to compare the sympathomimetic activity of the false transmitter with that of norepinephrine. The factors involved are rather complex and at least the following aspects have to be considered:

(a) relationship between the diminution of the norepinephrine content in the adrenergic neurons and the reduction of the amount of norepinephrine liberated by nerve stimulation.

(b) extent of the stoichiometrical replacement of the missing norepinephrine by the false transmitter(s).

(c) relationship between the ratio of norepinephrine and false transmitter stored in adrenergic nerves and the ratio of these amines liberated by nerve impulses.

(d) direct and indirect sympathomimetic action of the false transmitter. Of the total sympathomimetic activity of false transmitters only the direct component is important for their action on the effector organs.

(e) interference of the false transmitter with the re-uptake of norepinephrine into the sympathetic nerve endings.

(f) interference of the false transmitter with norepinephrine at the receptors of the effector organs.

(g) interference of the false transmitter with the synthesis of norepinephrine.

The many factors determining the functional consequences of the replacement of norepinephrine by false transmitters amply demonstrate that predictions depending merely on the knowledge of the sympathomimetic activity of a false transmitter are very hazardous. For a series of false transmitters the different factors determining the functional consequences have been analyzed and the results have been reviewed recently (Thoenen, 1969; Muscholl, 1966; Kopin, 1968). For more detailed information the reader is referred to these reviews.

After having briefly surveyed the possibilities of how false transmitters can be formed and which factors determine the functional consequences, I would like to discuss in more detail the prerequisites necessary for an amine to act as a false adrenergic transmitter: The physiological transmitter norepinephrine is transported by an active, sodium-dependent mechanism through the neuronal membrane (Iversen, 1967; Iversen and Kravitz, 1966) and is then incorporated into the storage vesicles which are present in particularly high numbers in the adrenergic nerve terminals (Richardson, 1962; Burnstock et al., 1964; Tranzer et al., 1969). Studies of the subcellular distribution of norepinephrine in sympathetically innervated organs have shown that the main part of norepinephrine sediments with the microsomal fraction (von Euler and Hillarp, 1965; Potter, 1966; Stjärne, 1964; Gutman and Weil-Mal-

TABLE 1

RELATIONSHIP BETWEEN CHEMICAL COMPOSITION OF AMINES, THEIR TRANSPORT THROUGH THE NEURONAL MEMBRANE, ACCUMULATION IN THE MICROSOMAL FRACTION AND LIBERATION BY NERVE IMPULSES

| Amine | Transport though neuronal membrane | Accumulation in microsomal fraction | Liberated by nerve stimulation | References |
|---|---|---|---|---|
| norepinephrine | + | + | + | Potter, 1966; Stjärne, 1964; Burgen & Iversen, 1965; Kopin, 1966; Musacchio et al. 1965 |
| epinephrine | + | + | + | Potter, 1966; Burgen & Iversen, 1965 |
| isoproterenol | — | + | — | Von Euler & Lishajko, 1967; Andén et al., 1964; Hertting, 1964; Burgen & Iversen, 1965 |
| α-methylnorepinephrine | + | + | + | Haefely et al., 1967; Potter, 1965; Burgen & Iversen, 1965; Lundborg, 1967; Bondareff, 1966; Kopin, 1966; Philippu & Schümann, 1966. |
| α-methylepinephrine | + | + | + | Muscholl, 1966; Potter, 1966, Burgen & Iversen, 1965; Lindmar et al. 1967 |
| dopamine | + | + | + | Thoenen et al., 1967a; Potter, 1966; Burgen & Iversen, 1965; Kopin, 1966; Musacchio et al. 1965; Musacchio et al., 1966, 1967 |
| α-methyldopamine | + | + | + | Burgen & Iversen, 1965; Kopin, 1966; Musacchio et al., 1966; Thoenen et al., 1967b |

**TABLE I** *(continued)*

| Amine | Transport though neuronal membrane | Accumulation in microsomal fraction | Liberated by nerve stimulation | References |
|---|---|---|---|---|
| tyramine | + | − | − | Burgen & Iversen, 1965; Kopin, 1966; Musacchio *et al.*, 1964, 1965 |
| octopamine | + | + | + | Potter, 1966; Burgen & Iversen, 1965; Kopin, 1966; Musacchio *et al.*, 1964, 1965. |
| m-tyramine | + | − | − | Burgen & Iversen, 1965; Kopin, 1966, Musacchio *et al.*, 1965 |
| m-octopamine | + | + | + | Potter, 1966; Burgen & Iversen, 1965, Kopin, 1966; Musacchio *et al.*, 1965 |
| α-methylmetatyramine | + | − | − | Thoenen, 1969; Burgen & Iversen, 1965; Kopin, 1966 |
| α-methylmetoctopamine (metaraminol) | + | + | + | Thoenen, 1969; Crout *et al.*, 1964; Crout, 1966; Crout *et al.*, 1965; Potter, 1966; Burgen & Iversen, 1965; Lundborg, 1967; Kopin, 1966 |
| α-methyltyramine | + | − | − | Iversen, 1966; Burgen & Iversen, 1965; Kopin, 1966; Musacchio *et al.*, 1965; Thoenen *et al.*, 1966 |
| α-methyloctopamine | + | + | + | Potter, 1966; Burgen & Iversen, 1965; Kopin, 1966; Musacchio *et al.*, 1965; Thoenen *et al.*, 1966 |

**TABLE I** *(continued)*

| Amine | Transport though neuronal membrane | Accumulation in microsomal fraction | Liberated by nerve stimulation | References |
|---|---|---|---|---|
| phenethylamine | + | — | — | Potter, 1966; Burgen & Iversen, 1965; Kopin, 1966 |
| phenethanolamine | + | (+) | (+) | Potter, 1966; Burgen & Iversen, 1965; Kopin, 1966 |
| amphetamine | + | — | — | Burgen & Iversen, 1965; Kopin, 1966; Musacchio *et al.*, 1965; Thoenen *et al.*, 1966 |
| 5-hydroxydopamine | + | + | + | Thoenen *et al.*, 1967; Tranzer & Thoenen, 1967a; Tranzer *et al.*, 1969 |
| 6-hydroxydopamine | + | + | + | Thoenen & Tranzer, 1968; Bennett *et al.*, 1970 |
| 4-methoxy-3,5-dihydroxyphenethylamine | + | + | + | Thoenen *et al.*, 1967, 1968a, b |
| 5-hydroxytryptamine (serotonin) | + | + | + | Tranzer *et al.*, 1969; Thoa *et al.*, 1967, 1969; Snipes *et al.*, 1968; Jaim-Etcheverry & Zieher, 1969 |

herbe, 1967a), and it has been concluded that the sedimentation of an amine with this fraction can be equated with its localization in the ultramorphologically visualized granulated vesicles (Potter, 1966). However, if one imagines that the sympathetic nerve terminals represent only about 1/1000 to 1/10 000 of the total volume of a densely innervated organ and that the microsomal fraction, even after additional purification on a density gradient, is still rather heterogeneous both with respect to structure and origin of the elements (Taylor, *et al.* 1966; Gutman and Weil-Malherbe, 1967b), one can well appreciate the value of visualizing a false transmitter in intact tissues at the ultrastructural level. This possibility provides greater security in the interpretation of the cell fractionation experiments.

As already mentioned above, both the transport of amines through the neuronal membrane and the accumulation in the storage vesicles show no strict chemical specificity, and the physiological transmitter norepinephrine shares these properties with a great number of other amines (for references see Table 1). The question now arises of whether the transport by the neuronal membrane pump is the sole and critical prerequisite for an amine to act as a false transmitter or whether an accumulation in the storage vesicles is also necessary. The answer to this question is not only important for the elucidation of the properties necessary for an amine to act as a false transmitter but it also has more general implications, *i.e.* whether the transmitter liberated from the sympathetic nerve ending originates from the axoplasm or from the storage vesicles.

A great number of phenethylamines have been shown by direct and indirect evidence to be transported into the adrenergic neuron by the same transfer system as the physiological transmitter norepinephrine (Table 1). The great variety of these amines demonstrates clearly that the chemical specificity of this transport system is low and that not only phenethylamines but also 5-hydroxytryptamine is accumulated. However, not all the amines transported into the adrenergic neuron also act as false transmitters, indicating that transport into the neuron by the amine pump is certainly not the only prerequisite. In contrast to the inconsistent correlation between the property of being transported and that of acting as a false transmitter, the correlation becomes perfect if the additional condition of being accumulated in the microsomal fraction is fulfilled (Table 1).

In general, the chemical prerequisites for accumulation in the microsomal fraction are more specific than those for membrane transport. From the experimental information so far available it can be deduced that at least two ring hydroxy groups or one ring hydroxy group and a hydroxy group on the $\beta$-C atom of the side chain are necessary for a phenethylamine to be accumulated in the microsomal fraction. Whether a single OH group in the side chain is sufficient is not yet definitively established (Thoenen, 1969). The prerequisites for an accumulation in the microsomal fraction are also fulfilled in the case of isoproterenol. This amine has been shown to be taken up into vesicles isolated from splenic nerves (von Euler and Lishajko, 1967). However, since it is not transported by the neuronal amine pump (Andén *et al.*, 1964; Hertting, 1964; Burgen and Iversen, 1965), it obviously cannot act as a false transmitter. It seems that the amine group is of primary importance for the transport through the neuronal membrane and that an increase in the size of the N-substitution of the phenethylamine decreases its affinity to the transport system. At least the affinity of the N-methyl-substituted epinephrine is smaller than that of norepine-phrine (Burgen and Iversen, 1965; Iversen, 1967) and the N-isopropyl-substitution of isoproterenol abolishes the affinity to the transport system virtually completely (Hertting, 1964; Burgen and Iversen, 1965). It therefore seems that the amine group is of critical importance for the transport through the neuronal membrane whereas the OH-substitutions on ring and side chain are of primary relevance for the accumulation in the microsomal fraction.

The substances acting as false adrenergic transmitters are not restricted to the phenethylamines as shown by the example of 5-hydroxytryptamine which is trans-ported into peripheral adrenergic nerves and is liberated by nerve impulses (Thoa et al., 1967, 1969). 5-Hydroxytryptamine is already present in the sympathetic nerves of the pineal gland under physiological conditions (Owman, 1964; Falck et al., 1966; Pellegrino de Iraldi and Guendet, 1969). It most probably originates from the pinealocytes which synthesize large amounts of 5-hydroxytryptamine (Falck et al., 1966) and which are in closest proximity to the adrenergic nerve endings. The func-tional implications of the presence of 5-hydroxytryptamine in the adrenergic nerves of the pineal gland are not yet established but the presence of a transmitter in a neuron which does not possess the necessary enzymatic machinery for its synthesis raises the more general question of whether this exchange of transmitter substances could not be of functional importance in the brain, where neurons with different transmitter substances are located in close proximity, so favoring the uptake of transmitters from other neurons, provided that the transport and storage properties of these transmitters are interchangeable. This exchange of transmitter substances could represent a further possibility for the modulation of the synaptic transmission in the central nervous system, above all, in view of the preferential release of newly synthesized and newly incorporated transmitters (Besson et al., 1969).

As already mentioned above, the microsomal fraction obtained from a sympathetic-ally innervated organ is rather heterogeneous and the overwhelming part of even a purified vesicular fraction does not originate from adrenergic nerves but from other tissues (Taylor et al., 1966; Gutman and Weil-Malherbe, 1967b). Therefore a direct localization of the physiological and false transmitters at the ultrastructural level in intact tissues would represent additional and more convincing evidence that the ac-cumulation of a substance in the microsomal fraction can be considered as a reliable criterion for its localization in the storage vesicles of the adrenergic neurons.

For the electronmicroscopic visualization of physiological and false transmitters the fixation procedure is of crucial importance (for references see Tranzer et al., 1969). After fixation with osmium tetroxide alone, the main part of the vesicles in the adre-nergic nerve terminals appear empty and only a few of them contain a small dense core (Fig. 2a). However, a much higher proportion of the vesicles contain electron-dense material after combined glutaraldehyde–osmium fixation (Fig. 2b), and a considerable further improvement was achieved by the triple fixation method using aldehydes, dichromate and osmium tetroxide (Tranzer and Snipes, 1968) (Fig. 2c). After this fixation virtually all the vesicles contain large quantities of electron-dense

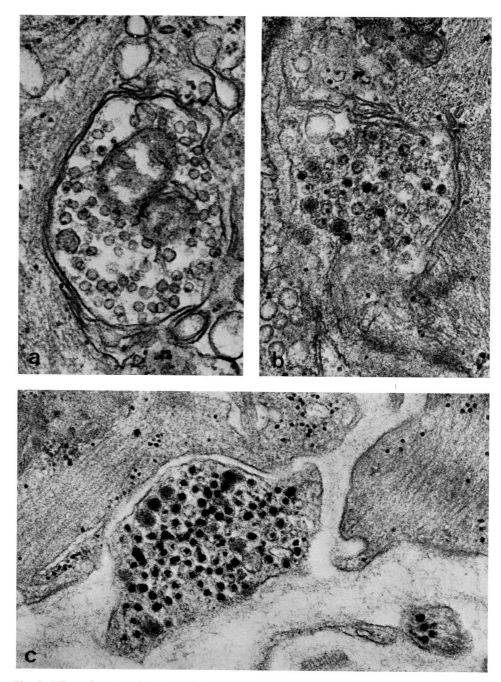

Fig. 2. Effect of various fixation techniques on the preservation of the physiological transmitter norepinephrine in adrenergic nerve terminals of the rat vas deferens; (a) osmium tetroxide fixation alone, (b) double fixation in glutaraldehyde and osmium tetroxide, (c) triple fixation sequence in glutaraldehyde-*p*-formaldehyde, dichromate and osmium tetroxide. Note the differences in the degree of filling of the vesicles with electron-dense material as well as the proportion of the dense core vesicles to those appearing empty. ($\times$ 50 000).

material, demonstrating that all the vesicles in adrenergic nerve endings are able to store norepinephrine and that the empty vesicles in the adrenergic nerve terminals do not represent a second population of vesicles with different functional properties, but that these differences result mainly from insufficient fixation in addition to a possible difference in the degree of amine filling of the vesicles (Tranzer *et al.*, 1969; Tranzer and Thoenen, 1967b). That the electron-dense material represents norepinephrine can be deduced from the fact that after depletion of norepinephrine by reserpine, the electron-dense material disappears. However, if a similar degree of norepinephrine depletion is produced by administration of 5-hydroxydopamine or its metabolic precursor 5-hydroxydopa the ultramorphological manifestation is quite different (Tranzer and Thoenen, 1967a; Tranzer *et al.*, 1969). All the vesicles are completely filled with dense osmiophilic material representing the fine structural localization of a

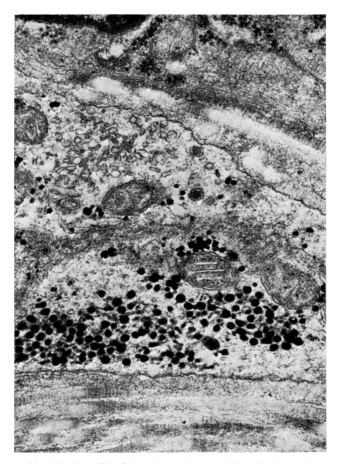

Fig. 3. Fine structural localization of the false adrenergic transmitter 5-hydroxydopamine (5-OH-DA) in the iris of a cat. All the vesicles of the adrenergic nerve terminals are completely filled with a dense core representing the injected amine 5-OH-DA, whereas the vesicles of a nearby cholinergic nerve terminal appear empty. × 40 000.

false transmitter (Fig. 3). The specificity of this localization is evident from micrographs of organs with a mixed adrenergic and cholinergic innervation. Only the vesicles of the adrenergic nerve terminals are filled with osmiophilic material whereas the vesicles of the cholinergic nerves remain empty. The micrographs obtained after administration of 5-hydroxydopamine are particularly impressive, and the peculiar properties of this amine make it suitable as a marker for the identification of adrenergic

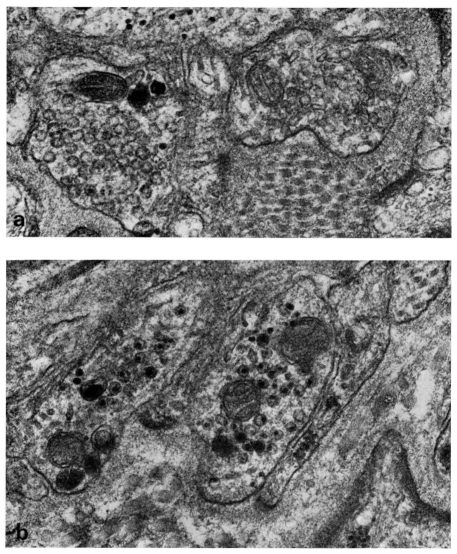

Fig. 4. Fine structural localization of the false transmitter 5-hydroxytryptamine (5-HT) in the iris of a cat; (a) nerve terminals after pretreatment of the animal with α-methylmetatyrosine. Almost all the vesicles of all the nerve terminals appear empty whereas in (b), after additional incubation of the iris in a solution containing 5-HT, most of the vesicles now contain a dense core representing the storage of 5-HT. × 50 000.

neurons in regions where the fixation of the physiological transmitter norepinephrine has proven to be very difficult (Tranzer and Thoenen, 1967a; Tranzer *et al.*, 1969). In addition to 5-hydroxydopamine a series of other amines acting as false transmitters can be visualized by electron microscopy, although the demonstration is not as impressive as for 5-hydroxydopamine. In addition to various phenethylamines such as α-methylnorepinephrine (Bondareff, 1966), 4-methoxy-2,5-dihydroxyphenethylamine (Tranzer, unpublished observation) and 6-hydroxydopamine (Bennett *et al.*, 1970) (immediately after injection before the destructive effects become evident), 5-hydroxy-tryptamine (Tranzer *et al.*, 1969; Snipes *et al.*, 1968; Jaim-Etcheverry and Zieher, 1969) can also be visualized in adrenergic nerve terminals (Fig. 4).

In conclusion, the fine structural localization of the physiological and of some false adrenergic transmitters in the vesicles of the adrenergic neurons provides sound and realistic support for the view that the accumulation of amines in the microsomal fraction of sympathetically innervated organs can be equated with an accumulation in the storage vesicles of the adrenergic nerve terminals. Furthermore, the accumulation in the storage vesicles is an indispensable prerequisite for an amine to act as a false transmitter which also gives additional support to the view, deduced from other observations (van Orden *et al.*, 1966, 1967; Farnebo and Hamberger, 1970), that adrenergic transmitter substances are liberated directly from the storage vesicles and not from the free transmitter pool in the axoplasm.

## REFERENCES

ANDÉN, N. E. (1964) *Acta pharmacol. (Kbh.)*, **21**, 260.

ANDÉN, N. E., CORRODI, H., ETTLES, M., GUSTAFSSON, E. AND PERSSON, H. (1964) *Acta pharmac. tox.*, **21**, 247.

BENNETT, T., BURNSTOCK, G., COBB, J. L. S. AND MALMFORS, T. (1970) *Brit. J. Pharmacol.*, **38**, 802.

BESSON, M. J., CHERANNY, A. A., FELTZ, P. AND GLOWINSKI, J. (1969) *Proc. natl. Acad. Sci. (Wash.)*, **62**, 741.

BONDAREFF, W. (1966) *Exptl. Neurol.*, **16**, 131.

BURGEN, A. S. V. AND IVERSEN, L. L. (1965) *Brit. J. Pharmacol.*, **25**, 34.

BURNSTOCK, G., HOLMAN, M. E. AND MERRILLEES, N. C. R. (1964) *Pharmacology of the Smooth Muscle*, Pergamon Press, Oxford.

CARLSSON, A. AND LINDQVIST, M. (1962) *Acta physiol. scand.*, **54**, 87.

CARLSSON, A., LINDQVIST, M., FUXE, K. AND HÖKFELT, T. (1966) *J. Pharm. Pharmacol.*, **18**, 60.

CROUT, J. R. (1966) *Circulat. Res.*, **18**, Suppl. I, 120.

CROUT, J. R. ALPERS, H. S., TATUM, E. L. AND SHORE, P. A. (1964) *Science*, **145**, 828.

CROUT, J. R., JOHNSTON, R. R., WEBB, W. R. AND SHORE, P. A. (1965) *Clin. Res.*, **13**, 204.

DAY, M. D., AND RAND, M. J. (1963) *J. Pharm. Pharmacol.*, **15**, 221.

EULER, U. S. VON AND HILLARP, N.-Å. (1956) *Nature (Lond.)*, **177**, 43.

EULER, U. S. VON AND LISHAJKO, F. (1967) *Int. J. Neuropharmacol.*, **6**, 431.

FALCK, B., OWMAN, CH. AND ROSENGREN, E. (1966) *Acta physiol. scand.*, **67**, 300.

FARNEBO, L.-O. AND HAMBERGER, B. (1970) *J. Pharmacol. exptl. Ther.*, **172**, 332.

FISCHER, J. E., HORST, W. D. AND KOPIN, I. J. (1965) *Brit. J. Pharmacol.*, **24**, 477.

GOLDSTEIN, M. AND ANAGNOSTE, B. (1965) *Biochim. biophys. Acta*, **107**, 166.

GUTMAN, Y. AND WEIL-MALHERBE, H. (1967a) *Brit. J. Pharmacol.*, **30**, 4.

GUTMAN, Y. AND WEIL-MALHERBE, H. (1967b) *J. Neurochem.*, **14**, 619.

HAEFELY, W., HÜRLIMANN, A. AND THOENEN, H. (1967) *Brit. J. Pharmacol.*, **31**, 105.

HAGEN, P. (1962) *Brit. J. Pharmacol.*, **18**, 175.

HERTTING, G. (1964) *Biochem. Pharmacol.*, **13**, 1119.

IVERSEN, L. L. (1966) *J. Pharm. Pharmacol.*, **18**, 481.

IVERSEN, L. L. (1967) *The Uptake and Storage of Noradrenaline in Sympathetic Nerves*, University Press, Cambridge.

IVERSEN, L. L. AND KRAVITZ, E. A. (1966) *Mol. Pharmacol.*, **2**, 360.

JAIM-ETCHEVERRY, G. AND ZIEHER, L. M. (1969) *J. Pharmacol. exptl. Ther.*, **166**, 264.

KOPIN, I. J. (1968) *Ann. Rev. Pharmacol.*, **8**, 377.

KOPIN, I. J. (1966) *Pharmacol. Rev.*, **18**, 513.

LINDMAR, R., MUSCHOLL, E. AND SPRENGER, E. (1967) *Naunyn-Schmiedebergs Arch. exptl. Path. Pharmak.*, **256**, 1.

LUNDBORG, P. (1967) *Acta physiol. scand.*, **72**, Suppl. 302.

McDONALD, R. H., GOLDBERG, L. I., McNAY, J. L. AND TUTTLE, E. P. (1964) *J. clin. Invest.*, **43**, 1116.

McNAY, J. L. AND GOLDBERG, L. I. (1966) *J. Pharmacol. exptl. Ther.*, **151**, 23.

MOLINOFF, P. AND AXELROD, J. (1969) *Science*, **164**, 428.

MUSACCHIO, J. M., FISCHER, J. E. AND KOPIN, I. J. (1966) *J. Pharmacol. exptl. Ther.*, **152**, 51.

MUSACCHIO, J. M., KOPIN, I. J. AND SNYDER, S. (1964) *Life Sci.*, **3**, 769.

MUSACCHIO, J. M., KOPIN, I. J. AND WEISE, V. K. (1965) *J. Pharmacol. exptl. Ther.*, **148**, 22.

MUSCHOLL, E. (1966) *Ann. Rev. Pharmacol.*, **6**, 107.

MUSCHOLL, E. AND MAÎTRE, L. (1963) *Experientia (Basel)*, **19**, 658.

OBIANWU, H. O., STITZEL, R. AND LUNDBORG, P. (1968) *J. Pharm. Pharmacol.*, **20**, 585.

ORDEN, L. S. VAN, BENSCH, K. G. AND GIARMAN, N. J. (1967) *J. Pharmacol. exptl. Ther.*, **155**, 428.

ORDEN, L. S. VAN, BLOOM, F. E., BARNETT, R. J. AND GIARMAN, N. J. (1966) *J. Pharmacol. exptl. Ther.*, **154**, 185.

OWMAN, CH. (1964) *Int. J. Neuropharmacol.*, **2**, 105.

PELLEGRINO DE IRALDI, A. AND GUENDET, R. R. (1969) *Int. J. Neuropharmacol.*, **8**, 9.

PHILIPPU, A. AND SCHÜMANN, H. (1966) *Experientia (Basel)*, **22**, 119 .

POTTER, L. T. (1966) *Pharmacol. Rev.*, **18**, 439.

RICHARDSON, K. C. (1962) *J. Anat. (Lond.)*, **96**, 427.

SEIDEN, L. S. AND CARLSSON, A. (1964) *Psychopharmacologia (Berl.)*, **5**, 178.

SNIPES, R. L., THOENEN, H. AND TRANZER, J. P. (1968) *Experientia (Basel)*, **24**, 1026.

STJÄRNE, L. (1964) *Acta physiol. scand.*, **62**, Suppl. 228.

TAYLOR, P. W., CHIDSEY, C. A., RICHARDSON, K. C., COOPER, T. AND MICHAELSON, I. A. (1966 *Biochem. Pharmacol.*, **15**, 681.

THOA, N. B., AXELROD, J. AND ECCLESTON, D. (1967) *Pharmacologist*, **9**, 251.

THOA, N. B., ECCLESTON, D. AND AXELROD, J. (1969) *J. Pharmacol. exptl. Ther.*, **169**, 68.

THOENEN, H. (1969) *Bildung und funktionelle Bedeutung adrenerger Ersatztransmitter*, Springer-Verlag Berlin-Heidelberg-New York.

THOENEN, H., GEROLD, M., HAEFELY, W. AND HÜRLIMANN, A. (1968a) *Experientia (Basel)*, **24**, 158.

THOENEN, H., HAEFELY, W., GEY, K. F. AND HÜRLIMANN, A. (1965) *Life Sci.*, **4**, 2033.

THOENEN, H., HAEFELY, W., GEY, K. F. AND HÜRLIMANN, A. (1967) *Naunyn-Schmiedebergs Arch. exptl. Path. Pharmak.*, **259**, 17.

THOENEN, H., HAEFELY, W., GEY, K. F. AND HÜRLIMANN, A. (1967a) *J. Pharmacol. exptl. Ther.*, **156**, 246.

THOENEN, H., HAEFELY, W., GEY, K. F. AND HÜRLIMANN, A. (1967b) *Naunyn-Schmiedebergs Arch. exptl. Path. Pharmak.*, **258**, 181.

THOENEN, H., HÄUSLER, G. AND HÜRLIMANN, A. (1968b) *J. Pharmacol. exptl. Ther.*, **162**, 70.

THOENEN, H., HÜRLIMANN, A., GEY, K. F. AND HAEFELY, W. (1966) *Life Sci.*, **5**, 1715.

THOENEN, H. AND TRANZER, J. P. (1968) *Naunyn-Schmiedebergs Arch. exptl. Path. Pharmak.*, **261**, 271.

TRANZER, J. P. AND SNIPES, R. L. (1968) *Fourth European Regional Conference on Electron Microscopy*, Rome, 519.

TRANZER, J. P. AND THOENEN, H. (1967a) *Experientia (Basel)*, **23**, 743.

TRANZER, J. P. AND THOENEN, H. (1967b) *Experientia (Basel)*, **23**, 123.

TRANZER, J. P. THOENEN, H., SNIPES, R. L. AND RICHARDS, J. G. (1969) *Progr. Brain Res.*, **31**, 33.

UDENFRIEND, S. AND ZALTZMAN-NIRENBERG, P. (1963) *J. Pharmacol. exptl. Ther.*, **138**, 194.

# IV. RELEASE, UPTAKE, STORAGE AND METABOLISM OF TRANSMITTER SUBSTANCES

# Observation on Chromogranins, the Satellite Proteins of the Catecholamines in Chromaffin Cells and Adrenergic Neurones

H. BLASCHKO*

*University Department of Pharmacology, Oxford (U.K.)*

The chief contribution that the biochemists have made to the study of adrenergic mechanisms lies in the support that they have adduced for the idea that humoral transmission at nerve endings is related to the process of secretion of a hormone from an endocrine cell. The catecholamines serve as both hormones and transmitter substances.

The tissues from which these amines are released share, as has been known for a long time, a common origin. In recent years it has become clear that chromaffin cells and adrenergic neurones also contain a number of similar, possibly identical, macromolecular compounds. The first of these to be studied were the enzymes which serve as catalysts of the chemical reactions that constitute the steps of the biosynthetic pathway, but we now know that the same is true for what we might at present best call *satellite proteins*. This term is meant to imply that they accompany the messenger, at the level of the storage site, and possibly also in the event of release. These are the two properties of the satellite proteins around which attention has centred so far, but one hopes that one day these macromolecules may also be studied for any intrinsic properties of physiological significance. Too little is known at present of systems other than the adrenergic ones, but it may be timely to remind ourselves here of the fact that the neurophysins, macromolecules present in the neurones that terminate in the posterior lobe of the pituitary gland, represent satellite proteins of an analogous kind.

The study of the compounds that we now call the *chromogranins* (Blaschko *et al.*, 1967) began in Oxford in 1962, in co-operation with Mrs. Karen Helle (Blaschko and Helle, 1963). This study was undertaken because it appeared that the water-soluble proteins of the chromaffin granules were present in these particles in quantities that made it possible for the protein to participate, possibly together with adenosine triphosphate (ATP), in a storage complex. Although subsequent work has not revealed any particular affinity of the protein for the catecholamines, we cannot exclude that there may be some sequestration of the low-molecular-weight compounds, in a protein matrix. Smith and Winkler (1967) have reported that solutions of chromogranin in high concentration form a thixotropic gel.

---

* Visiting Professor, Institute of Physiology, University of Bergen (Norway).

The early work showed that chromogranin was a mixture of proteins, with one constituent preponderant (Blaschko and Helle, 1963); this compound which has been highly purified in several laboratories (Smith and Winkler, 1967; Smith and Kirshner, 1967; Geffen *et al.*, 1969a) is now called chromogranin A. It seems possible that chromogranin A is an oligomer, possibly a dimer or a tetramer; this idea is supported by the observation that the amino acid composition of the soluble lysate obtained from chromaffin granules is very similar to that of chromogranin A (Schneider *et al.*, 1969); moreover, the protein that is eluted in the peak following chromogranin A has a molecular weight about one-half that of chromogranin A and an amino acid composition very similar to that of chromogranin A (Smith and Kirshner, 1967).

Recent findings that some of the enzyme dopamine-$\beta$-hydroxylase appears in the water-soluble protein fraction raise the question as to what is chromogranin. Until recently, most authors have used the term for all the water-soluble constituents of the chromaffin granules. Eventually it might become useful to restrict the use of the term to compounds similar in chemical composition. However, this will have to wait until more is known of the chemistry of the minor constituents.

Our knowledge of the localization of chromogranin A has been greatly advanced when it was established that the highly purified protein had antigenic properties (Helle, 1966; Sage *et al.*, 1967; Geffen *et al.*, 1969a).

In 1965, Banks and Helle discovered that chromogranin was released from the perfused bovine adrenal gland when amine secretion was induced by adding carbamylcholine. We now know that under these conditions all water-soluble constituents of the granules appear in the perfusate (Schneider *et al.*, 1969), including also the water-soluble portion of the enzyme dopamine-$\beta$-hydroxylase (Viveros *et al.*, 1968). Chromogranin is also secreted into the adrenal venous blood when the splanchnic nerve is electrically stimulated *in vivo* (Blaschko *et al.*, 1967).

These findings have taught us that the secretory abilities of the chromaffin cells are much greater than was known. The release of the chromogranins is a true secretion; like the release of the catecholamines, chromogranin A release is dependent upon the presence of calcium ions (Schneider *et al.*, 1969).

These new findings have given strong support to the idea, first proposed by De Robertis and his colleagues (1964), that catecholamine release from the chromaffin cells occurs by exocytosis. This idea was first proposed on the basis of anatomical observations, and these have been extended more recently (Blaschko and Smith, 1971). Also, ATP and its metabolites are released from the gland upon stimulation (Douglas, 1968; Banks, 1966). All these compounds occur extracellularly, in relation to the amounts of amine released, in proportions not very different from those that are found in the chromaffin granules, as obtained from a sucrose density gradient (Smith, 1968).

Nature has presented us in the adrenal medulla with a very convenient starting material for biochemical studies. We first made use of the bovine adrenal gland when Langemann (1951) demonstrated the presence of the enzyme L-dopa decarboxylase in this tissue. Subsequently the enzyme was also found in adrenergic neurones. This pattern has since been repeated, not only in the study of the other catalysts of the biosynthetic pathway but more recently also in the study of chromogranin.

The search for chromogranin in the nervous system depended upon immunological studies. Banks *et al.* (1969) prepared noradrenaline-carrying particles from bovine splenic nerve and found that they contained material that reacted with the antiserum against chromogranin (see also Hopwood, 1968; Geffen *et al.*, 1969a).

The work by Geffen, Livett and Rush (1969a) was carried out using an antibody against sheep chromogranin; they were able to show that in this species also the amine-carrying fraction contained the protein. They also used an immunofluorescence microscopic method for the study of the protein in sympathetic neurones. They showed that fluorescence was marked in the soma of the sympathetic ganglion cells. The axons were more feebly fluorescent, but the material was found to accumulate proximal to a point of constriction, suggesting that the site of origin of the chromogranin was the cell body. Similar observations were made using a specific antibody against dopamine-$\beta$-hydroxylase; there is evidence from several laboratories that in nerve tissue this enzyme is also located in the amine-carrying particles.

There has been a report that an antibody-binding protein is present in the brain stem of the ox (Hopwood, 1968).

The observations on release of chromogranins from the stimulated chromaffin cell have led in recent months to an enquiry into the events that occur when adrenergic neurones are stimulated. Two groups of workers have briefly reported on such experiments (Geffen *et al.*, 1969b; Potter *et al.*, 1969); both have reported that when stimulation of the splenic nerve leads to a release of noradrenaline, both chromogranin A and dopamine-$\beta$-hydroxylase are also set free and appear in the perfusate. Thus, the adrenergic neurones resemble the chromaffin cells also in their ability to mobilise macromolecules when the low-molecular-weight chemical messenger is set free. There is, however, an interesting difference between the two tissues in the quantitative relationship between the amounts of amines and of proteins that are liberated. The adrenal medulla releases chromogranin and amine in approximately the same ratio in which they are found in chromogranin granules isolated from a sucrose density gradient. On the other hand, the perfusates from stimulated splenic preparations contain only a few per cent of the amount of proteins that would be expected on the basis of the amount of amine that can be recovered. In assessing these results, we must remember that at adrenergic nerve endings the relationship between site of release and blood vessels are different from that in the adrenal medulla, where it is the hormone released into the circulation that is carrying the message. At the nerve endings, entry of material into the blood stream is not a phenomenon to which we can attribute any physiological significance at present.

If we consider the question of a possible function of chromogranin release from nerves we remember that for a very long time physiologists have discussed the so-called trophic function of nerves exerted upon the effector organ. There is some evidence that such actions are not exerted by the transmitter substances. There have been reports that nerve homogenates can promote regeneration in the limb bud of the newt, and that the factor responsible for this effect is heat-labile (Lebowitz and Singer, 1970). We shall have to remember that the specific biochemical abilities of nerves are not restricted to the low-molecular-weight mediators.

*References p. 242*

Release of hormones by exocytosis is a process believed to occur in endocrine tissues other than the adrenal medulla. In nerves, this process was first suggested in observations on the so-called miniature end plate potentials at the motor end plate by Katz and his colleagues (1962). Here the mediator is acetylcholine. No information on characteristic satellite proteins in cholinergic neurones is available. In adrenergic systems miniature end plate potentials have also been described (Burnstock and Holman, 1966). Taken together with the biochemical observations here reported, it seems likely that exocytosis is a mechanism that is common to the release of chemical messenger from both nerve endings and endocrine cells.

## ACKNOWLEDGEMENTS

I should like to acknowledge support from the Norwegian Research Council for Sciences and Humanities as well as from the Royal Society.

## REFERENCES

BANKS, P. AND HELLE, K. (1965) *Biochem. J.*, **97**, 40C.

BANKS, P. (1966) *Biochem. J.*, **101**, 536.

BANKS, P., HELLE, K. B. AND MAYOR, D. (1969) *Pharmacol.*, **5**, 210.

BLASCHKO, H. AND HELLE, K. (1963) *J. Physiol.*, *Lond.*, **169**, 120P.

BLASCHKO, H., COMLINE, R. S., SCHNEIDER, F. H., SILVER, M. AND SMITH, A. D. (1967) *Nature*, **215**, 58.

BLASHKO, H. K. F. AND SMITH, A. D. (1971) *Phil. Trans. Roy. Soc. Lond. B*, **261**, 273–435.

BURNSTOCK, G. AND HOLMAN, M. E. (1966) *Pharmacol. Rev.*, **18**, 481.

DOUGLAS, W. W. (1968) *Brit. J. Pharmacol.*, **34**, 451.

GEFFEN, L. B., LIVETT, B. G. AND RUSH, R. A. (1969a) *J. Physiol.*, *Lond.*, **204**, 593.

GEFFEN, L. B., LIVETT, B. G. AND RUSH, R. A. (1969b) *J. Physiol.*, *Lond.*, **204**, 58P.

HELLE, K. (1966) *Biochim. biophys. Acta*, **117**, 107.

HOPWOOD, D. (1968) *Histochemie*, **13**, 619.

KATZ, B. (1962) *Proc. Roy. Soc. Lond. B.*, **155**, 455.

LANGEMANN, H. (1951) *Brit. J. Pharmacol.*, **6**, 318.

LEBOWITZ, P. AND SINGER, M. (1970) *Nature, Lond.*, **225**, 824.

POTTER, W. P. DE, SCHAEPDRYVER, A. F. DE, MOERMAN, E. J. AND SMITH, A. D. (1969) *J. Physiol.*, *Lond.*, **204**, 102P.

ROBERTIS, E. D. P. DE (1964) *Histophysiology of Synapses and Neurosecretion*, Pergamon Press, Oxford, pp. 193–198.

SAGE, H. J., SMITH, W. J. AND KIRSHNER, N. (1967) *Molec. Pharmacol.*, **3**, 81.

SCHNEIDER, F. H., SMITH, A. D. AND WINKLER, H. (1969) *Brit. J. Pharmacol.*, **31**, 94.

SMITH, A. D., Biochemistry of Chromaffin Granules. In P. N. CAMPBELL (Ed.), *The Interaction of Drugs and Subcellular Components in Animal Cells*, Churchill, J. & A., London, 1968, pp. 239–292.

SMITH, A. D. AND WINKLER, H. (1967) *Biochem. J.*, **103**, 483.

SMITH, W. J. AND KIRSHNER, N. (1967) *Molec. Pharmacol.*, **3**, 52.

VIVEROS, O. H., ARQUEROS, L. AND KIRSHNER, N. (1968) *Life Sci.*, **7**, 609.

# Molecular Mechanisms of Nervous Transmission and Synaptic Plasticity

E. GIACOBINI

*Department of Pharmacology\*, Karolinska Institutet, Stockholm (Sweden)*

> When I remember memory, then is the memory itself present with me by itself: but when I remember forgetfulness, then is present both memory and forgetfulness; memory is present, by which I have remembered, forgetfulness is present, which I have remembered.
>
> St. Augustine, Confessions, X,
> (translation by W. Watts, 1631)

### WHAT IS SYNAPTIC PLASTICITY?

The synapse is not a static and fixed structure but may undergo relevant changes even in the fully developed adult nervous system.

The complex chemical, structural and functional changes which may take place in the synapse during development or under the influence of experimental conditions constitute the basis of its plasticity.

The neurophysiologist, when talking of plasticity, generally means reversible ("slow" or "fast") changes in the bioelectric properties of the synapse.

As a result of work in our laboratory, we would like instead to underline some phenomena involving a series of changes in the chemical structure of the synapse. The phenomena we are referring to are slow in nature as compared with those studied by physiologists (hours or days instead of milliseconds or seconds).

We feel, however, that both types of plasticity are important for understanding the development and function of the nervous system.

In this paper we shall consider only those plastic changes which are directly related to chemical transmission.

The final task and common pathway for both the neurochemist and neurophysiologist is to approach the problem of learning which involves storing and handling information. The neurochemist is looking for specific chemical changes in specific parts of the neuron following the handling of information.

We would like to learn among other things whether "to remember" and "to forget" represent two different biochemical-physiological processes or are the same one.

---

\* Present address: Research Laboratories, AB Draco, S-221 01 Lund, Sweden.

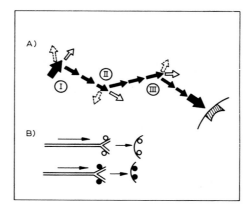

Fig. 1. Schematic diagram of growth of nerve fibers during development: A) In spite of different possibilities, the nerve fiber selectively chooses "one" direction of growth. B) Individual identification tags of a chemical nature selectively guide the nerve fiber to connect with the "correct" nerve cell. (See text.)

The problem is not particularly new, at least in philosophy, as we can see from the quotation of St. Augustine (354 A.D.). We should not forget that St. Augustine was an enthusiastic spokesman for the doctrine of predestination which, translated into neurobiological terms, implies that the differentiation of each neuronal pathway or connection depends on a decision taken *a priori* (divine = genetic). According to Attardi and Sperry (1963) patterning of synaptic connections must be handled by the growth mechanism directly, independently of function and with very great selectivity. According to the selectivity theory the establishment and maintenance of synaptic connections depends on highly specific cytochemical affinities ("similarities"). How is such a mechanism regulated? We can think of at least three different ways: (a) differentiation mechanisms (genetically directed), (b) induction by means of contact, (c) other effects, like embryonal gradient.

In other words, one could think that the cells in the CNS are marked at a very early stage of development by means of individual "identification tags" (Attardi and Sperry, 1963). These identification tags could be of a chemical nature. In this way millions of nerve cells can be "recognized" by other cells or neuronal processes (Attardi and Sperry, 1963) (Fig. 1).

We would like to suggest that these identification tags are identical with the specific proteins involved in the mechanism of chemical transmission, that is those enzymes participating in the synthesis, metabolism and inactivation of the transmitter molecules ("biosynthetic enzymes" or "satellite enzymes" according to Blaschko, this volume, see page 239).

The controversy concerning the significance of the appearance and development of enzymes related to transmission motivated a series of investigations in our laboratory (Giacobini G. *et al.*, 1970).

The autonomic and spinal ganglia of chick embryo are readily identifiable and separable as early as the 5th day of incubation. The nerve cells of these ganglia undergo

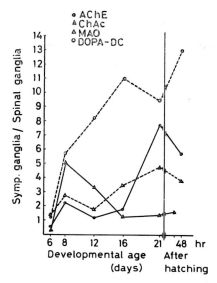

Fig. 2. Developmental changes of the ratio of sympathetic/spinal ganglia for AChE, ChAc, MAO and dopa-DC activity in chick embryo.

very marked changes of size and structure during embryonic life, during which time the synapse is formed (only in the sympathetic ganglia). Therefore embryonic autonomic ganglia represent an excellent material for studying the appearance and changes of specific proteins connected with transmission.

The transmitter, NA (noradrenaline), which is synthesized in the cell bodies of the sympathetic neurons can be demonstrated histochemically in the chick embryo of 3–4 days of incubation (Enemar et al., 1965). The variation in AChE (acetylcholinesterase), ChAc (cholineacetylase), MAO (monoamine oxidase) and dopa-DC (dopa-decarboxylase) activity in the two types of ganglia, "synaptic" (sympathetic) and "asynaptic" (spinal), can be compared better by studying the ratio between the two ganglia (symp/spinal) (Fig. 2). A distinct peak of activity is observed at the 8th day with a ratio of about 2, 3 and 5 for AChE, MAO and ChAc, respectively. This indicates that maximal activity of the three enzymes is reached during the period in which synaptic connections begin to form in the ganglion. This also corresponds to the moment of most intense neuronal maturational activity. Dopa-DC does not show the same pattern but instead its activity continues to increase progressively from the 6th day to the 15th day. The localization of these events is principally the synaptic site for AChE and ChAc and the cell body for MAO and dopa-DC. The specific fluorescence for NA and the NA content of the ganglia show similar pattern (Enemar et al., 1965).

In the ensuing days the ChAc and dopa-DC ratio shows a marked difference from that of AChE and MAO, and no second peak is apparent for these enzymes at the time of hatching (Giacobini G. et al., 1970).

In order to be able to interpret this difference we have to consider the fact that the neuron in this period is not only growing in size but also establishing functional connections with the periphery. Since only AChE, MAO and dopa-DC are present (Giacobini E. *et al.*, 1970s) in the postganglionic adrenergic pathway (that is in the cell body and the efferent fibers) the second peak of enzyme activity may coincide with the completion of the peripheral innervation and the commencement of the function at birth. The intermediary period between the two peaks probably corresponds to a period of migration of MAO, AChE and dopa-DC from the cell body toward the innervated region (Giacobini G. *et al.*, 1970a).

What are the factors of the selective "chemotactic guidance" governing the growth of new fibers in the sympathetic ganglia?

Some critical factors must determine the direction and the polarity of this growth. These factors may be of a chemical nature so that even if different possibilities are offered to the growing fiber and these are mechanically and morphologically feasible the fiber will always choose the "correct" direction and the "correct" connection on the basis of chemical affinity or selectivity (Fig. 1).

## PRINCIPLES GOVERNING SYNAPTIC PLASTICITY

On the basis of well established results reported in the literature and results which will emerge in the context of this paper, the following points can be suggested:

1. Nerve cells differ one from another functionally and chemically.

2. Synapses between different cells may be "different" functionally and chemically.

3. Nerve cells and axons carry identification tags starting at the beginning of development. In this way they reach the "correct" synaptic connection (genetic control) (Fig. 1).

4. The identification tags carried by the growing neuron might be constituted by specific proteins ("biosynthetic enzymes" or "satellite proteins" according to Blaschko, this volume, see page 239) involved in the process of chemical transmission at the synapse.

5. The identification tag system is active *only* during development. (See the part of this paper concerning experiments with heterologous anastomoses.)

6. *As a consequence of 5*, "wrong" connections (synapses) might be constructed under particular experimental or pathological conditions in the adult nervous system.

7. *As a consequence of 6*, "new" receptors can be formed or "silent" receptors can be activated.

8. The mechanisms responsible for storing information might use the plasticity of the synapse as a possibility for "remodeling" the synaptic connections. This "remodeling" involves "addition" or "subtraction" of fibers and connections between different neurons.

9. As a consequence of 8, synaptic plasticity might be involved in the mechanism of learning (handling or storing information).

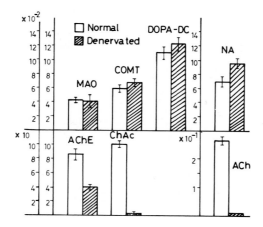

Fig. 3. The effect of preganglionic denervation on five enzymes and two transmitters in L7 sympathetic ganglia of the cat. The units are reported in the original papers.

## EXPERIMENTAL MODELS FOR STUDYING SYNAPTIC PLASTICITY

### *Importance of synaptic connections and impulse activity for the maintenance of transmitter metabolism in the neuron*

#### *(a) The effect of preganglionic denervation on ganglia*

The structural and morphological changes occurring during denervation have been carefully followed and described by electron microscopists (Hámori *et al.*, 1968). Both presynaptic fibers and synaptic boutons show signs of degeneration as early as 24 hours after denervation. The apparatus responsible for the synthesis and metabolism of the transmitter acetylcholine (ACh) is completely inactivated.

Preganglionic denervation of the L7 ganglion in the cat after three weeks results in a loss of both ChAc and AChE activity in the ganglia (Fig. 3) (Giacobini E. *et al.*, 1967; Buckley *et al.*, 1967b). The decrease in enzyme activity is about 98 % for ChAc but only 60 % for AChE, indicating that the former enzyme (ChAc) is located principally at the presynaptic site. The data in Fig. 3 show that in the presynaptically denervated L7 ganglia neither MAO nor COMT nor dopa-CD activity is significantly changed. It should be stressed that MAO and dopa-CD are selectively localized in the cell body of the adrenergic cells. The location of COMT is still obscure (Giacobini and Kerpel-Fronius, 1969). The NA content of the cervical superior ganglion cells is significantly increased 2–3 weeks after denervation, while ACh is markedly reduced to only 8 % of the original amount (Giacobini E. *et al.*, 1970).

Noradrenaline in the sympathetic ganglia of the cat originates almost exclusively from the somata and axons of the postganglionic adrenergic neurons and is several times higher in sympathetic ganglia than in most regions of the CNS.

ACh, on the other hand, is stored principally in the preganglionic nerve terminals.

From these data it is evident that sympathetic ganglia constitute an excellent ma-

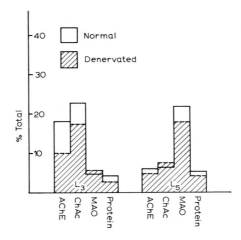

Fig. 4. Mean ChAc, AChE, MAO activity and protein content of at least ten values of synaptosomal (L3) and mitochondrial (L5) fractions of normal and denervated superior cervical ganglia of the cat.

terial for studying the plasticity of synthesizing and inactivating mechanisms of transmitters.

The morphological changes found by Hámori *et al.* (1968) consisting of clumping and agglutination of synaptic vesicles appears as early as 6 hours after the denervation. If the sensitivity of our assays were better, the changes in the content of transmitters and in enzyme activity could probably be seen at a much earlier stage than that reported in our biochemical studies. The changes described apply therefore to a kind of steady-state situation after complete degeneration of the synapse has been reached.

Studies performed on cells isolated from the same ganglia and under the same experimental conditions agree completely with the data obtained at the level of whole ganglia; however, they add important details about biochemical changes following denervation. Such details are described elsewhere (Buckley *et al.*, 1967b; Consolo *et al.*, 1968; Giacobini E. *et al.*, 1967; Giacobini E. *et al.*, 1970a).

*(b)  Changes in enzyme activity after synaptic deprivation in synaptosomal fractions of ganglia*

Subcellular fractions of single autonomic ganglia (1–2 mg w.w.) can be obtained by means of a newly described technique (Giacobini E. and Mitchard, 1969). The possibility of examining the subcellular constituents of cells in a small population of neurons is of great value because of the variability and functional differentiation of the nerve cells which is present not only in the CNS but also in autonomic ganglia.

In the synaptosomal fraction (L3 Fig. 4) it is apparent that both ChAc and AChE activity are strongly reduced after denervation while MAO and proteins are not changed. In the mitochondrial fraction (L5 Fig. 4) no changes are seen in MAO, AChE or ChAc activities. This agrees well with the results obtained at the level of whole ganglia homogenates or of single isolated cells.

## Conclusion

The deprivation of functional synaptic connections in sympathetic ganglia produces accumulation of the postganglionic transmitter (NA) in the cell body, almost complete disappearance of the preganglionic transmitter (ACh) and a slight increase of the activity of some inactivating enzymes (MAO, cell experiments, Giacobini E. *et al.*, 1970a).

Our study suggests that other biochemical changes may be detectable in the adrenergic neuron after denervation, and there is a need for further studies at the cellular level. It seems very unlikely that biochemical changes correlated to plastic changes of small and specific portions of the synapse in certain neurons along given pathways could be detected in chemical analysis of the *total* brain or even small portions of the brain.

### MICROCHEMICAL APPROACHES TO THE STUDY OF SYNAPTIC PLASTICITY

In view of the remarkable development of microtechniques in chemical analysis, significant progress in cellular neurochemistry is to be expected, and it is very likely that some biochemistry about neuronal plasticity will emerge in the next few years.

The application of methods of biochemical analysis to synaptic plasticity involves some precise requirements. These are: (a) quantitative significance of the results, (b) high specificity of the assay method employed, (c) high sensitivity allowing analysis at the cellular and subcellular level, that is high resolution power of the assay method, (d) the presence of drugs in the experiment should not interfere with the chemical assay, (e) the assay should be unaffected by side reactions, (f) there should be the possibility of *rapid* analysis of several samples at one time.

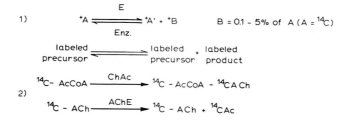

Fig. 5. Principle for microradiometric assay with quantitative recovery.

Isotopic techniques which have recently been introduced in cellular analysis (Buckley *et al.*, 1967a) have proved to be of great help. The principle of the microradiometric assay with quantitative recovery is shown in Fig. 5 together with two examples (AChE and ChAc activity measurement). A schematic diagram of the isotopic techniques developed in our laboratory for measuring different enzyme activities in $\mu$g or sub-$\mu$g quantities of nervous tissue is shown in Table 1 and Table 2. Table 3 shows that isotopic techniques may be more sensitive than both colorimetric and fluorimetric methods and as sensitive as gas-chromatographic techniques. On the other hand,

TABLE 1

QUANTITATIVE CELLULAR ASSAY OF ENZYME ACTIVITY RELATED TO CHOLINERGIC AND
ADRENERGIC TRANSMISSION

Methods used in the reported investigations

| Transmitter or precursor | Related enzyme | Micromethod | References |
|---|---|---|---|
| ACh | AChE | Cartesian-magnetic diver isotopic | Giacobini (1957) Mitchard *et al.* (1970) Koslow & Giacobini (1969) |
| | ChAc | isotopic | Buckley *et al.* (1967, b) |
| NA | MAO | isotopic | Consolo *et al.* (1968) |
| | COMT | isotopic | Giacobini & Kerpel-Fronius (1969) |
| | TH | isotopic | Park & Giacobini (1971) |
| Dopa | dopa-DC | isotopic | Giacobini & Noré (1971) |
| 5-HT | 5-HTP-DC | isotopic | Giacobini & Noré (1971) |

TABLE 2

PRINCIPLE OF RADIOMETRIC MICROASSAY FOR ENZYME ACTIVITY, TYPE OF LABELED
SUBSTRATE AND LABELED PRODUCT

Methods used in the reported investigations

| Enzyme | Principle | Labeled substrate | Labeled product |
|---|---|---|---|
| MAO | solvent extraction | [$^{14}$C]tyramine | 3-OH-indolacetaldehyde (acid) |
| COMT | solvent extraction | [5-$^{14}$C]adenosyl-methionine | 3-methoxy-4-OH-benzoate |
| Dopa-DC | diffusion volatilization | [$^{14}$C]dopa | $^{14}CO_2$ |
| Tyrosine hydroxylase | TLC-adsorption | [1-$^{14}$C]tyrosine | [1-$^{14}$C]dopa |
| AChE | precipitation | [$^{14}$C]acetylcholine | [$^{14}$C]acetate |
| ChAc | precipitation | [$^{14}$C]acetyl CoA | [$^{14}$C]acetylcholine |

TABLE 3

SENSITIVITY OF ISOTOPE PROCEDURE AND COMPARISON WITH THAT OF OTHER METHODS

| Technique | Sensitivity (moles of measurable substrate) |
|---|---|
| Colorimetric | $10^{-9}$–$10^{-10}$ |
| Fluorimetric | $10^{-11}$–$10^{-12}$ |
| Isotopic | $10^{-12}$–$10^{-13}$ |
| Gas chromatographic | $10^{-13}$–$10^{-14}$ |
| Micromanometric (Cartesian diver) | $10^{-12}$–$10^{-13}$ |
| Micromagnetic (magnetic diver) | $10^{-13}$–$10^{-14}$ |

the number of results obtained per experiment is much larger with isotopic than with micromanometric or magnetic diver techniques (Table 3).

Several enzymes related to the metabolism of transmitters or precursors of the ACh and NA system have been studied by means of the cytochemical techniques reported. The principle of these techniques is given in Table 2. The concentration of NA in single cells was determined by means of the technique described by Caspersson *et al.* (1966) by Giacobini E. *et al.* (1970).

*How can we explore synaptic plasticity in the adult? Construction of heterogenous synapses*

This problem involves the construction of a synapse in the adult animal using an "incorrect tag" (physiologically non existent, Fig. 1). Will this experimentally forced connection be accepted by the neuron or will it be rejected? This involves the question of how connections between neurons should be constructed in order to permit transmission of impulses.

One of the oldest approaches to this problem is the investigation of heterogenous anastomoses made by Langley (1898–99) and Langley and Andersson (1904). These authors tried to answer the above question by investigating whether nerve fibers could act as substitutes for one another.

The results of their observations were considered to provide the first strong support for the theory that transmission of nerve impulses across synapses is mediated by chemical factors which may be different from neuron to neuron.

TABLE 4

STRUCTURES IN WHICH HETEROGENOUS SYNAPSES HAVE BEEN CONSTRUCTED

(1) Sympathetic ganglia (cervical and lumbar)
(2) Central nervous system (spinal cord)
(3) Striated and smooth muscles

On the basis of data available in the literature it can be seen that three structures have been mainly exploited for the construction of heterogenous synapses (Table 4): (a) sympathetic ganglia, (b) spinal cord, and (c) striated and smooth muscles.

The prevalent connecting fibers used in experiments with sympathetic ganglia have been cholinergic fibers. However, sensory fibers from the vagus have been connected to cholinergic fibers (De Castro, 1934; Baron, 1934; Hillarp, 1946; Matsumura and Koelle, 1961).

Regarding the construction of heterogenous synapses in muscles and effector organs, the connections have previously been made between similar fibers, principally between cholinergic fibers, with the exception of the reinnervation of the nictitating membrane with the hypoglossal nerve (Vera *et al.*, 1957; Lennon *et al.*, 1967).

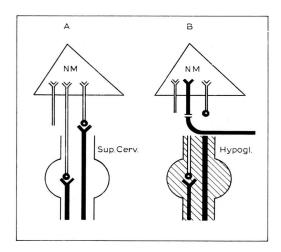

Fig. 6. Schematic diagram of the anastomosis between the hypoglossal nerve and the postganglionic fibers of the superior cervical ganglion. A. normal condition, B. after the anastomosis, NM = nictitating membrane. Dark fibers = cholinergic fibers, white fibers = adrenergic fibers. For details see the text.

### Construction of heterogenous synapses in effector organs
### The nictitating membrane

We used (Giacobini E. *et al.*, 1971) the nictitating membrane of the cat as a model for the construction of heterogenous synapses in effector organs.

Normally the nictitating membrane is mainly innervated by postganglionic fibers originating from the superior cervical ganglion. The great majority of these fibers are adrenergic and fluoresce intensely for NA. Most of the cell bodies giving rise to the postganglionic fibers are located inside the ganglion but a few are found in the preganglionic trunk (Fig. 6).

The operation performed by us is shown schematically in Fig. 6. The superior cervical ganglion was excised and part of the preganglionic trunk was sutured to the hypoglossal nerve (containing mostly cholinergic fibers). After 6–9 months the nictitating membrane as well as the hypoglossal nerve were examined. As a result of the operation the nictitating membrane appears to be completely devoid of the rich net of terminals strongly fluorescent for catecholamines which is normally found (Giacobini E. *et al.*, 1971).

The results of the biochemical and histochemical analyses are summarized in Table 5. ChAc activity, which is generally very low, was highly increased. MAO activity on the contrary was strongly decreased after denervation and subsequent reinnervation. AChE was slightly increased. This strongly suggests the absence of the normal adrenergic fibers and the presence of new cholinergic fibers.

By stimulating the hypoglossal trunk it was possible to elicit (in about 90% of the operated cats) a contraction of the nictitating membrane indicating a functional reinnervation of the organ.

TABLE 5

BIOCHEMICAL AND HISTOCHEMICAL CHANGES IN NORMAL AND HYPOGLOSSAL REINNER-
VATED NICTITATING MEMBRANES OF THE CAT

| Assay | Enzyme transm. | Normal | Reinnervated |
|---|---|---|---|
| Biochem. | MAO | +++ | (0) |
| | ChAc | (0) | +++ (+ 70%) |
| | AChE | (+) | + (+ 25%) |
| Histochem. | NA (fluor.) | +++ | 0 |
| | AChE (Koelle) | (+) | 0 |

This study leaves little doubt about the possibility of reinnervating a peripheral organ with nerve fibers of different origin and establishing completely new and heterogenous synaptic connections and brings up many questions about the function of receptors in reinnervated organs. As demonstrated by the studies of Guth and Bernstein (1961) and Garrett (this volume, see page 475), when a choice is given for a structure (sympathetic ganglia or salivary glands, respectively) to be reinnervated by their own or "foreign" fibers or by one or the other division (adrenergic or cholinergic fibers), the correct functional connection is selected whenever possible. This could indicate: (a) the maintenance of a "specific" affinity in the adult or (b) the possibility of inhibition of the incorrectly growing fiber by the correctly growing fiber.

*Construction of heterogenous synapses in the peripheral nervous system*

In the investigation by Koslow and coll. (1971a and b) an attempt was made for the

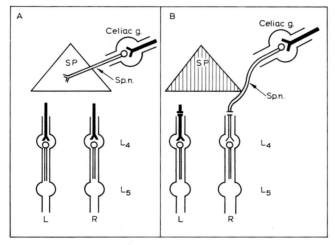

Fig. 7. Schematic diagram of the splenic nerve–L4 ganglion anastomosis. A. normal connections, B. after the anastomosis, SP = spleen, Sp.n. = splenic nerve. Dark fibers = cholinergic fibers, white fibers = adrenergic fibers. For details see the text.

*References pp. 257–258*

TABLE 6

BIOCHEMICAL AND HISTOCHEMICAL CHANGES IN NORMAL AND SPLENIC REINNERVATED
L4 SYMPATHETIC GANGLIA OF THE CAT

| Assay | Enzyme transm. | Normal | Reinnervated |
|-------|----------------|--------|--------------|
| Biochem. | MAO | + | +++ (× 10) |
|  | ChAc | +++ | (+) (10%) |
|  | AChE | +++ | + (30%) |
| Histochem. | NA (fluor.) | ++ | +++ |
|  | AChE (Koelle) | ++ | ++ |

first time to substitute the normally connecting preganglionic cholinergic fibers in the ganglia with adrenergic fibers and to challenge the formation of new synapses completely different and incorrect with respect to their physiological and biochemical nature. That is, we attempted to build an adrenergic–cholinergic anastomosis in the sympathetic ganglia. The operation which was attempted in 44 cats is shown schematically in Fig. 7.

The postsynaptic adrenergic fibers originating from the celiac ganglion and constituting the main part of the splenic nerve innervating the spleen were sutured with the preganglionic cholinergic fibers entering the L4 (or L5) ganglion in the cat and made to reinnervate these ganglia.

The controls were constituted by contralateral either normally innervated ganglia or ganglia denervated and subsequently reinnervated with homologous preganglionic cholinergic fibers. The biochemical and histochemical results of this investigation are summarized in Table 6. The histochemical (fluorescence) test performed in the reinnervated ganglia shows a large number of new fibers entering the ganglia and establishing connections with the neurons. The resolution of the fluorescent method in light microscopy does not allow a clear discrimination of fine synaptic connections. However, it can be seen that the fibers entering the ganglia are highly fluorescent for catecholamines and can be traced back to the anastomosis with the splenic nerve. Their identity is therefore to be referred to the adrenergic fibers originated from the connected splenic nerve (Koslow et al., 1971 a and b). The biochemical results (Table 6) show that MAO activity increased almost 10 times in the reinnervated ganglia while ChAc diminished to about 10% of the original values. AChE diminished by about 70% (Table 6). These results agree with previous findings in the same ganglia after denervation, however, the increased MAO activity can only be explained by the presence of new adrenergic fibers entering the ganglion. AChE activity, demonstrated by means of Koelle's reaction, was not changed as far as the number of positive fibers and intensity of staining. The neurophysiological data obtained by such experiments are shown in Fig. 8 (Koslow et al., 1971 a and b).

Recording of the compound action potential obtained in normal unoperated preparations show that some preganglionic fibers synapse in the ganglion while other

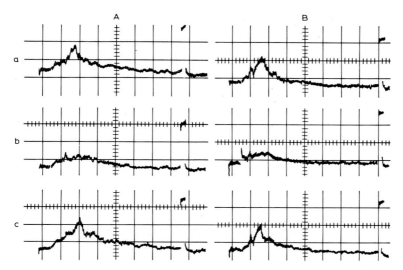

Fig. 8. Dopa-dependent response. Evoked potential from the splenic reinnervated ganglion activated by orthodromic stimulation of the splenic nerve. A, B represent one ganglion. A-a Control response, 2 h after isolation. A-b Following 60 min repetitive stimulation and successive 70 min rest. A-c 30 min after the addition of 25 ng/ml dopa to the bath. B-a Control response, 7 h after the isolation, twice restored by dopa. B-b Following 30 min repetitive stimulation and successive 30 min rest. B-c 10 min after the addition of 125 ng/ml dopa to the bath (Koslow *et al.*, 1971a).

fibers pass directly through. In about half of the successfully reinnervated ganglia the electrical response was similar to normal control ganglia. In the other group of reinnervated ganglia, the electrical response showed very peculiar characteristics. Pharmacological studies aiming to establish whether the two groups of ganglia could be differentiated on the basis of their pharmacological response showed that complete restoration of the postganglionic response to electrical stimulation after repetitive supramaximal stimulation (30–60 min) could be accomplished after the addition of dopa to the bath medium (Fig. 8). Dopa was capable of restoring the abolished ganglionic response several times; however, the combined addition of dopa and pyridoxal phosphate (Fig. 8) was able to restore the response regularly. The dopa-dependent ganglionic transmission was blocked by the ganglionic blocker, hexamethonium.

These data suggest that when the L4 ganglion is reinnervated with fiber originating from the splenic nerve, new excitatory synapses are formed. The action of dopa and pyridoxal phosphate on the electrophysiological response suggests that these sympathetic neurons may now have made connections with "adrenergic" preganglionic fibers. A cholinergic component (receptor?) cannot be ruled out, and the action of hexamethonium cannot be easily interpreted as an action of the monoaminergic transmitter on a nicotinic receptor. The significance of these data has to be interpreted in the light of the present conception of the physiological role of catecholamines in ganglionic transmission mechanisms.

*References pp. 257–258*

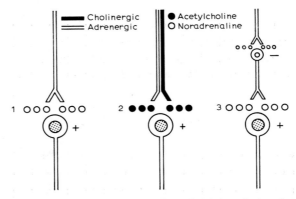

Fig. 9. Different explanations for the excitatory effect of NA in splenic reinnervated sympathetic ganglia: 1, direct excitatory effect of NA; 2, the few cholinergic fibers present in the splenic nerve exert an excitatory effect; 3, short interneurons of an adrenergic nature exert an inhibitory effect. The result is disinhibition.

The role of catecholamines and the "normal" presence of adrenergic components in sympathetic ganglia can be explained according to the following:

(a) presence of postganglionic adrenergic fibers originating from so-called accessory ganglia present outside the sympathetic ganglia in the chain.

(b) vasoconstrictor fibers originating from adrenergic fibers in the cervical superior ganglion releasing amines in the blood stream (capillaries). From such sites the amines reach the ganglion cells.

(c) chromaffin cells or small interneurons (Williams's interneurons). According to Eränkö (this volume, see page 39) in the rat, small neurons with short fibers branching inside the ganglion and near the vessels are present. Their number is approximately 500–600 per ganglion, that is a ratio of 1:50 with respect to the other neurons. In the cat they contain dopamine but no noradrenaline or 5-HT.

(d) postganglionic collaterals of adrenergic fibers (responsible for recurrent inhibition).

(e) possibility of "leakage" of NA from the adrenergic cell bodies after preganglionic stimulation (self-inhibition).

For references about the above points, see Haefely (1969).

In order to explain the excitatory effect of NA found in the reinnervated ganglia, different hypotheses should be taken into account (Fig. 9):

(a) a direct excitatory effect of the "new" adrenergic fibers entering the ganglia.

(b) the few cholinergic fibers present in the splenic nerve could exert a direct excitatory effect (however this can not explain the fact that transmission is re-established only after dopa and pyridoxal phosphate). Cholinergic fibers could release NA according to the interaction theory proposed by Ehinger et al. (1968). This hypothesis does not explain the effect of NA (See (a) above).

(c) the presence of short interneurons (interneurons of an adrenergic nature exerting an inhibitory effect). The result would be a disinhibition. This hypothesis is difficult to understand at present.

How can one explain the presence and identity of "adrenergic" receptors on the membrane of the "adrenergic" cell after reinnervation? Is it still the same kind of receptor or a "double-face" or "bivalent" receptor (NA/ACh) or are two separate receptors present? How does NA affect the nicotinic receptor (hexamethonium experiments)?

### GENERAL CONCLUSIONS

The conclusions of this study may be summarized as follows:

1. It can be demonstrated that in the adult nervous system it is possible to establish not only "new" but even "wrong" synaptic connections between neurons. This indicates a high degree of plasticity of the neuron in the adult stage and that the identification-tag mechanism may be "inactivated" in the adult under certain conditions.

2. Noradrenaline which is generally considered to exert an inhibitory effect within the sympathetic ganglia may under certain conditions, be capable of acting as an excitatory transmitter. This situation is similar to that encountered in invertebrate ganglia where ACh or NA can act both as excitatory and inhibitory molecules (Gerschenfeld *et al.*, 1967).

3. "New" receptors can be developed on the membrane under certain conditions or "old" receptors can be changed and adapted in such a way that they can react with more than one transmitter.

The question can be asked (see the introductory part of this paper) of how much we can manipulate the neuron with its membrane receptors, and whether the synapse under special conditions can lose its "memory" (anastomosis experiments). Finally, are the mechanisms of plasticity which have been discovered under special experimental conditions relevant to the understanding of the process of learning?

### ACKNOWLEDGMENT

The work performed in our laboratory and reported in this paper was supported by grants from the U.S. Public Health Service, National Institute of Health, NB 04561-06, and from the Swedish Medical Research Council projects Nos. 12X-246-06 and B71-14X-246-07 to E.G.

### REFERENCES

ATTARDI, D. AND SPERRY, R. W. (1963) *Exp. Neurol.*, **7**, 46–64.
BARON, M. (1934) *Zeitung Mikroskop.-Anatomischen Forschung*, **35**, 331.
BLASCHKO, H., this volume, page 239.
BUCKLEY, G., CONSOLO, S., GIACOBINI, E. AND McCAMAN, R. (1967a) *Acta Physiol. Scand.*, **71**, 341–347.
BUCKLEY, G., CONSOLO, S., GIACOBINI, E. AND SJÖQVIST, F. (1967b) *Acta Physiol. Scand.*, **71**, 348–356.
CASPERSSON, T., HILLARP, N. Å. AND RITZEN, M. (1966) *Exp. Cell Res.*, **45**, 415.
CONSOLO, S., GIACOBINI, E. AND KARJALAINEN, K. (1968) *Acta Physiol. Scand.*, **74**, 513–520.
DE CASTRO, F. (1934) *Trav. Lab. Rech. Biol. Univ. Madrid*, **29**, 397.
EHINGER, B., FALCK, B. AND PERSSON, H. (1968) *Acta Physiol. Scand.*, **72**, 139–147.

ENEMAR, A., FALCK, B. AND HÅKANSSON, R. (1965) *Develop. Biol.*, **11**, 268.

ERÄNKÖ, O. AND ERÄNKÖ, L., this volume, page 39.

GARRETT, J. R., this volume, page 475.

GERSCHENFELD, H. M., ASCHER, P. AND TAUC, L. (1967) *Nature*, **213**, 358–359.

GIACOBINI, E. (1957) *J. Neurochem.*, **1**, 234.

GIACOBINI, E., PALMBORG, B. AND SJÖQVIST, F. (1967) *Acta Physiol. Scand.*, **69**, 355–361.

GIACOBINI, E. AND KERPEL-FRONIUS, S. (1969) *Acta Physiol. Scand.*, **75**, 523–529.

GIACOBINI, E. AND MITCHARD, M. (1969) *Brit. J. Pharmacol.*, **35**, 370.

GIACOBINI, E., KARJALAINEN, K., KERPEL-FRONIUS, S. AND RITZEN, M. (1970) *Neuropharmacology*, **9**, 59–66.

GIACOBINI, E., KERPEL-FRONIUS, S., KOSLOW, S., OLSSON, L. AND STEPITA-KLAUCO, M. (1971), *J. Pharm. Exp.* Therap., In press.

GIACOBINI, E. AND NORÉ, B. (1971) *Acta Physiol. Scand.*, In press.

GIACOBINI, G., MARCHISIO, P. C., GIACOBINI, E. AND KOSLOW, S., (1970) *J. Neurochem.*, **17**, 1177–1185.

GIACOBINI, G., FILOGAMO, G., GIACOBINI, E. AND NORÉ, B. (1971) *J. Neurochem.*, In press.

GUTH, L. AND BERNSTEIN, J. J. (1961) *Exp. Neurol.*, **4**, 59–69.

HAEFELY, W. E. (1969) In AKERT, K. AND WASER, P. G. (Eds.), *Mechanisms of Synaptic Transmission (Progress in Brain Research, Vol. 31)*, Elsevier, Amsterdam, pp. 61–72.

HÁMORI, J., LÁNG, E. AND SIMON, L. (1968) *Z. Zellforsch. Mikroskop. Anat.*, **90**, 37–52.

HILLARP, N. Å. (1946) *Acta Anatomica, Suppl. IV*, 1–153.

KOSLOW, S. AND GIACOBINI, E. (1969) *J. Neurochem.*, **16**, 1523–1528.

KOSLOW, S., STEPITA-KLAUCO, M., OLSSON, L. AND GIACOBINI. E. (1971a), *Experientia (Basel)*, In press.

KOSLOW, S., STEPITA-KLAUCO, M., OLSSON, L. AND GIACOBINI, E. (1971b) To be published.

LANGLEY, J. N. (1898–99) *J. Physiol.*, **23**, 240.

LANGLEY, J. N. AND ANDERSSON, K. K. (1904) *J. Physiol.*, **30**, 439.

LENNON, A. M., VERA, V. L., REX, A. L. AND LUCO, J. V. (1967) *J. Neurophysiol.*, **30**, 1523.

MATSUMURA, M. AND KOELLE, G. B. (1961) *J. Pharmacol. Exp. Therap.*, **134**, 28.

MITCHARD, M., GIACOBINI, E. AND CARLSSON, B., (1970) *Anal. Biochem.*, **37**, 112–124.

PARK, J. AND GIACOBINI, E. (1971) To be published.

VERA, C. L., VIAL, J. D. AND LUCO, J. V. (1957) *J. Neurophysiol.*, **20**, 365.

# Preferential Secretion of Newly Formed Catecholamines: Comparison Between Sympathetic Nerves and Adrenal Medulla

L. STJÄRNE

*Department of Physiology, Karolinska Institutet, Stockholm (Sweden)*

The finding that the rate of formation of noradrenaline (NA), as calculated from the conversion of labelled tyrosine to NA, exceeds the estimates of the rate of NA synthesis based on the rate of disappearance of labelled NA, led to the concept of preferential secretion of newly formed neurotransmitter (Sedvall *et al.*, 1968). Results obtained by a variety of techniques in several species have lent considerable experimental support to this concept, both for noradrenergic (Kopin *et al.*, 1968; Thierry *et al.*, 1970), dopaminergic (Besson *et al.*, 1969) and cholinergic (Collier, 1969) nerves. Recently, similar preferential resting secretion of newly formed catecholamines (CA) has been observed in adrenal medulla (Hempel and Männl, 1969).

While the concept of a small, fast functional transmitter pool, mainly supported by *de novo* synthesis, coexisting with a large, relatively inert 'storage' pool, has gained widespread acceptance, the basic evidence obtained by direct techniques still appears controversial. Thus direct determination of the fate of NA newly formed from labelled tyrosine in the isolated perfused cat spleen led Kopin *et al.* to the conclusion that newly formed NA, during prolonged high-frequency nerve stimulation, is preferentially secreted and may represent as much as two thirds of the total NA secreted. On the other hand Blakeley *et al.* (1969) were unable to find evidence for preferential secretion of newly formed NA during intermittent high-frequency nerve stimulation in the same tissue. Furthermore, results obtained in a balance study in the isolated perfused cat spleen led Hedqvist and Stjärne (1969) to conclude that reuptake and reuse of transmitter are major factors in the maintenance of transmitter output during prolonged nerve stimulation, and that the NA synthesis capacity of sympathetic nerves appears to be regulated to cover only the small, unavoidable transmitter deficit resulting, in spite of the highly active recapture mechanism, from chemical degradation, extraneuronal binding or washout into the circulation.

In view of this apparent controversy, and since the available evidence of preferential secretion of newly formed CA from adrenal medulla concerns resting secretion only, the present experiments were carried out to compare the effects of secretory stimulation on newly formed CA in sympathetic nerves and adrenal medulla. The details of this study are reported elsewhere (Stjärne and Wennmalm, 1971a; Stjärne, 1971).

*References p. 267*

METHODS

*Perfusions*

*Sympathetic nerves*: The isolated, sympathetically innervated rabbit heart, perfused according to Langendorff with Tyrode's solution containing 20 $\mu$g/ml of ascorbate and aerated with 6.5% $CO_2$ in $O_2$ (Löffelholtz and Muscholl, 1969), was selected for the study of the fate of newly formed NA in sympathetic nerves. Heart rate and contractile force were recorded with the aid of commercial Grass equipment, as previously described (Hedqvist *et al.*, 1970). [14]C-labelled tyrosine, 50 $\mu$C (New England Corp., uniformly labelled, specific activity 446 mC/mmole), diluted with unlabelled tyrosine to give final concentrations of $2.5 \times 10^{-7}$ M or $2 \times 10^{-5}$ M, was infused at a constant rate during 10 min. After 4 min both left and right sympathetic nerve trunks were electrically stimulated supramaximally and continuously at 5 or 10/sec for 4 to 6 min. The effluent, which was immediately acidified, was collected separately for each 2-min period. At the end of the stimulation period the heart was rapidly homogenized in 0.4 M perchloric acid.

*Adrenal*: The study of the fate of newly formed CA in adrenal medulla was carried out on the isolated cat adrenal gland, perfused in a retrograde manner at a rate of 1 ml/min with Krebs–Henseleit medium containing ascorbate and gassed as in the heart experiments. [14]C-labelled tyrosine, 50 $\mu$C, diluted with unlabelled tyrosine to give final concentrations of $5 \times 10^{-6}$ M or $2 \times 10^{-5}$ M, was infused for a period of about 30 min. At intervals of about 8 min secretion was induced by rapid injection into the inflow cannula of acetylcholine or carbachol. The dosage was adjusted to give approximately equal secretory responses, and thus rose stepwise from 25 $\mu$g to 100 $\mu$g. The effluent was collected at 2-min intervals and immediately acidified. After the third stimulation the adrenal was rapidly homogenized. In some experiments the distribution of radioactive material was determined in whole homogenate extracted with 0.4 M perchloric acid, and in other experiments in different subcellular fractions. The gland was then homogenized in 0.25 M sucrose in a Potter–Elvehjem apparatus with a perspex pestle. Nuclei, unbroken cells and debris were removed by centrifugation at 1000 $\times$ *g* for 10 min. The supernatant was further centrifuged at 15 000 $\times$ *g* for 20 min to sediment the bulk of the amine storage particles. This supernatant was centrifuged at 286 000 $\times$ *g* for 30 min, and the final high-speed supernatant as well as the particulate fractions, was extracted with perchloric acid.

*Analysis*

The effect of secretory stimulation in the adrenal perfusions was monitored fluorimetrically by direct oxidation of small aliquots of the effluent fractions. The pooled fractions representing each stimulation period were then analysed separately.

Catechol compounds in the different extracts were adsorbed on alumina columns at pH 8.3. Non-catechols including tyrosine were removed by careful washing. Catechols were then eluted with 0.3 M acetic acid. Separation of the various catechol compounds in the eluate was carried out by ion-exchange column chromatography (Amberlite CG-120, sodium form, column size usually 4 $\times$ 50 mm, flow rate about

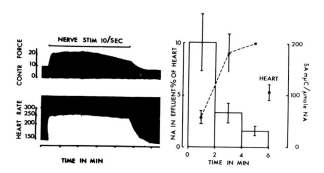

Fig. 1. Left panel: Typical record of effect of prolonged nerve stimulation at 10/sec on contractile force and on heart rate in the rabbit heart. Right panel: Effect of nerve stimulation for 4–6 min during infusion of [¹⁴C]tyrosine, $2 \times 10^{-5}$ M, on efflux of NA. Specific activity of NA in effluent and in heart at the end of the experiment. All values represent means $\pm$ S.E.M. of 7–9 observations, except for the 4–6-min period (1–2 observations).

3 ml/h). After removal of acid material including DOPA and metabolites by washing with 0.25 M sodium acetate, pH 4, NA and dopamine (DA) were separated by elution with 1 N HCl. In order to determine the possible occurrence of labelled adrenaline (A) formed during the adrenal perfusion, taller columns were occasionally used (4 × 180 mm).

The radioactivity in 1-ml aliquots of the different chromatographic fractions was determined by counting in 10 ml of Instagel (Packard Corp.) in a Packard Liquid Scintillation Spectrometer. Due to the low activity level in the samples, the apparatus was adjusted to count for 20 min or a minimum of 2000 impulses. In spite of the low activity, the values obtained on repeated counting showed good agreement. Fluorimetrically determined NA defined the position of the labelled NA in the chromatograms. The position of labelled DA was checked occasionally by determining the native fluorescence of non-labelled DA added as carrier.

Fluorimetric assay of NA and A was carried out by a modification of the method of von Euler and Lishajko (1961). In the adrenal experiments A was separately estimated by oxidation at pH 2 (Anton and Sayre, 1962), and NA by fluorimetric assay according to Merrills (1962), replacing ascorbate with thioglycolic acid (final concentration 0.2%).

## RESULTS

### Heart

Nerve stimulation produced a distinct increase in heart rate and contractile force. The chronotropic response was usually well maintained throughout the stimulation period, while the inotropic response exhibited variable degrees of fading (Fig. 1). During resting periods, NA in the effluent was below a measurable level. During the first 2 min of stimulation, NA efflux equalled about 10% of the NA finally remaining in the heart, only to fall progressively to very low levels during continued stimulation.

*References p. 267*

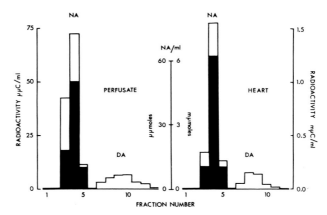

Fig. 2. Typical chromatogram demonstrating separation of NA from DA in heart and perfusate extracts.

Thus the decline in NA efflux far exceeded that in mechanical response to nerve stimulation.

Chromatographic analysis of the heart revealed the presence of labelled NA as well as of small amounts of DA formed from the labelled tyrosine (Fig. 2). In view of the lack of information concerning the degree of equilibration of exogenous tyrosine with endogenous tyrosine in that intraneuronal compartment which serves as the immediate source of tyrosine for NA formation, the activity levels were not used for calculation of the absolute rates of synthesis or of secretion of newly formed amines.

Newly formed NA, and in some experiments small amounts of labelled DA, were also found in the perfusate. The specific activity of NA in the perfusate rose during the stimulation period and towards the end was consistently about twice as high $(1.81 \pm 0.24, n = 9)$ as that in the heart (Fig. 1).

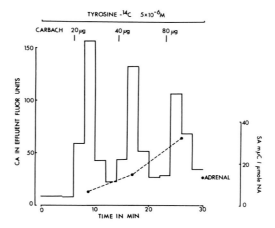

Fig. 3. Typical example of secretory effect of carbachol on perfused cat adrenal. Specific activity of NA in effluent and adrenal at the end of the experiment.

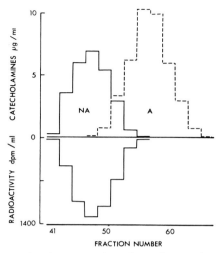

Fig. 4. Typical chromatogram showing separation of NA from A in perfused adrenal tissue, and absence of radioactivity in A peak.

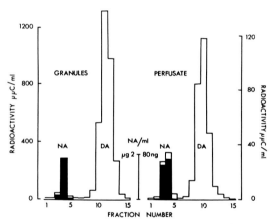

Fig. 5. Chromatogram, typical of several experiments showing separation of NA from DA in extracts of the 15 000 × *g* sediment from perfused adrenal and in effluent. Note predominance of DA in effluent.

*Adrenal*

Successively increased dosage of acetylcholine or carbachol was required to maintain about equal secretory response from the perfused cat adrenal (Fig. 3). The relative proportion of NA to total catecholamines (A + NA) in the effluent was considerably higher (1.80 ± 0.25, $n = 4$) than that in the adrenal, indicating that the secretory stimulus used induces preferential secretion of NA.

Chromatographic analysis revealed the formation of DA and NA, but not A (Fig. 4), from the labelled tyrosine, suggesting that the A formation is slow, that newly formed A is not preferentially secreted, or that newly formed NA has a distribution which prevents it from serving as an immediate precursor of A.

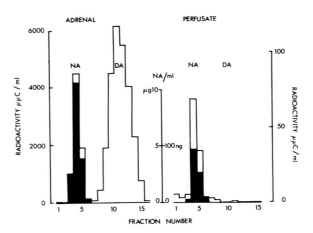

Fig. 6. Chromatogram, typical of several experiments, showing separation of NA from DA in extracts
of adrenal and perfusate. Note absence of DA in effluent.

Labelled DA accumulated in the adrenal in every experiment, making up $80.4 \pm 4.4$ ($n = 4$) % of the total labelled CA (NA + DA) in the gland, even including the 'large granule fraction' (Fig. 5). However, while the labelled DA appeared in the effluent during secretory stimulation in several experiments, it was completely absent from the perfusate in others (Fig. 6). Thus the type of stimulus used produced preferential secretion of NA, the relative proportion of labelled NA to total labelled CA (NA + DA) in the effluent as compared with that in adrenal tissue being $2.94 \pm 0.56$ ($n = 4$).

The specific activity of the NA secreted rose during the infusion of labelled tyrosine and repeated secretory stimulation, to reach a level during the last stimulation period considerably higher than that in adrenal tissue at the end of the experiment ($2.29 \pm 0.27$, $n = 4$).

### DISCUSSION

The experiments were designed to study the fate of newly formed CA in sympathetic nerves and adrenal medulla. Some incidental observations were made which appear to deserve a brief comment.

In the rabbit heart experiments newly formed DA was found in tissue as well as in effluent. The DA efflux might represent 'leakage' of precursor, secretion of DA as 'false transmitter' by the same mechanism which normally secretes NA (Thoenen and Tranzer, 1971), or secretion of DA as 'true' transmitter from dopaminergic neurons possibly existing in the heart (Angelakos *et al.*, 1963) and accidentally included in the nerve stimulation.

In adrenal medulla newly formed DA was also found to accumulate, even in the 'large granule fraction'. Part of this DA might be located in the postulated separate DA-storing particles (Lishajko, 1968). However, it seems possible that some accumulated in the NA-forming vesicles, in that case indicating latency in the DA $\beta$-hydroxylation process, possibly even product inhibition of this reaction by accumulation in this particular 'compartment' of newly formed NA (Laduron, 1969).

The variable appearance of DA in the effluent from the adrenal, following secretory stimulation, might represent 'leakage', secretion of DA as 'false hormone' by a mechanism which normally secretes NA, or specific secretion of DA as a 'true hormone', from separate 'dopaminergic' subcellular or cellular units (Lishajko, 1970). In agreement with the observations of Hempel and Männl (1969), in some instances DA was found to make up a very considerable proportion of the newly formed CA appearing in the effluent from the adrenal. However, in both studies the relative proportion of newly formed DA to NA was even higher in the tissue, suggesting selective retention of DA or preferential mobilization of NA.

In regard to the main issue, the results clearly show preferential secretion of newly formed NA, in adrenal medulla as well as in sympathetic nerves. The findings in the rabbit heart thus confirm the observations of Kopin *et al.* (1968), although the specific activity ratio of perfusate/tissue for NA was not as high in the present study. The observed preference for newly formed NA clearly emphasizes the importance of *de novo* synthesis of NA, not primarily for replacement of the NA secreted and thus lost from the stores, but for the maintenance of transmitter output during prolonged stimulation.

However, this should not obscure the probable role of recapture and reuse of preformed as well as of newly synthesized NA in this process (Hedqvist and Stjärne, 1969), as suggested by recent results obtained in the rabbit heart indicating that recapture of NA released by nerve stimulation in this tissue may be as high as 75% (Stjärne and Wennmalm, 1971).

In the cat adrenal gland Hempel and Männl (1969) previously reported preferential resting secretion of newly formed DA and NA. The present results show that this is true for the secretion induced by acetylcholine and its analogues as well.

The question now arises of how these findings can be reconciled with the hypothesis of secretion by exocytosis, which implies the simultaneous appearance in the effluent from stimulated adrenal gland or sympathetically innervated tissue of CA, the enzyme protein dopamine $\beta$-hydroxylase (DBO) (Viveros *et al.*, 1968; De Potter *et al.*, 1969) and the 'structural' protein chromagranin (CG) (De Potter *et al.*, 1969; Banks and Helle, 1965; Blaschko *et al.*, 1967), as well as of ATP or its metabolites (Douglas *et al.*, 1965). It has recently been proposed that such discharge of all soluble components of the CA vesicles, at least in adrenal medulla, may be an all-or-none process, forming the basis of 'quantal' secretion in this tissue (Viveros *et al.*, 1969; Kirshner and Viveros, 1970). This might be understood to imply that the amine vesicles represent disposable 'bags', prepackaged with their load of different secretory products, which might therefore be assumed to have the same turnover rate. Obviously preferential secretion of newly formed amines makes such an assumption unlikely, since the macromolecules of the vesicles most probably are formed in the perinuclear region, while ATP might be derived, possibly from mitochondria, at various levels in the cell, and the very presence of the enzyme DBO in the amine vesicles indicates that at least part of the amine formation occurs 'peripherally' in the cells (Fig. 7).

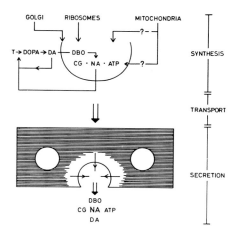

Fig. 7. Diagram representing features in synthesis and turnover of the amine vesicle membrane in sympathetic nerves and adrenal medulla, of the intravesicular macromolecules, dopamine β-hydroxylase (DBO) and chromogranin (CG), of adenine nucleotides, mainly ATP, and of CA. Formation of membranes and of macromolecules is assumed to occur in the perinuclear region of the cell body, while the intravesicular ATP involved in the storage complex is assumed to be generated in mitochondria, possibly at both central and peripheral parts of the cell. CA formation is indicated to occur at all levels, presumably in nerve tissue mainly in the periphery, while in adrenal medulla much of the amine synthesis may occur at an earlier stage, closer to the area of vesicle formation. The vesicles are transported to the 'periphery' to secrete their material directly onto the cell surface. CA formation is shown to be controlled by end-product inhibition of the rate-limiting initial hydroxylation of tyrosine (degree of shading, lower part of the figure) by extravesicular CA (including DA?). In the immediate vicinity of the secreting vesicle the tyrosine hydroxylation step is disinhibited, resulting in local acceleration of CA synthesis and in preferential secretion of the newly formed amine.

It thus seems that any hypothesis for CA secretion, in sympathetic nerves as well as in adrenal medulla, would have to allow for differences in turnover rates between the CA and other soluble intravesicular components, particularly the macromolecules, and for logistic reasons, especially in the nerves. While there is considerable experimental evidence that exocytosis is involved in the secretory mechanisms in adrenal medulla (Viveros *et al.*, 1968, 1969; Banks and Helle, 1965; Blaschko *et al.*, 1967; Douglas *et al.*, Kirshner and Viveros, 1970), and possibly also in sympathetic nerves (De Potter *et al.*, 1969), this may not be the whole story. Exocytosis, defined as the discharge of the various soluble components of the vesicles directly onto the cell surface, may be a process required for the simultaneous, focal secretion of the intravesicular micro- and macromolecules to the extracellular space (Stjärne, 1970). Persistence for some time of the 'gate' providing facilitated communication between the interior of the vesicles and the extracellular medium might allow continued secretion of amines, preformed and drawn from the immediate vicinity of the secreting vesicle, or newly synthesized. The resulting local disinhibition of the tyrosine hydroxylation process by local reduction in end-product inhibition of NA synthesis (Kopin, 1968) might explain the local acceleration of NA formation and the preferential secretion of the newly formed amine (Fig. 7).

ACKNOWLEDGEMENT

This work was in part carried out together with Dr. Å. Wennmalm, with the skilful technical assistance of Mrs. Maud Arwidsson and Miss H. Darbäck. It was supported by research grants from the Magnus Bergvall Foundation and the Knut and Alice Wallenberg Foundation.

REFERENCES

ANGELAKOS, E. T., FUXE, K. AND TORCHIANA, M. L. (1963) *Acta Physiol. Scand.*, **59**, 184.
ANTON, A. H. AND SAYRE, D. F. (1962) *J. Pharmacol. Exp. Therap.*, **138**, 360.
BANKS, P. AND HELLE, K. (1965) *Biochem. J.*, **97**, 40.
BESSON, M. J., CHERAMY, A., FELTZ, P. AND GLOWINSKI, J. (1969) *Proc. Natl. Acad. Sci. U.S.*, **62**, 741.
BLAKELEY, A. G. H., BROWN, G. L., DEARNALEY, D. P. AND HARRIS, V. (1969) *J. Physiol.*, **200**, 59P.
BLASCHKO, H., COMLINE, R. S., SCHNEIDER, F. H., SILVER, M. AND SMITH A. D. (1967) *Nature*, **215**, 58.
COLLIER, B. (1969) *J. Physiol.*, **205**, 341.
DE POTTER, W. P., DE SCHAEPDRYVER, A. F., MOERMAN, E. J. AND SMITH, A. D. (1969) *J. Physiol.*, **204**, 102P.
DOUGLAS, W. W., POISNER, A. M. AND RUBIN, R. P. (1965) *J. Physiol.*, **179**, 130.
VON EULER, U. S. AND LISHAJKO, F. (1961) *Acta Physiol. Scand.*, **51**, 348.
HEDQVIST, P. AND STJÄRNE, L. (1969) *Acta Physiol. Scand.*, **76**, 270.
HEDQVIST, P., STJÄRNE, L. AND WENNMALM, Å. (1970) *Acta Physiol. Scand.*, **79**, 139.
HEMPEL, K. AND MÄNNL, H. F. K. (1969) *Naunyn-Schmiedebergs Arch. Pharmakol.*, **264**, 363.
KIRSHNER, N. AND VIVEROS, O. H. (1970) In: G. KRONEBERG AND J. J. SCHÜMANN (Eds.) *Bayer Symposium II, 1969*, Springer, Verlag, Berlin.
KOPIN, I. J., BREESE, G. R., KRAUSS, K. R. AND WEISE, V. K. (1968) *J. Pharmacol. Exp. Therap.*, **161**, 271.
LADURON, P. (1969) *Biosynthèse, Localisation Intracellulaire et Transport des Catécholamines*, Vander, Louvain.
LISHAJKO, F. (1968) *Acta Physiol. Scand.*, **72**, 255.
LISHAJKO, F. (1970) *Acta Physiol. Scand.*, **79**, 405.
LÖFFELHOLTZ, K. AND MUSCHOLL, E. (1969) *Naunyn-Schmiedebergs Arch. Pharmakol.*, **265**, 1.
MERRILLS, R. J. (1962) *Nature*, **193**, 988.
SEDVALL, G. C., WEISE, V. K. AND KOPIN, I. J. (1968) *J. Pharmacol. Exp. Therap.*, **159**, 274.
STJÄRNE, L. (1971) to be published.
STJÄRNE, L. (1970) In: G. KRONEBERG AND H. J. SCHÜMANN (Eds.), *Bayer Symposium II, 1969*, Springer Verlag, Berlin.
STJÄRNE, L. AND WENNMALM, Å. (1971a) *Acta Physiol. Scand.*, **80**, 428.
STJÄRNE, L. AND WENNMALM, Å. (1971b) *Acta Physiol. Scand.*, **81**, 286.
THIERRY, A. M., BLANC, G. AND GLOWINSKI, J. (1970) *Europ. J. Pharmacol.*, **10**, 139.
THOENEN, H. AND TRANZER, J. P. (1971) this volume, p. 223.
VIVEROS, O. H., ARQUEROS, L. AND KIRSHNER, N. (1968) *Life Sci.*, **7**, 609.
VIVEROS, O. H., ARQUEROS, L. AND KIRSHNER, N. (1969) *Science*, **165**, 911.

# Blood Platelet as a Model for Monoaminergic Neurons

M. K. PAASONEN, LIISA AHTEE AND E. SOLATUNTURI

*Department of Pharmacology and Electron Microscope Laboratory, University of Helsinki*
*Helsinki (Finland)*

Blood platelets from various species contain or accumulate 5-hydroxytryptamine (5-HT), adrenaline, noradrenaline and dopamine, and rabbit platelets contain high amounts of histamine. There are certain similarities in the transfer, storage and metabolism of these amines in platelets and some other tissues, *e.g.* nerve endings and chromaffin cells. Therefore the platelet has become a model cell frequently employed by neuroscientists from different disciplines. Since in this symposium our report is the only one dealing with platelets, a considerable part of it will be devoted to giving a general picture of the platelet and its biogenic amines. For references and further details, recent reviews on this subject are available (Paasonen, 1965, 1968; Markwardt, 1968; Pletscher, 1968; Pletscher *et al.*, 1968).

## *Platelet morphology and storage of biogenic amines*

The ultrastructure of platelets has been studied since the beginning of electron microscopy (Wolpers and Ruska, 1939), and reviews on this topic have been published (Schulz, 1968; Michal and Firkin, 1969; Mustard and Packham, 1970). Mammalian blood platelets are small anuclear cells which change their shape easily in response to various stimuli such as a decrease in temperature, contact with foreign surfaces and the action of many drugs and agents. The shape of the platelets seen by electron microscopy also depends on the method of preparation. Normal platelets which have been rapidly fixed in plasma with glutaraldehyde and then with osmium tetroxide are usually disc-shaped with a diameter of about 1 to 3 $\mu$m (Fig. 1). Often they have pseudopod-like cytoplasmic protrusions.

The cell membrane of platelets is similar to many other cell membranes. It is composed of the usual unit membrane having a total thickness of about 8 nm. The platelet membrane adsorbs on its outer surface various materials such as plasma proteins and mucopolysaccharides (Nakao and Angrist, 1968) which form an extracellular coat.

Typical of blood platelets is a marginal bundle of microtubules lying along the cell membrane in the equatorial plane of the cell. The diameter of the platelet microtubules is about 20 to 30 nm, and they are composed of about 12 filamentous subunits (Behnke and Zelander, 1967). These subunits resemble the filaments or microfibrils that are seen in platelets crossing in the cytoplasm (Sixma and Molenaar, 1966). The micro-

*References pp. 277–279*

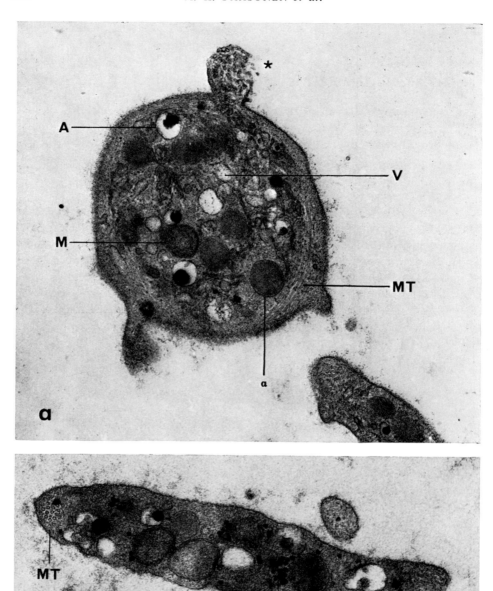

Fig. 1. Normal rabbit platelet sectioned in the equatorial plane (a) and in the transverse plane (b). Amine granules (A), α-granules (α), a mitochondrion (M), a bundle of microtubules (MT), vacuoles (V) and glycogen particles (G) are visible. Sometimes there are protrusions (*) containing circular structures of approximately the same diameter as the microtubules. Glutaraldehyde fixation in platelet-rich plasma at 25°C, postfixation with osmium tetroxide and lead citrate staining. × 50 000.

fibrils have been suggested to be thrombosthenin, the contractile protein of platelets (Zucker-Franklin and Bloomberg, 1969). The main function of the microtubules in platelets is probably to provide the shape of these cells. Platelet microtubules are labile structures and disappear when platelets become spherical in cold or when incubated with rather high concentrations of various agents such as colchicine, vinca alkaloids (White, 1968) and chlorpromazine (Fig. 2). Microtubules are also seen in platelet pseudopods where they may be newly formed during the pseudopod formation. The marginal bundle of microtubules also seems to take part in the movement of platelet granules during aggregation processes (White, 1969).

In normal platelets the intracellular organelles and inclusions are randomly distributed in the cytoplasm. Among them there are a few small and poorly developed mitochondria with few christae. Nevertheless, they may have an important role in the energy metabolism of platelets, especially in the production of ATP, of which there are great amounts in platelets (Gross, 1967). The platelets of man, rabbit, cattle and dog also exhibit considerable monoamine oxidase (MAO) activity, while this is missing in cat, horse and rat platelets (Paasonen and Solatunturi, 1965a). At least in rabbit platelets this MAO activity is limited solely to mitochondria (Solatunturi and Paasonen, 1966). An important part of the energy metabolism in platelets is based on glycolysis (Gross, 1967). The main energy store in these cells is glycogen which appears in platelets, as in many other cells, as small particles with a diameter of about 30 nm.

Platelets contain usually a number of vacuoles of various shapes and dimensions. These organelles can be involved in the phago- and exocytotic activities of platelets. Vacuoles, small vesicles and fine channels seen in platelets have been theorized as forming a canalicular system with connections to the cell surface (Firkin, 1968).

Platelets have two types of osmiophilic granules. The rather large (200 to 300 nm in diameter) $\alpha$-granules seem to be surrounded by a double membrane (Rodman, 1967) with a total thickness of about 20 nm. They contain hydrolytic enzymes and it has been suggested that they are platelet lysosomes (Day *et al.*, 1969).

In glutaraldehyde and osmium-fixed normal rabbit platelets there is another type of granule. These granules have a diameter of about 100 to 230 nm and are surrounded by a single membrane. They have a highly osmiophilic core which usually is somewhat smaller than the whole organelle. In most cases this core seems to be homogeneous in its electron density, but sometimes some inner granulations or density differences can be seen in it, especially in platelets fixed at room temperature for the preservation of microtubules. There is much evidence that the platelet 5-HT (and in rabbit platelets also histamine) is localized in these granules (Solatunturi and Paasonen, 1966; Tranzer *et al.*, 1966; Bak *et al.*, 1967; Solatunturi and Tuomisto, 1968) which are therefore called amine granules or 5-HT organelles. After incubation of these cells with 5-HT the amine granules can also be demonstrated in the platelets of species having very little or no 5-HT in their platelets (guinea pig, rat). Pletscher and coworkers (for references, see Born, 1970) have observed that in 5-HT organelles isolated in a pure form from rabbit platelets the proportion of 5-HT to ATP is about 2.3:1. The concentration of these two components within the organelles is incredibly high: 40 to 50% w/v, while the protein content is less than 1%.

*References pp. 277–279*

ATP and 5-HT when cooled in the above-mentioned molecular ratio, form micelles having a molecular weight of several hundreds of thousands (Berneis *et al.*, 1969; see also Born, 1970). Addition of $Mg^{2+}$ or $Ca^{2+}$ in low concentrations increases the molecular weight while higher concentrations have the opposite effect. ATP + noradrenaline + $Ca^{2+}$ also form micelles which are disrupted by increasing $Ca^{2+}$ or adding tyramine. It is tempting to assume that these phenomena work in the amine storage sites of the platelets, adrenal medulla and nerve endings.

### *Uptake, release and metabolism of biogenic amines*

Platelets do not synthesize their amines with the possible exception of histamine in the rabbit (Tuomisto, 1970). Therefore the amines must come from outside, and it is well established that 5-HT is taken up by platelets against a concentration gradient of several hundreds (Stacey, 1961). This concentration mechanism functions in two parts, firstly the amine is transferred through the cell membrane and secondly taken up by the granule. The initial rate of uptake of 5-HT into platelets follows Michaelis–Menten kinetics (Born and Gillson, 1959). The uptake involves a carrier mechanism of limited capacity which is temperature dependent and inhibited by various metabolic poisons. Sodium is necessary for this uptake, and it has been suggested that the hypothetical carrier forms a complex with 5-HT and sodium (Sneddon, 1969). When platelets are incubated with 5-HT there is an increased exchange of $K^+$ (Born, 1967) which could mean that the supposed carrier returns to the outside of the membrane associated with potassium (Sneddon, 1969). In addition to the energy-requiring mechanism passive diffusion of 5-HT also occurs when the concentration of amine outside the platelets is higher than about 20 $\mu$g/ml (Born and Bricknell, 1959).

Platelets accumulate adrenaline and noradrenaline, too, but this occurs at a much lower rate than the uptake of 5-HT and never reaches a high platelet/plasma ratio. Although diffusion may be a predominant mechanism of accumulation for these amines, an active process may also operate (Born and Smith, 1970). The uptake of dopamine by human platelets, on the other hand, has been recently demonstrated to be rather similar to that of 5-HT (Boullin and O'Brien, 1970). In contrast to 5-HT, dopamine is lost rapidly from platelets, although dopamine has a high affinity for the 5-HT storage granules (Da Prada and Pletscher, 1969). Metaraminol, which has a high affinity for noradrenaline storage sites is taken up by human and rabbit platelets against a concentration gradient of at least 40 (Ahtee and Saarnivaara, in press). The rate of uptake of histamine by rabbit platelets resembles that of adrenaline. There is reason to believe that active transport is involved. It has been emphasized, however, that the limiting step here, and perhaps with other amines as well, is the platelet membrane and not the concentrating mechanism of the storage granules (Tuomisto, 1968a).

5-HT is released from platelets by various rauwolfia alkaloids and related agents without a clear change in platelet structure. The main point of action of these agents is in the amine storage sites (Pletscher *et al.*, 1968). Reserpine also liberates histamine from rabbit platelets both *in vivo* and *in vitro* although this release is slower than

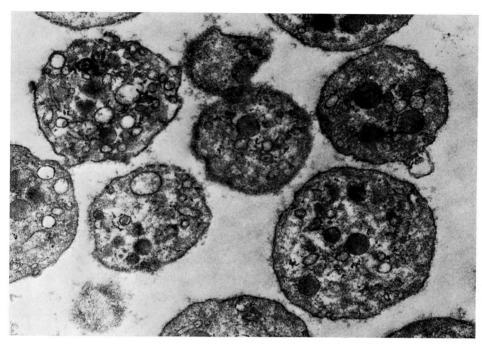

Fig. 2. Rabbit platelets which have been incubated in plasma at 37°C for 1 h with $10^{-3}$ M chlorpromazine are without microtubules and electron-dense amine granules. Their cell membranes are broken. Preparation for electron microscopy as in Fig. 1. × 20 000.

5-HT release, probably due to the poor membrane permeability of histamine (Tuomisto, 1968b). A number of phenothiazine derivatives such as chlorpromazine have been found in our laboratory to cause 5-HT and histamine release from rabbit and human platelets *in vitro*, as will be discussed later. Various aliphatic and aromatic amines liberate 5-HT by displacing it at the storage sites (May *et al.*, 1969). The release of histamine by these amines, however, is the result of cytolysis. Generally compounds releasing 5-HT also release histamine from platelets as well as catecholamines after their accumulation in the platelets.

It is assumed that platelets retain their 5-HT, or some portion of it, for as long as they exist. However, if 5-HT is released *in vitro* by tetrabenazine for example, due to their MAO the platelets metabolize their 5-HT. 5-Hydroxyindoleacetaldehyde is first formed, and in the presence of red cells which supply aldehyde dehydrogenase (ADG), this is transformed to 5-hydroxyindoleacetic acid (Paasonen and Airaksinen, 1965). If ADG is not available the aldehyde is reduced to 5-hydroxytryptophol. Isolated platelets metabolize exogenous dopamine in a way related to that of 5-HT,

Platelet destruction including 5-HT and histamine release is also caused by cytolytic agents, proteolytic enzymes such as thrombin and trypsin, bacterial endotoxins, some animal venoms, antigen–antibody reactions, glycogen and several long-chain saturated fatty acids. The reaction is always very fast and often requires calcium (Markwardt, 1968).

*i.e.* into 3,4-dihydroxyphenylethanol and 3,4-dihydroxyphenylacetic acid (Pletscher, 1968). There is no catechol-*O*-methyl transferase in human platelets, but MAO, at least in rabbit platelets, under certain circumstances can inactivate adrenaline (Lahovaara *et al.*, 1968).

*Platelet as a model in pharmacology*

It has been found in our laboratory that chlorpromazine and related drugs cause release of 5-HT and histamine from blood platelets *in vitro*. In contrast to reserpine chloropromazine causes morphological changes in platelets damaging the plasma membrane and inducing the leakage of other cellular constituents (Paasonen, 1964; Telkkä *et al.*, 1964; Paasonen and Solatunturi, 1965b; Ahtee, 1966; Solatunturi, 1968). Chlorpromazine also has an affinity for the amine-storing granules which its non-tranquillizing analogue chlorpromazine sulphoxide does not possess (Solatunturi and Ahtee, 1968), although both of these phenothiazine derivatives are taken up by platelets to a similar degree (Ahtee and Paasonen, 1966). However, no change could be found in the subcellular distribution of 5-HT in chlorpromazine-treated platelets except when more than half of the 5-HT was released (Solatunturi and Ahtee, 1968).

The 5-HT release by chlorpromazine *in vitro* could be due to its membrane effects (Guth and Spirtes, 1964). In doses lower than that causing 5-HT release chlorpromazine prevents the hypotonic release of 5-HT from platelets (Ahtee, 1966) probably by stabilizing the platelet membrane similarly as it inhibits the hypotonic haemolysis of red cells. However, the haemolytic activity and 5-HT release could not be completely correlated, *e.g.* the demethylated derivatives caused more 5-HT release from platelets but were less active haemolysers than their tertiary amine derivatives (Ahtee and Paasonen, 1965, 1968a; Ahtee, 1966).

The membrane mechanism for 5-HT uptake into platelets in many ways resembles the uptake of noradrenaline into sympathetic nerve endings and synaptosomes. In sympathetic tissues in addition to the uptake into nerve endings there is another uptake mechanism which most probably represents the uptake into extraneuronal tissues. The second uptake process has been named 'uptake₂' to distinguish it from the neuronal process, 'uptake₁' (Iversen, 1967). In the perfused rat heart these two concentrating mechanisms, one of which operates at very low concentrations of noradrenaline (uptake₁) and the other (uptake₂) at higher ones, are inhibited differently by various drugs.

We studied human platelets to see whether the same inhibitor specificity could be found in the platelets, too, when both low and high noradrenaline concentrations are employed. The uptake of noradrenaline in a modified Tyrode solution was linear for about an hour when either a $10^{-7}$ M or $10^{-4}$ M noradrenaline concentration was used. Table 1 summarizes the effects of some drugs on the uptake of noradrenaline in the rat heart and human platelets. The results demonstrate clear differences in noradrenali-line uptake inhibitor specificity between rat adrenergic neurons and human platelets (Lahovaara *et al.*, 1970).

Imipramine is a more effective inhibitor of 5-HT uptake into human platelets than

TABLE 1

CONCENTRATIONS OF SOME DRUGS PRODUCING 50% INHIBITION OF NORADRENALINE
UPTAKE BY RAT HEART (see Iversen, 1967) AND HUMAN PLATELETS

| Heart | | Platelets | |
|---|---|---|---|
| Uptake$_1$ | | [$^3$H]NA $10^{-7}$M | |
| Desipramine | $1.3 \times 10^{-8}$M | Metaraminol | $2.3 \times 10^{-6}$M |
| Metaraminol | $7.6 \times 10^{-8}$M | Metanephrine | $3.5 \times 10^{-5}$M |
| Cocaine | $3.8 \times 10^{-7}$M | Desipramine | $5.0 \times 10^{-4}$M |
| Metanephrine | $4.3 \times 10^{-5}$M | Cocaine | $\sim 5.0 \times 10^{-2}$M |
| Uptake$_2$ | | NA $10^{-4}$M + [$^3$H]NA $10^{-7}$M | |
| Metanephrine | $2.9 \times 10^{-6}$M | Desipramine | $\sim 5.0 \times 10^{-5}$M |
| Desipramine | $\leq 1.0 \times 10^{-4}$M | Cocaine | $6.0 \times 10^{-5}$M |
| Cocaine | $>2.0 \times 10^{-4}$M | Metaraminol | $\sim 2.0 \times 10^{-4}$M |
| Metaraminol | $>5.0 \times 10^{-4}$M | Metanephrine | $\sim 7.0 \times 10^{-4}$M |

desipramine, although desipramine as well as other antidepressants containing secondary amine structures are more active 5-HT releasers than the tertiary analogues (Ahtee *et al.*, 1968). This agrees with the findings of Carlsson and co-workers (1969a) that imipramine and tertiary amines in general were more potent in blocking the uptake of 5-HT into neurons.

There is a great deal of evidence that the antidepressants containing secondary amine structures, such as desipramine and protriptyline, are potent inhibitors of noradrenaline uptake (Iversen, 1967; Carlsson *et al.*, 1969b) both in the central and peripheral neurons. When we compared the abilities of some antidepressants to inhibit the uptake of metaraminol and 5-HT into human blood platelets, it was found that imipramine was by far the most potent inhibitor of 5-HT uptake. However, when the uptake of metaraminol was studied, compounds with a secondary amine structure were 15 to 30 times more potent than imipramine (Ahtee and Saarnivaara, in press).

6-Hydroxydopamine (6-OHDA) accumulates in the peripheral sympathetic neurons causing noradrenaline depletion and destruction of amine storage sites (Thoenen and Tranzer, 1968). After intraventricular administration of 6-OHDA Uretsky and Iversen (1970) demonstrated a clear depletion of dopamine and noradrenaline but not of 5-HT in the rat brain. 6-OHDA is a competitive inhibitor of noradrenaline uptake in rat hypothalamus and striatum *in vitro*, but does not interfere with 5-HT uptake under similar conditions (Iversen, 1970). In our experiments 6-OHDA did not release 5-HT from platelets *in vitro* except when platelets were incubated with 10 mM concentrations for several hours. Neither did it release 5-HT from rabbit platelets *in vivo* in a significant amount. We also studied whether it inhibits the uptake of 5-HT or noradrenaline into human platelets *in vitro*. Not until present in a concentration of 10 mM did it have a significant inhibitory effect on 5-HT uptake. Under similar conditions noradrenaline uptake was inhibited by a 1 mM concentration. However, these amounts of 6-OHDA are far above the 10 $\mu$M concentration

TABLE 2

BIOGENIC AMINES IN PLATELETS, CHROMAFFIN CELLS AND NERVE TERMINALS

|  | Platelets | Chromaffin cells | Nerve terminals |
|---|---|---|---|
| Synthesis of amines | No | Yes | Yes |
| Storage of amines | Yes | Yes | Yes |
| Storage granules | 100–230 nm | 100–300 nm | 40–60, 80–120 nm |
| Granular amine stability *in vitro* | Moderate | Good | Poor |
| Ratio: Amine/ATP | 2.3 | 4–5 | 4–5 |
| Amine-uptake inhibitors (*e.g.*) | Ouabain, Cocaine, Imipramine, Desipramine, Reserpine, Prenylamine | Ouabain, Cocaine, Desipramine, Imipramine, Reserpine, Prenylamine | Ouabain, Cocaine, Despramine, Imipramine, Reserpine, Prenylamine |
| Amine releasers (*e.g.*) | Reserpine, Prenylamine, Chlorpromazine, Tyramine, Thrombin | Reserpine, Prenylamine, Chlorpromazine, Tyramine, Acetylcholine, Thrombin | Reserpine, Prenylamine, 6-OHDA, Tyramine, Nerve impulse |
| $Ca^{2+}$ required for release by | Thrombin | Acetylcholine | Nerve impulse |

found to be effective by Iversen. Most probably these differences result from the fact that platelets take up predominantly 5-HT and the uptake of other monoamines is more difficult and less frequent.

### General remarks

Table 2, a major part of which has already been discussed above, gives a short summary of biogenic amines in blood platelets, chromaffin cells and nerve terminals. One of the main differences between these three locations is that platelets do not synthesize their amines while the others do. Another difference is a morphological one. The amine granules of platelets are of about the same size as the amine storage granules of adrenomedullary cells (Wetzstein, 1957), the enterochromaffin cells of the intestinal mucosa (Penttilä, 1968) and the granulated vesicles of nerve cells in the hypothalamus (Pellegrino de Iraldi *et al.*, 1963). They are larger than the 'small granulated vesicles' in postganglionic adrenergic axons (Potter, 1966) and smaller than the amine-containing 'large granules' in mastocytoma cells (Hagen *et al.*, 1959). From all the amine organelles mentioned, the platelet amine granules seem to have the greatest equilibrium density (2.0 to 2.6 M) in sucrose density gradient experiments.

The ratio of cholesterol to phospholipids in the platelet membrane is lower than in red cells or muscle cells (Marcus *et al.*, 1967) and is quite similar to this ratio in adrenal medulla and synaptosomes. This may be important because monoamines such as 5-HT and noradrenaline are absorbed by phospholipids by a saturable process (Norlander, 1950; Ahtee and Johnson, unpublished) which might be influenced by the proportion of cholesterol.

The amine-uptake inhibitors include at least two types of compounds. Imipramine and desipramine are typical 'membrane pump' inhibitors. The main site of action, but not necessarily the mechanism of action, of cocaine and ouabain is probably the membrane, too. Reserpine-like drugs and prenylamine act on the intracellular stores. The uptake of monoamines into platelets can also be increased. Pretreatment with lithium increases monoamine uptake into platelets as it increases the uptake of noradrenaline into synaptosomes (Colburn *et al.*, 1967; Murphy *et al.*, 1969).

Agents belonging to several groups most probably acting by different mechanisms are mentioned as amine releasers. Here certain differences among the three locations are obvious.

The results obtained for platelets have often been applied to other tissues. The most active releasers of 5-HT from the platelets have been found to be the most active catecholamine releasers from the perfused adrenal gland and even, at high doses, to cause a release of 5-HT from rabbit lung (Ahtee and Paasonen, 1968b; Vapaatalo *et al.*, 1966). On the other hand, contrary to the psychotropic phenothiazine derivatives, we found some derivatives with little or no central action to be inactive as releasers of 5-HT from platelets and not to prevent the oxygen consumption by and ATPase in platelets (Ahtee and Paasonen, 1968c; Ahtee, 1970). Like sympathetic neurons platelets accumulate debrisoquin (Pocelinko and Solomon, 1970) and guanethidine (Boullin and O'Brien, 1969). It is also interesting that in some pathological states, *e.g.* mongolism, certain types of cerebral palsy and parkinsonism, the behaviour of monoamines in the platelets is changed and may reflect changes in the nervous system.

The usefulness of platelets as a pharmacological model for adrenergic neurons has been emphasized by Solomon and co-workers (1969) among others. This cell may be even more suitable for use as a model for 5-HT-neurons.

## ACKNOWLEDGEMENTS

The authors' present studies have been supported in part by the Sigrid Jusélius Foundation, Finland, and the National Research Council for Medical Sciences, Finland.

## REFERENCES

AHTEE, L. (1966) *Ann. Med. Exp. Fenniae*, **44**, 431–452.
AHTEE, L. (1970) Effect of substituted phenothiazines and related compounds on the Na+, K+-activated adenosine triphosphatase activity in blood platelets. *Abstracts of the Meeting for the 150 Anniversary of Prof. R. Bucheim, Tartu*, pp. 13–14.
AHTEE, L. AND PAASONEN, M. K. (1965) *Ann. Med. Exp. Fenniae*, **43**, 101–105.
AHTEE, L. AND PAASONEN, M. K. (1966) *J. Pharm. Pharmacol.*, **18**, 126–128.
AHTEE, L. AND PAASONEN, M. K. (1968a) *Acta Pharmacol. Toxicol.*, **26**, 213–221.
AHTEE, L. AND PAASONEN, M. K. (1968b) *Ann. Med. Exp. Fenniae*, **46**, 45–48.
AHTEE, L. AND PAASONEN, M. K. (1968c) *Ann. Med. Exp. Fenniae.*, **46**, 423–428.
AHTEE, L., TUOMISTO, J., SOLATUNTURI, E. AND PAASONEN, M. K. (1968) *Ann. Med. Exp. Fenniae*, **46**, 429–434.
BAK, I. J., HASSLER, R., MAY, B. AND WESTERMANN, E. (1967) *Life Sci.*, **6**, 1133–1146.
BEHNKE, O. AND ZELANDER, T. (1967) *J. Ultrastruct. Res.*, **19**, 147–165.
BERNEIS, K. H., DA PRADA, M. AND PLETSCHER, A. (1969) *Agents and Actions*, **1**, 35–38.

BORN, G. V. R. (1967) *J. Physiol.*, **190**, 273–280.
BORN, G. V. R. (1970) In: R. EIGENMANN (Ed.), *Proc. IVth Intern. Congr. Pharmacol.*, *Vol. II, Basel, 1969*, Schwabe & Co., Basel, pp. 38–58.
BORN, G. V. R. AND BRICKNELL, J. (1959) *J. Physiol.*, **147**, 153–161.
BORN, G. V. R. AND GILLSON, R. E. (1959) *J. Physiol.*, **146**, 472–491.
BORN, G. V. R. AND SMITH, J. B. (1970) *Brit. J. Pharmacol.*, **39**, 765–778.
BOULLIN, D. J. AND O'BRIEN, R. A. (1969) *Brit. J. Pharmacol.*, **35**, 90–102.
BOULLIN, D. J. AND O'BRIEN, R. A. (1970) *Brit. J. Pharmacol.*, **39**, 779–788.
CARLSSON, A., CORRODI, H., FUXE, K. AND HÖKFELT, T. (1969a) *Europ. J. Pharmacol.*, **5**, 357–366.
CARLSSON, A., CORRODI, H., FUXE, K. AND HÖKFELT, T. (1969b) *Europ. J. Pharmacol.*, **5**, 367–373.
COLBURN, R. W., GOODWIN, F. K., BUNNEY, W. E. JR. AND DAVIS, J. M. (1967) *Nature*, **215**, 1395–1397.
DA PRADA, M. AND PLETSCHER, A. (1969) *Life Sci.*, **8**, 65–72.
DAY, H. J., HOLMSEN, H. AND HOVIG, T. (1969) *Scand. J. Haematol.*, *Suppl.* **7**, 1–35.
FIRKIN, B. G. (1968) In G. V. R. BORN (Ed.), *Proc. Third Intern. Pharmacol. Meeting*, Vol. 6, Pergamon Press Ltd., London, pp. 67–73.
GROSS, R. (1967) In: K. M. BRINKHOUS, J. S. WRIGHT, J. P. SOULIER, H. R. ROBERTS AND S. HINNOM (Eds.), *Platelets: Their Role in Hemostasis and Thrombosis*, F. K. Schattauer-Verlag, Stuttgart, pp.143–154.
GUTH, P. S. AND SPIRTES, M. A. (1964) *Intern. Rev. Neurobiol.*, **7**, 231–278.
HAGEN, P., BARRNETT, R. J. AND LEE, F.-L. (1959) *J. Pharmacol. Exp. Therap.*, **126**, 91–108.
IVERSEN, L. L. (1967) *The Uptake and Storage of Noradrenaline in Sympathetic Nerves*, University Press, Cambridge.
IVERSEN, L. L. (1970) *Europ. J. Pharmacol.*, **10**, 408–410.
LAHOVAARA, S., NEUVONEN, P. AND PAASONEN, M. K. (1970) *Scand. J. Clin. Lab Invest.*, **25**, *Suppl.* 113, 18.
LAHOVAARA, S., PAASONEN, M. K. AND AIRAKSINEN, M. M. (1968) *Ann. Med. Exp. Fenniae*, **46**, 453–456.
MARCUS, A. J., BRADLOW, B. A., SAFIER, L. B. AND ULLMAN, H. L. (1967) *Thromb. Diath. Haemorrhag.*, *Suppl.* **26**, 43–52.
MARKWARDT, F. (1968) *Ann. Med. Exp. Fenniae*, **46**, 407–415.
MAY, B., MENKENS, I. AND WESTERMANN, E. (1969) *Naunyn-Schmiedeberg's Arch. Pharmakol.*, **265**, 24–48.
MICHAL, F. AND FIRKIN, B. G. (1969) *Ann. Rev. Pharmacol*, **9**, 95–118.
MURPHY, D. L., COLBURN, R. W., DAVIS, J. M. AND BUNNE.Y, W. E. JR. (1969) *Life Sci.*, **8**, 1187–1193.
MUSTARD, J. F. AND PACKHAM, M. A. (1970) *Pharmacol. Rev.*, **22**, 97–187.
NAKAO, K. AND ANGRIST, A. A. (1968) *Nature*, **217**, 960–961.
NORLANDER, O. (1950) *Acta Physiol. Scand.*, **21**, 325–331.
PAASONEN, M. K. (1964) *Naunyn-Schmiedeberg's Arch. Exp. Pathol. Pharmakol.*, **248**, 223–230.
PAASONEN, M. K. (1965) *J. Pharm. Pharmacol.*, **17**, 681–697.
PAASONEN, M. K. (1968) *Ann. Med. Exp. Fenniae*, **46**, 416–422.
PAASONEN, M. K. AND AIRAKSINEN, M. M. (1965) *Ann. Med. Exp. Fenniae*, **43**, 236–240.
PAASONEN, M. K. AND SOLATUNTURI, E. (1965a) *Ann. Med. Exp. Fenniae*, **43**, 98–100.
PAASONEN, M. K. AND SOLATUNTURI, E. (1965b) *Ann. Med. Exp. Fenniae*, **43**, 241–244.
PELLEGRINO DE IRALDI, A., FARINI DUGGAN, H. AND DE ROBERTIS, E. (1963) *Anat. Rec.*, **145**, 521–531.
PENTTILÄ, A. (1968) *Ann. Med. Exp. Fenniae*, **46**, 457–465.
PLETSCHER, A. (1968) *Brit. J. Pharmacol.*, **32**, 1–16.
PLETSCHER, A., DA PRADA, M. AND TRANZER, J. P. (1968) *Ann. Med. Exp. Fenniae*, **46**, 399–406.
POCELINKO, R. AND SOLOMON, H. M. (1970) *Biochem. Pharmacol.*, **19**, 697–703.
POTTER, L. T. (1966) *Pharmacol. Rev.*, **18**, 439–451.
RODMAN, N. F. (1967) In: BRINKHOUS, K. M., WRIGHT, J. S., SOULIER, J. P., ROBERTS, H. R. AND HINNOM, S. (Eds.), *Platelets: Their Role in Hemostasis and Thrombosis*, F. K. Schattauer-Verlag, Stuttgart, pp. 9–19.
SCHULZ, H. (1968) *Thrombocyten und Thrombose im elektronenmikroskopischen Bild*, Springer-Verlag, Berlin.
SIXMA, J. J. AND MOLENAAR, I. (1966) *Thromb. Diath. Haemorrhag.*, **16**, 153–162.
SNEDDON, J. M. (1969) *Brit. J. Pharmacol.*, **37**, 680–688.
SOLATUNTURI, E. (1968) *Ann. Med. Exp. Fenniae*, **46**, 435–440.

SOLATUNTURI, E. AND AHTEE, L. (1968) *J. Pharm. Pharmacol.*, **20**, 289–292.

SOLATUNTURI, E. AND PAASONEN, M. K. (1966) *Ann. Med. Exp. Fenniae*, **44**, 427–430.

SOLATUNTURI, E. AND TUOMISTO, J. (1968) *Ann. Med. Exp. Fenniae*, **46**, 447–452.

SOLOMON, H. M., ASHLEY, C., SPIRT, N. AND ABRAMS, W. B. (1969) *Clin. Pharmacol. Therap.*, **10**, 229–238.

STACEY, R. S. (1961) *Brit. J. Pharmacol.*, **16**, 284–295.

TELKKÄ, A., NYHOLM, M. AND PAASONEN, M. K. (1964) *Experientia*, **20**, 27–28.

THOENEN, H. AND TRANZER, J. P. (1968) *Naunyn-Schmiedeberg's Arch. Pharmakol.*, **261**, 271–288.

TRANZER, J. P., DA PRADA, M. AND PLETSCHER, A. (1966) *Nature*, **212**, 1574–1575.

TUOMISTO, J. (1968a) *Ann. Med. Exp. Fenniae*, **46**, 330–339.

TUOMISTO, J. (1968b) *Ann. Med. Exp. Fenniae*, **46**, 441–446.

TUOMISTO, J. (1970) *Ann. Med. Exp. Fenniae*, **48**, 164–167.

URETSKY, N. J. AND IVERSEN, L. L. (1970) *J. Neurochem.*, **17**, 269–278.

VAPAATALO, H. J., AHTEE, L. AND PAASONEN, M. K. (1966) *Ann. Med. Exp. Fenniae*, **44**, 464–468.

WETZSTEIN, R. (1957) *Z. Zellforsch.*, **46**, 517–576.

WHITE, J. G. (1968) *Amer. J. Pathol.*, **53**, 281–291.

WHITE, J. G. (1969) *Amer. J. Pathol.*, **54**, 467–478.

WOLPERS, C. AND RUSKA, H. (1939) *Klin. Wochschr.*, **23**, 1077–1081 and 1111–1117.

ZUCKER-FRANKLIN, D. AND BLOOMBERG, N. (1969) *J. Clin. Invest.*, **48**, 165–175.

# Mast Cell as a Model for Uptake and Storage of 5-Hydroxytryptamine

S.-E. JANSSON

*Department of Anatomy, University of Helsinki, Helsinki (Finland)*

Mast cells contain large amounts of histamine and, in rat and mouse, 5-hydroxytryptamine (5-HT). Uvnäs and his group (1970) have clarified the process of binding and release of histamine in mast cells. Green and Furano (Green, 1966) and Day and Stockbridge (1964) studied the uptake of several amines using neoplastic ascites tumour mast cells, Eränkö and Kauko (1965) mesenteric, Eränkö and Jansson (1967) peritoneal mast cells.

Because of the high endogenous content of 5-HT (some 0.6 $\mu$g/$10^6$ mast cells) and because of the ease with which the cells can be handled, the uptake and storage of 5-HT in normal mast cells, investigated by the present author, show that the mast cell serves as a useful comparative model for the adrenergic neurons.

### Uptake of 5-HT in mast cells in vitro

Day and Stockbridge (1964) demonstrated that neoplastic mast cells take up 5-HT by two mechanisms: firstly, passive diffusion and secondly, active uptake dependent on energy from cellular metabolism.

Observations by the present author suggest that normal mast cells handle the amine in a similar way, *i.e.* at low concentrations of exogenous 5-HT the amine is taken up by an active mechanism, while at high concentrations of 5-HT the amine is incorporated by a passive mechanism.

(1) The uptake showed the following saturation characteristics (Jansson, 1970a): maximum uptake during 1 h at 37° C was achieved at about 0.5 $\mu$g/ml of exogenous 5-HT, and higher concentrations in the medium did not accelerate the uptake during the first hour. The amine was readily taken up from low concentrations (0.1 to 0.44 $\mu$g/ml) and was concentrated in the cell more than 1000 times. The uptake was fairly rapid during the first hour but was slower during succeeding hours.

(2) The uptake was highly temperature dependent (Jansson, 1970a): at 0° C little uptake occurred; at room temperature the uptake was dependent on the 5-HT concentration of the medium (Fig. 1).

(3) The uptake was depressed by uncouplers of oxidative phosphorylation (dinitrophenol and carbonyl cyanide *p*-trifluoromethoxy phenylhydrazone); metabolic inhibitors such as sodium cyanide and sodium azide had no significant effect on the uptake (Jansson, 1970a).

*References pp. 289–290*

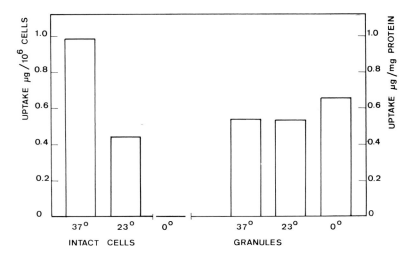

Fig. 1. Effect of temperature on the uptake of 5-HT by intact mast cells and isolated mast cell granules. Samples incubated for 1 h at a 5-HT concentration of 0.44 μg/ml (intact cells) of 4.4 μg/ml (granules).

(4) The uptake was dependent on calcium and magnesium ions; it dropped to about 40% of the control uptake if these ions were omitted (Jansson, 1970a).

(5) The uptake was depressed by drugs such as reserpine, prenylamine, imipramine, mepyramine, chlorpromazine, cocaine, amitriptyline and ouabain at concentrations which had little effect on the endogenous 5-HT content of the intact cells (Jansson, 1970a, b, c).

TABLE 1

EFFECT OF VARIOUS DRUGS ON THE UPTAKE OF 5-HT BY INTACT MAST CELLS

Samples were incubated with the drug for 30 min at 37° C before 0.44 μg/ml 5-HT was added. The uptake with drug (difference between original and 5-HT content reached in μg) is expressed in per cent of the control uptake observed under identical conditions but without drug.

| Drug | Molar concentration | Uptake in the presence of drug (per cent of control uptake) |
|---|---|---|
| Prenylamine | $10^{-5}$ | 0* |
| Reserpine | $10^{-5}$ | 17 |
| Chlorpromazine | $10^{-5}$ | 1 |
| Imipramine | $10^{-5}$ | 16 |
| Mepyramine | $10^{-4}$ | 0** |
| Ouabain | $10^{-5}$ | 57 |
| Cocaine | $10^{-5}$ | 2 |
| Amitriptyline | $10^{-5}$ | 9 |

\*   5-HT content 23% below original level.
\*\* 5-HT content 32% below original level.

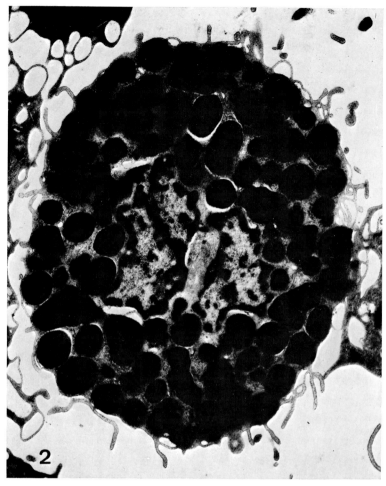

Fig. 2. Normal rat peritoneal mast cells incubated for 1 h in the Krebs–Ringer–glucose solution. Note the highly osmiophilic granules which fill up the cytoplasm. Electron micrograph. × 8000.

This apparently active uptake resulted in an increase of the 5-HT content of the mast cells with about 0.6 $\mu$g/$10^6$ mast cells during 1 h at 37° C at an exogenous 5-HT concentration of 0.44 $\mu$g/ml. No correlation to the endogenous 5-HT content was noted. During a long incubation in a medium with a high concentration of 5-HT (4.4 $\mu$g/ml) the uptake increased for at least 4 h (Jansson, 1970a). This raises the problem of the binding site of 5-HT. It therefore seemed of interest to study the distribution of 5-HT within the mast cells after incubation in this amine.

### Distribution of 5-HT in mast cells in vitro

Fluorescence microscopy using semi-ultrathin Epon sections revealed that the specific fluorescence of 5-HT was limited to the granules (Fig. 5), indicating that 5-HT is

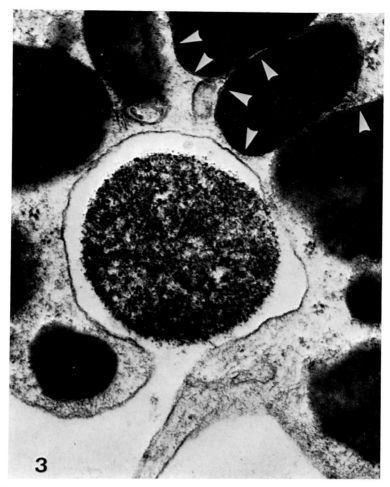

Fig. 3. Higher magnification of a rat peritoneal mast cell showing that a tight perigranular membrane surrounds intracellular granules (arrowheads). One granule (centre) shows a particulate internal structure and is situated inside a vacuole communicating with the surrounding medium, suggesting exocytosis. Electron micrograph. × 70 000.

principally bound to the granules and that normally there is no free 5-HT in the cytoplasm (Jansson, 1970b).

Incubation in 5-HT made the granules more intensely fluorescent, but the intergranular cytoplasm was still non-fluorescent. This indicates that the major part of the exogenous 5-HT was incorporated into the granules (Fig. 6).

Confirmation of these results was obtained by measuring the 5-HT content in the different fractions after freezing and thawing and differential centrifugation. The percentage of 5-HT recovered from the supernatant of the experimentally treated cells was the same as that which could be recovered from the supernatant of control material.

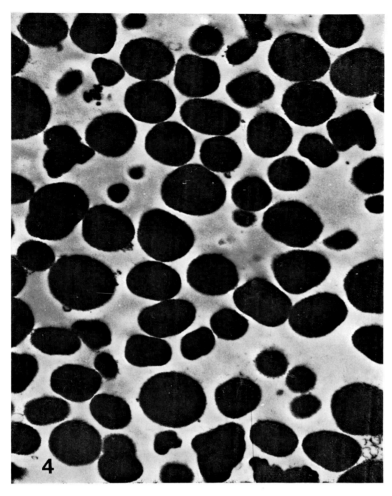

Fig. 4. The granule-containing sediment obtained after differential centrifugation of frozen and thawed mast cell suspension. The sediment consists of a virtually pure mast cell granule fraction. Note that the granules are not surrounded by any membrane. Electron micrograph. × 8500.

Release experiments with drugs and pH variations also indicated that exogenous and endogenous 5-HT are similarly bound to the granules (Jansson, 1970b).

Reserpine and imipramine depressed 5-HT uptake by intact mast cells, but these drugs were not able to alter the normal granular location of 5-HT. The percentage of 5-HT recovered from the supernatant after freezing and thawing and differential centrifugation of cells incubated with drug and 5-HT was the same as that which could be recovered from the supernatant of cells incubated with 5-HT only (Jansson, 1970b). This observation was also confirmed by fluorescence microscopy which revealed that 5-HT taken up despite drug block was incorporated into the granules. In order to study the reserpine-resistant granular uptake of 5-HT, experiments with isolated mast cell granules were performed.

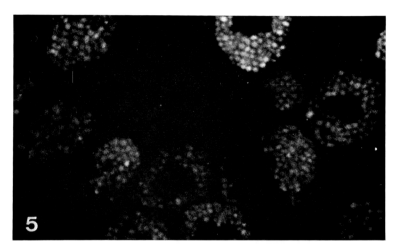

Fig. 5. Fluorescence photomicrographs of rat peritoneal mast cells after exposure to formaldehyde vapour. 1 $\mu$ Epon section. The mast cells show a distinct fluorescence due to their 5-HT content which is exclusively distributed among the granules, leaving the intergranular cytoplasm virtually non-fluorescent. $\times$ 1200.

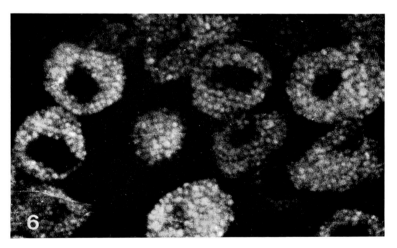

Fig. 6. Fluorescence photomicrograph of another sample from the same batch of cells as in Fig. 5 but incubated in a medium containing 0.44 $\mu$g/ml 5-HT. Formaldehyde-induced fluorescence. 1 $\mu$ Epon section. Note the increased fluorescence intensity as compared with Fig. 5. The fluorescence is still granularly distributed despite the 5-HT uptake. $\times$ 1200.

### Uptake of 5-HT by isolated mast cell granules

Isolation of mast cell granules was performed according to Lagunoff *et al.* (1964) and Thon and Uvnäs (1966). After freezing and thawing of the peritoneal cell suspension in isotonic sucrose, pH 6.9, differential centrifugation produced two par-

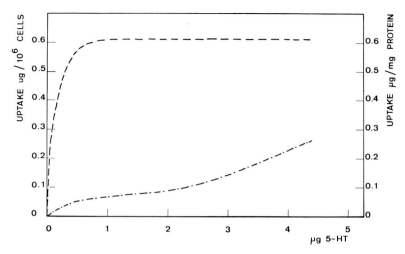

Fig. 7. Uptake of 5-HT by intact mast cells (- - -) and isolated mast cell granules (— . - . —).

ticulate sediments, the lighter of which consisted of an almost pure fraction (Fig. 4). Electron microscopically, it was observed that the granules were non-delimited, *i.e.* no membranes were observed around the granules.

The uptake by this granule fraction was low at low concentrations in the medium (0.22 and 0.44 $\mu$g/ml) (Jansson, 1970c), but the uptake increased with the concentration of 5-HT in the medium and showed little tendency to saturation at the same range tested for intact mast cells (Fig. 7). At 4.4 $\mu$g/ml the uptake increased with incubation time, reaching a level about 270% over the original 5-HT content after 6 h.

The uptake was independent of temperature between 5-HT concentrations of 0.4 and 4.4 $\mu$g/ml (Fig. 1) and was not accelerated by the addition of ATP and/or ions (Jansson, 1970c), which in themselves induced a rapid release of 5-HT, as has also been found for histamine by Lagunoff *et al.* (1964) and Thon and Uvnäs (1966). Metabolic inhibitors had no significant effect on the uptake.

These results suggest that the uptake of 5-HT by isolated, membrane-free mast cell granules is passive, as has been previously shown for histamine by Thon and Uvnäs (1966) and Bergendorff and Uvnäs (1967).

The effect of some drugs studied with intact mast cells was also studied on isolated granules.

Reserpine and guanethidine clearly depressed the uptake without great effect on the endogenous 5-HT content (Jansson, 1970c). Prenylamine and amitriptyline depressed the uptake in some experiments but the endogenous content was also drastically lowered. Cocaine, imipramine and ouabain had no notable effect on either the endogenous content or the uptake of 5-HT by the granules (Jansson, 1970c).

The effects of reserpine and prenylamine were further studied in combined *in vivo–in vitro* experiments. Granules separated from mast cells of reserpine-injected rats showed a decreased ability to take up 5-HT, while mast cell granules of prenylamine-treated rats had an uptake which did not differ from the uptake of granular fractions prepared from untreated rats.

### Comparison of mast cell and nervous tissue

In the brain the first step in the synthesis of 5-HT is the hydroxylation of tryptophan (Grahame-Smith, 1964; Weber and Horita, 1965), while in mast cells this hydroxylase is missing, the only enzyme in the synthesis chain being the 5-hydroxytryptophan decarboxylase (Slorach and Uvnäs, 1968). Another dissimilarity is that in the brain 5-HT is mainly metabolized by monoamine oxidase (Ecclestone et al., 1966) while in the mast cell 5-HT is not oxidized (see Green, 1966).

5-HT is stored in the mast cells as well as in the nervous system in intracellular storage granules. There are, however, great differences between the mast cell granules and the 5-HT-storing synaptic vesicles. The mast cell granule has a diameter of some 500 nm (Smith, 1963) while the small granular (dense-cored) vesicles are about 30–60 nm in diameter (see Whittaker, 1965, 1969; Potter, 1967). Vesicles with a diameter up to 200 nm were reported after homogenization (see Potter, 1967), and Wesemann (1969) isolated 5-HT-storing vesicles with a diameter of 50–130 nm.

The dense core of the vesicles contains ATP and a special protein (see Blaschko in the present volume) and thus differs greatly from the mast cell granules which are made up of a protein–heparin complex (Uvnäs et al., 1970). The mechanism of binding of 5-HT or noradrenaline in the synaptic vesicles is not known, but an amine–ATP complex has been postulated (Potter, 1967). In the mast cells histamine and probably 5-HT are bound to weak carboxylic groups in the protein part of the protein–heparin complex (Uvnäs et al., 1970). Intracellularly the mast cell granules as well as the dense-cored vesicles have a unit membrane (Fig. 3), but as the dense-cored vesicles lose their dense core during isolation (Potter, 1967) while retaining their vesicle (i.e. the membrane bag), no isolation procedure has as yet been described by which extracellular mast cell granules surrounded by membrane could be obtained. Thus, the protein–heparin–amine complex of extracellular mast cell granules is directly exposed to the surrounding medium.

The role of the small granular vesicles in the release mechanism of nervous amines is unknown; in the mast cells the release takes place by exocytosis, by which the granular material and the amines leave the cell by a reverse pinocytosis (Fillion et al., 1970; see also Fig. 3), and in this the mast cells resemble the adrenal medulla in which the release is also apparently due to exocytosis (Douglas, 1968). While the extracellular mast cell granules are exposed to the ions in the surrounding medium, the amines are liberated by an ion-exchange mechanism (Uvnäs et al., 1970).

The consensus to date is that the adrenergic neuron possesses two main uptake mechanisms, one located at the cell membrane, the other at the amine-storing vesicles (Sachs, 1970). Although it has not been possible to demonstrate uptake of amines in the adrenergic neuron or in any synapse model against an electrochemical gradient (Iversen and Born, 1968), the two uptake mechanisms exhibit features which suggest that they are of an active nature (Iversen, 1963; Dengler *et al.*, 1961; Hamberger, 1967; Carlsson *et al.*, 1963; Philippu *et al.*, 1969; Sachs, 1970). In the intact mast cell it was shown (Jansson, 1970a) that there is apparently an active component in the uptake of 5-HT. The uptake mechanism has been postulated as being located at the cell membrane (Jansson, 1970c) because isolated mast cell granules took up 5-HT passively (Jansson, 1970c). It should, however, again be pointed out that intracellularly the granules are surrounded by membranes (Fig. 3), whereas isolated granules were without any limiting membrane. Therefore, the possibility cannot be excluded that in the intact mast cell an active uptake also takes place at the perigranular membranes.

The endogenous amine content of the central nervous system and the 5-HT content of mast cells are affected by the same drugs (Carlsson, 1966; Jansson, 1970). Moreover, the uptake of 5-HT by both intact mast cells and isolated mast cell granules is affected by drugs which also act on amine uptake in nervous tissue (Carlsson, 1966). It has been shown that drugs such as imipramine and cocaine which affect the membrane pump in the nervous tissue (Carlsson, 1966) also apparently exert a blocking action on the cell membrane in the mast cells (Jansson, 1970c). On the other hand, reserpine and guanethidine were the only drugs clearly affecting the uptake of 5-HT by isolated mast cell granules, and these drugs also affect the granular uptake of amines in nervous tissue (Carlsson, 1966; Lundborg and Stitzel, 1968).

In conclusion, despite obvious dissimilarities, the mast cell resembles the adrenergic neuron in many respects, having a high endogenous amine content which can be affected by the same type of drugs affecting the amine content in nervous tissue, and having an efficient amine uptake mechanism which can be modulated by the same kinds of drugs known to act on amine uptake in the central nervous system. The mast cells therefore undoubtedly serve as an interesting model for nervous monoaminergic synapses in addition to being in themselves exciting objects of scientific investigation.

## REFERENCES

BERGENDORFF, A. AND UVNÄS, B. (1967) *Acta Pharmacol. Toxicol.*, **25**, Suppl. **4**, 32.
CARLSSON, A. (1966) In: U. S. VON EULER, S. ROSELL AND B. UVNÄS (Eds.), *Mechanisms of Release of Biogenic Amines*, Pergamon Press, Stockholm.
CARLSSON, A., HILLARP, N.-Å. AND WALDBECK, B. (1963) *Acta Physiol. Scand.*, **59**, Suppl. **215**.
DAY, M. AND STOCKBRIDGE, A. (1964) *Brit. J. Pharmacol.*, **23**, 405.
DENGLER, H. J., SPIEGEL, E. H. AND TITUS, E. O. (1961) *Science*, **133**, 1072.
DOUGLAS, W. W. (1968) *Brit. J. Pharmacol.*, **34**, 451.
ECCLESTONE, D., MOIR, A. T. B., READING, H. W. AND RITCHIE, I. M. (1966) *Brit. J. Pharmacol.*, **28**, 367.
ERÄNKÖ, O. AND JANSSON, S.-E. (1967) *Acta Physiol. Scand.*, **70**, 449.
ERÄNKÖ, O. AND KAUKO, L. (1965) *Acta Physiol. Scand.*, **64**, 283.
FILLION, G. M. B., SLORACH, S. A. AND UVNÄS, B. (1970) *Acta Physiol. Scand.*, **78**, 547.
GRAHAME-SMITH, D. G. (1964) *Biochem. J.*, **92**, 52.
GREEN, J. P. (1966) In: U. S. VON EULER, S. ROSELL AND B. UVNÄS (Eds.), *Mechanisms of Release of Biogenic Amines*, Pergamon Press, Stockholm.
HAMBERGER, B. (1967) *Acta Physiol. Scand.*, Suppl. **295**.
IVERSEN, L. L. (1963) *Brit. J. Pharmacol.*, **21**, 523.

IVERSEN, L. L. AND BORN, G. V. R. (1968) In: G. E. W. WOLSTENHOLME AND M. O'CONNOR (Eds.), *Adrenergic Neurotransmission, Discussion*, J. & A. Churchill Ltd., London.

JANSSON, S.-E. (1970a) *Acta Physiol. Scand.*, **78**, 420.

JANSSON, S.-E. (1970b) *Acta Physiol. Scand.*, in press.

JANSSON, S.-E. (1970c) *Acta Physiol. Scand.*, in press.

LAGUNOFF, D., PHILLIPS, M. T., ISERI, O. A. AND BENDITT, E. P. (1964) *Lab. Invest.*, **13**, 1331.

LUNDBORG, P. AND STITZEL, R. (1968) *Acta Physiol. Scand.*, **72**, 100.

PHILIPPU, A., BURKAT, V. AND BECKE, H. (1969) *Europ. J. Pharmacol.*, **6**, 96.

POTTER, L. T. (1967) In: R. READER (Ed.), *Catecholamines in Cardiovascular Physiology and Disease*, American Heart Association, New York.

SACHS, CH. (1970) *Noradrenaline Uptake Mechanisms*, Kungl. Boktryckeriet, P. A. Norstedt & Söner, Stockholm.

SMITH, D. E. (1963) *Ann. N.Y. Acad. Sci.*, **103**, 40.

SLORACH, S. A. AND UVNÄS, B. (1968) *Acta Physiol. Scand.*, **73**, 457.

THON, I.-L. AND UVNÄS, B. (1966) *Acta Physiol. Scand.*, **67**, 455.

UVNÄS, B., ÅBORG, G.-H. AND BERGENDORFF, A. (1970) *Acta Physiol. Scand.*, Suppl. **336**.

WEBER, L. J. AND HORITA, A. (1965) *Biochem. Pharmacol.*, **14**, 1141.

WESEMANN, W. (1969) *FEBS Letters*, **3**, 80.

WHITTAKER, V. P. (1965) *Progr. Biophys. Mol. Biol.*, **15**, 39.

WHITTAKER, V. P. (1969) In: A. LAJTHA (Ed.), *Handbook of Neurochemistry*, Plenum Press, New York, London.

# Effects of Inorganic Electrolytes on the Membrane Transport and Metabolism of Serotonin and Norepinephrine by Synaptosomes

ANJA H. TISSARI* AND DONALD F. BOGDANSKI

*Laboratory of Chemical Pharmacology, National Heart and Lung Institute, National Institutes of Health, Bethesda, Md. 20014 (U.S.A.)*

Isolated nerve endings (synaptosomes) prepared from brain homogenates were described by De Robertis *et al.* (1961) and by Gray and Whittaker (1962). Comprehensive reviews of the morphological and biochemical properties of synaptosomes have been published (Whittaker, 1965; De Robertis, 1966, 1967; Maynert and Kuriyama, 1964; Bogdanski *et al.*, 1968a).

Morphologically, synaptosomes are characterized by their content of storage vesicles and small mitochondria enclosed by a plasma membrane. The identity of such particles with nerve endings is confirmed by the occasional presence of thickened pre- and post-synaptic membranes with attached sub-synaptic web. Synaptosomes distribute on a sucrose gradient together with potassium ion and lactic dehydrogenase, considered to be soluble cytoplasmic markers.

Much biochemical evidence indicates that synaptosomes carry on general metabolic activities as well as specific metabolic functions appropriate for their normal functions as nerve endings *in vivo*. Synaptosomes contain endogenous stores and manufacture the neurohormones acetylcholine (Whittaker, 1965; De Robertis *et al.*, 1962, 1963), norepinephrine (NE) (De Robertis, 1967; Laverty *et al.*, 1963; Potter and Axelrod, 1962, 1963), 5-hydroxytryptamine (5-HT) (Potter and Axelrod, 1962; Michaelson and Whittaker, 1962; Zieher and De Robertis, 1963; Rodriquez de Lores Arnaiz and De Robertis, 1964a),dopamine (De Robertis, 1967; Laverty *et al.*, 1963) and histamine (Michaelson, 1968). Of particular interest is the ability of synaptosomes to manufacture labeled NE from labeled tyrosine (Bogdanski *et al.*, 1968a), a process involving a chain of enzyme reactions, and to maintain steady-state levels of 5-HT (synthesis and loss of 5-HT being in balance) from endogenous substrates (Bogdanski *et al.*, 1968b). Synaptosomes contain the enzymes that destroy amines, monoamine oxidase (Rodriquez De Lores Arnaiz and De Robertis, 1962) and catechol-*O*-methyltransferase (Alberici *et al.*, 1964). The process of membrane transport of amines has been well established for 5-HT, NE and dopamine (Bogdanski *et al.*, 1968b; Tissari *et al.*, 1969; Colburn *et al.*, 1967, 1968; Snyder and Coyle, 1969). Synaptosomes contain ATP (Nyman and Whittaker, 1963) and synthesize ATP from inorganic phosphate

---

* Present address: Department of Pharmacology, University of Helsinki, Siltavuorenpenger 10A, Helsinki 17, Finland.

(Bradford, 1969), and contain $(Na^+ + K^+)$–ATPase activity (Tissari *et al.*, 1969; Kurokawa *et al.*, 1965; Hosie, 1965; Abdel-Latif *et al.*, 1967). Synaptosomes maintain a $K^+$ gradient across the plasma membrane, a gradient which can be reduced by ouabain (Marchbanks, 1967; Bogdanski *et al.*, 1970). The existence of $Na^+$ gradient has not been established and may not exist *in vitro*, at least not throughout the cytoplasm as a whole (Bogdanski *et al.*, 1970). Preparations containing synaptosomes respire in the presence of various substrates (Bradford, 1969), synthesize protein (Autilio *et al.*, 1968) and contain adenyl cyclase activity (De Robertis *et al.*, 1967). It is reasonable to conclude from the above list of functions that morphologically and metabolically, synaptosomes show properties of viable nerve endings.

An important early finding in experiments with synaptosomes was that the autolysis of synaptosomes incubated at 37°, with release of acetylcholine, was decreased if the synaptosomes were suspended in Krebs–Ringer (Clementi, 1966). One of us had independently reported that rat heart slices stored NE only in the presence of $Na^+$ (Bogdanski, 1965), findings that were subsequently extended to synaptosomes and expanded to include 5-HT (Bogdanski *et al.*, 1968b). The discovery of the $Na^+$ requirement for the storage of amines by central and peripheral nerve endings led to our studies on the effect of this ion on the uptake process for NE and 5-HT for which a $Na^+$ requirement was also found by ourselves (Bogdanski *et al.*, 1968b; Bogdanski and Brodie, 1966) and by others (Iversen and Kravitz, 1966; Gillis and Paton, 1967). This $Na^+$-dependent uptake is important for the economy of the cell, for recent studies by Hedqvist and Stjärne (1969) are in accord with earlier assumptions that the action of neurotransmitters on post-synaptic receptors was terminated by the recapture of neurotransmitters by the nerve endings that released it. Hence, the same amine store can be used more than once, particularly during rapid firing of the nerves.

The present report summarizes the results of our experiments on the ion requirements for transport and storage of amines by synaptosomes. Many of the findings to be described in this article parallel those found earlier in the adrenergic nerve endings in heart slices. Most findings have been previously reported or are in press.

Synaptosomes were prepared from homogenates of rat or rabbit brain stem using discontinuous sucrose gradients essentially as described by Rodriquez de Lores Arnaiz and De Robertis (1964), modified according to Tissari *et al.* (1969). During the preparation other cell fractions are isolated, including the soluble and mitochondrial fractions and membrane fragments. Several findings define the functional integrity of synaptosomes. Radioactive 5-HT or NE previously injected into the brain ventricles *in vivo* localize chiefly in the synaptosomal fraction (Bogdanski *et al.*, 1968a). Given sufficient time for absorption and metabolism of exogenous [³H]NE to proceed *in vivo* (18 h) about half of the [³H]NE present on the gradient was recovered in the synaptosomal fraction (Fig. 1). Most of the remainder can probably be attributed to contamination of these fractions by synaptosomes. Synaptosomes transport, accumulate, store and metabolize more amines than any other fraction (Bogdanski *et al.*, 1968b). An important point in establishing specificity of synaptosomes is that parallel measurements of accumulation (the ratio of internal/external amine concentrations) and metabolism of amines by synaptosomes show parallel responses to experimental

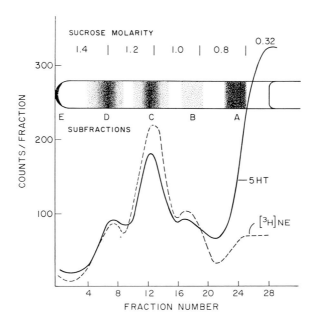

Fig. 1. Localization of [³H]NE and [5-¹⁴C]HT injected *in vivo* (intraventricular) by various rat brain fractions. Top line refers to sucrose molarity. A, B, C, D and E refer to brain fractions. Synaptosomes are found in B, C and D. A is myelin. The solid line refers to counts of [5-¹⁴C]HT. The broken line refers to counts of [³H]NE. Synaptosomes were prepared 120 min after the intraventricular injection of [5-¹⁴C]HT and 17 h after [³H]NE. Reproduced by courtesy of the U.S. Government Printing Office.

TABLE 1

THE EFFECT OF VARIOUS MEDIA ON ACCUMULATION AND METABOLISM OF [5-¹⁴C]HT BY SYNAPTOSOMES

Control media, including that labeled 143 mM $Na^+$, were Krebs–bicarbonate solution, 95% $O_2$–5% $CO_2$. Experiments with $Na^+$-deficient media (sucrose) contained 0.84 mg protein/ml, accounting for the greater metabolism seen here than in the remaining experiments in which the protein concentration was about 0.2 mg/ml. "Accumulation ratio" is the ratio (intracellular [5-¹⁴C]HT)/(extracellular [5-¹⁴C]HT). "Uptake and metabolism" gives accumulated 5-HT and metabolized 5-HT expressed as the percent of [5-¹⁴C]HT originally present in the incubation medium. Courtesy Pergamon Press, Oxford, England.

| Medium | Incubation time (min) | Accumulation ratio | Uptake and metabolism (%) |
|---|---|---|---|
| 143 mM $NA^+$ | 15 | 18 | 95 |
| 25 mM $Na^+$ | 15 | 10 | 77 |
| 0 mM $Na^+$ | 15 | 2 | 15 |
| Control | 15 | 16 | 42 |
| Reserpine | 15 | 2.9 | 50 |
| Reserpine and Pargyline | 15 | 29 | 12 |
| Control | 25 | 31 | 69 |
| Ouabain $10^{-3}$ M | 25 | 4.8 | 21 |

*References pp. 301–302*

TABLE 2

ACCUMULATION AND UPTAKE OF [5-$^{14}$C]HT IN SYNAPTOSOMAL AND IN MITOCHONDRIAL LAYERS

The accumulation ratios, and uptake and metabolism defined as in Table 1. MAOI, Pargyline, 50 mg/kg i.v. 1 hour earlier.

|  | Accumulation ratio | Uptake and metabolism (%) |
|---|---|---|
| Rat C layer (synaptosomes) | | |
| Krebs–HCO$_3$ | 20 | 72 |
| O Na | 5 | 8 |
| Rat D layer (mitochondria) | | |
| Krebs–HCO$_3$ | 14 | 77 |
| O Na | 5 | 29 |
| Rabbit C layer (synaptosomes) | | |
| Krebs-HCO$_3$ | 28 | 90 |
| Rabbit D layer (mitochondria) | | |
| Krebs–HCO$_3$ | 3 | 75 |
| Krebs–MAOI | 12 | 10 |

manipulation. For example, blocking the inward transport of amine by ouabain or a Na$^+$-deficient medium inhibits both processes. In contrast, reserpine, which prevents storage by the intracellular vesicles but does not block transport, prevents accumulation by increasing the deamination of amines by monoamine oxidase within the cell. Blocking monoamine oxidase by means of the injection of monoamine oxidase inhibitor *in vivo* restores accumulation of amine in the reserpinized synaptosomes (Bogdanski *et al.*, 1968b; Tissari *et al.*, 1969) (Table 1).

The above evidence indicates that synaptosomes accumulate amine and also metabolize it. In contrast, the mitochondrial fraction metabolizes 5-HT at a rate that is largely, but not entirely, independent of Na$^+$, indicating that a Na$^+$-dependent transport process is not involved. Moreover, the mitochondrial fraction does not accumulate 5-HT or NE (Table 2).

It is now well known that Na$^+$ is essential for the storage of NE by heart and brain nerve endings and that Na$^+$ is also essential for the inward transport of exogenous NE and 5-HT (see introduction). The Na$^+$ requirement for uptake, the facilitation of uptake by low [K$^+$] and inhibition by high [K$^+$], and the blockade of uptake by ouabain (Bogdanski *et al.*, 1968b, 1970a; Tissari *et al.*, 1969; Colburn *et al.*, 1968) are all factors previously discovered to be essential for the uptake of amino acids and sugars by a variety of other tissues. We therefore adopted, as a working hypothesis, the ion gradient hypothesis of membrane transport suggested by Riggs *et al.* (1958) and later extended and modified by Crane (1965), Vidaver (1964b), Schultz and Zalusky (1965), Curran *et al.* (1967), Eddy (1968) and Jacquez and Schaeffer (1969). The work of Crane (1965) has been most helpful to us in this regard. Briefly stated, transport is visualized as being mediated by a mobile carrier which has access to the inside and

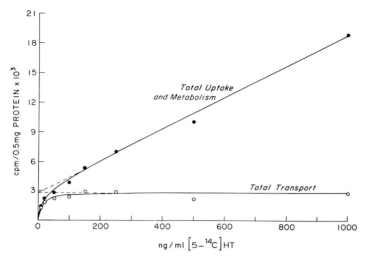

Fig. 2. Initial rates of uptake as a function of [5-¹⁴C]HT concentration. Uptake and metabolism include [5-¹⁴C]HT accumulated by the synaptosomes and metabolites formed intracellularly and released into the incubation medium. Various concentrations of [5-¹⁴C]HT were incubated 6.5 min with synaptosomes suspended in Krebs–bicarbonate medium at 37°. ●——●, observed uptake and metabolism. The linear portion of the curve represents amine that had penetrated the cell membrane by passive diffusion superimposed upon amine that was transported into the cell. Upon extrapolation of the linear portion to the y-axis (dashed line), the y-intercept represents O uptake by passive diffusion at O concentration. Subtraction of this amount from the linear curve at any concentration represents the amount of amine that entered the cell by passive diffusion at that concentration. Subtraction of passive diffusion from total uptake represents the amount of amine entering the cell by the membrane transport mechanism, and is indicated by ○——○. Data of Bodganski et al. (1970b).

outside of the cell membrane. The affinity of the carrier for amine is determined by the ionic environment, and is high at the outside surface of the membrane where the [Na⁺] is high and [K⁺] is low. The affinity is decreased at the interior surface of the membrane where the relative ionic concentrations are the reverse of the external concentrations. The carrier, amine and Na⁺ enter the cell stoichiometrically, as a ternary complex, the amine being released inside the cell to be stored or metabolized. The intracellular ionic environment is restored by the outward pumping of Na⁺ by the Na⁺ pump, thought to be related to the (Na⁺ + K⁺)–ATPase system (Bogdanski et al., 1968b; Bogdanski and Brodie, 1969b).

In addition to the similarities in the properties of the systems that transport various organic solutes we have previously mentioned, including amines, we can now make the following points. (1) The initial rate of transport of low concentrations of 5-HT is a saturable process (Fig. 2), suggesting that transport of amine involves a separate carrier or binding mechanism. Since transport of 5-HT comprises mostly amine that has been metabolized within the synaptosome (Bogdanski et al., 1968b; Tissari et al., 1969), the evidence is in accord with the concept that transport is mediated by a saturable carrier and not a binding mechanism elsewhere in the synaptosome (Bogdanski et al., 1970b). (2) Double-reciprocal plots of the initial rate of accumulation (1/v) of 5-HT or NE against substrate concentration (1/c) produced straight lines

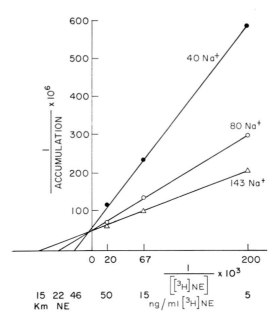

Fig. 3. Lineweaver–Burk plots of accumulation *vs.* [³H]NE conc. as related to Na conc. Various [³H]NE concentrations were incubated 7 min with synaptosomes suspended in Krebs–bicarbonate solution, pH 7.4, at 37°. The actual [³H]NE conc. in ng/ml and reciprocals and the various Na⁺ concentrations are given on the figure. Averages of 4 experiments. Data of Bogdanski *et al.* (1970b).

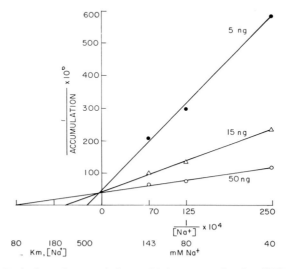

Fig. 4. Lineweaver–Burk plots of accumulation *vs.* Na⁺ conc. as related to [³H]NE conc. The data are the same as those plotted in Fig. 3. The actual Na⁺ conc. and reciprocals and the various [³H]NE concentrations are given in the figure. Data of Bogdanski *et al.* (1970b).

which are also in accord with the concept that transport is mediated by a saturable carrier mechanism that obeys Michaelis–Menten kinetics. When the data representing experiments run in the presence of various [Na$^+$] were plotted (Fig. 3), a series of straight lines of various slopes were formed, the lines intersecting the $y$ axis at approximately the same point, indicating that the maximum velocity of accumulation of NE was nearly unchanged. The various slopes indicated that Na$^+$ reduced the apparent $K_m$, or the concentration of amine at which the velocity of transport is half maximal, suggesting that Na$^+$ increases the affinity of the carrier for amine. In the case of 5-HT, $V_{max}$ was also altered by various [Na$^+$] but only about 20% as much as the $K_m$ (Bogdanski et al., 1970b). (3) The same data were used to plot $1/v$ against $1/[Na^+]$ with various concentrations of 5-HT and NE. A series of lines was formed (Fig. 4) which indicated that $K_m$ was altered but not $V_{max}$ (Bogdanski et al., 1970b). According to the concepts of Vidaver (1964) and Kipnis and Parrish (1965), the data are in accord with the concept that the mobile carrier, amine and metal ion form a stoichiometric ternary complex which moves to the interior of the cell. The concept of a stoichiometric relationship between Na$^+$, organic solute and carrier has been proposed by a number of investigators in the field of amino acid and glucose transport (Crane, 1965; Curran et al., 1967; Vidaver, 1964; Kipnis and Parrish, 1965) and appears to apply to amine transport as well (Bogdanski and Brodie, 1969; Sugrue and Shore, 1969). (4) The affinity of the carrier for amine in the presence of Na$^+$ is antagonized by high [K$^+$] (Bogdanski et al., 1968b; Colburn et al., 1968; Bogdanski and Brodie, 1966). Double

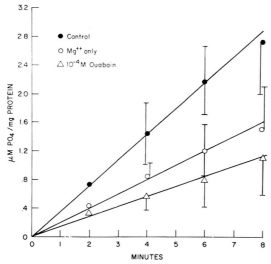

Fig. 5. Effects of ouabain on (Na$^+$ + K$^+$)–ATPase activity in synaptosomes in the presence of Na$^+$ and K$^+$. Synaptosomes were first warmed for 5 min before ATP was introduced into the suspension. ●——●, control synaptosomes were incubated in 0.15 M Tris buffer, pH 7.2, containing 1 mM EDTA, 4 mM Mg$^{2+}$, 120 mM Na$^+$, and 20 mM K$^+$. △——△, ATP and ouabain were added together at final concentrations of 3 mM and 10$^{-4}$M. ○——○, effect of Na$^+$ + K$^+$ omission. (Na$^+$ + K$^+$)–ATPase activity is expressed as micromoles of phosphate released from ATP per min per milligram of protein. The curves represent the average and standard deviation of four experiments.
Data of Tissari et al. (1969), courtesy of Academic Press.

reciprocal plots of previous experiments with heart slices showed that high [K⁺] increased the $K_m$ but had no effect on $V_{max}$ suggesting that K⁺ is a competitive antagonist of Na⁺ (Bogdanski and Brodie, 1969).

All the preceding kinetic data affirm the view that amines are transported by a carrier whose affinity for amine is increased by Na⁺ and decreased by K⁺.

Another approach to the problem of transport has been the study of the relationship of temporal inhibition of transport to the temporal inhibition of the energy-producing enzyme (Na⁺ + K⁺)–ATPase which is thought to maintain ion gradients in cells. Ouabain and K⁺-free media have been used to inhibit (Na⁺ + K⁺)–ATPase (Bogdanski *et al.*, 1968b, 1970a; Tissari *et al.*, 1969; Tissari and Bogdanski, 1971). The K⁺-free medium offers the advantage that it represents the absence of an essential component of the environmental fluid, and any delay found in the development of transport inhibition cannot be explained by the time required for the attachment of inhibitor, such as ouabain, to receptor (Bogdanski *et al.*, 1970a). (1) We have reported (Tissari *et al.*, 1969) that ouabain and lack of K⁺ blocks (Na⁺ + K⁺)–ATPase almost instantaneously (Fig. 5) but that the blockade of accumulation of 5-HT occurs after a measurable time lag (Tissari *et al.*, 1969; Bogdanski *et al.*. 1970a) (Fig. 6). (2) The development of

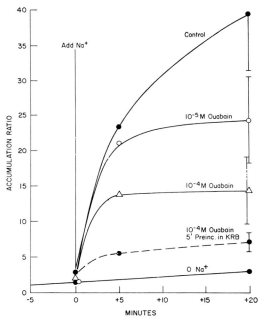

Fig. 6. Effect of Na⁺-free medium containing various concentrations of ouabain. Synaptosomes were incubated for 5 min with ouabain in a Na⁺-free solution (isotonicity maintained by sucrose) containing all other electrolytes normally present in Krebs–bicarbonate solution (KRB). At zero time, Na⁺ and/or [5-¹⁴C]HT was added at a final concentrations of 20 ng/ml or 143 mM respectively. Accumulation of [5-¹⁴C]HT in the Na⁺-free medium without subsequent addition of Na⁺ is also shown (bottom curve, designated O Na⁺). For comparison, the dashed curve shows the effect of a 5-min preliminary incubation of synaptosomes with Na⁺ and ouabain on accumulation of [5-¹⁴C]HT added at zero time. The curves represent the average and standard deviation of five experiments. Data of Tissari *et al.* (1969), courtesy of Academic Press.

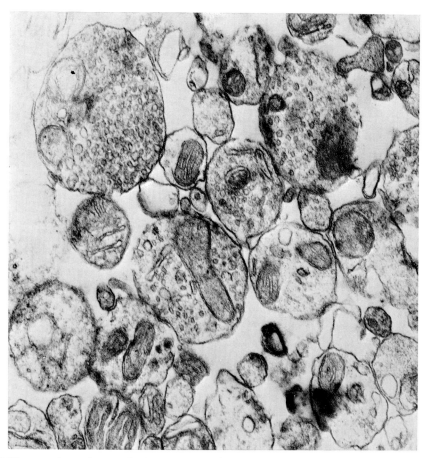

Fig. 7. Electron photomicrograph of synaptosomes incubated 15 min in Krebs–bicarbonate solution, pH 7.4 at 37°. × 20 000.

transport block apparently requires the presence of $Na^+$ in the medium (Tissari *et al.*, 1969) (Fig. 6). If the inhibition of $(Na^+ + K^+)$–ATPase is the main direct action of ouabain, it follows that ouabain blocks transport by a secondary process that is dependent upon the presence of $Na^+$ in the medium. An important secondary response to the blockade of $(Na^+ + K^+)$–ATPase is the redistribution of ions across the cell membrane. We have reported data that are in accord with that view. Synaptosomes maintain an ouabain-sensitive $K^+$ gradient with respect to the extracellular fluid (Escueta and Appel, 1969; Bogdanski *et al.*, 1970a), but probably do not maintain a $Na^+$ gradient unless the large amounts of $Na^+$ measured in preparations of synaptosomes that were incubated in Krebs–bicarbonate solution are not in solution in the cytoplasm (Bogdanski *et al.*, 1970a). In agreement with Escueta and Appel (1969), this laboratory has shown (Bogdanski, unpublished) that the $K^+$ gradient depends in part upon extracellular $Na^+$, which has entered the cell by diffusion and is probably extruded from the cell in exchange with extracellular $K^+$ (Ling and Abdel-Latif, 1968),

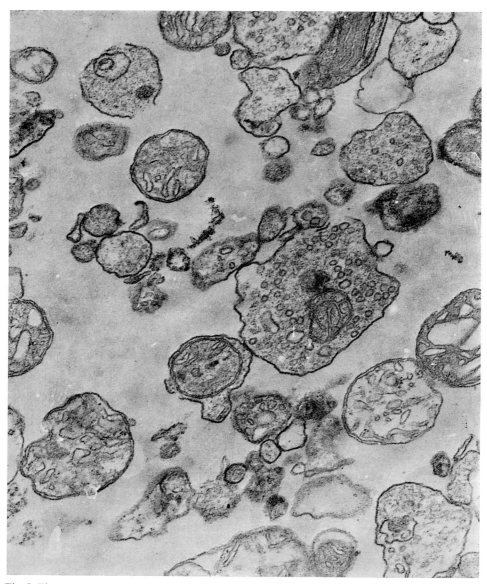

Fig. 8. Electron photomicrograph of synaptosomes incubated 60 min in a Na+-free solution, (pH 7.4, isotonicity maintained by sucrose, 37°), containing all other cations normally contained in Krebs–bicarbonate solution. × 20 000.

the conventional mode of operation of the electrolyte pump. This line of evidence raises the possibilities that local Na+ gradients exist in the immediate vicinity of the membrane pump, or, in any event, the carrier for amine can be kept free of Na+ at the interior of the membrane by being in close proximity to the electrolyte pump. Presumably, the local accumulation of intracellular Na+ at the carrier is one of the secondary processes responsible for the $Na^+$-dependent inhibition of transport by ouabain and by $K^+$-free media. The effect of this accumulation of intracellular $Na^+$ is to increase the affinity of the carrier for amine inside the membrane, thus reducing the carrier affinity gradient that normally exists between the inside and the outside of the membrane. The reduction in affinity gradient decreases the rate of transport. Another effect of the inhibition of electrolyte transport by ouabain and $K^+$-free media is the reduction of the $K^+$ gradient. Potassium ion helps maintain an affinity gradient by decreasing the high affinity produced in the presence of $Na^+$. The $K^+$ gradient itself may participate in the transport process (Bogdanski, 1965; Bogdanski and Brodie, 1966).

Sugrue and Shore (1969) recently reported data at variance with ours. They indicated that $Na^+$ affects the $V_{max}$ for transport not the $K_m$. A possible reason for the discrepancy is their use of relatively large concentrations of the non-physiological substrate metaraminol for their experiments, whereas we used smaller concentrations of 5-HT or NE which are physiological substrates.

White and Keen (1970) reported that transport of $[^3H]NE$ by synaptosomes was blocked by metabolic inhibitors even though a $Na^+$ gradient was established by adding more $Na^+$ to the incubation mixture. Since electrolytes were probably not transported in the presence of the metabolic inhibitors used in their experiments (Escueta and Appel, 1969), their findings with $[^3H]NE$ are probably very similar to ours in which we failed to observe accumulation of $[^3H]NE$ in ouabain-treated synaptosomes to which $Na^+$ was subsequently added (Tissari *et al.*, 1969; Bogdanski *et al.*, 1970a). This result was in contrast to the normal accumulation of 5-HT under identical conditions. The reason for the apparent differences between the transport process for 5-HT and NE is not known, although several possibilities come to mind. We feel that on the basis of available data, similarities should be stressed although the differences are interesting and potentially significant.

We are indebted to Dr. John W. Crayton for the following electron microscopic histological studies of synaptosomes at the National Institute of Mental Health. The essential results of preliminary studies indicate that synaptosomes incubated in Na-deficient media (as compared with those incubated in Krebs–bicarbonate medium) show a time-dependent swelling of their mitochondria and vesicles. These changes appear to be minimal and involve only a few scattered synaptosomes at 15 min., which is longer than the time interval used in the initial rate studies (7 min). At 2 h, most synaptosomes were involved; the vesicles and mitochondria were generally greatly swollen or lysed. Even at 2 h however, a few synaptosomes appeared to be histologically normal. On the basis of histological and biochemical data, we conclude that inhibition of uptake by $Na^+$-free, $K^+$-free or ouabain-containing media up to at least 20 min is mainly the result of impairment of the membrane transport mechanism, and not the disruption of cellular contents.

## REFERENCES

ABDEL-LATIF, A. A., BRODY, J. AND RAMAHI, H. (1967) *J. Neurochem.*, **14**, 1133.
ALBERICI, M., RODRIGUEZ DE LOREZ ARNAIZ, G. AND DE ROBERTIS E. (1964) *Life Sci.*, **4**, 1951.

AUTILIO, L. A., APPEL, S. H., PETTIS, P. AND GAMBETTI, P. L. (1968) *Biochemistry*, **7**, 2615.
BOGDANSKI, D. F. (1965) *Pharmacologist*, **7**, 168.
BOGDANSKI, D. F., BLASZKOWSKI, T. P. AND TISSARI, A. H. (1970a) *Biochim. Biophys. Acta*, **211**, 521.
BOGDANSKI, D. F. AND BRODIE, B. B. (1966) *Life Sci.*, **5**, 1563.
BOGDANSKI, D. F. AND BRODIE, B. B. (1969) *J. Pharmacol. Exp. Therap.*, **165**, 181.
BOGDANSKI, D. F., TISSARI, A. H. AND BRODIE, B. B. (1968a) in EFRON *et al.* (Eds.), *Psychopharmacology, Review of Progress 1957–1967*, U.S. Publ. Health Serv., Publ. 1836, Washington.
BOGDANSKI, D. F., TISSARI, A. H. AND BRODIE, B. B. (1968b) *Life Sci.*, **7** (Part 1), 419.
BOGDANSKI, D. F., TISSARI, A. H. AND BRODIE, B. B. (1970b) *Biochim. Biophys. Acta*, **219**, 189.
BRADFORD, H. F. (1969) *J. Neurochem.*, **16**, 675.
CLEMENTI, F. (1966) quoted by V. P. WHITTAKER, in U. S. VON EULER, S. ROSELL, AND B. UVNÄS (Eds.), *Mechanism of Release of Biogenic Amines*, Pergamon Press, London, p. 147–164.
COLBURN, R. W., GOODWIN, F. K., BUNNEY, JR., W. E. AND DAVIS, J. M. (1967) *Nature*, **215**, 1395.
COLBURN, R. W., GOODWIN, F. K., MURPHY, D. L., BUNNEY, JR., W. E. AND DAVIS, J. M. (1968) *Biochem. Pharmacol.*, **17**, 957.
CRANE, R. K. (1965) *Federation Proc.*, **24**, 1000.
CURRAN, P. F., SCHULTZ, S. G., CHEZ, R. A. AND FUISZ, R. E. (1967) *J. Gen. Physiol.*, **50**, 1261.
DE ROBERTIS, E., DE LORES, ARNAIZ, G. R., SALGANICOFF, L., PELLEGRINO DE IRALDI, A. AND ZIPHER, L. M. (1963) *J. Neurochem.*, **10**, 225.
DE ROBERTIS, E., PELLEGRINO DE IRALDI, A. AND DE LORES ARNAIZ, G. R. (1962) *J. Neurochem.*, **9**, 23.
DE ROBERTIS, E., PELLEGRINO DE IRALDI, A., RODRIGUEZ, G. AND GOMEZ, J. (1961) *J. Biophys. Biochem. Cytol.*, **9**, 229.
EDDY, A. A. (1968) *Biochemistry*, **108**, 489.
ESCUETA, A. V. AND APPEL, S. H. (1969) *Biochemistry*, **8**, 725.
GILLIS, G. N. AND PATON, D. M. (1967) *Brit. J. Pharmacol. Chemotherap.*, **29**, 309.
GRAY, E. G. AND WHITTAKER, V. P. (1962) *J. Anat.*, **96**, 79.
HEDQVIST, R. AND STJÄRNE, L. (1969) *Acta Physiol. Scand.*, **76**, 270.
HOSIE, R. J. A. (1965) *Biochem. J.*, **96**, 404.
IVERSEN, L. L. AND KRAVITZ, E. A. (1966) *Mol. Pharmacol.*, **2**, 360.
JACQUEZ, J. A. AND SCHAEFER, J. A. (1969) *Biochim. Biophys. Acta*, **193**, 368.
KIPNIS, D. M. AND PARRISH, J. E. (1965) *Federation Proc.*, **24**, 1051.
KUROKAWA, M., SAKAMOTO, T. AND KATO, M. (1965) *Biochem. J.*, **97**, 833.
LAVERTY, R., MICHAELSON, I. A., SHARMAN, D. F. AND WHITTAKER, V. P. (1963) *Brit. J. Pharmacol.*, **21**, 482.
LING, C. M. AND ABDEL-LATIF, A. A. (1968) *J. Neurochem.*, **15**, 721.
MARCHBANKS, R. M. (1967) *Biochem. J.*, **104**, 148.
MAYNERT, E. W. AND KURIYAMA, K. (1964) *Life Sci.*, **3**, 1067.
MAYNERT, E. W., LEVI, R. AND DE LORENZO, A. J. D. (1964) *J. Pharmacol.*, **144**, 385.
MICHAELSON, I. A. (1968) *Biochem. Pharmacol.*, **17**, 2435.
MICHAELSON, I. A. AND WHITTAKER, V. P. (1962) *Biochem. Pharmacol.*, **11**, 505.
NYMAN, M. AND WHITTAKER, V. P. (1963) *Biochem. J.*, **87**, 248.
POTTER, L. T. AND AXELROD, J. (1962) *Nature*, **194**, 581.
POTTER, L. T. AND AXELROD, J. (1963) *J. Pharmacol.*, **142**, 291.
RIGGS, T. R., WALKER, L. M. AND CHRISTENSEN, H. N. (1958) *J. Biol. Chem.*, **233**, 1479.
RODRIQUES DE LORES ARNAIZ, G. R. AND DE ROBERTIS, E. (1962) *J. Neurochem.*, **9**, 503.
RODRIQUES DE LORES ARNAIZ, G. R. AND DE ROBERTIS, E. (1964) *J. Neurochem.*, **11**, 213.
RODRIQUES DE LORES ARNAIZ, G. R. AND DE ROBERTIS, E. (1966) *Pharm. Rev.*, **18**, 413.
RODRIQUES DE LORES ARNAIZ, G. R. AND DE ROBERTIS, E. (1967) *Science*, **156**, 907.
RODRIQUES DE ARNAIZ, G. R., DE ROBERTIS, E., ALBERICI, M., BUTCHER, R. W. AND SUTHERLAND, E. W. (1967) *J. Biol. Chem.*, **242**, 3487.
SCHULTZ, S. G. AND ZALUSKY, R. (1965) *Nature*, **205**, 292.
SNYDER, S. N. AND COYLE, J. T. (1969) *J. Pharmacol.*, **165**, 78.
SUGRUE, M. F. AND SHORE, P. A. (1969) *J. Pharmacol. Exp. Therap.*, **170**, 239.
TISSARI, A. H. AND BOGDANSKI, D. F. (1971) *Pharmacology*, **5**, 225.
TISSARI, A. H., SCHÖNHÖFFER, P. S., BOGDANSKI, D. F. AND BRODIE, B. B. (1969) *Mol. Pharmacol.*, **5**, 593.
VIDAVER, G. A. (1964a) *Biochemistry*, **3**, 663.
VIDAVER, G. A. (1964b) *Biochemistry*, **3**, 795.
WHITE, T. D. AND KEEN, P. (1970) *Biochim. Biophys. Acta*, **196**, 285.
WHITTAKER, V. P. (1965) *Prog. Biophys. Mol. Biol.*, **15**, 39.
ZIEHER, L. M. AND DE ROBERTIS, E. (1963) *Biochem. Pharmacol.*, **12**, 596.

# V. HISTOCHEMISTRY OF CHOLINERGIC NERVOUS TRANSMISSION

# ZIO-positive and ZIO-negative Vesicles in Nerve Terminals*

K. AKERT, E. KAWANA** AND C. SANDRI

*Brain Research Institute of the University of Zürich, Zürich (Switzerland)*

## INTRODUCTION

The Champy–Maillet method (Maillet, 1962, 1968) has been successfully used in revealing unmyelinated nerve plexus at the light-microscopic level (Jabonero, 1964; Taxi, 1965). The essential reagent consists of a zinc iodide–osmium tetroxide mixture which is henceforth designated ZIO in this paper. Akert and Sandri (1968) and Akert *et al.* (1968) have introduced this method to electron microscopy and described its high affinity to synaptic vesicles in the nerve terminals of the subfornical organ and in the neuromuscular junctions of striated and smooth muscles. This affinity to synaptic vesicles is interesting for three reasons: (1) it may open a new approach to the problem of a 'synaptic stain', (2) it indicates a relationship with transmitter substances and/or with subcellular components relevant to transmitter functions, and (3) it may demonstrate relationships between synaptic vesicles and vesicle-forming cell constituents on the basis of common cytochemical properties.

An important technical improvement was achieved by Martin *et al.* (1969) who introduced the prefixation of neuropil with glutaraldehyde, thus providing superior preservation and more consistent impregnation of the tissue.

Initially, high hopes with respect to transmitter specificity were entertained on the basis of ZIO positivity in cholinergic nerve endings (Akert and Sandri, 1968). However, it was soon discovered that the synaptic vesicles of non-cholinergic systems, *e.g.* pineal nerves, retinal synapses (Pellegrino de Iraldi and Gueudet, 1968, 1969), all of the spinal cord nerve terminals (Kawana *et al.*, 1969), likewise responded to ZIO treatment. Thus, it became unlikely that the ZIO reagent is *a priori* specific for any one class of transmitter substances. The findings of Pellegrino de Iraldi and Gueudet (1969) of a ZIO-positive substrate in the inter- and intra-disk spaces of the outer segment of retinal photoreceptors suggested that possibly more than one category of substances could be implicated.

The following report is a summary of results from our own laboratory, where an attempt was made to differentiate between ZIO-positive and -negative components of the mammalian neuron. A similar study was carried out in the *Octopus* and published by Barlow and Martin (1970).

---

* With the aid of Grants Nr. 3.133.69 and Nr. 3.134.69 of the Swiss National Foundation for Scientific Research.
** On leave from the Brain Research Institute of the University of Tokyo, Japan.

*References p. 317*

## A. ZIO-POSITIVE SYNAPTIC VESICLES

Previous reports have dealt with ZIO-positive vesicles in terminals of motoneurons (Akert and Sandri, 1968) and preganglionic (Matus, 1970) and postganglionic sympathetic (Mallet, 1968; Pellegrino de Iraldi and Gueudet, 1968) and parasympathetic (Akert *et al.*, 1968) neurons. Intensive studies have since been made in our laboratory on nerve terminals in the following regions of the brain: spinal cord of monkey, cat and rat (Kawana *et al.*, 1969); caudate nucleus of the rat (Kawana *et al.*, 1971); Deiters' nucleus of monkey, cat and rat; subfornical organ of monkey (Akert *et al.*, 1969), cat and rat; optic tectum of the pigeon; pineal gland of the rat.

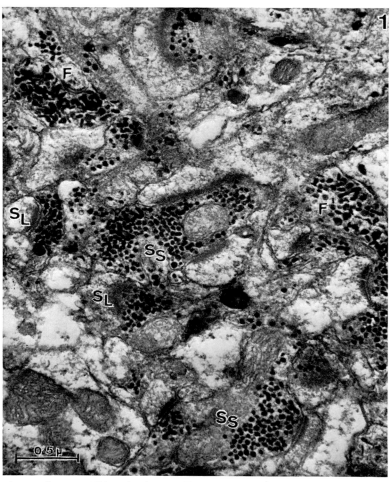

Fig. 1. Caudate nucleus, rat. ZIO-stained neuropil. Positive reaction is almost exclusively restricted to synaptic vesicles. Three types of terminals may be differentiated: F-type (with flattened vesicle profiles), $S_S$-type (with small-size spheric vesicle profiles), $S_L$-type (with larger-size spheric vesicle profiles). Note that synaptic vesicles are ZIO-positive regardless of their respective shape and size. Primary magnification × 20 000.

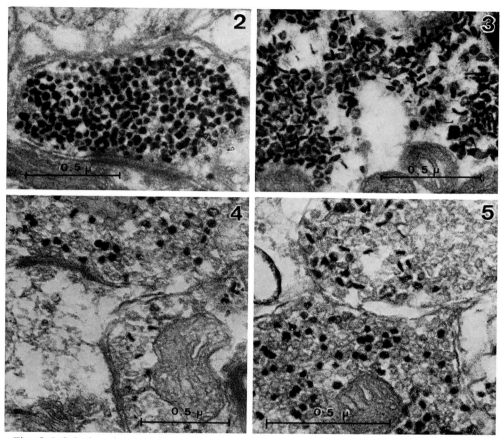

Figs. 2–5. Spinal cord, rat. ZIO-stained neuropil. Primary magnification × 40 000. Note the almost 100% positive staining of S-type vesicles in Fig. 2 and F-type vesicles in Fig. 3. The circular profiles in Fig. 3 are often less opaque than the elongated ones. This may be due to the disc shape of F-type vesicles rather than to incomplete impregnation. Figs. 4 and 5 show S- and F-type endings, which contain a fairly large proportion of unstained synaptic vesicles.

*Agranular synaptic vesicles* of the 300–600 Å range may give a positive ZIO reaction irrespective of form and size (S-type, F-type, see Fig. 1), and without regard to their association with peripheral or central, somatic or autonomic nervous systems. The ZIO reactivity of clear synaptic vesicles is an *all-or-none* phenomenon. This is particularly evident in the spheric vesicles which are consistently ZIO positive (*i.e.* the entire profile is solidly electron opaque) or altogether negative (Figs. 2 and 4). Endings with compressible vesicles seem to be an exception, since the staining is not uniform. However, the seemingly incomplete ('half-tone') staining of circular vesicle profiles in F-type terminals may have to do with geometry and optics rather than with diffusion and reactivity (Kawana *et al.*, 1969) since the flattenable vesicles are disks which present less than a 100 Å contrast layer to the electron beam. The presence of a reinforced margin (similar to erythrocytes) may explain the appearance of a lighter core and of an outer ring with increased opacity (Fig. 3).

*References p. 317*

The fact that some terminals contain an almost purebred ZIO-positive population of vesicles and other terminals may include more than 50% unstained elements, is illustrated in Figs. 2–5. An explanation of this differential reactivity is not readily available. It may reflect a real dichotomy: two types of vesicles or vesicles in two biochemically different functional states. If confirmed, this would be of considerable importance to those interested in the problems of transmitter functions because 'active' vesicles and 'storage' forms may be differentiated at the cytochemical level. On the other hand, experiences with ZIO reagent reveal that the impregnation intensity within a small tissue block decreases along an inward gradient. For the moment, it is safe to consider the possibility that the unstained vesicles reflect an artefactual failure of impregnation although the lack of a clear-cut reactivity gradient (all-or-none) seems to favour the physiological interpretation.

*Granular synaptic vesicles* of the 300–600 Å range seem to represent an additional exception to the all-or-none law of ZIO staining, since a large proportion of the reactive vesicles contain a pale core in a predominantly excentric position. This finding was made in pineal nerves (Pellegrino de Iraldi and Gueudet, 1968) as well as in other postganglionic sympathetic nerves (neuromyal junctions in spleen capsule and vas deferens of rat and cat). Fig. 7 gives an example. It seems quite safe to assume that the spacing occurs in the region of the granular area of these vesicles.

On the other hand, it seems important to note that prefixation with glutaraldehyde results in a uniform staining of all vesicles in sympathetic nerve endings, thus suggesting that ZIO affinity of the granule is by no means lacking. It is, however, easily lost unless protection is provided by preceding glutaraldehyde treatment. If this precaution is taken, the granulated vesicles seem to return to the all-or-none law of ZIO staining.

## B. OTHER ZIO-POSITIVE ORGANELLES

*Multivesicular bodies (mvb)* have been found in axons and axon terminals as well as in postsynaptic regions, including cell bodies and dendrites (see also Peters *et al.*, 1970). The majority contained ZIO-positive vesicles of varying size and shape. These vesicles may be flattened or spheric and their diameter corresponds approximately to the range of synaptic vesicles (Fig. 9A-D). In a very few cases, we have found mvb to be ZIO negative (Fig. 9E). A large number of ZIO-positive mvb were found in endothelial cells of cerebral blood vessels (Fig. 9C-D).

*Golgi complex:* Positive (Barlow and Martin, 1970) and negative (Matus, 1970) ZIO staining results have been reported to date. Light-microscopic investigations by Maillet and his school (1968) have revealed more consistent positive results. Yet, by citing Champy ('Le réactif osmium–iodure colore souvent quelques grains de la région Golgienne, mais jamais le réseau dans son ensemble') they point out certain variations and inconsistencies which we have been able to confirm at the electron microscopic level. Perhaps the most consistent finding is that of Matus (1970), who described (in sympathetic ganglion cells) an aggregation of ZIO-positive vesicles in the immediate vicinity of the Golgi complex. A ZIO-positive Golgi apparatus is shown in Fig. 10 and

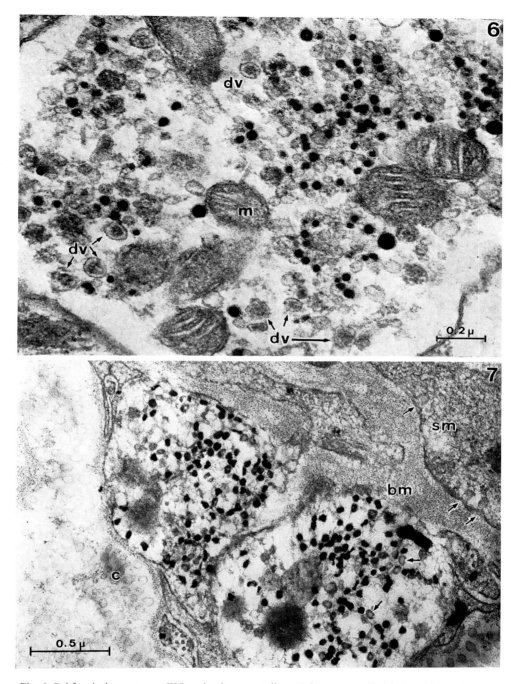

Fig. 6. Subfornical organ, cat. ZIO-stained nerve endings. Primary magnification × 20 000. Stained and unstained clear vesicles with circular profiles. Note that large dark-cored vesicles (dv) are consistently ZIO negative. m = mitochondria.

Fig. 7. Vas deferens, rat. ZIO staining of two nerve terminals. Note that a majority of vesicles are ZIO positive; a number of mostly unstained vesicles contain an electron-translucent core (arrow). c = collagen, bm = basement membrane, sm = smooth muscle cell with pinocytosis (arrows). Primary magnification × 20 000.

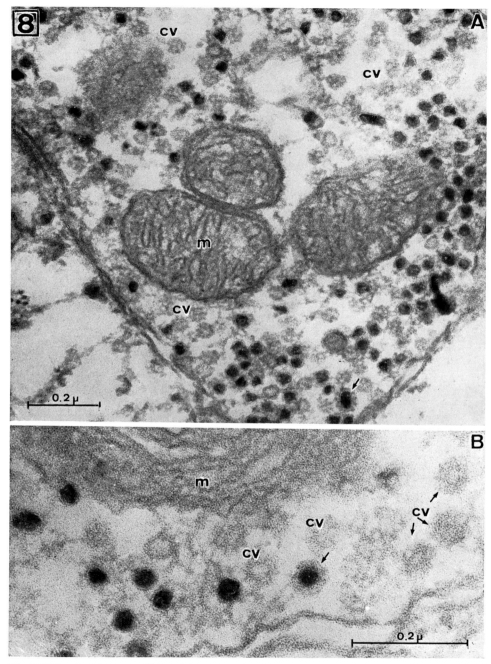

Fig. 8. Deiters' nucleus, cat. ZIO staining of nerve terminal. A: The majority of ZIO-positive vesicles are spheric and have a smooth surface. Many if not most of the ZIO-negative vesicles are of the coated (alveolate) type. Only one coated vesicle (cv) is ZIO positive (arrow). m = mitochondria. Primary magnification × 40 000. B: Similar preparation at × 80 000 primary magnification. The coated vesicles (cv) are ZIO negative with one exception (arrow).

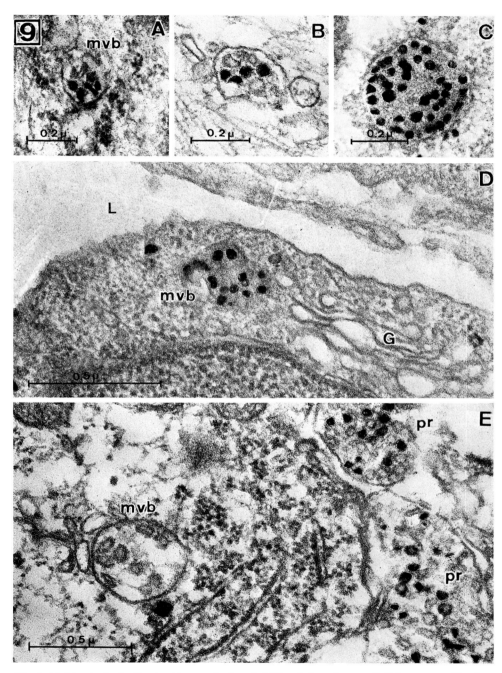

Fig. 9. Multivesicular bodies (mvb), rat spinal cord. ZIO staining of neuropil. Primary magnification × 40 000. A: Motoneuron, cell body. B: Axon. C and D: Capillary endothelium cell. Note the ZIO-negative Golgi complex (G). L = lumen. E: Motoneuron, cell body with ZIO-negative multivesicular body. pr = presynaptic terminals.

a negative one in Fig. 9D. Mak and Jersild (personal communication) have found ZIO-positive reactivity in Golgi complexes of intestinal epithelial cells after phospholipid ingestion, while examination prior to this treatment was negative. Prefixation with glutaraldehyde facilitated this reaction (Mak, 1969). Most of the positive findings in our material stem from Schwann cells and glia rather than from neurons. We have been unable thus far to define the conditions which are most favorable for obtaining a positive result.

*Smooth endoplasmic reticulum:* The continuity of rough and smooth endoplasmic reticulum in neuron perikarya can be easily demonstrated according to Peters *et al.* (1970). Smooth endoplasmic reticulum (SR) consists of tubular and cisternal elements which extend into dendrites and axons. ZIO-positive structures were found in axons and proximal portions of nerve terminals which consisted of irregular small profiles that seemed to form a continuous membrane-bound system (Fig. 12 and 13). In the longitudinal axonal profile one may recognize ZIO-positive elements interconnected like loosely strung beads. Other longitudinally arranged elements such as the microtubules and the neurofilaments are consistently ZIO negative. These findings lead to the conclusion that the ZIO-positive structure in the axon is SR and conversely that the SR of axons has a relatively high affinity for the ZIO stain.

Occasionally, we have observed SR in perikarya to be ZIO positive. A perinuclear cistern is shown to have reacted in Fig. 11. This observation is from a satellite cell in the cat spinal ganglion. A similar ZIO-positive effect has been reported in the nerve cells of the superior lobe of octopus (Barlow and Martin, 1970). We have been unable as yet to confirm this in mammalian neurons.

Friend (1969) has found an interesting affinity of multivesicular bodies and certain components of the Golgi complex to the prolonged incubation with unbuffered $OsO_4$ solution at 40° C. This prompted us to investigate the reactivity of nerve terminals to the same procedure (Kawana, unpublished). It was noted that synaptic vesicles were solidly stained — an effect which is not seen in conventionally osmicated sections. This observation shows that synaptic vesicles, mbv, Golgi and SR may have more than one cytochemical reaction in common. It reopens the speculation concerning the origin of synaptic vesicles.

## C. ZIO-NEGATIVE VESICLES AND GRANULES

*Dense-cored vesicles:* The fact that certain categories of vesicles which occur regularly in nerve terminals are ZIO negative was discovered during the initial phase of these investigations (Akert and Sandri, 1968; Akert *et al.*, 1968). The large-sized dense-cored vesicle is consistently unaffected by the reagent (Fig. 6), and this has been confirmed by several subsequent observers who investigated different types of terminals in different systems and species (Barlow and Martin, 1970; Martin *et al.*, 1969; Matus, 1970; Pellegrino de Iraldi and Gueudet, 1969). This negative finding is important from two points of view: (1) it illustrates the specificity — although of unknown nature — of the ZIO reagent, (2) it demonstrates the differential composition (and function) of dense-cored vesicles. Recent studies have added positive evidence by demonstrating

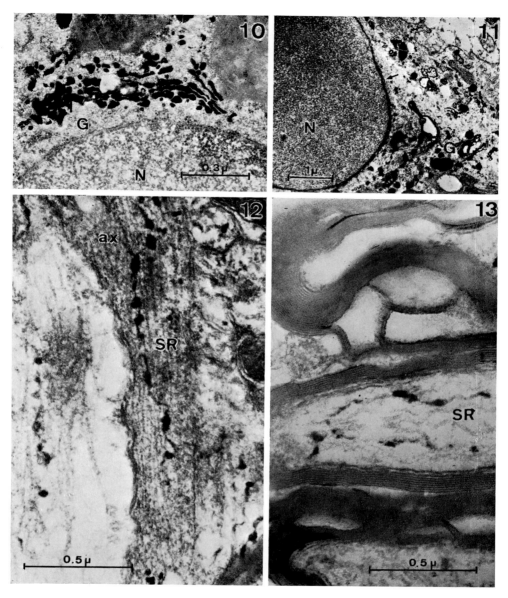

Fig. 10. Monkey Deiters' nucleus, oligodendrocyte. ZIO-positive Golgi complex (G). N = nucleus. Primary magnification × 40 000.

Fig. 11. Cat spinal ganglion, satellite cell. ZIO-positive Golgi complex (G). Note the ZIO-positive reaction of the perinuclear cistern (arrow). N = nucleus. Primary magnification × 8 000.

Fig. 12. Pigeon optic tectum. Initial axon (ax) segment with ZIO-positive smooth endoplasmic reticulum (SR). Microtubules are ZIO negative. Primary magnification × 40 000.

Fig. 13. Pigeon optic tectum. Myelinated axons. ZIO-positive smooth endoplasmic reticulum (SR). Primary magnification × 40 000.

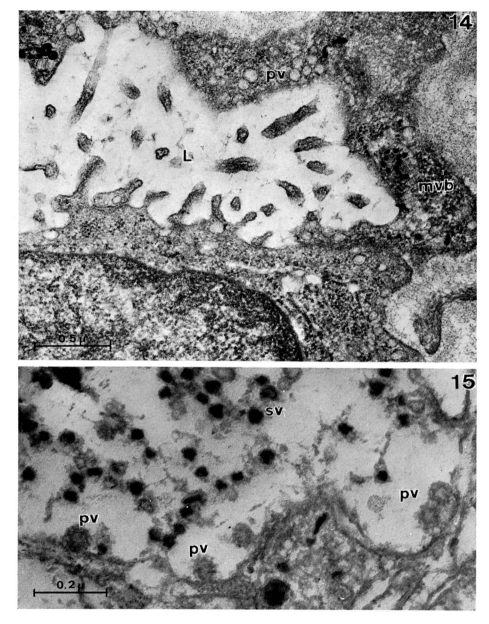

Fig. 14. Vas deferens, rat. Capillary endothelial cell. ZIO stain. Primary magnification × 20 000 .
Pinocytotic vesicles (pv) are ZIO negative (see also Fig. 7). mvb = multivesicular body with ZIO-
positive vesicles. L = lumen.
Fig. 15. Deiters' nucleus, cat. ZIO-stained nerve terminal with ZIO-positive synaptic vesicles (sv).
Note that plasmalemmal vesicles (pv) are ZIO negative.

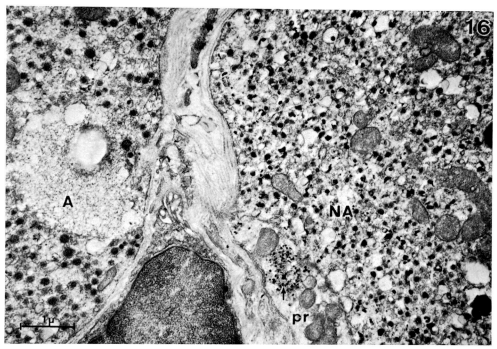

Fig. 16. Adrenal medulla, rat. Two adjacent cells which differ with respect to ZIO reactivity of chromaffin granules. At left, the chromaffin granules are predominantly non-reactive. The majority of cells belong to this type. At right, the chromaffin granules are vacuolated and many show ZIO-positive core. pr = nerve terminal with ZIO-positive synaptic vesicles (arrow). Primary magnification × 8 000. A = Adrenaline-producing cell. NA = Noradrenaline-producing cell.

that the core may be stained by the phosphotungstic acid (Bloom and Aghajanian, 1966; Jaim-Etcheverry and Zieher, 1969) and bismuth iodide (Pfenninger *et al.*, 1969) techniques while the clear synaptic vesicles are not impregnated.

*Neurosecretory granules:* A second category of ZIO-negative vesicles is represented by the neurosecretory granules which are characteristic of nerve terminals in the neurohypophysis, where they occur in association with clear spheric vesicles of the usual (300–600 Å) type. Rufener and Dreifuss (1970) have recently subjected these nerve endings to ZIO stain and obtained a consistently negative reaction of the neurosecretory granules and an equally consistent ZIO-positive staining result for the regular synaptic vesicles.

*Chromaffin granules:* The situation is more complex with regard to chromaffin granules. Matus (1970) noted that the catecholamine-containing granules of chromaffin cells in the superior cervical ganglion responded at least partially. In the adrenal medulla we found two types of cells: the more frequently occurring type contained largely ZIO-negative granules, whereas the rare type contained predominantly ZIO-positive granules. One is tempted to conclude that a differential ZIO affinity exists between adrenaline- and noradrenaline-producing elements (Fig. 16).

*Plasmalemmal vesicles* are derived from the cell membrane by a process of fission or pinocytosis. This phenomenon has been observed on the cell surface of nerve terminals by means of the freeze-etching technique (Akert *et al.*, 1969) as well as by conventional electron microscopy (Andres, 1964; Westrum, 1965). There is no room here to discuss the problems and mechanisms which relate plasmalemmal vesicles and the so-called *coated vesicles* (other names: complex, spiny, alveolate (Palay, 1963)) to each other and to synaptic functions. An excellent experimental contribution and review of this subject was recently published by Kanaseki and Kadota (1969). Several investigators have suggested that coated vesicles may be derived from the plasmalemma of nerve terminals and that they in turn may liberate the synaptic vesicles (Chalazonitis, 1970; Gray and Willis, 1971). In this context it is interesting to compare the ZIO-staining properties of plasmalemmal, coated and synaptic vesicles within the same nerve ending. Coated vesicles could be readily found in the boutons of spinal cord and caudate neuropil, but most frequently in Deiters' nucleus. Their site of predilection was away from the synapse at or near the axoplasmic membrane. The vast majority were ZIO negative, but in rare instances ZIO-positive coated vesicles could be seen (Figs. 8, 15).

The ZIO reactivity of pinocytotic vesicles was also examined in capillary endothelium (Fig. 14) and in smooth muscle cells (Fig. 7). The vesicles were consistently ZIO negative.

From these observations it may be concluded that a clear-cut difference between plasmalemmal and synaptic vesicles seems to exist with respect to their affinity to ZIO stain. This does not preclude the existence of functional relationships between the two types of vesicles, but adds to the complexity of the problem.

### ACKNOWLEDGEMENT

The technical assistance by Miss R. Emch, Miss L. Decoppet, Miss H. Bruppacher as well as many helpful discussions with Mr. K. Pfenninger are gratefully acknowledged. Special thanks are due to Miss U. Fischer for her untiring efforts in preparing the typescript and bibliography.

### SUMMARY

1. Terminals of peripheral and central, autonomic and somatic nerve fibres were studied using the Champy–Maillet method (ZIO stain) at the electron-microscopic level.

2. The ZIO stain shows a high affinity to synaptic vesicles regardless of their shape and size.

3. Large dark-cored vesicles (800–1500 Å) as well as neurosecretory granules of neurohypophyseal nerve endings (the latter according to Rufener and Dreifuss (1960) are consistently ZIO negative, while chromaffin granules may be ambivalent.

4. Positive ZIO reactivity may be observed under certain (as yet ill-defined) conditions in the following organelles: vesicles within multivesicular bodies, Golgi vesicles,

Golgi cisterns and smooth endoplasmic reticulum. The ZIO reactivity of the latter is particularly evident in longitudinal profiles of axons.

5. Predominantly negative results are seen in plasmalemmal vesicles and coated vesicles at or near the surface of nerve terminals.

## REFERENCES

AKERT, K. AND SANDRI, C. (1968) *Brain Res.*, **7**, 286–295.
AKERT, K., SANDRI, C. AND PFENNINGER, K. (1968) In: D. S. BOCCIARELLI (Ed.), *Electronmicroscopy*, Vol. 2, Roma Tip. Pol., Vaticana, pp. 521–522.
AKERT, K., MOOR, H., PFENNINGER, K. AND SANDRI, C. (1969) In: K. AKERT AND P. G. WASER (Eds.), *Mechanisms of Synaptic Transmission, Progress in Brain Research*, Vol. 31, Elsevier Amsterdam, pp. 223–240.
ANDRES, K. H. (1964) *Z. Zellforsch.*, **64**, 63–73.
BARLOW, J. AND MARTIN, R. (1970) *Brain Res.*, **24**, 129–168.
BLOOM, F. E. AND AGHAJANIAN, G. K. (1966) *Science*, **154**, 1575–1577.
CHALAZONITIS, N. (1970) In: S. H. BARONDES (Ed.), *Cellular Dynamics of the Neuron*, Academic Press, New York, pp. 229–243.
FRIEND, D. S. (1969) *J. Cell Biol.*, **41**, 269–279.
GRAY, E. G. AND WILLIS, R. A. (1971) *Brain Res.*, **25**, 231–253.
HILLARP, N. Å. (1959) *Acta Anat.*, **38**, 379–384.
JABONERO, V. (1964) *Acta Neuroveg.*, **26**, 184–210.
JAIM-ETCHEVERRY, G. AND ZIEHER, L. M. (1969) *J. Cell Biol.*, **42**, 855–860.
KANASEKI, T. AND KADOTA, K. (1969) *J. Cell Biol.*, **42**, 202–220.
KAWANA, E., AKERT, K. AND SANDRI, C. (1969) *Brain Res.*, **16**, 325–331.
KAWANA, E., AKERT, K. AND BRUPPACHER, H. (1971) *J. Comp. Neurol.*, in press.
MAILLET, M. (1962) *Trab. Inst. Cajal Invest. Biol.*, **54**, 1–36.
MAILLET, M. (1968) *Bull. Assoc. Anat.*, **53**, 233–394.
MAK, K. M. (1969) *Anat. Rec.*, **163**, 224.
MARTIN, R., BARLOW, J. AND MIRALTO, A. (1969) *Brain Res.*, **15**, 1–16.
MATUS, A. I. (1970) *Brain Res.*, **17**, 195–203.
PALAY, S. L. (1963) *J. Cell Biol.*, **19**, 89A–90A.
PELLEGRINO DE IRALDI, A. AND GUEUDET, R. (1968) *Z. Zellforsch.*, **91**, 178–185.
PELLEGRINO DE IRALDI, A. AND GUEUDET, R. (1969) *Z. Zellforsch.*, **101**, 203–211.
PETERS, A., PALAY, S. L. AND WEBSTER, H. F. (1970) *The Fine Structure of the Nervous System. The Cells and their Processes*, Harper and Row, New York, Evanston and London.
PFENNINGER, K., SANDRI, C., AKERT, K. AND EUGSTER, C. H. (1969) *Brain Res.*, **12**, 10–18.
RUFENER, C. AND DREIFUSS, J. J. (1970) *Brain Res.*, **22**, 402–405.
TAXI, J. (1965) *Ann. Sci. Nat. Zool.*, **7**, 413–674.
WESTRUM, L. E. (1965) *J. Physiol.*, **179**, 4.

# Dense Contents in Synaptic Vesicles Produced by Sequential Cation Binding, Alcohol Treatment and Osmium Tetroxide Fixation

A. KOKKO** AND R. J. BARRNETT

*Department of Anatomy, Yale University School of Medicine, New Haven, Connecticut (U.S.A.)*

Since the introduction of fine structural cytochemistry for localizing acyl transferases by the demonstration of acetylcarnitine transferase (Higgins and Barrnett, 1970), and subsequently the monoglyceride and the $\alpha$-glycerophosphate pathways of lipid synthesis (Higgins and Barrnett, 1971), other acyl transfer systems have been examined including choline acetyltransferase (Feigenson *et al.*, unpublished). In these experiments one type of final product was obtained when heavy metal salts were used as capture reagents to precipitate coenzyme A (CoA) by mercaptide formation as this was released from acetyl-CoA by the action of the transferase. Condition for the production of final product was compatible with the activity of partially purified choline acetyltransferase in the presence of any of several heavy metals; however, the cytochemical experiments were not satisfactory because a dense product not only occurred in the contents of 'clear' synaptic vesicles under incubating conditions in which choline acetyltransferase was active biochemically, but a similar density occurred in the absence of substrate, acetyl-CoA. In these experiments both control and experimental tissues were refixed in alcoholic osmium tetroxide because the mercaptides of CoA (experimental) are soluble in aqueous osmium tetroxide.

The above results, though more striking, were similar to those obtained by Bloom and Barrnett (1966) who also found that a variety of metal capture reagents bound to the contents of synaptic vesicles during experiments in which acetylcholinesterase was localized at fine structural level in the electroplax of electric eel. For these reasons, and because some synaptic vesicles which ordinarily contain electron-lucent contents can be made to appear dense after prolonged fixation in a mixture of osmium tetroxide, iodine and zinc chloride (Akert and Sandri, 1968), it was decided to initiate an investigation of the retention of material in synaptic vesicles which could be made opaque to electrons by various incubation and refixation of aldehyde-fixed tissue.

## MATERIALS AND METHODS

The ventral grey matter of the cervical spinal cord of albino rats fixed by perfusion

* This work was supported by USPHS grants AM-03688 and TICA-05055.
** Present address: Bioacoustic Research Laboratory, Dept. of Electrical Engineering, University of Illinois, Urbana, Ill.

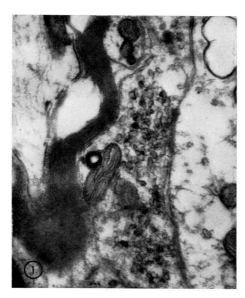

Fig. 1. Density obtained in "clear" synaptic vesicles after incubating of aldehyde-fixed section in cacodylate-buffered solution of $Pb^{2+}$, followed by refixation in alcoholic osmium tetroxide. In some vesicles material adjacent to the inner aspect of the vesicle membrane shows an increase in density. Some of the vesicles are partly or completely filled with dense material. $\times$ 50000.

through the left ventricle with a mixture 2 % glutaraldehyde and 1 % formaldehyde in cacodylate buffer (0.05 M, pH 7.4) for 15 min was used as the experimental tissue. After perfusion, the tissue was washed in cacodylate buffer for 15 min to 24 h either as sections, or small blocks of tissue which were sectioned after washing. The sections (50–100 $\mu$, produced with a tissue chopper) were incubated in various metal salt solutions (approximately 5 mM) with cacodylate buffer (0.05 M). Although 15 different metallic salts ($AgNO_3$, $HAuCl_4$, $BaCl_2$, $Cd(NO_3)_2$, $FeSO_4$, $Fe_2(SO_4)_3$, $HgCl_2$, $La(NO_3)_2$, $Pb(NO_3)_2$, $PtCl_2$, $PtCl_4$, $K(SbO)C_4H_4O$, $SnCl_2$, $UO_2(C_2H_3O_2)_2$, $Zn(NO_3)_2$), were tested, the most prominent results were obtained with three; $Cd^{2+}$, $Pb^{2+}$ and $Zn^{2+}$, and this report shall be confined to the experiments using these metals.

Various buffers were tested and the best results were obtained by using cacodylate. In addition pH's from 3 to 8 were also tested. It was found that the effect of metal incubation per unit time, as judged by the subsequent density developed in synaptic vesicles, occurred between pH 5.5 and 6.5. When incubations were conducted at pH's below 5, the subsequent density of vesicle contents decreased markedly; the decrease in density was not so marked at pH's above 6.5. In the final experiments, satisfactory results were obtained with incubations of 1 h at pH 6 at room temperature.

The subsequent density which developed in synaptic vesicles after incubation in solutions of metal ions was found to be also dependent on treatment with alcohol and on osmium tetroxide refixation. Therefore, various combinations of incubation in metal salts and buffer, treatment with different concentrations of alcohol and refixation in aqueous or alcoholic osmium tetroxide were also tested. In all instances,

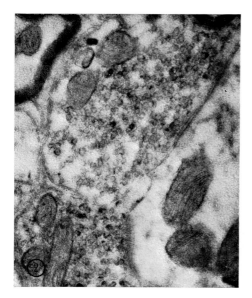 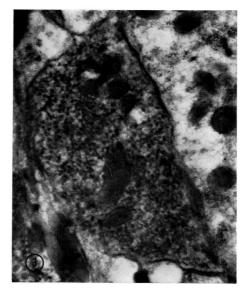

Fig. 2. Density obtained in synaptic vesicles after incubation in $Cd^{2+}$ solution followed by refixation in alcoholic $OsO_4$. The contents, partly filling some synaptic vesicles, show increased density and crescent forms are seen. $\times$ 80000.

Fig. 3. Density obtained in synaptic vesicles after aldehyde fixed tissue was incubated in buffered $Pb^{2+}$ medium, immersed in absolute ethanol, and refixed in alcoholic $OsO_4$. Almost all synaptic vesicles are filled with dense contents; the size of the vesicles is smaller than those not subjected directly to absolute alcohol. $\times$ 46000.

after final dehydration, the tissues were embedded in Epon–Araldite and examined after thin sectioning with an RCA EMU 3F electron microscope. No additional staining was used on the thin sections to enhance contrast.

## RESULTS

Dense contents occurred in synaptic vesicles in sections of spinal cord incubated in cacodylate-buffered solutions of $Cd^{2+}$, $Pb^{2+}$ and $Zn^{2+}$ (Figs. 1–3), providing the sections were refixed, directly after incubation, in alcoholic osmium tetroxide (1 % $OsO_4$ in 50 % ethanol) or immersed in absolute ethanol, followed by refixation in either alcoholic or aqueous osmium tetroxide. Although the vesicles, which ordinarily contain clear contents on routine fixation, showed increased density as a result of the above treatment in *all* synaptic endings, not all vesicles in a given ending reacted to the same extent. In most endings a substantial number of vesicles were unreactive and these were mixed in a random fashion with vesicles containing reactive or semireactive contents (Figs. 1 and 2).

The production and retention of dense contents in the synaptic vesicles varied depending on the treatment. Incubation in a buffered solution containing a metal salt, followed by fixation in alcoholic osmium tetroxide usually resulted in profiles in which only part of the contents of some vesicles were dense, especially portions adjacent to the

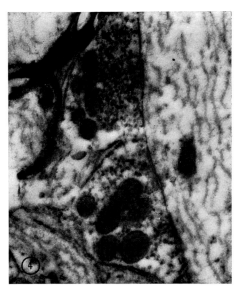

Fig. 4. Density obtained in synaptic vesicles by treating aldehyde-fixed tissue in absolute ethanol, refixing in alcoholic OsO$_4$, followed by dehydration in only absolute ethanol. A large number of the vesicles show increased density in the contents. The vesicle size is again small. × 40000.

interior of the limiting membrane, resulting in crescent or doughnut configurations (Figs. 1 and 2). When incubation in buffer containing the metal salt was followed by immersion in absolute ethanol before osmium tetroxide treatment, more vesicles reacted and these were usually more filled with dense contents (Fig. 3). Treatment with concentrated alcohol before refixation in osmium tetroxide impaired the fine structural preservation.

Significantly less density than observed in Figs. 1 and 2 occurred in synaptic vesicles if a 1–2 h buffer wash preceded refixation in alcoholic osmium tetroxide. Refixation of sections incubated in buffer containing metal salt direct in aqueous osmium tetroxide produced no dense vesicle contents (Fig. 6). This indicates that whatever vesicle contents, retained by aldehyde fixation and metal salt incubation for subsequent reaction with alcoholic osmium tetroxide, were resolubilized by aqueous solutions of either buffer alone or fixative. It also emphasizes a little appreciated fact that routine osmium tetroxide fixation extracts much of the contents of the hyaloplasm and of cell organelles.

If the sections incubated in metal salt solutions were dehydrated through lower concentrations of alcohol (10–30 %) prior to refixation in alcoholic osmium tetroxide, the vesicle contents also did not appear dense. This finding emphasizes the solvent action of dilute alcohol on material presumably retained as a result of aldehyde fixation and metal salt incubation. Aldehyde-fixed sections incubated in buffer containing a metal salt and dehydrated routinely or immersed directly in absolute ethanol without refixation in osmium tetroxide, showed no density in synaptic vesicles. It is apparent, therefore, that the density developed, as described in the

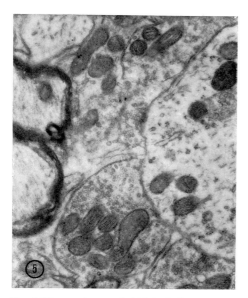 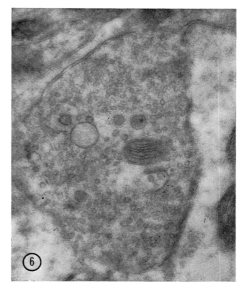

Fig. 5. No metal control. Aldehyde-fixed tissue, incubated in buffer alone, refixed in alcoholic osmium tetroxide followed by absolute alcohol dehydration. Synaptic vesicles have no dense contents. × 42000.

Fig. 6. After incubation in a $Pb^{2+}$-containing medium, the section was refixed in aqueous osmium tetroxide and dehydrated in absolute alcohol. Synaptic vesicles show no density. × 60000.

foregoing results, was directly due to osmium tetroxide and not the metal salts, the deposits of which on the basis of previous cytochemical experiments can be clearly distinguished from that produced by the refixation. It should be noted, however, that conspicuous density developed in neurotubules when $Pb^{2+}$ was used as the incubation metal. Mitochondria showed increased density of the matrix and of the content of spaces between membranes, but this depended on both the direct dehydration in absolute alcohol after incubation in metal salt solution, and refixation in alcoholic osmium tetroxide.

Thus, incubation in metallic solutions was important in developing density in synaptic vesicle contents only if the tissue was refixed in alcoholic osmium tetroxide, or treated with absolute ethanol prior to refixation in aqueous osmium tetroxide. In both instances of refixation, if the metal salt incubation was omitted, no density in synaptic vesicles occurred (Fig. 5). Since the increased density of the contents of the clear synaptic vesicles appeared also to be related to the concentration of alcohol used prior to refixation in osmium tetroxide, we explored the possibility of developing density in synaptic vesicles without the use of the buffered metal salt incubation. If aldehyde-fixed tissue sections were immersed directly in absolute ethanol, refixed in alcoholic osmium tetroxide, followed by dehydration in only absolute ethanol, vesicle contents were as dense as with metal treatment (Fig. 4). The vesicles were, however, shrunken, and often distorted in shape. The degree of density developed was significantly less if aqueous osmium tetroxide was used after the absolute alcohol

TABLE 1

THE EFFECT OF INCUBATION WITH METAL SALT SOLUTIONS, RINSES, DEHYDRATIONS AND REFIXATION IN OSMIUM TETROXIDE ON DENSITY OF SYNAPTIC VESICLE CONTENTS

| Incubation with | Rinse in buffer after incubation | Rinse in ethanol series after incubation | Rinse in absolute ethanol after incubation | No rinse after incubation | Alcoholic osmication | Aqueous osmication | No osmication | Dehydration in alcohol series | Dehydration in absolute ethanol only | Vesicles and vesicle contents |
|---|---|---|---|---|---|---|---|---|---|---|
| Cd, Pb, Zn | — | — | — | + | + | — | — | — | + | Dense contents partly filling vesicles, normal size. |
| Cd, Pb, Zn | — | — | + | — | + | — | — | + or | + | Dense contents filling vesicles, smaller size. |
| Cd, Pb, Zn | — | — | + | — | — | + | — | + or | + | Dense contents filling vesicles, shrunken. |
| No metal | — | — | + | — | + | — | — | — | + | Dense contents filling vesicles, shrunken. |
| Cd, Pb, Zn | + | — | — | — | + | — | — | — | + | No density in contents, normal size. |
| Cd, Pb, Zn | — | + | — | — | + | — | — | — | + | No density in contents, normal size. |
| Cd, Pb, Zn | — | — | + | + | — | + | — | + or | + | No density in contents, normal size. |
| Cd, Pb, Zn | — | — | — | — | — | — | + | — | + | No density in vesicles, shrunken. Neurotubules show dense contents with Pb. |
| Cd, Pb, Zn | — | + or | — | — or | — | — | + | — | — | No density in vesicles, normal size. Neurotubules show dense contents with Pb. |
| No metal | — | — | + | — | — | + | — | + or | + | No density in vesicles, shrunken. |
| No metal | — | — | + | — | + | — | — | + | — | No density in vesicles, shrunken. |
| No metal | — | — | — | + | + | — | — | — | + | No density in vesicles, normal size. |

treatment, or if routine dehydration through lower concentrations of ethanol were instituted after the alcoholic osmium refixation. Thus, it appeared that the contents of 'clear' synaptic vesicles are maintained by higher concentrations of alcohol for subsequent densification with alcoholic osmium tetroxide; dilute alcohol solubilized the material either before or after the osmium tetroxide treatment. Parenthetically, it should be noted that the marked shrinking effect of absolute alcohol on the synaptic vesicles was not as noticeable on the fine structural elements in perikarya of the neurons. The 'dense core' vesicles present in some synaptic endings were not affected by any of the treatments that caused increased density in the clear vesicles. (The results concerning density in the clear synaptic vesicles are summarized in Table I).

## DISCUSSION

It may be pertinent to the above experiments that all the conditions enumerated above which retained contents, subsequently appearing dense, in synaptic vesicles, were conditions in which acetylcholine (ACh) and CoA were precipitated, remained insoluble, and possibly reacted with osmium tetroxide although the precipitates do not become black. The insoluble mercaptides of CoA, formed with heavy metals, are soluble in aqueous solutions in the absence of excess metal, are soluble in dilute alcohol and aqueous osmium tetroxide but are insoluble in absolute alcohol or in alcoholic osmium tetroxide. Although this might at first hand suggest that the contents of synaptic vesicles contained ACh and CoA, this is not justified by the present experiments alone. It may be more significant that the reactions that increased the density of the contents of some 'clear' vesicles, occurred in all the synaptic endings in the neuropil of the gray matter of the ventral cervical cord. In a brief survey the same results occurred in the clear vesicles of synaptic endings of nine other areas of the central nervous system (olfactory bulb, frontal and occipital cortex, caudate nucleus, thalamus, hypothalamus, cerebellar cortex, and two regions of the brain stem) and the implications stated above, like the zinc–iodine–osmium reaction, are not justified for all synapses on the basis of present knowledge.

What seems more feasible is to hypothesize a component in the vesicle contents that has an excess of negative charges. The basis for this suggestion is the present experiments which indicate that in some circumstances reaction with cations is necessary for the subsequent retention of the material and when an excess of cationic choline was included in the metal salt-incubating media, no density subsequently developed after refixation with alcoholic osmium tetroxide. The identity of this presumed anionic material and its occurrence in vesicles of all synaptic terminals requires further experimentation.

## REFERENCES

AKERT, K. AND SANDRI, C. (1968) *Brain Res.*, **7**, 286.
BLOOM, F. E. AND BARRNETT, R. J. (1966) *J. Cell Biol.*, **29**, 475.
FEIGENSON, M., HIGGINS, J. A. AND BARRNETT, R. J., unpublished results.
HIGGINS, J. A. AND BARRNETT, R. J. (1970) *J. Cell Sci.*, **6**, 29.
HIGGINS, J. A. AND BARRNETT, R. J. (1971) *J. Cell Biol.*, in press.

# The Histochemical Localization of Choline Acetyltransferase*

ALVIN M. BURT

*Department of Anatomy, Vanderbilt University School of Medicine, Nashville, Tennessee (U.S.A.)*

## INTRODUCTION

The enzyme choline acetyltransferase catalyzes the following reaction:

$$\text{Acetyl-CoA} + \text{Choline} \rightleftharpoons \text{Acetylcholine} + \text{CoA}$$

The role of acetylcholine in nervous transmission and in membrane excitation has been the focal point of numerous studies in the field of neurobiology for many years. For over 20 years, procedures have been available for the localization of acetyl-cholinesterase (Koelle and Friedenwald, 1949), and since that time a number of modifications have been introduced which have improved the localization and specificity of this histochemical reaction. Recently, a similar evolutionary process began for the histochemical localization of choline acetyltransferase (Burt, 1969, 1970; Hebb *et al.*, 1970; Kása *et al.*, 1970). These procedures have been based upon the precipitation of CoA as a lead mercaptide and the subsequent conversion of this mercaptide to the visible PbS. An alternate approach to the histochemical localization of CoA has utilized the reducing property of the –SH group on CoA to reduce potassium ferricyanide. The potassium ferrocyanide thus formed will combine with uranyl ions to form an electron-dense precipitate. This procedure has been utilized by Higgins and Barrnett (1970) for the localization of carnitine transferase. This basic principle should be applicable for the localization of other acyl transferases, in particular choline acetyltransferase.

There are, however, four major points which must be considered in the histochemical localization of choline acetyltransferase. First, any enzymes capable of releasing CoA under the selected conditions of incubation will give a positive reaction. Second, we have not found a satisfactory histochemical inhibitor of choline acetyltransferase, one which can be used in defining the specificity of the reaction under the histochemical conditions employed. Third, our data suggest that choline acetyltransferase, under the conditions required for the histochemistry, can hydrolyze acetyl-CoA in the absence of choline. And finally, choline acetyltransferase is released from a tissue-bound state

* This investigation was supported by U.S. Public Health Service Research Career Development Award 1-K03-GM-10132 and Research Grant 1-R01-NB-07441 from the National Institutes of Health.

*References p. 335*

in direct proportion to the salt concentration of the incubation medium (Fonnum, 1967). This property is retained after formalin fixation (Burt, 1970). Our interpretation, therefore, of the histochemical data at this time has been based upon a number of criteria, no one of which is specific for choline acetyltransferase alone.

## HISTOCHEMICAL PROCEDURES

Procedures for the histochemical localization of choline acetyltransferase activity in rat central nervous tissue has been described in detail elsewhere (Burt, 1970; Kása et al., 1970). Although the procedure of Kása et al. is based on the same basic principle, the formation of a lead mercaptide, it differs in several important respects from the one developed in our laboratory and described below.

The nervous tissue for this study was frozen rapidly and sectioned in a cryostat. The sections were fixed in 2% formaldehyde (prepared fresh from paraformaldehyde) prior to incubation. The basic incubation medium used is as follows: 25 mM HEPES ($N$-2-hydroxyethylpiperazine-$N$-2-ethanesulfonic acid) buffer at a final pH of 6.0 with 4 mM choline, 0.2 mM acetyl-CoA, 1.8 mM $Pb(NO_3)_2$ and $1 \times 10^{-3}M$ DFP (diisopropyl fluorophosphate). These conditions are nearly optimal with respect to pH and lead concentration for the trapping of CoA as the lead mercaptide (Burt, 1970). In addition, we have found that the results are more consistent and reproducible if the fixed tissue sections are treated for 1 h with a $1 \times 10^{-3}M$ DFP solution prior to incubation. Kása et al. (1970) have shown that acetylcholinesterase will hydrolyze acetyl-CoA and this treatment with DFP is similar to that used in their laboratory. The use of DFP provides more consistent results than phospholine iodide which was used in our earlier studies (Burt, 1970). Following incubation at 37°C for 1.5 to 3 h the sections are washed briefly, placed in dilute ammonium sulfide, and subsequently mounted on slides with an aqueous mounting medium.

## SPECIFICITY OF THE REACTION

The localization of choline acetyltransferase activity with any procedure which involves the capture or precipitation of the reaction product, CoA, is going to be complicated by several factors. First, any enzymatic activity associated with the hydrolysis of acetyl-CoA or with the transfer of the acetyl group to another acyl acceptor endogenous to the system will give a positive reaction in this technique. The treatment with DFP leads to an eight-fold reduction in the rate of free acetate formation but it does not alter the rate of acetylcholine synthesis significantly. This reduction in acetate formation is apparently due to the inhibition of acetylcholinesterase (Kása et al., 1970) as well as other esterases and hydrolases. A second complicating factor is that choline acetyltransferase, in formalin-fixed tissue and under the incubation conditions described herein, appears to catalyze the hydrolysis of acetyl-CoA in the absence of choline (Burt, 1970). Thus, the elimination of choline from the incubation medium is not a satisfactory control. This conclusion was based upon the following observations: (1) When choline was not included in the incubation medium, the rate of acetate formation was doubled. (2) When $Cu^{2+}$ ($1 \times 10^{-4}M$) was added to the complete medium, acetylcholine synthesis was inhibited and the rate of acetate formation was reduced to one-fourth the initial level. This level of acetate formation was not altered by the removal of choline from the incubation medium (*i.e.*, in the presence of $Cu^{2+}$, choline had no effect on the rate of acetate formation). Choline acetyltransferase, and acyltransferases in general, are inhibited by low concentrations of $Cu^{2+}$ (Potter *et al.*, 1968; White and Cavallito, 1970). (3) The histological distribution of the reaction product in tissue incubated both with and without choline was identical although in the absence of choline, the deposition of reaction product may have been less intense. The fact that acetate formation is reduced by the addition of $Cu^{2+}$ further suggests that some of the acetate formation in the complete medium is related to choline acetyltransferase activity or to a $Cu^{2+}$-sensitive acetyl-CoA hydrolase.

Studies on rat brain choline acetyltransferase (Potter *et al.*, 1968) have indicated that both choline and acetyl-CoA must combine with the enzyme before either product is released; however, Schuberth (1966), in a study of placental choline acetyltransferase, has suggested that the reaction proceeds in two steps with the formation of an acetyl–enzyme intermediate. The more recent studies of White and Cavallito (1970) have suggested that the reaction proceeds by the Theorell–Chance ordered sequential mechanism (Cleland, 1963). This latter mechanism also would be compatible with the recent isotopic exchange data of Morris and Grewaal (1969b). If, under the conditions of incubation, an acetyl–enzyme intermediate were not stable or if this intermediate could accept water as an acetyl receptor in place of choline, then choline acetyltransferase would appear to split or hydrolyze acetyl-CoA. The studies of White and Cavallito (1970) further suggest that an imidazole moiety on the enzyme is part of the active center in the acetyl transfer reaction, both as an acceptor of the acetyl group and as a catalyst for the removal of a proton from the acetyl receptor. If an imidazole moiety is involved in the acetyl reaction, it should be noted that functions of the imidazole nucleus, such as acylation, are greatly affected by changes in pH (Barnard and Stein, 1958). The *N*-acetyl imidazole is readily hydrolyzed in water, especially at acid pHs and, for the optimal histochemical trapping of CoA with lead, we must of necessity work in the acid pH range.

The compound chloroacetylcholine, synthesized initially as an AChE inhibitor (Chiou and Sastry, 1968) has proved to be a rather potent inhibitor of choline acetyltransferase (Morris and Grewaal, 1969a). This compound has been used by Kása *et al.* (1970) in defining the specificity of their procedure for the histochemical localization of choline acetyltransferase. The results from our limited use of this inhibitor have not been conclusive and, at the present time, we are unable to make a definitive statement concerning the usefulness of this compound for the selective inhibition of choline acetyltransferase activity under our histochemical conditions. The development and use of a specific inhibitor is the most critical problem in the development of a more satisfactory procedure for the localization of choline acetyltransferase activity at this time.

Additional problems in the interpretation of histochemical data are associated with

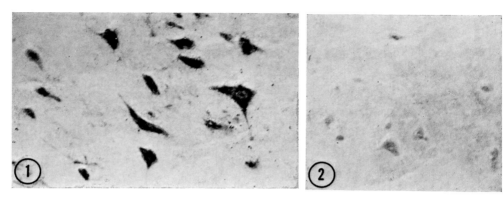

Fig. 1. Neurons of the rat brain medullary reticular formation. The section, 10 $\mu$ thick, was incubated for 150 min in the complete incubation medium. Note the heavy staining of the neuronal perikaryon. No counter stain. × 195.

Fig. 2. Neurons of the rat brain medullary reticular formation. The section, 10 $\mu$ thick, was incubated for 120 min in the complete incubation medium plus 0.1 M $KNO_3$. Note that the residual staining is confined primarily to the nuclei of the neurons; there is also some residual staining in the neuronal perikaryon. No counter stain. × 195.

the fact that choline acetyltransferase is selectively released from the tissue when the salt concentration in the medium is increased (Fonnum, 1967). Approximately 56 % of the enzyme in formalin-fixed tissue is soluble under the incubation conditions employed in this study (Burt 1970). Is the *in vivo* locus of the soluble fraction of the enzyme the same as that which remains bound to the tissue? This is one of the many questions which future investigations must seek to answer. When the salt concentration of the incubation medium was raised by the addition of $KNO_3$ (to a final concentration of 0.1 M), there was no change in the rate of acetylcholine synthesis, however, the enzyme was released from the tissue section and became soluble. We have used this property of choline acetyltransferase to advantage in attempting to define the histochemical localization of the enzymatic activity (Burt, 1970).

The following criteria have been used in the interpretation of the histochemical data. (1) In the complete incubation medium, approximately 2 moles of acetylcholine are synthesized for every mole of free acetate formed (Burt, 1970); hence, at least two-thirds of the reaction product is associated with choline acetyltransferase activity. (2) Choline acetyltransferase is selectively solubilized with $KNO_3$ and is inhibited by $Cu^{2+}$; however, the histological distribution of the remaining reaction product is identical for either treatment. This residual activity has been interpreted as nonspecific enzymatic activity. (3) The histological distribution of the reaction product, which has been interpreted as choline acetyltransferase activity is similar to that suggested by the microchemical studies of McCaman and Hunt (1965) and Goldberg and McCaman (1967). (4) The general distribution of the reaction product in the neuronal perikaryon and in the boutons terminaux is in agreement with the suggested intracellular distribution of the enzyme based on cell fractionation studies (Michael-

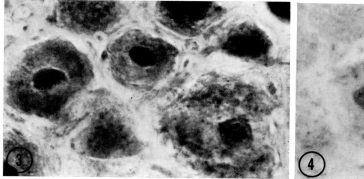
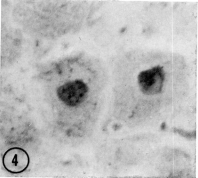

Fig. 3. Neurons of the rat dorsal root ganglion. Section, 8 $\mu$ thick, was incubated for 210 min in the complete incubation medium. No counter stain. $\times$ 620.

Fig. 4. Neurons of the rat dorsal root ganglion. Section, 8 $\mu$ thick was incubated for 200 min in the complete incubation medium plus 0.1 $M$ KNO₃. Note the residual staining in the neuronal nuclei with some faint staining in the perikaryon. No counter stain. $\times$ 620.

son, 1967). Although no one of these criteria is specific for choline acetyltransferase, the combination of all four strongly suggests that we are localizing choline acetyltransferase activity.

### DISTRIBUTION OF ENZYME ACTIVITY

The deposition of reaction product was confined essentially to the neuronal elements. Large motor neurons showed a heavy deposition of reaction product in the perikaryon, in the nucleus and in the form of small black granules on the surface of the cell. A similar distribution of reaction product was noted for neurons of numerous brain stem nuclei, such as the medullary reticular formation (Fig. 1) and the vestibular nuclei (Fig. 5). When either $Cu^{2+}$ (1 $\times$ 10⁻⁴M) or KNO₃ (0.1 M) was added to the incubation medium the heavy deposition of reaction product occurred only in the nuclei of the neurons; the perikaryon occasionally exhibited some light staining (Figs. 2, 4 and 6). This residual activity has been interpreted as non-specific enzymatic activity. Neurons such as the dorsal interneurons and many of the neurons of the neocortex showed little or no staining, while others, such as the caudate neurons and large pyramidal cells of the neocortex exhibited moderate to low levels of activity. The small dense granules (absent with either $Cu^{2+}$ or KNO₃ treatment) were visible on the surface of neurons in all categories (Fig. 5). As anticipated, these granular structures, interpreted as boutons terminaux (Burt, 1970), were absent in preparations of dorsal root ganglia (Figs. 3 and 4).

Choline acetyltransferase activity has been localized at the ultrastructural level with the electron microscope (Kása *et al.* 1970 and Fig. 8). In confirmation of light microscopic findings, the reaction end product was localized in the cell body, dendrites and axons of motor neurons. In some axon terminals, presumably cholinergic a heavy

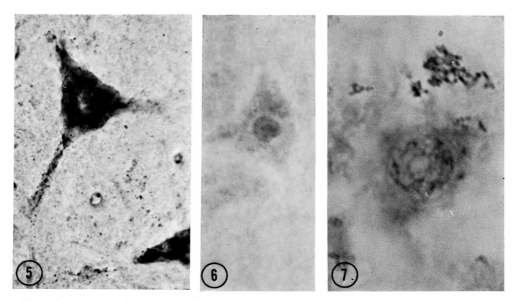

Fig. 5. Large neuron from a rat vestibular nucleus. Section, 10 $\mu$ thick, was incubated for 120 min in the complete incubation medium. Note the dense deposit of reaction product in the neuronal peri-karyon. Heavily stained boutons terminaux are visible on the surface of the neuron, especially on the proximal segments of the dendritic processes. Structures with similar staining properties are also visible in the surrounding neuropil. No counter stain. $\times$ 775.

Fig. 6. Large neuron from the same nucleus as in Fig. 5. Section, 10 $\mu$ thick, was incubated for 120 min in the complete incubation medium plus 0.1 $M$ KNO$_3$. Note the residual staining in the nucleus with some faint staining in the cytoplasm. The boutons terminaux, prominent in Fig. 5 are not stained. No counter stain. $\times$ 775.

Fig. 7. Neuron from the rat caudate nucleus. Section, 10 $\mu$ thick, was incubated for 120 min in the complete medium. The neuronal perikaryon is stained very lightly; the non-specific nuclear staining is also visible. Many heavy stained structures, resembling boutons terminaux, are present throughout the neuropil. Occasionally these structures appear to be in large clusters as illustrated directly above the neuron. This pattern is characteristic of the caudate nucleus (see text). $\times$ 1950.

concentration of enzyme reaction product was visible (axon 2, Fig. 8) whereas other axon terminals showed little or no evidence of enzymatic activity (axon 1, Fig. 8). Some of the reaction product in the extracellular spaces may represent diffusion artifact. Although the precise subcellular localization of choline acetyltransferase within the neuron and its processes will require further study, it is significant that discrete populations of boutons terminaux can be identified as being either choline acetyltransferase positive or choline acetyltransferase negative. All of the choline acetyltransferase-positive boutons contained the round clear synaptic vesicles whereas the boutons containing either ovoid or dense core vesicles were always negative. These findings add support to the idea that morphological differences between synaptic vesicles may be a reflection of differences in the chemical transmitter (see Kása et al., 1970).

A few observations can be made at this time concerning some of the regional dis-

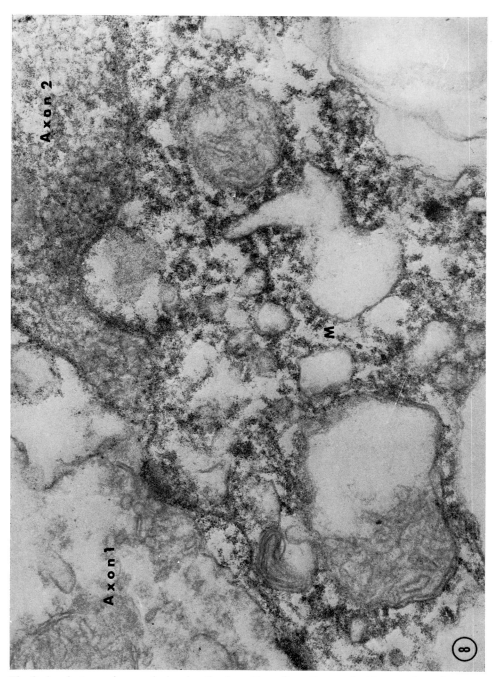

Fig. 8. An electron micrograph showing the deposition of reaction product in a portion of a motor neuron (M) and in one axon terminal (axon 2). An adjacent axon terminal (axon 1) is negative. The incubation medium contained acetyl-CoA, choline, DFP and lead nitrate in a cacodylate buffer, pH 5.9 (see Kása *et al.*, 1970). × 70000. The electron micrograph was provided through the courtesy of Drs. Peter Kása and Catherine Hebb.

tribution of choline acetyltransferase in the CNS of the rat. As might be anticipated, the motor neurons stain very heavily. This is true not only for spinal motor neurons, but for those motor neurons located in various brain stem nuclei as well. The neurons of the medullary reticular formation and the vestibular nuclei also stain intensely. Contrary to the findings of Kása et al. (1970) our studies indicate the presence of choline acetyltransferase activity in the neurons of the dorsal root ganglia (Figs. 3 and 4). The amount of activity, however, is much less than that of the motor neurons.

Our histochemical data on choline acetyltransferase activity in the cerebellum is in good agreement with the quantitative study of Goldberg and McCaman (1967). The subcerebellar nuclei, such as the dentate, are heavily stained. The molecular layer is nearly devoid of activity, the granular layer has a moderate level of activity and the soma of the Purkinje cells stains very lightly. A relatively large number of dense staining boutons terminaux are visible on and in the immediate vicinity of the Purkinje cell. It is of interest that most of the data of Goldberg and McCaman do not include samples of the Purkinje cell layer, however, in a l mited study of the guinea pig cerebellum the Purkinje cell layer was found to be more than three times as active as the molecular layer and nearly 50% more active than the granular layer. The positive boutons terminaux which we were able to demonstrate in the Purkinje cell layer may be related to the choline acetyltransferase-positive neurons which are demonstrable in the pontine and inferior olivary nuclei. Although Goldberg and McCaman found a moderate level of activity in the cerebellar white matter, the histochemical staining was essentially negative. However adequate diffusion of the reactants may be impaired by the heavy myelinization of the nerve fibers. Similar problems have been encountered in the localization of acetylcholinesterase activity (Tennyson et al., 1967). Kása et al. (1970), however, did not find histochemical evidence of choline acetyltransferase activity in the Purkinje cell layer. Their histochemical procedure was somewhat different from that of our laboratory and further study may resolve this question.

The caudate nucleus has been traditionally a rich source of choline acetyltransferase. However, our histochemical studies indicate that the relatively small neurons of the rat caudate nuclei have very little enzymatic activity in the neuronal perikaryon. The neuropil on the other hand contains many dense staining granules which resemble boutons terminaux. These granular structures are scattered throughout the neuropil both singly and clustered in groups (Fig. 7). This distribution of enzymatic activity would support the idea that the caudate neurons are not cholinergic, but cholinoceptive instead. The distribution of choline acetyltransferase activity in the caudate nucleus may be further resolved through the use of the electron microscope.

Neurons of the neocortex are nearly devoid of choline acetyltransferase activity, although the large pyramidal neurons of the primary motor and sensory areas stain lightly. Dense staining granular structures resembling boutons terminaux are present in the cortical neuropil. These boutons are most abundant in the large pyramidal cell layers both in the neuropil and on the surface of the pyramidal neurons.

## CONCLUSION

Basic histochemical procedures for the localization of choline acetyltransferase activity have been developed. These procedures, based upon the precipitation of a lead mercaptide, are applicable to both light and electron microscopic studies. The inherent weakness of these procedures resides in the lack of specificity in the reaction for the localization of only choline acetyltransferase activity. A number of observations, including parallel analytical studies, indicate that much of the non-specific activity can be eliminated and that we are indeed localizing the activity of choline acetyltransferase. However, specific inhibitors of choline acetyltransferase activity, which are suitable for the histochemical conditions, are needed for the improvement of these procedures. The application of these procedures to the study of the CNS will provide further insight into the organization and distribution of cholinergic and cholinoceptive neurons.

## ACKNOWLEDGEMENTS

The author would like to extend his appreciation to Dr. Catherine Hebb, ARC Institute of Animal Physiology, Babraham, Cambridge, England, and to Dr. Peter Kása, Department of Anatomy, Medical University, Szeged, Hungary, for their cooperation during the preparation of this manuscript and for providing the electron micrograph used herein.

## REFERENCES

BARNARD, E. A. AND STEIN, W. D. (1958) *Advan. Enzymol.*, **20**, 51–110.
BURT, A. M. (1969) *Anat. Rec.*, **163**, 162.
BURT, A. M. (1970) *J. Histochem. Cytochem.*, **18**, 408–415.
CHIOU, C.-Y. AND SASTRY, B. V. R. (1968) *Biochem. Pharmacol.*, **17**, 805–815.
CLELAND, W. W. (1963) *Biochim. Biophys. Acta*, **67**, 104–137.
FONNUM, F. (1967) *Biochem. J.*, **103**, 262–270.
GOLDBERG, A. M. AND MCCAMAN, R. E. (1967) *Life Sci.*, **6** 1493–1500.
HEBB, C., KÁSA, P. AND MANN, S. P. (1970) *J. Physiol.*, **208**, 1P–2P.
HIGGINS, J. A. AND BARRNETT, R. J. (1970) *J. Cell Sci.*, **6**, 29–51.
KÁSA, P., MANN, S. R. AND HEBB, C. (1970) *Nature*, **226**, 812–816.
KOELLE, G. B. AND FRIEDENWALD, J. B. (1949) *Proc. Soc. Exp. Biol. Med.*, **70**, 617–622.
MCCAMAN, R. E. AND HUNT, J. M. (1965) *J. Neurochem.*, **12**, 253–259.
MICHAELSON, I. A. (1967) *Ann. N.Y. Acad. Sci.*, **144**, 387–407.
MORRIS, D. AND GREWAAL, D. S. (1969 a) *Life Sci.*, **8**, 511–516.
MORRIS, D. AND GREWAAL, D. S. (1969 b) *Biochem. J.*, **114**, 85p.
POTTER, L. T., GLOVER, V. A. S. AND SAELENS, J. K., (1968) *J. Biol. Chem.*, **243**, 3864–3870.
SCHUBERTH, J. (1966) *Biochim. Biophys. Acta*, **122**, 470–481.
TENNYSON, V. M., BRZIN, M. AND DUFFY, P., (1967) *Progr. Brain Res.*, **29**, 41–61.
WHITE, H. L. AND CAVALLITO, C. J. (1970) *Biochim. Biophys. Acta*, **206**, 343–358.

# Ultrastructural Localization of Choline Acetyltransferase and Acetylcholinesterase in Central and Peripheral Nervous Tissue

P. KÁSA

*Department of Anatomy, University Medical School Szeged (Hungary)*

## INTRODUCTION

Cholinergic neuronal transmission has now been extensively studied by histochemical localization of acetylcholinesterase for 20 years (Koelle, 1949, 1963, 1969; Lewis and Shute, 1965; Kása and Csillik, 1966, 1968; Eränkö *et al.*, 1967; Csillik and Knyihár, 1968). It has been felt, however, that the histochemical demonstration of choline acetyltransferase (ChAc) which is a specific component of the cholinergic system (ChAc, ACh, and AChE) would give much more valuable information about cholinergic neuronal transmission while at the same time such a technique might also help the biochemist in analyzing the fine structural localization of the enzyme.

In order to find the sites of synthesis of ACh we have been working for some time on a histochemical technique for the localization of ChAc (Hebb *et al.*, 1970), the principle of which (Barrnett, 1968; Burt, 1969) is to precipitate the coenzyme A–SH group which is released during the formation of ACh. This is achieved by forming a mercaptide using a heavy metal such as lead.

Using our technique we have been able to demonstrate the morphological sites of ACh synthesis. These sites are different from that where AChE activity is present. To demonstrate these differences electron microscopic cytochemical research was undertaken to determine and compare the fine structural localization of ChAc and AChE in the rat spinal cord, cerebellar cortex, sciatic nerve and motor end-plate.

## MATERIAL AND METHODS

Rat spinal cord, cerebellar cortex, sciatic nerve and diaphragm were fixed by perfusion (5–7 min) with 1–2% freshly prepared formaldehyde in sodium cacodylate buffer (0.1 M, pH 7.5) containing 0.16–0.32 M sucrose. The samples were removed and

* Results described were obtained at the ARC Institute of Animal Physiology, Babraham, Cambridge, England, where the author was Wellcome Research Fellow for two years.

Abbreviations used: ChAc: choline acetyltransferase (acetyl-CoA: choline-O-acetyltransferase, E.C. 2.3.1.6); AChE: acetylcholinesterase (acetylcholine hydrolase E.C. 3.1.1.7); ACh: acetylcholine; AcCoA: acetylcoenzyme; DFP: di-isopropylphosphorfluoridate; ClACh: chloroacetylcholine-perchlorate; BrACh: bromoacetylcholine-perchlorate.

*References p. 344*

immersed (30–60 min at 0° C) in a similar fixative and finally washed in sodium cacodylate buffer (pH 7.0) for 2–3 h. Small pieces of fixed tissues were prepared free hand, using a razor blade.

*Electron histochemical demonstration of ChAc activity (Kása et al., 1970)*

All tissue samples were pre-incubated in $10^{-3}$M DFP (60 min) at room temperature and then incubated at 39° C in a medium containing:

| | | |
|---|---:|---|
| sodium cacodylate buffer (pH 5.9) | 30 | mM |
| DFP | 1 | mM |
| [$^{14}$C]acetyl-CoA | 0.67 | mM |
| choline chloride | 10 | mM |
| lead nitrate | 0.1 | mM |
| (Cl- or Br-acetylcholine, inhibitors for ChAc (Morris and Grewaal, 1969) | 10 | mM |

After DFP treatment, control sections were given a further incubation for 30 min at 0° C in 10 mM ClACh perchlorate and then incubated at 39° C in the main incubation medium supplemented with the same concentration of inhibitor. Other control tissue samples were incubated either in the absence of choline or with the omission of AcCoA and choline from the main incubation medium. Samples were incubated for 4 h and after incubation the medium was removed and the amount of [$^{14}$C]ACh which had been formed and released into it was estimated according to Hebb *et al.* (1970). After incubation the samples were rinsed in 0.1 sodium acetate buffer, developed in sodium sulphide (pH 7.5), postfixed in 1% OsO$_4$ solution, dehydrated and embedded in Araldite in the usual way. Sections were cut with a Reichert ultramicrotome and photographed in a Siemens 'Elmiskop' electron microscope.

To study the transport mechanism of ChAc and AChE from the cell body to the nerve endings, sciatic nerves of rats were ligated and after 24, 41, 48 and 65 h were examined biochemically and histochemically for accumulation of ChAc and AChE proximal and distal to the ligature.

*Electron histochemical localization of AChE activity*

The spinal cord, cerebellar cortex, diaphragm and sciatic nerve were fixed for 2–3 h in a mixture of 2% glutaraldehyde, 4% formaldehyde and 0.3 M sucrose in 0.1 M sodium cacodylate. Samples were washed in sucrose solution for at least 2–3 h and pre-incubated for 45–60 min in 0.3 M sucrose solution containing either $10^{-4}$M ethopropazine HCl or $10^{-4}$M BW 284 C51. Tissues were then incubated 5–10 min for the diaphragm and 30–60 min for other samples in a copper–lead–thiocholine medium (Kása and Csillik, 1966) which consisted of:

|                          |       |       |        |
|--------------------------|-------|-------|--------|
| acetylthiocholine iodide |       |       | 7.0 mg |
| sodium acetate           | 0.1   | M     | 2.2 ml |
| glycine                  | 3.75  | %     | 0.1 ml |
| CuSO$_4$                 | 0.1   | M     | 0.1 ml |
| lead nitrate             | 0.5   | %     | 0.1 ml |
| acetic acid              |       |       |        |
| (to adjust the pH)       | 0.1   | N     | 0–0.3 ml |

After incubation the samples were rinsed and treated with H$_2$S-saturated sucrose solution, postfixed in 1% OsO$_4$ solution, dehydrated and embedded in Araldite. Sections were cut on a Huxley ultramicrotome and were viewed and photographed on the Siemens 'Elmiscop' electron microscope.

## RESULTS

*ChAc activity in the spinal cord, sciatic nerve and motor end-plate*

Biochemical investigations have shown that these structures have a high ChAc content (Hebb and Silver, 1956; Hebb *et al.*, 1964). Histochemical demonstration of the enzyme revealed that ChAc activity occurs in all parts of cholinergic neurons. In the cell body and dendrites of motoneurons and possibly some other cells (lumbar region) enzyme activity appeared to be connected with the ribosomes and was deposited on the outer surface of other structural components – vesicles, tubules and the inner surface of the cell membrane – as well as free in the cytoplasm. In general, the reaction end-product was widespread throughout the cytoplasm (Figs. 1, 5) and never occurred inside the endoplasmic reticulum, tubules, vesicles or mitochondria.

In the *axons* of motoneurons, the reaction appeared to be attached to the axon filaments and to the outer surface of vesicles and was free in the axoplasm. At the *terminals*, lead precipitate occurred in the axoplasm and on the outer surface of synaptic vesicles and reaction product was present on the inner surface of the axon membrane (Figs. 1, 2, 4). Some lead precipitate was also found in between the membranes in the extracellular space. However, this is probably a diffusion artifact.

It must be emphasized that reaction end-product is present in those terminals where spherical (empty) vesicles are present, and not in those terminals where the vesicles are ovoid or elongated.

At the motor end-plate lead precipitate was found in the axon terminal. The distribution of the end-product here is similar to the localization that can be found in other terminals of cholinergic axons.

Preliminary results on the localization of ChAc in the archicerebellar cortex of the rat shows that end-product can be found in terminal parts of some mossy fibres and in a few axons (undetermined as yet) in the molecular layer.

Tissue samples pre-incubated in ClACh and incubated in the complete incubation medium did not show any specific reaction end-product, and there was only a small amount of lead precipitate where the choline was omitted from the incubation medium

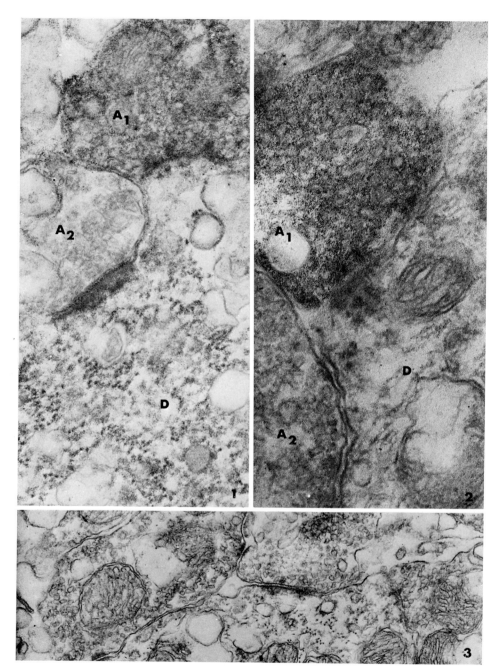

Fig. 1. Ultrastructual demonstration of ChAc activity in the spinal cord of the rat. Electron-dense precipitate is present both in the axon terminal ($A_1$) and in the dendrite (D). Note another nerve terminal ($A_2$) where no end-product is present. $\times$ 53 400.

Fig. 2. Sample incubated for ChAc. Heavy reaction end-product is present in the axon terminal (top left corner) while the precipitate is missing from the dendrite (D) and another nerve terminal ($A_2$). ChAc activity appears here and in Fig. 1 on the outer surface of synaptic vesicles, on the axon membrane and free in the axoplasm. $\times$ 92 000.

Fig. 3. Control sample pre-incubated in DFP ($10^{-3}$M) and incubated with the omission of choline from the incubation medium. $\times$ 30 000.

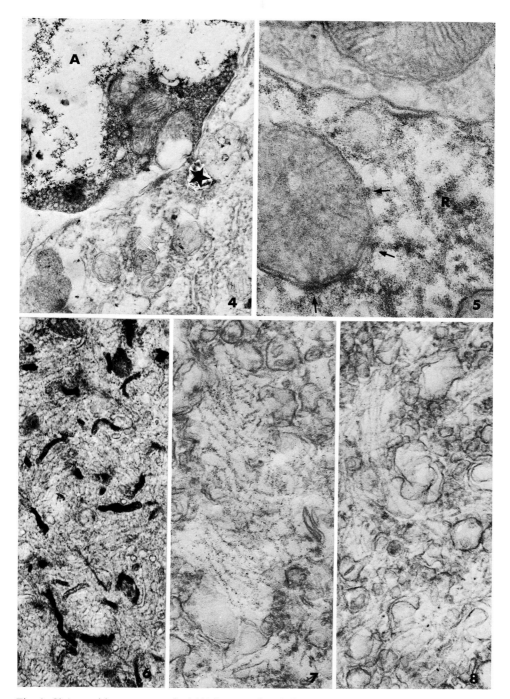

Fig. 4. ChAc-positive nerve terminal (A) in synaptic relationship (arrow) with a ChAc-negative cell body. (The * indicates an artifact.) × 35 000.

Fig. 5. High magnification of a portion of a ChAc-positive dendrite. The reaction product is present on the dendrite membrane, attached to the ribosomes (R) and to the outer surface of the mito-chondrium (arrows). × 68 500.

Fig. 6. AChE-active tubules and vesicles accumulated inside the axon (sciatic nerve) after ligature for 24 h. × 32 400.

Fig. 7. ChAc activity in the sciatic nerve at the end proximal to the lesion. Reaction product is present free in the axoplasm and attached to the axon filament. × 55 000.

Fig. 8. Control sample incubated with the omission of choline from the main incubation medium. Note the absence of reaction end-product × 45 000.

(Fig. 3). Some reaction product was present in the cytoplasm of glia cells when the samples were incubated in the absence of AcCoA and choline.

AChE activity can be found in the cell body of some cells in the spinal cord (lumbar segment) and in the Golgi cells of the cerebellar cortex. At the fine structural level, this activity appears to be in the endoplasmic reticulum, Golgi lamellae and inside some vesicles. Other structures– axons and dendrites – show reaction products on their surfaces.

When the sciatic nerve was ligated for 24, 41, 48 and 65 h, AChE and ChAc accumulated proximal to the lesion. AChE activity was present on the outer surface of the axon membrane and in tubules and vesicles inside the axon (Fig. 6). On the other hand, ChAc reaction end-product was present on the filaments and microtubules and could never be demonstrated inside the vesicles and tubules (Fig. 7). There was no reaction end-product in the control samples where choline was omitted from the incubation medium (Fig. 8).

## DISCUSSION

During the last decade the focus of attention has shifted to the biochemical and electron-histochemical analyses of cholinergic neuronal transmission. Biochemical results (Hebb and Smallman, 1956; Hebb and Whittaker, 1958; Toschi, 1959; De Robertis et al., 1963; Whittaker, 1965) show that the ACh system (ChAc, ACh and AChE) can be found in different fractions of brain homogenate. According to these studies, AChE activity is always associated with the particulate fractions, while ACh and ChAc can be found in both particulate and soluble fractions. Specially ChAc shows a great variability depending on the ionic concentration and pH of the solution used. Fonnum (1970) has shown that this enzyme is easily solubilized by increasing the pH and ionic strength of the incubation solution. McCaman et al. (1965) described species differences which exist in the pigeon and the guinea pig. Biochemical studies on the ACh system, however, cannot identify the exact cells that are cholinergic. In tissue slices where the neurons appear to maintain histological integrity and functional activity, the cholinergic neurons and cholinergic synaptic transmission can be analysed. Electron histochemical demonstration of ChAc (Kása et al., 1970; Kása, 1970) has permitted a clear picture of the distribution of this enzyme in different cells and axon terminals and therefore shed some light on the distribution of cholinergic neurons in the central and peripheral nervous tissue (see also Burt, 1969; 1970).

Choline acetyltransferase activity localized electron histochemically shows the morphological sites of the ACh production. It seems relevant to ask, however, on what basis we can assert that we are demonstrating ChAc activity with this histochemical technique? We can suppose this because:

(a) there is no reaction end-product, or very little, when choline is omitted from the main incubation medium;

(b) pre-incubation of tissue samples with haloacetylcholines (ClACh or BrACh) and incubation in the main incubation medium produced marked reduction of the reaction end-product;

(c) fixed samples incubated with the omission of AcCoA and choline in the presence of lead nitrate give negative results.

One may also ask what the presence of reaction end-product on the different structural components (vesicles, filaments, ribosomes and membranes) of the cell means? Does this mean that the enzyme is present in all of these structures? The answer is open to debate. It seems, however, that reaction end-product free in the cytoplasm of the cell body, dendrite and axon could represent the soluble part, while precipitate on structures might demonstrate the bound part of the enzyme. Fonnum (1970) also recently described the binding ability of ChAc to synaptosomes and other membranes due to the fact that ChAc has a positive surface charge. The ionic strength and the pH of the incubation medium as well as the surface charge of the enzyme could certainly modify the real distribution of the enzyme. Therefore we are only able to demonstrate cholinergic nerve cells while the fine structural localization of the enzyme remains questionable.

The electron histochemical demonstration of AChE by a modified Koelle method (Kása and Csillik, 1966) confirmed the biochemical results according to which AChE is present in a membrane-bound form. This enzyme is localized in the endoplasmic reticulum, vesicles, tubules, and on the outer surface of axons and dendrites, while the ChAc reaction end-product can never be demonstrated in these places. This probably means that the site of synthesis of ACh is different from that where the transmitter substance is hydrolysed.

Histochemical demonstration of ChAc revealed most reaction end-products in the cell body, where the enzyme is possibly synthesized. The main function of the enzyme, however, is at the nerve terminal. The question arises, therefore, of how this enzyme is transported from the cell body to the nerve terminal. Is there any structural component in the cell that might be responsible for the enzyme transport or does the ChAc migrate freely inside the axon? Experiments carried out on sciatic nerve have provided valuable information about the transport mechanism of ChAc and AChE. When the sciatic nerve was ligated, AChE accumulated more rapidly at the proximal end of the lesion than did the ChAc. AChE activity was present inside tubules and vesicles (Kása, 1968; Kreutzberg, 1969), while ChAc activity always occurred outside of these structures and was present free in the axoplasm or attached to axon filaments and microtubules. These electron-histochemical investigations revealed, therefore, that ChAc and AChE are localized and transported from the cell body to the nerve terminal with different structural components of the cell.

### CONCLUSIONS

Electron-histochemical demonstration of ChAc and AChE in different parts of nervous tissue show that the components of the ACh system are localized in different structures of the cholinergic nerve cells. AChE is present in the endoplasmic reticulum, Golgi lamellae, vesicles, tubules and on the outer surface of the axon and dendrite membrane, while ChAc activity occurs free in the cytoplasm or bound to the outer surface of vescicles and is attached to ribosomes, filaments and microtubules. The structural bases of the transport of these enzymes are different, too. AChE is possibly transported inside the axon tubules and vesicles, while ChAc is transported via axon filaments, on the outer surface of vesicles and possibly free in the cytoplasm.

These electron-microscopic histochemical studies confirm those biochemical results according to which the components of the ACh system (ChAc, ACh and AChE) are localized in structurally different places of the cholinergic nerve cell.

## ACKNOWLEDGEMENTS

The author wishes to express his gratitude to Dr. C. O. Hebb for the hospitality of her laboratory and for continuous stimulating interest. He is also most grateful to the Trustees of the Wellcome Trust for the fellowship which made his work in Babraham possible. Electron-microscopic facilities were provided by the Wellcome Trust.

## REFERENCES

BARRNETT, R. J. AND HIGGINS, J. A. (1968) *Proc. Electron Microscopy Soc. Amer., 26th Ann. Meeting*, p. 1.
BURT, A. M. (1969) *Anat. Rec.*, **163**, 162.
BURT, A. M. (1970) *J. Histochem. Cytochem.*, **18**, 408–415.
CSILLIK, B. AND KNYIHÁR, E. (1968) *J. Cell Sci.*, **3**, 529–538.
ERÄNKÖ, O., RECHARDT, L. AND HÄNINEN, L. (1967) *Histochemie*, **8**, 369–376.
FONNUM, F. (1970) *J. Neurochem.*, **17**, 1095–1100.
HEBB, C. O. AND SILVER, A. (1956) *J. Physiol.*, **134**, 718–728.
HEBB, C. O. AND SILVER, A. (1963) *J. Physiol.*, **169**, 41–42.
HEBB, C. O. AND SMALLMAN, B. N. *J. Physiol.*, **134**, 385–392. (1956)
HEBB, C. O. AND WHITTAKER, V. P. (1958) *J. Physiol.*, **142**, 187–196.
HEBB, C. O., KÁSA, P. AND MANN, S. P. (1970) *J. Physiol.*, **208**, 1P–2P.
HEBB, C. O., KRNJEVIC, K. AND SILVER, A. (1964) *J. Physiol.*, **171**, 504–513.
HEBB, C. O., MANECKJEE, A. AND MORRIS, D. (1970) in preparation.
KÁSA, P. (1970) *J. Physiol.*, **210**, 89P–90P.
KÁSA, P. (1968) *Nature*, **218**, 1265–1276.
KÁSA, P. AND CSILLIK, B. (1966) *J. Neurochem.*, **13**, 1345–1349.
KÁSA, P. AND CSILLIK, B. (1968) *Histochemie*, **12**, 175–183.
KÁSA, P., MANN, S. P. AND HEBB, C. O. (1970) *Nature*, **226**, 812–814.
KÁSA, P., MANN, S. P. AND HEBB, C. O. (1970) *Nature*, **226**, 814–816.
KOELLE, G. B. AND FRIEDENWALD, J. S. (1949) *Proc. Soc. Exp. Biol.*, **70**, 617–622.
KOELLE, G. B. (1963) *Handbuch der experimentellen Pharmakologie, Ergänzungswerk*, Berlin-Göttingen-Heidelberg, Springer, Bd. **15**, 187–298.
KOELLE, G. B. (1969) *Federation Proc.*, **28**, 95–100.
KREUTZBERG, G. W. (1969) *Proc. Natl. Acad. Sci. U.S.A.*, **62**, 722–728.
LEWIS, P. R. AND SHUTE, C. C. P. (1965) *J. Anat. (Lond.)*, **99**, 941.
McCAMAN, R. E., RODRIGUEZ DE LORES ARNAIZ, G., AND DE ROBERTIS, E. (1965) *J. Neurochem.*, **12**, 927–935.
MORRIS, D. AND GREWAAL, D. S. (1969) *Life Sci.*, **8**, 511–516.
DE ROBERTIS, E., RODRIGUEZ DE LORES ARNAIZ, G. SALGANICOFF, L., PELLEGRINO DE IRALDI, A. AND ZIEHER, L. M. (1963) *J. Neurochem.*, **10**, 225–235.
TOSCHI, G. (1959) *Exp. Cell Res.*, **16**, 232–235.
TUČEK, S. (1966) *J. Neurochem.*, **13**, 1317–1327.
WHITTAKER, V. P. (1965) *Progr. Biophysics Mol. Biol.*, **15**, 39–96.

# The Significance of Cholinesterase in the Developing Nervous System

ANN SILVER

*Agricultural Research Council Institute of Animal Physiology, Babraham, Cambridge (England)*

If it is accepted as a working hypothesis that nerve fibres which contain acetylcholinesterase (AChE) may be cholinergic, then studies on the acquisition of AChE in the developing nervous system might be expected to provide some guide to the more complex organization of possibly cholinergic and non-cholinergic neurones seen in the adult. Although useful information has been derived from work of this sort (see Krnjević and Silver, 1966; Silver, 1967), it is clear that during ontogenesis AChE may have functions that are unconnected with any role it may eventually have in transmission. For instance, certain cells which are devoid of AChE activity in the adult contain the enzyme at some stage of their development. The question is, what is the role of the AChE in these cells? Most of the views about the function of AChE during development are conjectural but nevertheless, this is perhaps an appropriate time to review them. With the advent of histochemical techniques for demonstrating choline acetyltransferase (choline acetylase; ChAc) it should no longer be so necessary to study the distribution of AChE simply as an indicator of possibly cholinergic pathways: more attention can be given to the enzyme in its own right.

In this paper the significance of AChE in the developing nervous system will be considered from two aspects. The first part will deal with some histochemical experiments on foetal brains which were done with the primary object of getting data on the distribution of possibly cholinergic elements in the adult. Quantitative experiments on AChE development will also be discussed. In the second part the emphasis will be on some of the speculations that have been put forward about the role of AChE during ontogenesis. The function of butyrylcholinesterase (BuChE) is little understood in the adult, let alone in the developing animal and will not, therefore, be dealt with.

## I. OCCURRENCE OF AChE-CONTAINING ELEMENTS DURING DEVELOPMENT

Work with Krnjević on the distribution of AChE in the forebrain of the adult cat (Krnjević and Silver, 1965) suggested that, with the possible exception of polymorph cells of Layer VI, few cholinergic cells are present in the cortex itself. Histochemical studies on the development of AChE in foetal kittens (Krnjević and Silver, 1966) provided further evidence that most of the AChE-containing fibres were processes of subcortically situated cells. First, at no stage of development was AChE activity ever

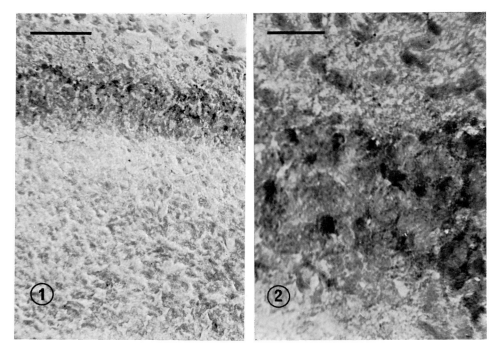

Fig. 1. AChE activity in cortical plate of foetal lamb, 35 days gestation. Counterstain: cresyl violet and eosin. Scale bar: 100 $\mu$.

Fig. 2. High-power view of AChE activity shown in Fig. 1. Scale bar: 25 $\mu$.

seen in the suprastriatal ependyma from which the cortical cells are derived. Second, the cortex remained free of stain until penetrated by AChE-containing fibres which could be traced to well-stained foci in the region of the lenticular and septal nuclei. Just before birth the white matter was suddenly invaded by large numbers of spindle-shaped cells which showed AChE activity in both cell bodies and processes. At least some of these cells, which appeared to be neuroblasts, orientated themselves round the sulcal troughs and seemed to give rise to the U-shaped system of AChE-containing fibres which is such a prominent feature of the adult cortex.

The general pattern of AChE development was surprisingly similar, particularly in the older foetuses, in a number of species including sheep, cat, guinea-pig and wallaby. This agrees with biochemical evidence (see later). Despite this overall similarity, there are differences in detail between different species. Whereas, in the kitten, forebrain enzyme appears initially right at the ventricular surface of the striatal germinal layer (identified by mitotic figures), enzyme in the chick optic lobe (Gerebtzoff, 1959) appears in the peripheral zone of the germinal layer and never in the central zone where mitosis occurs. In the foetal lamb neither the striatal nor the suprastriatal ependyma appeared to stain at any stage of development and the lenticular focus suddenly acquired AChE activity at 32 days gestation. At the same stage, deposits of end-product were seen in the lateral wall of the telencephalon, on the surface of the developing cortical plate (Figs. 1 and 2). At 70 days gestation, this cortical plate activity was still apparently independent of the lenticular projection but on the medial side of the forebrain, the superficial staining was in continuity with the strongly stained induseum griseum, exactly as in the kitten. The occurrence of staining in the cortical plate from an early stage might suggest that cholinergic cells are present in this layer but it was not possible to recognise any likely cells in the adult cortex. From 65 to 90 days gestation stained neuroblasts became increasingly common (Figs. 3 and 4) but then they decreased in number and were absent at birth. It is not clear how many of these cells retained AChE activity in their mature form. Although there was a rich network of stained fibres in the adult cortex very few of the cells seemed to be stained (Fig. 5). The system of U-fibres round the sulci was less well developed than in the cat and no orientation of neuroblasts was seen in this area.

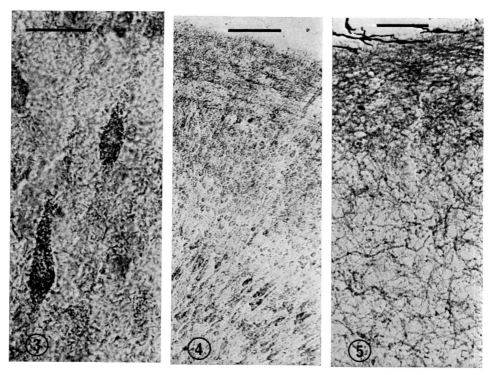

Fig. 3. AChE activity in migrating neuroblasts in cortex of foetal lamb, 100 days gestation. Scale bar:25 $\mu$.

Fig. 4. Part of marginal gyrus of foetal lamb, 121 days gestation. Note AChE activity in neuroblasts Scale bar: 100 $\mu$.

Fig. 5. Part of marginal gyrus of lamb, 1 month old. Note AChE activity in fibres but paucity of AChE-containing cells. The pia mater is pigmented. Scale bar: 100 $\mu$.

In view of the apparent paucity of stained cells in the adult sheep it seems very likely that most of the neuroblasts lose their enzyme as they mature. Such a loss of enzyme has been observed in the chick dorsal root ganglion (Strumia and Baima-Bollone, 1964; Tennyson *et al.*, 1968) and it occurs in cerebellar Purkinje cells of a number of species (Joó *et al.*, 1963; Csillik *et al.*, 1964; Sakharova, 1966). In sheep (Silver, 1967; 1969), stained Purkinje cells appeared in some folia between 66 and 75 days gestation and by 90 days activity was particularly strong (Figs. 6 and 7). From about 100 days onwards fewer cells stained but a small number of stained cells persisted in the adult. The question of loss of enzyme from cells will be discussed more fully later.

### Stability and lability in the development of AChE

Numerous quantitative studies have been made on the time-course of the development of cholinesterases in spinal cord and brain of a variety of species (Maletta *et al.*, 1966; Kling *et al.*, 1969; for earlier references see Silver, 1967). During development the concentration of AChE in some parts of the brain may exceed the concentration found in the same areas in the adult. This does not necessarily mean that these

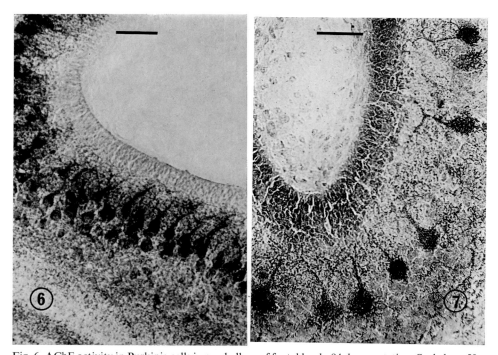

Fig. 6. AChE activity in Purkinje cells in cerebellum of foetal lamb, 94 days gestation. Scale bar: 50 $\mu$.

Fig. 7. AChE activity in Purkinje cells in cerebellum of foetal lamb, 100 days gestation. Scale bar: 50 $\mu$.

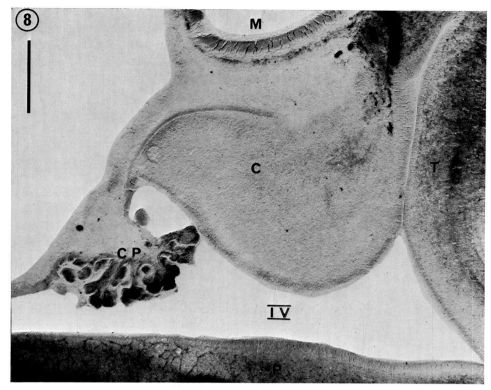

Fig. 8. Developing cerebellum (C) of foetal lamb, 38 days gestation. Note reaction for AChE in choroid plexus (CP). M, cavity of mesencephalon; IV, fourth ventricle; P, pons; T, tegmentum. Scale bar: 500 $\mu$.

structures actually lose enzyme as they mature — the fall in concentration may result from a dilution of cholinesterase-containing elements by the later development of elements which lack the enzyme. It should, however, be mentioned that certain cells are present only during development and eventually atrophy. Cajal-Retzius cells are of this type and Duckett and Pearse (1968) have shown that in the human brain these do contain AChE.

Evidence is available from several species to indicate that the time of onset of foetal movement can be correlated with the appearance of AChE. Hamburger and Balaban (1963) observed spontaneous muscular activity in the legs and wings of the chick embryo on day 7, the day on which AChE shows its first rapid increase. Similarly, Duckett and Pearse (1969) found histochemically demonstrable AChE in the anterior horn of the lumbar cord of 8 to 10 week old human foetuses and they pointed out that the sole reflex can be elicited during the 10th–11th week of foetal life. It is interesting that neurones of the posterior horn did not show activity until the 18th to 20th week although cutaneous sensation is apparently established between the 8th and 12th week.

In both spinal cord (see Duckett and Pearse, 1969) and brain, AChE appears first in the more caudal parts. McCaman and Aprison (1964) emphasized this caudal–rostral gradient of maturation in rabbit brain and showed that it holds for several enzymes in addition to AChE and choline acetylase. The caudal–rostral gradient does not, however, apparently apply to the posterior horns of the human foetal cord; Duckett and Pearse (1969) observed a gradient in the anterior horns but found that in the posterior horns, AChE activity appeared simultaneously at all levels in 18- to 20-week foetuses. The dorsal root ganglia of the chick are also an exception since the rostral ganglia possess histochemically detectable activity before the more caudal ones (Strumia and Baima-Bollone, 1964).

Evidence is accumulating which shows that during development AChE levels can be influenced by certain processes which do not affect the over-all protein concentration. Both pre- and post-natal exposure to x-rays appear to affect the rate of increase of AChE activity (on a wet weight basis) in rat brain (Maletta and Timiras, 1966; Maletta et al., 1967; Nair and Bau, 1969). It is difficult, at this stage, to draw meaningful conclusions from these results because it is not yet clear that the observed changes result from a specific effect on systems concerned with AChE. As Maletta and Timiras (1966) point out, the reactions might be part of a general metabolic response to radiation. Various groups of workers (Rosenzweig et al., 1962; Tapp and Markowitz, 1963; Kling et al., 1965; 1969) have reported that the cholinesterase levels can be influenced by the 'environment' of the developing animal. The changes found are generally small and results obtained by different workers do not always agree. Karczmar (1969) and Russell (1969) have both discussed the problems involved in interpreting data from this type of experiment.

*Electron microscopy of foetal AChE activity*

Using electron microscopic histochemistry, Tennyson et al. (1968) examined AChE activity in the rabbit dorsal root ganglion up to the 17th day of gestation. Activity was detectable earlier with the electron microscope than with the light microscope. Stain appeared first in the perikaryon, then in the axolemma of Lissauer's tract (this is the tract formed in the spinal cord by incoming dorsal root fibres) and finally in the agranular reticulum of the axons in the dorsal root. In the context of axon transport, this is a very interesting observation since it might suggest that the axolemmal enzyme in Lissauer's tract actually arises there and has not been transported from the cell body. In discussing these findings, Elliott (1968) raised the question of whether the enzyme was, in fact, present on the agranular reticulum but could not be demonstrated histochemically owing to some property of the lipoprotein complex with which it was associated during transport. This suggestion introduces a very pertinent point: inability to demonstrate AChE activity may reflect the inadequacy of the technique rather than lack of enzyme. Immature enzyme in transit may, perhaps, be particularly susceptible to inhibition during processing or, as Elliott suggests, the active group may be involved in binding and so be unable to react with the substrate. It is worth considering the possibility that reappearance of histochemically demonstrable AChE in Purkinje cells, following cerebellar lesions, could represent a change in binding of 'occult' enzyme and not a reactivation of enzyme synthesis.

## II. THE ROLE OF AChE DURING DEVELOPMENT

### *Metabolic function*

The appearance and disappearance of AChE activity during development is interesting: it is particularly so in cells such as those of the dorsal root ganglia which are definitely not cholinergic and in Purkinje cells where cholinergic transmission is, to say the least, doubtful.

One of the questions to ask is whether the AChE present in these developing cells does in fact have any function at all. Both Zacks (1954) and Gerebtzoff (1959) make the point that in the chick CNS, biochemical differentiation, *i.e.* acquisition of enzyme activity, occurs before morphological differentiation of migrating neuroblasts. Tennyson *et al.* (1968) have made a similar observation at the ultra-structural level in rabbit spinal cord. It could be that these undifferentiated cells are endowed, unselectively, with a whole range of systems which may be retained or lost depending on what the cell needs in its ultimate situation. This sort of arrangement would ensure a high degree of plasticity amongst the cells but is unlikely to apply to the dorsal root ganglia cells which apparently develop their activity once they are in their final position (Strumia and Baima-Bollone, 1964). Duckett and Pearse (1965) have evidence from studies of acid phosphatase in human foetal brain that Purkinje cells develop from ependymal cells which are, in turn, derived from the choroid plexus. In sheep, the choroid plexus stained for AChE (Fig. 8) but there was no obvious progression of stained elements from the ependyma to the Purkinje cell layer and the impression was that activity developed (or possibly, redeveloped) after the Purkinje cells had arrived from their site of origin. Results which suggest that the enzyme has a definite role in the Purkinje cells have come from experiments in which lesions are made in the adult cerebellum. Kása *et al.* (1966) found that AChE activity reappeared in the Purkinje cells of the rat archicerebellum when it was undercut in such a way that it was isolated from the rest of the cerebellum but its blood supply remained intact. They postulated that this might indicate that in the developing cell, AChE played some role in protein metabolism and this same system could be reactivated to take part in attempts to repair the cell. Against this is the finding of Phillis (1968) that in the cat, the reappearance of Purkinje cell AChE can be produced not only by lesions which axotomize the cells but also by peduncular lesions. Since most Purkinje cell axons terminate in the cerebellar nuclei, section of the peduncles would not cause direct damage to many of the cells themselves but it would destroy their afferent innervation. Phillis thought that deafferentation, by disturbing the normal pattern of activation, might have changed cellular metabolism. It is tempting to extend this view and suggest that the change involves a reversion to the situation which may have existed during development, before the cells had received their afferent input.

Any speculation about a possible metabolic role for AChE must include the question of whether or not acetylcholine (ACh) is its substrate. Crawford *et al.* (1966) have put forward the idea that the natural substrate for AChE might, in fact, be something other than ACh. This is an unconventional view but it serves as a reminder that cholinesterases can hydrolyse a large number of non-choline esters (Adams, 1949; see also Augustinsson, 1963). Developing cells which contain AChE in culture (Hösli and Hösli, 1970; Kim, 1970) might be useful tools in further biochemical studies.

Some preliminary experiments (Silver, 1969) on the choline acetyltransferase level in folia from the cerebellum of foetal sheep indicated that those folia which contained many well-stained Purkinje cells had a higher choline acetyltransferase activity than those with fewer stained cells. However, it seemed likely that the difference in ChAc levels was associated with differences in the number of AChE-containing fibres in the white matter, rather than with differences in the Purkinje cells themselves. More rigorous experiments are necessary to determine whether in the cerebellum, ACh is present within those cells which contain AChE. Marchisio and Consolo (1968) have such evidence in the case of chick spinal ganglia. Using a radiochemical method, they observed two peaks of ChAc activity which corresponded with previously reported (Levi-Montalcini and Levi, 1943) peaks for histogenesis of ganglion cells and they concluded that ACh synthesis and cell maturation proceeded in parallel. They pointed out that Hokin (1965) had shown that ACh stimulates the synthesis of certain phospholipid components of cell membranes and they suggested this observation might have some bearing on the role of ACh in the developing nerve cell. If the function of ACh in these sensory cells (and, by extrapolation, in developing and injured Purkinje cells) is to produce membrane (see also Hokin, 1967) then AChE could be necessary to control the process. One could argue that in the mature cell, AChE in the endoplasmic reticulum of cholinoceptive, but non-cholinergic, cells might have a similar controlling function, if, as Larrabee (1967) has postulated, a transmitter not only turns on the mechanism which produces depolarization but simultaneously sets up reactions to reconstitute the membrane.

Further evidence of a metabolic function for ACh in development is provided by Marchisio and Giacobini (1969) who found that changes in levels of ChAc in various parts of the brain of the developing chick were not clearly related to the times of onset of spontaneous and reflex electrical activity described by Corner et al., (1967). They also found that in all areas except the optic lobe, the level of ChAc fell sharply on hatching.

*Substrate induction of enzyme*

Work on cultures of non-nervous tissues such as lung and heart have produced results which may have some bearing on AChE in developing neurones. Burkhalter *et al.* (1957) found that addition of ACh to explants of chick lung caused an increase in AChE but not of BuChE. Since the effect was not produced by sodium chloride, choline or acetate they concluded that ACh had caused the appearance of AChE by substrate induction. On the other hand, Burdick and Strittmatter (1965) found no evidence of substrate induction of AChE in cultures of whole chick brain. They measured AChE, ChAc and ACh and found a sudden increase in AChE activity per mg protein on the 16th day of incubation but ChAc activity did not increase until a day later and the increase of ACh content, which occurred on the 18th day, was only slight. More recently, Turbow and Burkhalter (1968) showed that when ACh was added to cultures of chick spinal cord, the fall in AChE which normally occurred was prevented. The authors point out that although ACh may produce this effect by the mechanism of substrate induction, an alternative possibility is that ACh may, by increasing cell permeability, improve the intracellular milieu for protein synthesis.

### Control of receptor sites

Roberts et al. (1965) obtained results from the chick heart which suggested that the presence of cholinomimetics could stimulate the formation of cholinoceptive sites. They cultured explanted embryos (0–7 somite blastomeres) for 20 h on nutrient agar containing methacholine, neostigmine, physostigmine, atropine or arecoline and then recorded the change in frequency of heart beat produced by applications of ACh. Hearts of embryos grown on media containing atropine or arecoline behaved much as those of controls but in embryos grown in the presence of the cholinomimetics or anticholinesterases, the depression of heart rate (% change) produced by ACh was much greater. The authors suggested that the increased sensitivity to ACh occurred because the drugs had stimulated the development of extra acetylcholine receptors. Atropine and arecoline apparently lacked the stereochemical specificity necessary for this effect. The hypothesis that the increase in sensitivity is due to an increase in receptor sites is not the only explanation for the observation; nevertheless, the fact that the presence of certain drugs can alter the sensitivity of cells to ACh prompts further speculation about developing neurones. In the light of these results it seems possible that an immature neurone might develop a sensitivity to ACh if it were located in or migrated through an area where ACh was present. Since such sensitivity would be inappropriate unless the neurones were destined to be cholinoceptive, it could be that AChE in non-cholinoceptive cells has a protective function, preventing the development of bizarre sensitivity in susceptible cells. The reappearance of AChE activity in Purkinje cells following cerebellar and penduncular lesions might perform a similar role if the structural disorganization in some way exposed the cells to ACh.

Further observations made on chick hearts indicate that the AChE activity may be high compared with ACh levels. Paff et al. (1966) have shown that in 50–60 h chick embryos ACh, AChE and eserine have marked effects on the electrocardiogram and they conclude that ACh is essential for the spontaneous rhythmic contractions of the uninnervated heart (see also Karnovsky, 1964; Hagopian et al., 1970), but that in some regions, e.g. the atrio-ventricular junction, the AChE level may be high and the ACh level, low. The presence of the 'excess' AChE may ensure, as discussed above, that the development of sensitivity to ACh follows a controlled pattern. Vlk and Tuček (1962) showed that in the dog atria, the ACh level rose as the vagal innervation matured but at the same time, the AChE activity fell. Such a fall might be expected if the 'regulating' role of AChE were no longer needed, perhaps because the vagus nerve itself imposes some sort of restraint on the development of receptors. It may be relevant to mention in this context that Guth and Zalewski (1963) showed, in rats, that when the hypoglossal nerve is implanted into the normally innervated sternomastoid muscle virtually no new end-plates are developed. If the muscle is first denervated, then the implanted hypoglossal is able to form new end-plates.

SUMMARY

The first part of the paper is concerned with histochemistry of foetal material and is illustrated with reference to sheep. The time-course of AChE development and reports that quantitative changes can be produced by environmental factors are also discussed. Electron microscopy of developing AChE is mentioned briefly. In the second part the question whether AChE has any special role during development is considered and the possibilities of metabolic function, substrate induction and control of receptor sites are discussed.

REFERENCES

ADAMS, D. H. (1949) *Biochim. Biophys. Acta*, **3**, 1–14.
AUGUSTINSSON, K.-B. (1963) In G. B. KOELLE (Ed.), *Cholinesterases and Anticholinesterase Agents*, Springer-Verlag, Berlin, pp. 89–128.
BURDICK, C. J. AND STRITTMATTER, C. F. (1965) *Arch. Biochem. Biophys.*, **109**, 293–301.
BURKHALTER, A., JONES, M. AND FEATHERSTONE, R. M. (1957) *Proc. Soc. Exp. Biol. Med.*, **96**, 747–750.
CORNER, M. A., SCHADÉ, J. P., SEDLÁČEK, J., STOECKART, R. AND BOT, A. P. C. (1967) In C. G. BERNHARD AND J. P. SCHADÉ (Eds.), *Developmental Neurobiology, Progress in Brain Research*, Vol. 26, Elsevier, Amsterdam-New York, pp. 145–192.
CRAWFORD, J. M., CURTIS, D. R., VOORHOEVE, P. E. AND WILSON, V. J. (1966) *J. Physiol.*, **186**, 139–165.
CSILLIK, B., JOÓ, F., KÁSA, P., TOMITY, I. AND KÁLMÁN, GY. (1964) *Acta Biol. Hung.*, **15**, 11–17.
DUCKETT, S. AND PEARSE, A. G. E. (1965) *Rev. Can. Biol.*, **24**, 23–27.
DUCKETT, S. AND PEARSE, A. G. E. (1968) *J. Anat.*, **102**, 183–187.
DUCKETT, S. AND PEARSE, A. G. E. (1969) *Anat. Rec.*, **163**, 59–66.
ELLIOTT, K. A. C. (1968) Formal discussion. *Progr. Brain Res.*, **29**, p. 61.
GEREBTZOFF, M. A. (1959) *Cholinesterases*, Pergamon Press, London.
GUTH, L. AND ZALEWSKI, A. A. (1963) *Exp. Neurol.*, **7**, 316–326.
HAGOPIAN, M., TENNYSON, V. M. AND SPIRO, D. (1970) *J. Histochem. Cytochem.*, **18**, 38–43.
HAMBURGER, V. AND BALABAN, M. (1963) *Develop. Biol.*, **7**, 533–545.
HOKIN, L. E. (1965) *Proc. Natl. Acad. Sci. U.S.*, **53**, 1369–1376.
HOKIN, L. E. (1967) *Neurosci. Res. Program Bull.*, **5**, 26–31.
HÖSLI, E. AND HÖSLI, L. (1970) *Brain Res.*, **19**, 494–496.
JOÓ, F., KÁSA, P., KÁLMÁN, GY. AND CSILLIK, B. (1963) *Folia Histochem. Cytochem.*, **1**, Suppl., 1, 118.
KARCZMAR, A. G. (1969) *Federation Proc.*, **28**, 147–157.
KARNOVSKY, M. J. (1964) *J. Cell Biol.*, **23**, 217–232.
KÁSA, P., CSILLIK, B., JOÓ, F. AND KNYIHÁR, E. (1966) *J. Neurochem.*, **13**, 173–178.
KIM, S. U. (1970) *Experientia*, **26**, 292–293.
KLING, A., FINER, S. AND NAIR, V. (1965) *Intern. J. Neuropharmacol.*, **4**, 353–357.
KLING, A., FINER, S. AND GILMOUR, J. (1969) *Intern. J. Neuropharmacol.*, **8**, 25–31.
KRNJEVIĆ, K. AND SILVER, A. (1965) *J. Anat.*, **99**, 711–759.
KRNJEVIĆ, K. AND SILVER, A. (1966) *J. Anat.*, **100**, 63–89.
LARRABEE, M. (1967) Formal discussion. *Neurosci. Res. Program Bull.*, **5**, p. 43.
LEVI-MONTALCINI, R. AND LEVI, G. (1943) *Arch. Biol. (Liège)*, **54**, 189–206.
MALETTA, G. J. AND TIMIRAS, P. S. (1966) *J. Neurochem.*, **13**, 75–84.
MALETTA, G. J., VERNADAKIS, A. AND TIMIRAS, P. S. (1966) *Proc. Soc. Exp. Biol. Med.*, **121**, 1210–1211.

MALETTA, G. J., VERNADAKIS, A. AND TIMIRAS, P. S. (1967) *J. Neurochem.*, **14**, 647–652.
MARCHISIO, P. C. AND CONSOLO, S. (1968) *J. Neurochem.*, **15**, 759–764.
MARCHISIO, P. C. AND GIACOBINI, G. (1969) *Brain Res.*, **15**, 301–304.
McCAMAN, R. E. AND APRISON, M. H. (1964) In W. A. HIMWICH AND H. E. HIMWICH (Eds.), *The Developing Brain, Progress in Brain Research, Vol. 9*, Elsevier, Amsterdam-New York, pp. 220–233.
NAIR, V. AND BAU, D. (1969) *Brain Res.*, **16**, 383–394.
PAFF, G. H., BOUCEK, R. J. AND GLANDER, T. P. (1966) *Anat. Rec.*, **154**, 675–684.
PHILLIS, J. W. (1968) *J. Neurochem.*, **15**, 691–698.
ROBERTS, C. M., GIMENO, M. A. AND WEBB, J. L. (1965) *J. Cell. Comp. Physiol.*, **66**, 273–280.
ROSENZWEIG, M. R., KRECH, D., BENNETT, E. L. AND ZOLMAN, J. F. (1962) *J. Comp. Physiol. Psychol.*, **55**, 1092–1095.
RUSSELL, R. W. (1969) *Federation Proc.*, **28**, 121–131.
SAKHAROVA, A. V. (1966) *Tsitologiya*, **8**, 54–59.
SILVER, A. (1967) *Intern. Rev. Neurobiol.*, **10**, 57–109.
SILVER, A. (1969) *Experientia*, **25**, 63–64.
STRUMIA, E. AND BAIMA-BOLLONE, P. L. (1964) *Acta Anat.*, **57**, 281–293.
TAPP, J. T. AND MARKOWITZ, H. (1963) *Science*, **140**, 486–487.
TENNYSON, V. M., BRZIN, M. AND DUFFY, P. (1968) In A. LAJTHA AND D. H. FORD (Eds.), *Brain Barrier Systems, Progress in Brain Research, Vol. 29*, Elsevier, Amsterdam-New York, pp. 41–61.
TURBOW, M. M. AND BURKHALTER, A. (1968) *Develop. Biol.*, **17**, 233–244.
VLK, J. S. AND TUČEK, S. (1962) *Physiol. Bohemoslov.*, **11**, 53–57.
ZACKS, S. I. (1954) *Anat. Rec.*, **118**, 509–537.

# The Demonstration of Acetylcholinesterase in Autonomic Axons with the Electron Microscope

PETER M. ROBINSON*

*Agricultural Research Council, Institute of Animal Physiology, Babraham, Cambridge (U.K.)*

## INTRODUCTION

It has been known for some time that cell bodies and axons of some post-ganglionic autonomic neurons stain for acetylcholinesterase (AChE) activity (see Koelle, 1963). The first aim of the present paper is to review the evidence identifying AChE as a component of cholinergic function in post-ganglionic autonomic axons. The second aim is to discuss, from a functional viewpoint, the significance of the ultrastructural location of AChE activity and to report some new findings which relate to the interpretation of the function of the enzyme.

## SECTION I

### *The evidence relating AChE to acetylcholine release*

On the basis of classical pharmacological experiments, at least two types of efferent autonomic fibres have been distinguished, those which release acetylcholine (ACh) (cholinergic axons) and those which release noradrenaline (NA) (adrenergic axons) (see Ferry 1966; Campbell, 1970; Gershon, 1970). However, an alternative explanation which involves ACh in NA release, has been offered (see Burn and Rand, 1959; 1965). There is also evidence for other, as yet unidentified, transmitter substances in the autonomic nervous system (see Campbell, 1970). In addition, sensory fibres are undoubtedly present in nerve bundles supplying the viscera.

Pharmacological experiments are often hard to interpret and many workers have turned to histochemical techniques to study the problem of the identification of autonomic axons. Since the application of the formaldehyde–fluorescence technique to terminal autonomic axons (Falck, 1962) a method for the demonstration of catecholamine-containing axons has been available. An increasing number of workers are combining this method for catecholamines with AChE histochemical methods (to demonstrate cholinergic axons) on the assumption that axons which stain for AChE are cholinergic. The chemical and morphological reliability of the fluorescence technique is well documented (Corrodi and Jonsson, 1967) whereas the evidence relating AChE to ACh release is often conflicting. Re-examination of this field, in its application to the autonomic nervous system, forms the first part of the present paper.

---

* Present address: Department of Anatomy, University of Melbourne, Victoria (Australia).

*References pp. 369–370*

*The distribution of AChE in neurons known to be cholinergic*

Somatic motor neurons and preganglionic autonomic neurons are known to be cholinergic. The cell bodies that give rise to these axons stain for AChE (see Koelle, 1963; Soderholm, 1965) as do the preterminal and the terminal parts of the axons themselves (Koelle, 1963; Davis and Koelle, 1965, 1967; Schlaepfer and Torack, 1966; Bloom and Barnett, 1966, 1967; Brzin, Tennyson and Duffy, 1966, 1967; Schlaepfer, 1968).

Parasympathetic neurons which are known to be cholinergic, such as those in the ciliary ganglion, also show this pattern of staining for AChE (see Koelle, 1963).

The results imply that cholinergic neurons stain for AChE in the cell body and axon, but what remains in question is whether AChE is necessarily *only* associated with cholinergic fibres.

*The distribution of AChE in neurons known to be non-cholinergic*

Peripheral afferent (dorsal root) neurons do not possess significant levels of choline acetylase (ChAc) in the adult mammal (see Hebb, 1957) yet there are a number of reports of AChE activity in dorsal root ganglion cells (*e.g.* Giacobini, 1967; Koelle, 1963; Brzin, Tennyson and Duffy, 1967) in dorsal root fibres (Burgen and Chipman, 1951; Schlaepfer, 1968) and in some (but not all) sensory endings (see Koelle, 1963).

Unfortunately it is very difficult to distinguish sensory fibres amongst the terminal ramifications of autonomic motor axons with either the light or electron microscope at the present time, and unless special precautions to exclude sensory fibres have been taken, an unknown number of possibly AChE-positive afferent fibres may be present amongst efferent autonomic axons.

*Distribution of AChE in post-ganglionic autonomic neurons*

*AChE activity in cell bodies in autonomic ganglia*

Combined AChE and fluorescent histochemical techniques have been applied to sympathetic ganglia in a number of animals. In some cases these studies have been supplemented by histochemical analysis of individual isolated cells. In the cat (Hamberger *et al.*, 1963; Buckley *et al.*, 1967; Giacobini *et al.*, 1967), rat (Eränkö and Härkönen, 1964) and guinea pig (Bell and McLean, 1967) cholinergic ganglion cells have been identified on the basis of high AChE activity (and, when this has been done, high ChAc activity) and on the absence of catecholamine fluorescence. It is clear, however, that a number of fluorescent (noradrenaline-containing) cells also show AChE activity. Large numbers of cells show both activities in rat ganglion, whereas smaller number of cells show dual activities in guinea pig and cat. In addition, there are always some cells which contain catecholamine but which do not stain for AChE. All the cells in sympathetic ganglia are surrounded by AChE-stained neuropil.

## Interpretation of the function of AChE in noradrenergic cell bodies

It is generally agreed that sympathetic ganglion cells which stain for AChE and do not contain noradrenaline (which, in the cat, have been shown to also contain ChAc) are cholinergic in the normally accepted sense. That is to say they release ACh which then has a post-synaptic action.

It is also generally agreed that the fluorescent cells ultimately release noradrenaline, which then has a post-synaptic action. However, the role of the AChE which has been shown to be present in the cell bodies of catecholamine-containing cells is not settled.

One interpretation is based on the suggestion that the cholinergic system (ChAc, ACh and AChE) is present in all nerve tissue and is involved either in conduction of the action potential (Nachmansohn, 1959, 1961; Dettbarn, 1967) or in release of the final transmitter substance, whether it is ACh or not (Burn and Rand, 1959, 1965; Koelle, 1963; Eränkö, 1967).

If either of these suggestions is correct, adrenergic neurons should contain ChAc and the axon as well as the cell body of noradrenergic cells would be expected to stain for AChE.

Another interpretation of AChE in noradrenergic cell bodies is based on the function of AChE at cholinergic synapses. Since the great majority of, if not all, preganglionic autonomic axons are cholinergic (see Volle, 1966) all the adrenergic cell bodies in an autonomic ganglion will be cholinoceptive and would be expected to contain cell body, but not axonal, AChE (see Koelle, 1963; Shute and Lewis, 1965; Eränkö, 1967).

This first hypothesis is not supported by the results of assays of enzyme levels in sympathetic ganglion. In these experiments 98–100% of the ChAc activity in sympathetic ganglia was lost after preganglionic denervation (Hebb and Waites, 1956) yet about 20% of the AChE remains behind in the denervated ganglion cells (Sawyer and Hollinshead, 1945). The ChAc surviving denervation is associated with a small number of presumably cholinergic cells, while the remaining AChE is associated with a greater number of presumably adrenergic cells (Buckley et al., 1967; Giacobini, 1967).

## AChE activity in autonomic axons

There is a considerable body of pharmacological evidence for the presence of a functional cholinesterase in noradrenergic nerve trunks (see Ferry, 1966) and a number of workers have studied the distribution of AChE-staining axons in smooth muscle tissue by combined AChE/catecholamine–fluorescence techniques, however, as the workers concerned pointed out, the resolution of the combined techniques was not sufficient to allow the examination of single axons and only nerve trunks could be studied.

In the majority of tissues examined in this series of experiments, there was a striking similarity between the patterns of distribution of catecholamine-containing and AChE-positive nerve trunks. However, in a few cases, individual trunks which showed only one activity were noted (Jacobowitz and Koelle, 1965; Eränkö and Räisänen, 1965). In more recent years a great number of studies have been made using the combined techniques and a number of tissues have now been described in which CA-containing and AChE-positive fibres are found in different patterns (*e.g.* El-Bermani *et al.*, 1970; Hebb and Linzell, 1970).

One investigation with the light microscope has been reported which did not suffer from the particular disadvantages of the combined AChE–fluorescence techniques. In this series of experiments rat iris was examined for AChE staining and CA-fluorescence (under optimum conditions for each) after sympathetic and parasympathetic denervation. The results obtained indicated that the CA-containing fibres from the superior cervical ganglion of the rat did not stain for AChE (Ehinger and Falck, 1966).

Confirmation of this result has come from electron microscope studies on cat autonomic axons. In these experiments, axons which accumulated [³H]noradrenaline (and were subsequently associated with silver grains after autoradiography), which were presumably adrenergic axons, also did not stain for AChE. Of the axons which did not take up [³H]noradrenaline, some stained for AChE and some did not (Esterhuizen *et al.*, 1968; Graham *et al.*, 1968).

None of these results exclude the possibility that *some* adrenergic axons may stain for AChE. Also an unknown amount of enzyme inhibition has undoubtedly occurred during the preparation of the tissue in all the histochemical techniques used to study this problem, therefore, while it is well established that some non-adrenergic axons possess high AChE activity it cannot be taken as proven that adrenergic axons themselves do not possess any AChE activity at all. This point is dealt with further later in this review.*

SECTION 2

This section of the present paper reviews the methods available at each stage of the histochemical procedures suitable for electron microscopy, as they relate to the discussion in the first section.

Smaller quantities of stain (and therefore lower enzyme activities) and greatly improved resolution have followed the use of suitably controlled electron microscope methods for AChE.

Nevertheless, unless suitable conditions are employed at all stages in the process, interpretation of the staining pattern is very difficult.

*Fixation*

The two fixatives most commonly used for electron-microscopic histochemistry, formaldehyde and glutaraldehyde, have both been shown to produce excellent morphological preservation (either used alone, or in combination) over a wide range of conditions, but there is very little quantitative information about the effect of these fixatives on enzyme activity (see Hopwood, 1969 and Pearse, 1968).

---

* Note added in proof: Since this manuscript was prepared, AChE has been reported on axons containing small granular vesicles in the rat pineal gland (Eränkö *et al.*, Histochem. J. 1970, 479).

## Purity of the fixatives

Formaldehyde can be used either as a diluted sample (usually 1 in 4) from a stock formalin solution (this fixative is usually referred to as 10% formalin) or as a solution of formaldehyde made from paraformaldehyde. There seems to be little doubt that the latter is the only form of formaldehyde suitable for electron microscope histochemistry (see Pease, 1964).

Glutaraldehyde, which appears to be made only by Union Carbide, can be obtained from laboratory suppliers in various 'grades' (of purity). A number of methods have been suggested to further purify the stock solution in the laboratory, e.g. Fahimi and Drochmans (1965) developed a method of vacuum distillation, Hopwood (1967a) used filtration through Sephadex G-10 and Anderson (1967) tested activated charcoal.

The degree of purity of the glutaraldehyde solution may have little effect on morphology (Robertson and Schultz, 1970) but according to data published by Anderson (1967), it has a major effect on the enzyme activity retained by fixed tissue. In these experiments Anderson compared the cholinesterase activity remaining in rat skeletal muscle slices after fixation in 4% commercial grade glutaraldehyde (approx. 20% enzyme activity remaining) and glutaraldehyde purified with activated charcoal (approx. 45% activity remaining) or distillation (approx. 75% activity remaining). These results underline the need to use purified glutaraldehyde in cholinesterase histochemistry.

Anderson also tested the effect of 4% formaldehyde (presumably prepared from paraformaldehyde) on rat skeletal muscle cholinesterase activity (approx. 70% activity remaining). Therefore from the viewpoint of the retention of cholinesterase enzyme activity, distilled glutaraldehyde is the fixative of choice. If this is unavailable, formaldehyde is preferable to charcoal-purified glutaraldehyde.

## Concentration of fixative

Taxi (1952) tested the action of various concentrations of formalin on the activity of cholinesterases at 18° C and found that the cholinesterase activity remaining in fixed tissue decreased with increased concentration of formalin. Walker and Seligman (1963) found a similar effect on dehydrogenase activity.

A series of experiments were carried out in this laboratory to test the effect on cholinesterase activity of treating brain slices with 0.5, 1, 2 and 4% formaldehyde (prepared from paraformaldehyde) for 1 h at 0–4° C. The results are shown in Table 1 (Robinson and Mann, unpubl. obs.).

Although Maunsbach (1966) found very little difference in the standard of structural preservation by glutaraldehyde at different concentrations down to 0.25% (provided the buffer system had the appropriate osmolality), Baker and McRae (1966) found 0.25% formaldehyde to be inadequate. They have shown that acceptable results can be obtained using 1% formaldehyde, and this has been confirmed for smooth muscle tissue in this laboratory (Robinson, unpubl. obs.).

*References pp. 369–370*

## TABLE 1

TOTAL CHOLINESTERASE ACTIVITY RETAINED IN RABBIT BRAIN SLICES AFTER TREATMENT
WITH FORMALDEHYDE

The formaldehyde was dissolved immediately before use in 0.075 M cacodylate–HCl buffer pH 7.2
containing 0.2 M sucrose. The slices were then washed in buffered sucrose at the same concentration
for 2 h and homogenized. The enzyme level remaining was determined by the Ellman *et al.* (1961)
method using acetylthiocholine iodide without inhibitors. (Robinson and Mann, unpublished
observation).

| Concentration of formaldehyde in g/100 ml | Percentage cholinesterase activity remaining |
|:---:|:---:|
| 0 | 100 |
| 0.5 | 78 |
| 1 | 70 |
| 2 | 56 |
| 4 | 47 |

### Temperature of fixation

It has been well known since the early reports of the use of formalin as a fixative for
histochemistry (Seligman *et al.*, 1951; Taxi, 1952) that more activity is retained in
fixed tissue when fixation is carried out at low temperatures. Once again, as Baker and
McRae (1966) found little difference in tissue morphology when formaldehyde
fixation was performed at any temperature between 0° and 45° C, continuing the
established practice of fixing at ice bath temperatures would seem advisable.

### Duration of fixation

Seligman *et al.* (1951), Taxi (1952), Janigan (1964) and Hopwood (1967b) have
studied the effect of the time of fixation on enzyme activity retained in fixed tissue and
found that with increasing length of fixation there is a greater loss of enzyme activity.

Preliminary experiments carried out in this laboratory indicate that the rate of
inactivation of enzyme activity decreases with duration of fixation (Robinson and
Mann, unpubl. obs.). The optimum duration of fixation will clearly depend on the rate
of diffusion of the fixative and the thickness of tissue to be fixed (*i.e.* shorter times
could be used after initial perfusion).

### Buffer and osmolality of fixative solution

The choice of buffer used in aldehyde fixation appears to have little effect on either
morphology or enzyme activity except that in some cases enzyme systems may be
susceptible to some anions [*e.g.* 0.1 M phosphate inhibits glucose-6-phosphate

dehydrogenase activity, Lohr and Waller (1963)] and the buffer may react with part of the incubation medium, *e.g.* phosphate with lead ions (see Hopwood, 1969).

### Effect of fixation on penetration of histochemical media

Brzin *et al.* (1966) and Tennyson *et al.* (1968) reported that *intracellular* enzyme activity was only detectable by microgasometric or cytochemical techniques after fixation or after damage to the cell membrane of the unfixed cell. They interpreted this result as indicating that fixation rendered the cell membrane more permeable to substrates and other constituents of the media. Jard *et al.* (1966) investigated the effect of various fixatives on cell membrane permeability and concluded that cell membranes remain impermeable to most molecules after aldehyde fixation (compared with osmium tetroxide) but that the membrane permeability was greater after glutaraldehyde than after formaldehyde.

Janigan (1964, 1965) has reported major differences between the degree of inactivation of different enzymes by the same fixative solution and significant differences between the inactivation of the same enzyme in different species. It would therefore be unwise to draw more than tentative conclusions about the effect of changes of fixation conditions from results on different enzymes. Precise values for enzyme activity after a given set of fixation conditions must be determined in each individual case.

To summarize, the general trends which emerge from this review of the results of altering fixation conditions are:
1. Substantial improvement in enzyme activity follows the use of purified glutaraldehyde, and distillation is the method of choice. If distilled glutaraldehyde is unavailable, then formaldehyde is the fixative of choice.
2. Substantial improvement in enzyme activity follows the use of reduced concentrations of fixative. A 50% increase in activity of rabbit brain ChE was achieved by decreasing formaldehyde concentration from 4% to 1%.
3. Greater enzyme activity is retained in tissue when fixation is carried out at low temperatures and for short durations. Because the rate of enzyme inactivation falls with time there is a good argument for decreasing the duration of fixation to the minimum necessary to obtain adequate structural preservation. Nevertheless, because fixation decreases barriers to penetration of media, there may well be an optimum time of fixation for the demonstration of enzyme activity. This latter factor would be more significant in electron microscopy where tissue slices and diced pieces are incubated than in light microscopy in which frozen sections are used.

### Histochemical incubation conditions

Because pseudocholinesterase (ChE) hydrolyses acetylcholine at a significant rate, ChE activity may produce stain when acetylthiocholine is used as a histochemical substrate. Because of the widespread distribution of ChE, steps are usually taken to

inhibit its activity in histochemical incubations designed to demonstrate AChE.
Inhibitors commonly used are:
Di-isopropylfluorophosphate (DFP) $10^{-6}$–$10^{-7}$M (see Koelle, 1950, 1963)
Ethopropazine hydrochloride (EP) $10^{-4}$M (Bayliss and Todrick, 1956)
Tetra-isopropylpyrophosphoramide (iso-OMPA) $10^{-5}$M (Bayliss and Todrick, 1956)

There are numerous reports of species differences in the response to cholinesterase inhibitors (see Holmstedt, 1963) and unless the effectiveness of the selected inhibitor has been checked on enzyme from the species to be examined, serious inaccuracies may result, particularly with long incubation times. For example, Table 2 compares the effectiveness of ethopropazine as an inhibitor of ChE in the rat (from Bayliss and Todrick, 1956) and in the chick (S.P. Mann, personal communication).

It is important that ChE activity be inhibited throughout the period of incubation. Substrates compete with inhibitors for enzyme sites and pre-incubation is usually employed to ensure the maximum effective inhibition (Koelle, 1950, 1963). It is also common practice to demonstrate that the enzyme activity remaining after ChE inhibition can be inhibited by a specific inhibitor such as BW284C51 (Bayliss and Todrick, 1956).

TABLE 2

PSEUDOCHOLINESTERASE ACTIVITY REMAINING IN ENZYME SAMPLES AFTER ETHOPROPAZINE

The figures for the rat were taken from Bayliss and Todrick, 1956. The figures for the chicken were supplied from unpublished work by S. P. Mann.

|  | Concentration of ethopropazine M | Percentage ChE activity remaining |
|---|---|---|
| Rat | $8 \times 10^{-5}$ | 5 |
| Chicken | $1 \times 10^{-4}$ | 55 |

*Visualization of AChE activity*

A number of modifications of the original copper–thiocholine technique (Koelle and Friedenwald, 1949) have been successfully applied to electron microscopy. These modifications can be grouped into categories:

(a) Methods in which the original conditions are essentially retained *e.g.* Lewis and Shute, 1966.

(b) Methods in which an additional metal ion is introduced *e.g.* Kása and Csillik, 1966

(c) Methods in which the sulphide step is omitted *e.g.*, Tennyson, Brzin and Duffy, 1965

(d) Methods in which a different capture reagent is used *e.g.*, Davis and Koelle, 1965

(e) Methods in which the thiocholine reacts with ferricyanide *e.g.*, Karnovsky, 1964.

Unfortunately, these variations, and *their* subsequent modifications have tended to remain the chosen method of the laboratory in which they were developed, and no systematic attempt has been made to compare a variety of methods on one tissue. In spite of this trend, two methods, that of Lewis and Shute (1966) and of Karnovsky (1964) have been used by a number of investigators and these two methods have, amongst others, also been applied to autonomic axons.

The remainder of this review will be restricted to discussing the location of AChE enzyme sites in post-ganglionic autonomic axons as demonstrated by electron-microscopic techniques.

*Axons:* All authors are in agreement that some post-ganglionic autonomic axons possess AChE on or in the axon membrane. This is usually indicated by dense deposits of stain particles lying between the axon and the Schwann cell (Robinson and Bell, 1967; Burnstock and Robinson, 1967; Hirano and Ogawa, 1967; Esterhuizen *et al.*, 1968), however stain particles lying on the axon membrane have been clearly shown by Robinson (1969). All stained axons in the cat appeared to possess about the same level of activity (Esterhuizen *et al.*, 1968; Graham *et al.*, 1968) but experiments using different incubation times have demonstrated axons with varying activities in the toad (Robinson and Bell, 1967 and guinea pig, Burnstock and Robinson, 1967; Robinson, 1969).

Very little intra-axonal activity has been demonstrated. Some axons contain small stain particles in axons examined with the Lewis and Shute method (Esterhuizen *et al.* 1968; Graham *et al.*, 1968) and some vesicles appeared to stain in a small number of axons examined with the Karnovsky method (Robinson and Bell, 1967; Robinson, 1969).

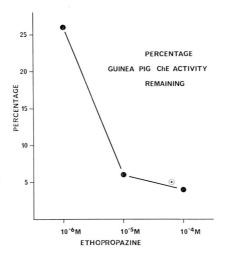

Fig. 1. The effect of various concentrations of ethopropazine hydrochloride on ChE activity in guinea pig brain homogenate after 1 h preincubation. These determinations were carried out by the Ellman *et al.* (1961) method using butyrylthiocholine iodide as substrate in the presence of $5 \times 10^{-5}$ M BW284C51. Spontaneous hydrolysis of substrate was measured and taken into account. The circled point is the activity quoted by Bayliss and Todrick (1956) for the rat.

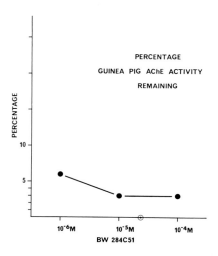

Fig. 2. The effect of various concentrations of BW284C51 on AChE activity in guinea pig brain homogenate after 1 h preincubation. These determinations were carried out by the Ellman *et al.* (1961) method using acetylthiocholine iodide as substrate in the presence of $10^{-4}$ M ethopropazine. Spontaneous hydrolysis of substrate was measured and taken into account. The circled point is the activity quoted by Bayliss and Todrick (1956) for the rat.

This lack of intra-axonal staining in autonomic nerves is surprising in view of the rapid transport of AChE down axons which has been associated with axoplasmic transport (see Lubinska, 1964) and the intra-axonal stain demonstrated by Brzin *et al.* (1966) and Tennyson *et al.* (1968) in preganglionic autonomic axons, and Schlaepfer and Torack (1966) and Schlaepfer (1968) in sciatic nerve and spinal roots.

*Schwann cells:* Schwann cells associated with AChE-positive axons also stain for AChE (Robinson, 1969).

*Muscle cells:* Post-synaptic, *i.e.* muscle membrane stain, has been demonstrated in toad bladder and guinea pig vas deferens with the Karnovsky technique in patches on smooth muscle cell membranes adjacent to AChE-stained axons (Robinson and Bell, 1967; Robinson, 1969).

The electron microscope can detect very small quantities of stain (particles of approx. 50–100 Å diameter) and it can therefore be used as a sensitive method for localizing low levels of enzyme activity. Because those electron microscope methods for AChE which have been applied to autonomic axons have either involved prolonged fixation in glutaraldehyde (*e.g.* Esterhuizen *et al.*, 1968) or have been restricted to relatively short incubation times by non-enzymic staining (*e.g.* Robinson, 1969) the question remains whether the electron microscope could detect stain due to AChE activity in noradrenergic axons under conditions of minimum enzyme inactivation and long incubation times.

To study this point the guinea pig vas deferens was fixed in 1% formaldehyde for $1\frac{1}{2}$ h and incubated for up to 8 h at 18° C in the medium of Kása and Csillik (1966) in the presence of ethopropazine $10^{-4}$M [this concentration of ethopropazine had been previously shown to inhibit guinea pig ChE by 796% (text Fig. 1)].

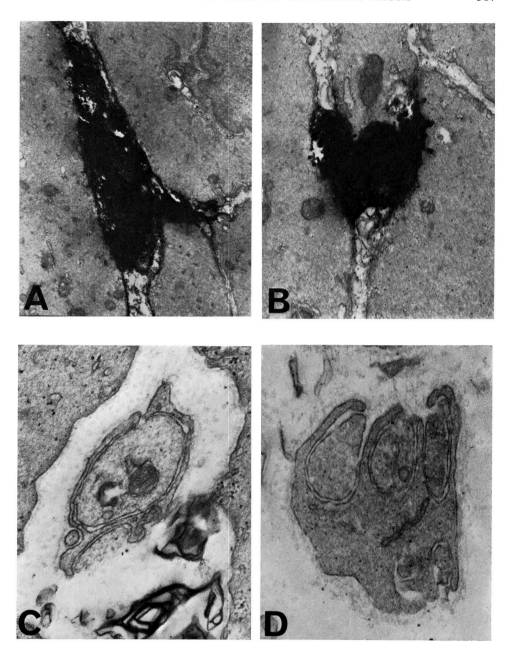

Fig. 3. Guinea pig vas deferens incubated for 8 h in Kása and Csillik (1966) medium using acetyl-thiocholine iodide as substrate in presence of $10^{-4}$ M ethopropazine. A & B, stained axons: C & D, unstained axons. Approximate magnification: A, × 10000; B, × 20000; C, × 40000; D, × 40000.

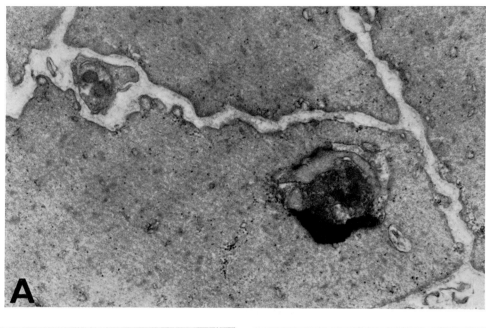

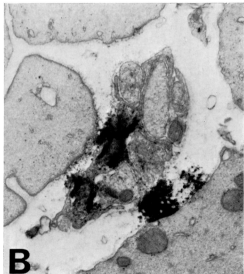

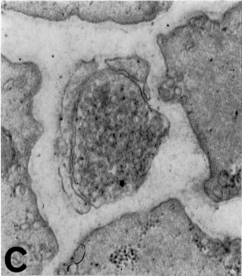

Fig. 4. Guinea pig vas deferens incubated for 8 h in Kása and Csillik (1966) medium using acetyl-thiocholine iodide as substrate in presence of $10^{-4}$ M ethopropazine. A, Stained axon (embedded in a muscle cell) and an unstained axon; B, A group of stained and unstained axons; C, An axon from tissue treated with $5 \times 10^{-5}$ M BW284C51 in addition to ethopropazine $10^{-4}$ M. Note the small amount of stain in this axon. This probably represents the 3% of AChE activity not inhibited by BW284C51 (see text Fig. 2). Approximate magnification: A, $\times$ 25000; B, $\times$ 20000; C, $\times$ 40000.

The results were clear-cut. The majority of axons remained unstained after 8 h incubation (Figs. 3 and 4) although CA-containing axons could not be identified after 1 % formaldehyde fixation, the majority of the axons in the guinea pig vas deferens are adrenergic (see Robinson, 1969, for a discussion).

## SUMMARY

AChE occurs with ChAc and ACh in the cell bodies and axons of known cholinergic neurons (ventral horn cells, pre-ganglionic autonomic and post-ganglionic cholinergic cells) but it also occurs *without* ChAc and ACh in some peripheral afferent (dorsal root ganglion) cell bodies and some adrenergic ganglion cell bodies. Other peripheral afferent and adrenergic ganglion cells do not contain AChE.

Some peripheral afferent axons stain for AChE.

It has been clearly demonstrated that the majority of adrenergic axons do not stain for AChE, yet the possibility that some adrenergic axons contain detectable levels of AChE cannot be excluded at the present time.

AChE in autonomic nerve fibres is located on axon membranes and on the membranes of some Schwann cells.

## ACKNOWLEDGEMENTS

I would like to thank Dr. C. Hebb for the opportunity to work in her laboratory and for her encouragement and advice during the preparation of this manuscript. I would also like to acknowledge financial support from the University of Melbourne and the British Council.

## REFERENCES

ANDERSON, P. J. (1967) *J. Histochem. Cytochem.*, **15**, 652.
BAKER, J. R. AND McRAE, J. M. (1966) *J. Roy. Microscop. Soc.*, **85**, 391.
BAYLISS, B. J. AND TODRICK, A. (1956) *Biochem. J.*, **62**, 62.
BELL, C. AND McLEAN, J. R. (1967) *J. Pharmacol.*, **157**, 69.
BLOOM, F. E. AND BARNETT, R. J. (1966) *J. Cell Biol.*, **29**, 475.
BLOOM, F. E. AND BARNETT, R. J. (1967) *Ann. N.Y. Acad. Sci.*, **144**, 626.
BRZIN, M., TENNYSON, V. M. AND DUFFY, P. E. (1966) *J. Cell Biol.*, **31**, 215.
BRZIN, M., TENNYSON, V. M. AND DUFFY, P. E. (1967) *Intern. J. Neuropharmacol.*, **6**, 265.
BUCKLEY, G., CONSOLO, S., GIACOBINI, E. AND SJOQVIST, F. (1967) *Acta Physiol. Scand.*, **71**, 348.
BURGEN, A. S. V. AND CHIPMAN, L. M. (1951) *J. Physiol.*, **114**, 296.
BURN, J. H. AND RAND, M. J. (1959) *Nature*, **184**, 163.
BURN, J. H. AND RAND, M. J. (1965) *Ann. Rev. Pharmacol.*, **5**, 163.
BURNSTOCK, G. AND ROBINSON, P. M. (1967) *Circulation Res.*, **20**, Suppl. III, 43.
CAMPBELL, G. (1970) In E. BULBRING, A. F. BRADING, A. W. JONES AND T. TOMITA (Eds.), *Smooth Muscle*, Edward Arnold, London, p. 451.
CORRODI, H. AND JONSSON, G. (1967) *J. Histochem. Cytochem.*, **15**, 65.
DAVIS, R. AND KOELLE, G. B. (1965) *J. Histochem. Cytochem.*, **13**, 703.
DAVIS, R. AND KOELLE, G. B. (1967) *J. Cell Biol.*, **34**, 157.
DETTBARN, W. D. (1967) *Ann. N.Y. Acad. Sci.*, **144**, 483.
EHINGER, B. AND FALCK, B. (1966) *Acta Physiol. Scand.*, **67**, 201.
EL-BERMANI, A. W., McNARY, W. F. AND BRADLEY, D. E. (1970) *Anat. Rec.*, **167**, 205.

ELLMAN, G. L., COURTNEY, K. D., ANDRES, V. AND FEATHERSTONE, R. M. (1961) *Biochem. Pharmacol.*, **7**, 88.

ERÄNKÖ, O. (1967) *Ann. Rev. Pharmacol.*, **7**, 203.

ERÄNKÖ, O. AND HÄRKÖNEN, M. (1964) *Acta Physiol. Scand.*, **61**, 299.

ERÄNKÖ, O. AND RÄISÄNEN, L. (1965) *Acta Physiol. Scand.*, **63**, 505.

ESTERHUIZEN, A. C., GRAHAM, J. D., LEVER, J. D. AND SPRIGGS, T. L. (1968) *Brit. J. Pharmacol.*, **32**, 46.

FAHIMI, H. D. AND DROCHMANS, P. (1965) *J. Microscopie*, **4**, 725.

FALCK, B. (1962) *Acta Physiol. Scand.*, **56**, Suppl. 197, 1.

FERRY, C. B. (1966) *Physiol. Rev.*, **46**, 420.

GERSHON, M. D. (1970) In E. BULBRING, A. F. BRADING, A. W. JONES AND T. TOMITA (Eds.), *Smooth Muscle*, Edward Arnold, London, p. 496.

GIACOBINI, E. (1967) *Ann. N.Y. Acad. Sci.*, **144**, 646.

GIACOBINI, E., PALMBORG, B. AND SJOQUIST, F. (1967) *Acta Physiol. Scand.*, **69**, 355.

GRAHAM, J. D., LEVER, J. D. AND SPRIGGS, T. L. (1968) *Brit. J. Pharmacol.*, **33**, 15.

HAMBERGER, B., NORBERG, K. A. AND SJOQVIST, F. (1963) In G. B. KOELLE, W. W. DOUGLAS AND A. CARLSSON (Eds.), *Intern. Pharmacol. Meeting*, Pergamon Press, Oxford, **3**, 41.

HEBB, C. (1957) *Physiol. Revs.*, **37**, 196.

HEBB, C. AND LINZELL, J. L. (1970) *Histochem. J.*, (in press).

HEBB, C. AND WAITES, G. (1956) *J. Physiol.*, **132**, 667.

HIRANO, H. AND OGAWA, K. (1967) *J. Electronmicroscopy (Tokyo)*, **16**, 3131.

HOLMSTEDT, B. (1963) *Handbuch der Experimentellen Pharmakologie*, *Vol. 15*, Springer-Verlag, Berlin, p. 328.

HOPWOOD, D. (1967a) *Histochemie*, **11**, 289.

HOPWOOD, D. (1967b) *J. Anat.*, **101**, 83.

HOPWOOD, D. (1969) *Histochem. J.*, **1**, 323.

JACOBOWITZ, D. AND KOELLE, G. B. (1965) *J. Pharmacol.*, **148**, 225.

JANIGAN, D. T. (1964) *Lab. Invest.*, **13**, 1038.

JANIGAN, D. J. (1965) *J. Histochem. Cytochem.*, **13**, *473*.

JARD, S., BOURGUET, V., CARASSO, N. AND FAVARD, P. (1966) *J. Microscopie*, **5**, 31.

KARNOVSKY, M. J. (1964) *J. Cell Biol.*, **23**, 217.

KÁSA, P., AND CSILLIK, B. (1966) *J. Neurochem.*, **13**, 1345.

KOELLE, G. B. (1950) *J. Pharmacol. Exp. Therap.*, **100**, *158*.

KOELLE, G. B. (1963) *Handbuch der Experimentellen Pharmakologie*, Vol. 15, Springer-Verlag, Berlin, p. 187.

KOELLE, G. B. AND FRIEDENWALD, J. S. (1949) *Proc. Soc. Exp. Biol.*, **20**, 617.

LEWIS, P. R. AND SHUTE, C. C. D. (1966) *J. Cell Sci.*, **1**, 381.

LOHR, G. W. AND WALLER, H. D. (1963) In H. U. BERGMEYER (Ed.), *Methods of Enzymatic Analyses*, Academic Press, New-York-London.

LUBINSKA, L. (1964) *Progr. Brain Res.*, **13**, 1.

MAUNSBACH, A. B. (1966) *J. Ultrastruct. Res.*, **15**, 283.

NACHMANSOHN, D. (1959) *Chemical and Molecular Basis of Nerve Activity*, Academic Press, New York-London.

NACHMANSOHN, D. (1961) *Science*, **134**, 1962.

PEARSE, A. G. E. (1968) *Histochemistry: Theoretical and Applied*, Vol. 1, 3rd ed., Churchill, London.

PEASE, D. C. (1964) *Histological Techniques for Electron Microscopy*, Academic Press, New York.

ROBERTSON, E. A. AND SCHULTZ, R. L. (1970) *J. Ultrastruct. Res.*, **30**, 275.

ROBINSON, P. M. (1969) *J. Cell Biol.*, **41**, 462.

ROBINSON, P. M. AND BELL, C. (1967) *J. Cell Biol.*, **33**, 93.

SAWYER, C. H. AND HOLLINSHEAD, W. H. (1945) *J. Neurophysiol.*, **8**, 137.

SCHLAEPFER, W. W. (1968) *Z. Zellforsch. Mikroskop. Anat.*, **88**, 441.

SCHLAEPFER, W. W. AND TORACK, R. M. (1966) *J. Histochem. Cytochem.*, **14**, 369.

SELIGMAN, A. M., CHAUNCEY, H. H. AND NACHLAS, M. M. (1951) *Stain Technol.*, **26**, 19.

SHUTE, C. C. AND LEWIS, P. R. (1965) *Nature*, **205**, 242.

SÖDERHOLM, U. (1965) *Acta Physiol. Scand.*, **65**, Suppl. 256.

TAXI, J. (1952) *J. Physiol. (Paris)*, **44**, 595.

TENNYSON, V. M., BRZIN, M. AND DUFFY, P. (1965) *J. Cell Biol.*, **27**, 105.

TENNYSON, V. M., BRZIN, M. AND DUFFY, P. (1968) *Progr. Brain Res.*, **29**, 41.

VOLLE, R. L. (1966) *Pharmacol. Rev.*, **18**, 839.

WALKER, D. G. AND SELIGMAN, A. M. (1963) *J. Cell Biol.*, **16**, 455.

# New Findings Concerning the Localization by Electron Microscopy of Acetylcholinesterase in Autonomic Ganglia*

GEORGE B. KOELLE, RICHARD DAVIS AND ELOISE GABEL SMYRL

*Department of Pharmacology, Medical School, University of Pennsylvania, Philadelphia, Pa. 19104*
*(U.S.A.)*

It is difficult, if indeed desirable, to embark upon a long-range investigation without harboring some preconceived notions as to the general nature of the results that will be obtained. In fact, one of the guiding principles in the design of experiments is the testing of hypotheses. It is therefore disconcerting when one obtains relatively direct evidence that is distinctly at variance with conclusions drawn previously from what had been assumed to be valid, although indirect, evidence. Such has been our recent experience in the course of electron microscopic studies of the localization of acetylcholinesterase (AChE) in autonomic ganglia of the cat. The sequence of these findings and the probable basis for the discrepancies noted will be presented briefly here.

## LIGHT MICROSCOPIC AND PHARMACOLOGICAL STUDIES

With the development of the copper thiocholine (CuThCh) histochemical method for acetylcholinesterase (AChE) and pseudocholinesterase (ChE) (Koelle and Friedenwald, 1949; Koelle 1950, 1951, 1955), it became possible to determine the localization of these enzymes in fresh frozen sections with high degrees of specificity and sensitivity, and to a reasonable degree of accuracy within the limits of resolution afforded by light microscopy. Early observations indicated that known cholinergic neurons contain relatively high concentrations of AChE throughout their lengths, whereas the concentrations of AChE in non-cholinergic (*e.g.*, adrenergic, sensory) neurons vary from moderate to essentially none, according to the particular site and species. Particularly high concentrations of AChE were noted at the motor endplates (MEP's) of skeletal muscle; here, the observations were convincing that most of the enzyme is located postjunctionally, at the surface and multiple invaginations of the subneural, modified sarcoplasmic membrane (Couteaux and Taxi, 1952; Couteaux, 1958).

In order to investigate the cytological localization of AChE in the superior cervical, ciliary, and other autonomic ganglia of the cat, beyond what could be seen by direct light-microscopic observation of stained sections, additional procedures were employed. Prior to staining, tissues were treated *in vitro* and *in vivo*, with various an-

* The original investigations from the authors' laboratory mentioned in this review were supported by National Institute of Neurological Diseases and Stroke Research Grant NB 00282.

*References pp. 374–375*

ticholinesterase (anti-ChE) agents, including reversible and irreversible, and lipid-soluble and -insoluble compounds, administered alone and in combination to both normal and preganglionically denervated cats. From the results obtained, it was postulated that the AChE of cholinergic neurons is distributed between an internal or reserve fraction (enzyme recently synthesized within the endoplasmic reticulum) and an external or functional fraction (enzyme incorporated within the surface of the neuronal membrane, with the functional groups oriented externally) (Koelle and Steiner, 1956; Koelle, 1957). This concept was supported by pharmacological evidence (McIsaac and Koelle, 1959). On the basis of the disappearance of essentially all the functional AChE from the superior cervical and stellate ganglia following preganglionic denervation, it was concluded that the enzyme is practically entirely presynaptic at those sites (Koelle and Koelle, 1959). A similar conclusion had been reached several years previously from studies of the AChE activities of homogenates of normal and denervated cat superior cervical ganglia (Sawyer and Hollinshead, 1945), and has been confirmed by subsequent histochemical studies (Holmstedt *et al.*, 1963; Gromadski and Koelle, 1965). Similar evidence indicated that the functional AChE of the two parasympathetic ganglia studied, the ciliary and the sphenopalatine, is both presynaptic and postsynaptic (Koelle and Koelle, 1959).

An investigation of the physiological function of AChE in the cat superior cervical ganglion suggested that the presynaptic membrane is more sensitive than the postsynaptic to the actions of acetylcholine (ACh) and carbachol, and that such drugs can release endogenous ACh from the presynaptic terminals (Volle and Koelle, 1961). From these and the foregoing histochemical findings, it was proposed that the ACh released initially by the preganglionic nerve impulse acts at the same presynaptic terminals to prolong briefly their depolarization, and hence amplify the amount of ACh released to effect synaptic transmission (Koelle, 1962). A similar proposal, of a cholinergic link in adrenergic transmission, had been made by Burn and Rand (1959); more recently, this concept has been extended to several sites of non-cholinergic transmission in the central nervous system (Koelle, 1969). These proposals have not gone unchallenged (Ferry, 1966; Brown, 1969; Collier, 1969).

The next logical histochemical step in these studies was to seek by electron microscopy more direct evidence of the precise location of AChE at ganglionic synapses.

### ELECTRON MICROSCOPIC HISTOCHEMISTRY OF AChE

Electron microscopic studies have been performed with modifications of the CuThCh method itself (Lewis and Shute, 1966; Brzin *et al.*, 1966) and with the related thiocholine–copper–ferricyanide method (Karnovsky and Roots, 1964; Phillis, 1965; Bell, 1966). However, as discussed previously (Koelle, 1970), this approach has inherent limitations to the accuracy of localization obtainable, namely, the quaternary and hence poorly penetrating nature of the substrate (acetylthiocholine), and the relatively large dimensions and low electron-density of the primary reaction products. The less specific lead–thiolacetic acid (Pb–TA) method is superior in both these respects (Crevier and Bélanger, 1955; Barrnett, 1962); by substituting aurous gold for lead as the capturing agent, a highly electron-dense reaction product (Au$_2$S) of still finer dimensions was obtained (Koelle and Foroglou-Kerameos, 1965; Koelle and Gromadzki, 1966). By means of the gold–thiolacetic acid (Au–TA) method, the AChE of the MEP of mouse intercostal muscle was localized with high precision at the pre- and postjunctional membranes (Davis and Koelle, 1967).

In attempting to refine the (Au–TA) method, it was discovered that the major substrate was actually acetyldisulfide, (CH$_3$COS)$_2$, a contaminant of the commercial preparation of *practical* thiolacetic acid employed (Koelle and Horn, 1968). The localization of AChE at the MEP was improved further with both a gold–acetyldisulfide method, and by the use of another derivative, bis-(thioacetoxy) aurate (Koelle *et al.*, 1968). However, none of these modifications afforded satisfactory localization of AChE at autonomic ganglia. Reasons for this probably included the lower absolute concentration of AChE, and the relatively higher concentrations of other hydrolytic enzymes at the ganglia in comparison with the MEP (Giacobini and Holmstedt, 1960; Denz, 1953). More recently, it has been found that the major factor responsible for the difficulty in localizing the ganglionic AChE is probably its solubility at that site. When fresh frozen sections of cat superior cervical ganglion were immersed in saline solution or 0.3 % Triton X-100 for 40 min at 37°C, subsequent staining for AChE showed that the former treatment caused marked diffusion of the enzyme, and the latter its nearly total loss from the ganglion; prior fixation in buffered (pH 7.3) 4 % formaldehyde solution for 8 h or longer prevented most of these effects, although there was some diminution in the intensity of staining (Koelle *et al.*, 1970). No detectable diffusion or loss of AChE from MEP's occurred following similar treatment of sections of intercostal muscle. Without speculating on the molecular or physical basis for the difference, it seems clear that most of the AChE of the ganglion is in a soluble, or 'lyo' form, whereas that at the MEP is largely in a fixed, or 'desmo' form (Eränkö *et al.*, 1964). Hence, the matter of optimal fixation assumes much greater importance for the former tissue to insure the prevention of diffusion of the enzyme while retaining demonstrable activity at all sites.

By employing various modifications of the acetyl disulfide and bis-(thioacetoxy) aurate methods with tissues fixed in 4 % formaldehyde for 8 h or longer, it has recently been possible to obtain marked improvement in the electron microscopic localization of AChE in the cat superior cervical and ciliary ganglia. Its distribution is now being studied in detail and will be reported subsequently. However, one pattern has been observed consistently: at synaptic sites in both ganglia, most of which are axo-dendritic, the AChE appears to be concentrated predominantly at the postsynaptic membranes, while at the corresponding presynaptic membranes the intensity of staining for AChE is generally lower or even absent. Thus, these observations indicate the reverse of the conclusions reached from the indirect studies described in the preceding section.

### CURRENT CONCLUSIONS

How can the discrepancy between the recent electron-microscopic and the earlier findings regarding the localization of AChE at autonomic ganglionic synapses be reconciled? Of the various possibilities, two seem most likely. First, in spite of the relatively prolonged fixation period now used, this may still be insufficient to render the AChE of the presynaptic membranes insoluble under the conditions of staining employed; in contrast, the postsynaptic AChE may exist originally at a lower concentration but in a less soluble form, like that of the MEP's. For several reasons an alternative explanation appears more plausible. The loss of nearly all the AChE of the superior cervical ganglion following preganglionic denervation was assumed earlier to indicate that under normal conditions the enzyme is associated almost exclusively with the preganglionic nerve fibres and their terminals (Koelle, 1951; Koelle and Koelle, 1959; Sawyer and Hollinshead, 1945). This assumption now seems unwarranted. From studies of the AChE at the MEP of skeletal muscle, it appears that the motor nerve fibre exerts an important 'trophic' influence in maintaining at least a substantial fraction of the AChE at the postjunctional membrane (reviewed in Guth, 1968). Whether the AChE-inducing factor is ACh itself or some other substance or substances released by the nerve terminal has not been established. Nevertheless, it now seems likely that the loss of ganglionic AChE following preganglionic denervation can reflect its disappearance from both preganglionic fibers, following their degeneration, and from postsynaptic structures, with the loss of the presynaptic trophic influence. These possibilities and their physiological implication are now under investigation.

## ACKNOWLEDGEMENT

We wish to acknowledge the recent collaborative participation of Dr. Winifred A. Koelle and the valuable technical assistance of Miss Ashley V. Fine, Mrs. Eileen R. Hathaway, and Mr. Stanley Tevis in the studies described.

## REFERENCES

BARRNETT, R. J. (1962) *J. Cell Biol.*, **12**, 247.
BELL, C. (1966) *J. Histochem. Cytochem.*, **14**, 567.
BROWN, D. A. (1969) *J. Physiol.*, **201**, 225.
BRZIN, M., TENNYSON, V. M. AND DUFFY, P. E. (1966) *J. Cell Biol.*, **31**, 215.
BURN, J. H. AND RAND, M. J. (1959) *Nature*, **184**, 163.
COLLIER, B. (1969) *J. Physiol.*, **205**, 341.
COUTEAUX, R. AND TAXI, J. (1952) *Arch. Anat. Microscop. Morphol. Exp.*, **41**, 352.
COUTEAUX, R. (1958) *Exp. Cell Res., Suppl.*, **5**, 294.
CREVIER, M. AND BÉLANGER, L. F. (1955) *Science*, **122** 256.
DAVIS, R. AND KOELLE, G. B. (1967) *J. Cell Biol.*, **34**, 157.
DENZ, F. A. (1953) *Brit. J. Exp. Pathol.*, **34**, 329.
ERÄNKÖ, O., HÄRKÖNEN, M., KOKKO, A. AND RÄISÄNEN, L. (1964) *J. Histochem. Cytochem.*, **12** 570.
FERRY, C. B. (1966) *Physiol. Rev.*, **46**, 420.
GIACOBINI, E. AND HOLMSTEDT, B. (1960) *Acta Pharmacol. Toxicol.*, **17**, 94.
GROMADSKI, C. G. AND KOELLE, G. B. (1965) *Biochem. Pharmacol.*, **14**, 1745.
GUTH, L. (1968) *Physiol. Rev.*, **48**, 645.
HOLMSTEDT, B., LUNDGREN, G. AND SJÖQVIST, F. (1963) *Acta Physiol. Scand.*, **57**, 235.
KARNOVSKY, M. J. AND ROOTS, L. (1964) *J. Histochem. Cytochem.*, **12**, 219.
KOELLE, G. B. (1950) *J. Pharmacol. Exp. Therap.*, **100**, 158.

KOELLE, G. B. (1951) *J. Pharmacol. Exp. Therap.*, **103**, 153.

KOELLE, G. B. (1955) *J. Pharmacol. Exp. Therap.*, **114**, 167.

KOELLE, G. B. AND STEINER, E. C. (1956) *J. Pharmacol. Exp. Therap.*, **118** 420.

KOELLE, G. B. (1957) *J. Pharmacol. Exp. Therap.*, **120**, 488.

KOELLE, G. B. (1962) *J. Pharm. Pharmacol.*, **14**, 65.

KOELLE, G. B. AND FOROGLOU-KERAMEOS, C. (1965) *Life Sci.*, **4**, 417.

KOELLE, G. B. AND GROMADZKI, C. G. (1966) *J. Histochem. Cytochem.*, **14**, 443.

KOELLE, G. B. AND HORN, R. S. (1968) *J. Histochem. Cytochem.*, **16**, 743.

KOELLE, G. B., DAVIS, R. AND DEVLIN, M. (1968) *J. Histochem. Cytochem.*, **16**, 754.

KOELLE, G. B. (1969) *Federation Proc.*, **28**, 95.

KOELLE, G. B. AND FRIEDENWALD, J. S. (1949) *Proc. Soc. Exp. Biol.*, **70**, 617.

KOELLE, W. A., SHARIFI HOSSAINI, K. AKBARZADEH, P. AND KOELLE, G. B. (1970) *J. Histochem. Cytochem.*, **18**, 812.

KOELLE, W. A. AND KOELLE, G. B. (1959) *J. Pharmacol. Exp. Therap.*, **126**, 1.

KOELLE, G. B. (1970) in *International Symposium on Drugs and Cholinergic Mechanisms in the Central Nervous System*, Skokloster, Sweden, Almqvist and Wiksell, Stockholm, p. 431.

LEWIS, P. R. AND SHUTE, C. C. D. (1966) *J. Cell Sci.*, **1**, 381.

McISAAC, R. J. AND KOELLE, G. B. (1959) *J. Pharmacol. Exp. Therap.*, **126**, 9.

PHILLIS, J. W. (1965) *Experientia*, **21**, 266.

SAWYER, C. H. AND HOLLINSHEAD, W. H. (1945) *J. Neurophysiol.*, **8**, 135.

VOLLE, R. L. AND KOELLE, G. B. (1961) *J. Pharmacol. Exp. Therap.*, **133**, 223.

# Spatial Relations between Acetylcholinesterase and the Acetylcholine-Synthesizing System in a Cholinergic Neuron

B. CSILLIK

*Department of Anatomy, University Medical School Szeged (Hungary)*

Acetycholine*, the orthodox transmitter substance in cholinergic synapses (Dale, 1914, 1955) is produced by the enzyme choline acetylase (choline acyltransferase, E.C. 2.3.1.6) from choline and active acetate, transported by coenzyme A. Synaptic transmission is thought to be mediated by a jet-like extrusion of ACh from the presynaptic terminal, ACh being bound to receptor moieties on the postsynaptic membrane (according to the classical theory of neurochemical transmission); or alternatively, ACh may exert two subsequent dual intracellular actions, first in the presynaptic and then in the postsynaptic cell, without ever traversing the synaptic cleft (as suggested by Nachmansohn, 1955). In any case, having been bound to receptor molecules, and having altered the stereochemical conformation of the latter resulting in an increased permeability of the membrane and in consequent depolarization (excitatory postsynaptic potential), ACh is rapidly hydrolysed by AChE (E.C. 2.1.1.7). Inactivation of ACh is a prerequisite for the reorganization of the receptor molecule, *i.e.* for the rearrangement of the membrane barrier thus enabling the cell to reestablish the membrane potential.

AChE has been reliably located first by Koelle and Friedenwald (1949) at the light-microscopic level and later (Davis and Koelle, 1967; Koelle *et al.*, 1967; Fukuda and Koelle, 1969) also electron microscopically. In the meantime, a number of practical modifications and adaptations of the Koelle principle have been developed at the ultrastructural level, *e.g.* those of Couteaux (1963), Lewis and Shute (1964), Csillik *et al.* (1966), Kása and Csillik (1966), Eränkö *et al.*, (1967) and Csillik and Knyihár (1968a, b). These techniques (substrate: acetylthiocholine) can be used more or less successfully in various parts of the nervous system. Other substrates (thiolacetic acid, naphthyl acetate, indoxyl acetate, etc.) were employed by various workers in attempts to locate AChE together with various less specific esterases (aliesterases, arylesterases, etc.) both at the light and electron microscope levels; the pertinent literature has been summarized (Csillik and Knyihár, 1968b). The specificity of these methods is inferior to that of the thiocholine procedure which can locate AChE so precisely in a close-to-molecular range that it has not yet been surpassed.

More difficult is the question of localizing the ACh-synthesizing system. From the theoretical point of view, the optimal technique would be an immunocytochemical

---

* Abbreviations used: ACh, acetylcholine; AChE, acetylcholinesterase; ChA, choline acetylase; HC-3, hemicholinium.

*References p. 385*

approach using fluorescein-labelled antibodies for light microscopy and ferritin (or horse-radish) marking of the antibody at the electron-microscopic level. Until now, unfortunately, such attempts have failed because of the difficulties inherent in the isolation of a chemically and immunologically pure enzyme preparation. Another possibility is locating the free –SH groups of Coenzyme A liberated after the donation of active acetate to ChA as proposed by Burt (1969) and adapted to electron micros-copy by Kása et al. (1970). Finally, enzymes can be located by autoradiographically demonstrating their specific isotope-labelled inhibitors injected in advance into the animals in vivo. In the present report, studies performed by means of this technique will be described.

Hemicholinium is known to inhibit acetylcholine synthesis by interfering with transport, activation or binding of choline in the synthesizing machinery. Thus, HC-3 is not a 'real' enzyme inhibitor (such as DFP for ChE: Ostrowski and Bernard, 1961, 1969); rather, it is a competitive antagonist. Therefore, in order to eliminate any negative artifacts (washing out by the fixative, dislocation during embedding, etc.) we used non-fixed cryostat sections that were applied to precoated microscope slides (Kodak AR-10 stripping film, emulsion side up). Localization of reduced silver grains was surprisingly good and could be seen under high power (Csillik and Knyihár, 1970).

In order to be concise, in this paper only the transmitter metabolism of the spinal motoneuron representing a clear-cut cholinergic neuron will be discussed. It was our aim to locate both synthesizing and inactivating systems of ACh within various parts of this particular neuron.

### MATERIAL AND METHODS

Studies were performed on albino rats, 150–220 g body weight. For electron-cyto-chemical purposes (AChE) the animals were perfused with a 4°C, pH 7.2 formaldehy-de–glutaraldehyde mixture through the left ventricle; samples of the spinal cord, dia-phragm and m.flexor digitorum brevis of the hind limb were used. (Muscles fixed by means of immersion yielded similar results.) Frozen sections (50–60 $\mu$) prepared from the aldehyde-fixed samples were incubated at pH 6.2 (muscles) or pH 6.3 (spinal cord) at room temperature (20°) for 10–60 minutes in the following solution (Csillik and Knyihár, 1968a):

| | |
|---|---|
| Acetylthiocholine, | 7 mg |
| Sodium acetate, 0.1 M, | 2.2 ml |
| Acetic acid, 0.1 M, | 0.3 ml |
| Glycine, 3.75 %, | 0.1 ml |
| $CuSO_4$, 0.1 M, | 0.1 ml |
| $PbNO_3$, 0.1 M, | 0.1 ml |
| Uranyl acetate, 0.1 M, | 0.1 ml |

After incubation, the sections were briefly rinsed in distilled water, and subsequently treated with an isohydric $(NH_4)_2S_2$ solution (1 %) obtained from commercial $(NH_4)_2S_2$, titrated with 1 $N$ acetic acid to obtain a neutral pH, and centrifuged. The supernatant was diluted to a final concentration of 1 %. After repeated rinsing in distilled water, the sections were trimmed under microscopic control and post-fixed in collidine–osmium (Luft, 1958) for 20 min. Dehydration was carried out in a graded series of alcohols and propylene oxide; samples were embedded in Durcupan (Fluka). Sections (silver or gray interference colours) were obtained on a Reichert ultratome, using glass knives. Inspection and photography of the sections was performed on a Tesla 513B electron microscope.

Autoradiographic localization of HC-3 was performed as follows:

[14C]HC-3 was injected intraperitoneally (0.3 mg/kg); 30–45 min later, *i.e.* after manifestation of the pharmacological symptoms of HC-3 poisoning, the rats were killed by decapitation; the spinal cord and various skeletal muscles were then frozen with dry ice to cryostat chucks. Sectioning was performed in a dark room, and the sections were immediately (*i.e.*, in the cold chamber of the cryostat) applied to the autoradiographic emulsion Kodak AR-10. Slides were precoated in advance (24 h earlier), emulsion side up and dried appropriately in a black box. These mounts were kept in the cryostat for 5–10 min in order to achieve attachment of the sections without any significant melting. Exposure was for 21–90 days; the slides were then developed in Kodak autoradiographic developer and studied without counterstaining under a conventional or a phase contrast microscope.

## RESULTS AND DISCUSSION

(i) In the spinal cord, AChE is concentrated in the cytoplasm of motoneurons (layer IX of Rexed), around large and medium nerve cells of layer VIII (ventromedial nucleus, most clearly visible in the lumbar segments) and in the nerve cells of the lateral column (preganglionic autonomic neurons, most distinctly apparent in the thoracic segments). In the posterior column, AChE activity is diffusely distributed in the neuropil, with the exception of the substantia gelatinosa Rolandi*.

Under the electron microscope, AChE reaction in the motoneurons is located within the lumina of the granular endoplasmic reticulum, concentrated in parallel arrays making up Nissl bodies. Mitochondria within Nissl granules or the lamellae of the Golgi system located as a rule in between Nissl granules, are devoid of any enzyme reaction.

This kind of localization of AChE in the endoplasmic reticulum was first hypothesized by Fukuda and Koelle (1959) based on the light-microscopic observation of AChE activity in the Nissl granules. All subsequent investigators employing various modifications of the Koelle technique (Lewis and Shute, 1965; Eränkö *et al.*, 1967; Kása and Csernovszki, 1967; Kása and Csillik, 1968) were able to confirm directly this early prediction. In addition, we found that the end-product of the enzyme reaction does not uniformly fill out the lumina of endoplasmic cisterns but outlines 320 Å 'endoplasmic units' located in the lumen (Csillik and Knyihár, 1968b). Endoplasmic units are thought to be concerned with the 'final step' in protein synthesis,

---

* This layer exerts a unique acid phosphatase activity (Gerebtzoff *et al.*, 1970).

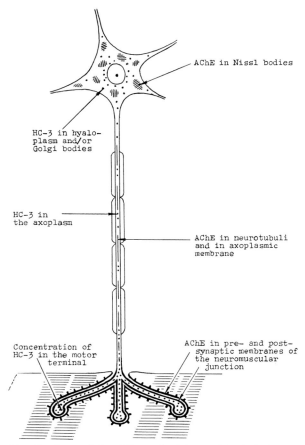

Fig. 1. Summary of localizations of the ACh-synthesizing and hydrolysing systems in the spinal motoneuronal unit. Sites of ACh synthesis as found by the autoradiographic localization of [$^{14}$C]-HC-3 are illustrated by dots; those of ACh hydrolysis, as seen in light- and electron-microscopic cytochemical sections, are shown by hatched areas and by heavy lines.

possibly with the elaboration of the tertiary structure responsible for enzyme activity.

The pattern obtained by the autoradiographic localization of [$^{14}$C]HC-3 is slightly different. Motoneurons show up clearly, containing numerous grains in their cytoplasm; under high power, the fine structural localization of the grains appears to leave out Nissl bodies, *i.e.* the grains are concentrated in the ground cytoplasm not occupied by clusters of endoplasmic reticulum. Electron-microscopic autoradiographic studies to prove this are being carried out in this laboratory.

Since HC-3 is not a 'real' enzyme inhibitor, but rather a competitive antagonist of the choline metabolism, it would be incorrect to equate the localization of reduced silver grains with the sites of choline acetylase. The exact localization of this enzyme remains unknown for the time being; the only fact that can be stated with certainty is that the intracellular transport and/or activation of choline takes place in between the Nissl bodies. By extrapolating these results it may be assumed that the site of the

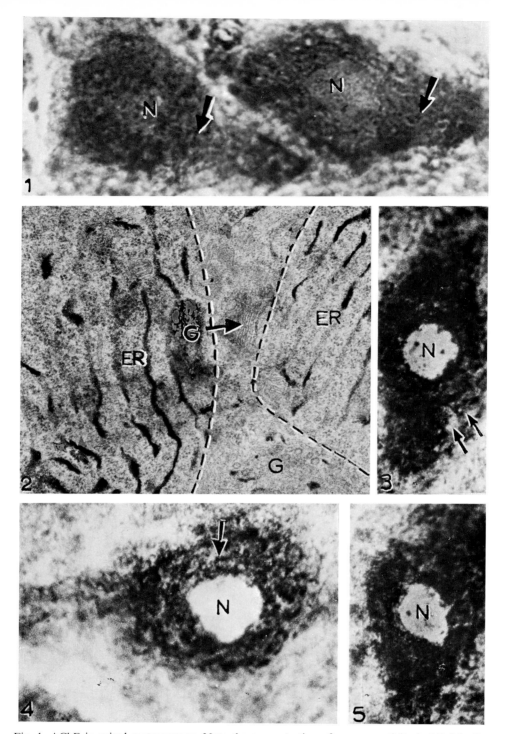

Fig. 1. AChE in spinal motoneurons. Note the concentration of enzyme activity in Nissl bodies (arrows) within the cytoplasm. N: nucleus. × 500.

Fig. 2. Electron-cytochemical localization of AChE in a nerve cell. Note the electron-dense deposit within the cisternae of the endoplasmic reticulum (ER) and the non-reacting area of hyaloplasm and Golgi system (G). Outlines of Nissl bodies are marked by dashed lines. × 40 000.

Figs. 3, 4 and 5. Autoradiographic localization of [$^{14}$C]HC-3 in spinal motoneurons. Note the concentration of silver grains in the hyaloplasmic area of the nerve cells, sparing out nuclei (N) and Nissl bodies (arrows). × 500.

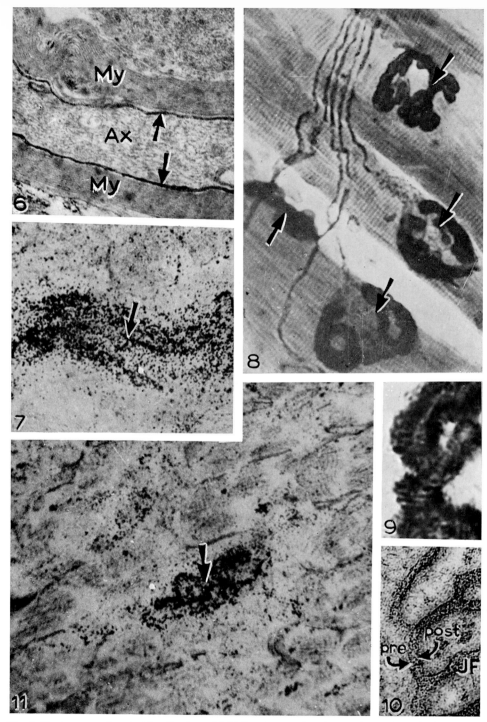

Fig. 6. Electron-cytochemical localization of AChE in the axoplasmic membrane (arrow) of a myelin-ated nerve fibre. Both axoplasm (Ax) and the myelin (My) are devoid of any enzyme reaction. × 25 000.

Fig. 7. Autoradiographic localization of [¹⁴C]HC-3 within an intramuscular nerve branch. × 500.

Fig. 8. Light-microscopic localization of AChE in motor end-plates (arrows). Nerve fibres proceeding to the subneural apparatuses are stained by silver proteinate. × 350.

Fig. 9. Light microscopic localization of AChE in the subneural apparatus of the motor end-plate. Note the enzyme activity of the 'organites', consisting of rows of submicroscopic junctional folds. × 1800.

Fig. 10. Electron-cytochemical localization of AChE in the motor end-plate. Enzyme activity is confined to pre- and postsynaptic membranes and to the walls of the junctional folds (JF). × 45 000.

Fig. 11. Autoradiographic localization of [¹⁴C]HC-3 in the flexor digitorum brevis muscle of the rat. Note the concentration of reduced silver grains in the motor end-plate (arrow) and the slight activity at the surfaces of muscle fibres. × 500.

ACh-synthesizing machinery of the nerve cell does not coincide with that of the AChE-synthesizing system.

(ii) In the axons of spinal motoneurons (*i.e.* in motor nerve fibres) AChE activity is weak; in formalin-fixed sections, this activity does not show up under the light microscope at all. In non-fixed cryostat sections, the activity can be readily visualized*. Under the electron microscope, activity appears to be concentrated in the axoplasmic membrane (Schlaepfer and Torack, 1966; Csillik *et al.*, 1968). In the proximal stump of transected axons a heavy AChE activity seen in axonal neurotubuli (Kása, 1968) has been interpreted as a sign that AChE is being transported through these organelles from the site of production (perikaryon: Nissl bodies) to the site of final destination (presynaptic membrane of the terminal).

[¹⁴C]HC-3 was found autoradiographically throughout the entire length of the motor axons; there is a higher concentration of silver grains in the non-myelinated preterminal part of the axon than in myelinated fibres of the nerve trunk.

Accordingly it appears that both AChE and ChA are transported from the peri-karyon *via* the axon to the terminal, supposing again that sites of choline transport (actually shown by the autoradiographic localization of [¹⁴C]HC-3) are closely related to those of ACh synthesis.

(iii) In the motor end-plate, AChE is evenly distributed on pre- and postsynaptic membranes. However, the postsynaptic membrane is thrown into multiple folds resulting in an at least 10-times larger surface area than that of the postsynaptic membrane. Accordingly, the postsynaptic AChE ('subneural apparatus') is predominant and, at least in light-microscopic histochemical sections, the pattern of axonal arborization is not apparent.

It should be kept in mind, however, that this 1:10 ratio between pre- and postsynaptic membranes holds good only for α-junctions ('terminaison en placque'), whereas in γ-junctions ('terminaison en grappe'), where the postsynaptic membrane is either entirely smooth or equipped with only a limited number of small folds, the presynaptic AChE is nearly equal to the postsynaptic one. Accordingly, in γ-junctions (*e.g.* in intrafusal motor endings of mammalian muscle spindles) light microscopy reveals a substantially weaker AChE activity than in extrafusal (α) motor endings.

[¹⁴C]HC-3 is concentrated in motor end-plates. The distribution of silver grains corresponds to the axonal arborization; no similarity to the subneural apparatus can be detected. Denervation (transection of the sciatic nerve or intramuscular transection of the phrenic nerve) results after 10 days in the complete disappearance of reduced silver grains from motor end-plates of the m.flexor digitorum brevis or in the hemidiaphragm subjected to surgery.

Accordingly, in the cholinergic terminal the sites of ACh synthesis and those of breakdown are again spatially divided; the former is located within the terminal axoplasm whereas the latter is confined to the pre- and postsynaptic membranes. These cytochemical observations agree with biochemical studies. The membrane-bound

---

* For reasons unknown at present, activity is markedly increased a few weeks after degeneration (Sávay and Csillik, 1956).

*References p. 385*

character of AChE is well-known (Lapetina *et al.*, 1967) whereas the localization of ChAc in axoplasmatic compartments has also been demonstrated unequivocally, in spite of the divergent views of De Robertis (1963) and Whittaker (1965).

Thus it appears that all the main parts of the cholinergic neuron (perikaryon, axon, terminal) contain the enzyme systems for both production and breakdown of ACh. These enzymes like other neuroproteins appear to be synthesized in the perikaryon and transported *via* axonal flow into the terminal. The different locations of AChE and [$^{14}$C]HC-3 within the perikaryon might reflect the fact that AChE activity shows up at the sites where the enzyme protein is ready to hydrolyse its specific substrate, whereas the location of [$^{14}$C]HC-3 may point to the site of the physiological action of the ACh-synthesizing system even though the enzyme protein (ChAc) is, in all probability, synthesized, as is any other protein, in the endoplasmic reticulum. At present, the spatial relation of AChE to ChAc in the axon is unknown; here, however, a difference may persist since AChE is confined to axolemmal membranes, whereas ChAc appears to be located within the axoplasm. In the axon, both activities are low due to their being *en voyage* to the terminal. Finally, both synthesizing and hydrolysing activities are most active in the terminal. AChE is distributed on the synaptolemmal surface; one is inclined to suppose that the presynaptic AChE activity somehow induces the production of the postsynaptic AChE contingent. The ACh-synthesizing machinery is definitely located within axoplasmatic structures of the terminal; it may be in the hyaloplasm as suggested by Whittaker (1965) or in the particulate (vesicular) fraction as proposed by De Robertis (1963).

What is the fate of the transmitter?

Since ACh is synthesized within the terminal axoplasm, it has to arrive at the presynaptic (axolemmal) membrane by means of a conveyor mechanism. Synaptic vesicles might be, as suggested by various investigators since De Robertis' first hypothesis, transporters of the newly synthesized transmitter. The fact that synaptic vesicles are *de facto* concentrated at the presynaptic membrane of the excited neuromuscular junction has been suggested by Hubbard and Kwanbunbumpen (1968) and by Jones and Kwanbunbumpen (1970) and shown by us by means of an objective geometric mathematical analysis (Csillik and Bense, 1970).

However, as soon as the ACh packets arrive at the presynaptic membrane, they are exposed to the hydrolysing capacity of AChE. Thus, there is very little chance that any ACh molecule could pass the synaptic cleft and become attached to the postsynaptic membrane. Accordingly, one is inclined to accept Nachmansohn's idea (1955) that both release *and* breakdown of ACh are intracellular events; in other words: ACh does *not* pass the synaptic cleft. We believe the arylesterase sandwiched in between pre- and postsynaptic membranes (Csillik and Knyihár, 1968a) is the factor responsible for an intermediary process, the details of which are unknown at present that links presynaptic events with postsynaptic ones.

Presently, we do not know the details of the postsynaptic process. At least in the motor end-plate, it might be assumed that both at the pre- and the postsynaptic membranes, ACh is bound by receptor molecules, the stereochemical conformation of which is altered by this binding in such a way as to promote the movement of various ions through reopened membrane channels. However, we do not know from where the postsynaptic acetylcholine is derived; neither do we know where postsynaptic AChE is synthesized. Observations on embryonic and early neonatal muscles suggest that the sarcoplasmic reticulum might be involved in the production of the appropriate enzymes. The fact that in the muscle fibres we found a 'background' [$^{14}$C]HC-3 reaction favours such an assumption.

## REFERENCES

BURT, A. M. (1969) cit. in P. KÁSA, S. P. MANN AND C. O. HEBB (1970).

COUTEAUX, R. (1963) *Proc. Roy. Soc. B*, **158**, 457–480.

CSILLIK, B. AND BENSE, S. (1970) *Acta Biol. Acad. Sci. Hung.*, (in the press).

CSILLIK, B., JOÓ, F., KÁSA, P. AND SÁVAY, G. (1966) *Acta Histochem.*, **25**, 58–70.

CSILLIK, B. AND KNYIHÁR, E. (1968a) *J. Cell. Sci.*, **3**, 529–538.

CSILLIK, B. AND KNYIHÁR, E. (1968b) *Acta Biochim. Biophys. Acad. Sci. Hung.*, **3**, 165–170.

CSILLIK, B. AND KNYIHÁR, E. (1970) *J. Histochem. Cytochem.*, **18**, 58.

CSILLIK, B., KNYIHÁR, E. AND HALÁSZ, N. (1968) *J. Neuro-Visceral Rel.*, **31**, 3–10.

DALE, H. H. (1914) *J. Pharmacol. Exp. Therap.*, **5**, 147–190.

DALE, H. H. (1955) *Proc. Mayo Clin.*, **30**, 5–20.

DAVIS, R. AND KOELLE, G. B. (1967) *J. Cell. Biol.*, **34**, 157–171.

DE ROBERTIS, E., ARNAIZ, G. R. DE L., SALGANICOFF, L., DE IRALDI, A. P. AND ZIEHER, L. M. (1963) *J. Neurochem.*, **10**, 225–235.

ERÄNKÖ, O., RECHARDT, L. AND HÄNNINEN, L. (1967) *Histochemie*, **8**, 369–376.

FUKUDA, T. AND KOELLE, G. B. (1959) *J. Biophys. Biochem. Cytol.*, **5**, 433–440.

GEREBTZOFF, M.-A., BUDO, C., PONCELET, G. AND SCHOENEN, J. (1970) *Bull. Assoc. Anat. 54e Congr., Sofia, 1969)*, No. 145.

HUBBARD, J. I., AND KWANBUNBUMPEN, S. (1968) *J. Physiol.*, **194**, 407–420.

JONES, S. F. AND KWANBUNBUMPEN, S. (1970) *J. Physiol.*, **207**, 31–50.

KÁSA, P. (1968) *Nature*, **218**, 1265–1267.

KÁSA, P. AND CSERNOVSZKY, E. (1967) *Acta Histochem.*, **28**, 274–285.

KÁSA, P., AND CSILLIK, B. (1966) *J. Neurochem.*, **13**, 1345–1349.

KÁSA, P. AND CSILLIK, B. (1968) *Histochemie*, **12**, 175–183.

KÁSA, P., MANN, S. P. AND HEBB, C. O. (1970) *Nature*, **226**, 814–816.

KOELLE, G. B., DAVIS, R. AND GROMADZKI, C. G. (1967) *Ann. N.Y. Acad. Sci.*, **144**, 613–622.

KOELLE, G. B. AND FRIEDENWALD, J. S. (1949) *Proc. Soc. Exp. Biol. Med.*, **70**, 617–622.

LAPETINA, E. G., SOTO, E. F. AND DE ROBERTIS, E. (1967) *Biochim. Biophys. Acta*, **135**, 33–43.

LEWIS, P. R. AND SHUTE, C. C. D. (1964) *J. Physiol.*, **175**, 5–7.

LEWIS, P. R. AND SHUTE, C. C. D. (1965) *J. Anat.*, **99**, 941.

LEWIS, P. R. AND SHUTE, C. C. D. (1966) *J. Cell Sci.*, **1**, 381–390.

MCCAMAN, R. E., DE LORES ARNAIZ, G. R. AND DE ROBERTIS, A. (1965) *J. Neurochem.*, **12**, 927–935.

NACHMANSOHN, D. (1955) *Ergeb. Physiol.*, **48**, 575–683.

OSTROWSKI, K. AND BERNARD, E. A. (1961) *Exp. Cell. Res.*, **25**, 465–468.

SÁVAY, GY. AND CSILLIK, B. (1956) *Acta Morph. Hung.*, **6**, 289–297.

SCHLAEPFER, W. W. AND TORACK, R. M. (1966) *J. Histochem. Cytochem.*, **14**, 369–378.

WHITTAKER, V. P. (1965) *Progr. Biophys. Mol. Biol.*, **15**, 41–96.

# VI. AUTONOMIC INNERVATION PATTERNS

# Fine-structural Identification of Autonomic Nerves and their Relation to Smooth Muscle

GEOFFREY BURNSTOCK AND TAKASHI IWAYAMA

*Department of Zoology, University of Melbourne, Parkville, Victoria (Australia)*

## GENERAL MODEL OF THE AUTONOMIC NEUROMUSCULAR JUNCTION

The application of modern cellular techniques has given a clearer picture of the nature of the autonomic neuro-effector junction. In particular, electron microscope and fluorescent histochemical studies of the precise relationship of individual nerves to single smooth muscle cells (see Burnstock, 1970) have supported and extended the earlier concept of the 'autonomic ground plexus' put forward by Hillarp (1946); these morphological results, together with studies of the electrophysiology of transmission (see Bennett and Burnstock, 1968) allow a model of the autonomic neuromuscular junction to be proposed, which is illustrated in Fig. 1. The essential features are: (1) smooth muscle cells, connected by low resistance pathways represented by specialised areas of close apposition or 'nexus' (Dewey and Barr, 1962) are arranged in *effector bundles*. (2) Transmitter is released 'en passage' from large numbers of

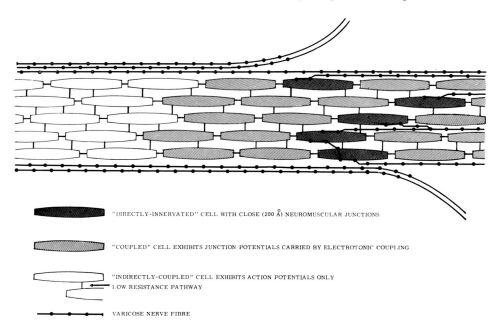

"DIRECTLY-INNERVATED" CELL WITH CLOSE (200 Å) NEUROMUSCULAR JUNCTIONS

"COUPLED" CELL EXHIBITS JUNCTION POTENTIALS CARRIED BY ELECTROTONIC COUPLING

"INDIRECTLY-COUPLED" CELL EXHIBITS ACTION POTENTIALS ONLY
LOW RESISTANCE PATHWAY

VARICOSE NERVE FIBRE

Fig. 1. Schematic representation of autonomic innervation of smooth muscle. For explanation see text.

preterminal varicosities as well as from the terminal varicosity. (3) In most organs, some, but not all, the smooth muscle cells are directly innervated, *i.e.* have close (less than 500 Å) apposition with axon varicosities naked of Schwann cell investment (Fig. 2); these have been termed '*directly-innervated cells*'. (4) The cells adjoining 'directly innervated cells' are coupled electrotonically to them by low resistance pathways, so that passive potential changes, in particular excitatory junction potentials, are observed in these cells, which have been termed '*coupled cells*'. (5) When the muscle cells in an area of the effector bundle become depolarised simultaneously, an all-or-none action potential is initiated which propagates through the tissue. Thus, in some tissues, many cells, called here '*indirectly-coupled*' cells, are neither directly innervated nor directly coupled to innervated cells, yet contract on stimulation of the nerves which supply the organ. It should be pointed out that it is unlikely that the three cell types described in this model are different in structure and properties; on the contrary it is probable that many cells might play the role of a 'directly-innervated', 'coupled' or 'indirectly-coupled' cell at different times during the normal physiological pattern of nervous control of the organ in the intact animal.

This model appears to be applicable to all systems, although there is considerable variation in the density of innervation of smooth muscle in different organs. For example, all the muscle cells of the mouse and rat vas deferens and probably some other organs, appear to be directly-innervated with at least one and probably up to six close (200 Å) neuromuscular junctions (Richardson, 1962; Taxi, 1965; Yamauchi and Burnstock, 1969b). In other organs, such as the guinea-pig vas deferens, urinary bladder, nictitating membrane and dog retractor penis, between one quarter and three-quarters of the muscle cell population appear to be directly-innervated (see Merrillees, 1968; Burnstock, 1970), so that only a small proportion of 'indirectly-coupled' cells are likely to be present. Finally, in systems such as the ureter, uterus, arteries and longitudinal muscle coat of the gut, only a small proportion of muscle cells are directly-innervated, so that a large number of cells are 'indirectly coupled' and are activated via a well developed nexus system for intermuscle fibre spread of activity.

SMOOTH MUSCLE AND SYMPATHETIC NERVES GROWN IN TISSUE CULTURE

*Nexus between smooth muscle cells*

Nexus are likely to form the morphological basis of the low resistance pathways which allow electrotonic coupling of activity in muscle effector bundles. They are a prominent feature in sparsely innervated organs, such as ureter and gut, where spread of activity between muscle cells is of considerable importance (see Burnstock, Holman and Prosser, 1963a). It was surprising that nexus were also found in the mouse and rat vas deferens, where every cell appears to be directly-innervated (Richardson, 1962; Lane and Rhodin, 1964; Yamauchi and Burnstock, 1969b), so that activation of cells by interfibre spread of current would not appear to be necessary. However, evidence for interfibre spread of activity has been demonstrated in the mouse vas deferens (Furness and Burnstock, 1969).

ment of synapses in the human gut (Read and Burnstock, 1970), and of autonomic neuromuscular junctions in anterior eye chamber transplants of vas deferens and taenia coli (Burnstock *et al.*, 1970b).

## SYNAPTIC CLEFT

There is considerable variation in the precise relationship of nerve varicosities and muscle cells in different organs, and the whole question of what constitutes the autonomic neuromuscular cleft needs resolution, particularly in view of the physiological and pharmacological evidence of 'en passage' release of transmitter from varicosities in extensive preterminal axons (Malmfors, 1965; Bennett and Burnstock, 1968; Furness, 1970).

Nerve–muscle separation in the regions of closest apposition in the vas deferens is about 200 Å (Richardson, 1962; Merrillees *et al.*, 1963; Lane and Rhodin, 1964; Yamauchi and Burnstock, 1969b; and Fig. 2a, c). From an analysis of a serial electron microscope study of the nervous environment of single smooth muscle cells in the guinea pig vas deferens (Merrillees, 1968), it was concluded that it was unlikely that transmitter released from varicosities further than 1000 Å away would have a significant effect on muscle cells (Bennett and Merrillees, 1966). This conclusion was supported by the results of an entirely different approach, namely, acetylcholinesterase (AChE) staining (Robinson, 1969). In this study it was shown that about 15–20 % of the axon profiles in the guinea pig vas deferens showed heavy positive staining for AChE, but that only muscle membranes within 1200 Å of these profiles showed matching AChE staining. Furthermore, Schwann cell processes intervened between muscle and nerve membranes in 80 % of all the cases where nerves were separated from muscle by greater than 1100 Å.

The closest apposition between nerves and smooth muscle in most blood vessels studied is consistently greater (500–800 Å) than in the vas deferens (see Burnstock, 1970). A study of AChE staining in the guinea pig uterine artery, comparable to that described above for the vas deferens, showed that in this case there was matching muscle staining for AChE within 10000 Å of stained nerve profiles (Bell, 1969). This could be taken as an indication that in blood vessels the effective neuromuscular cleft is about 10 000 Å (*i.e.* about 10 times wider than the neuromuscular cleft in the vas deferens).

In the longitudinal muscle coat of the alimentary tract most varicose nerves are confined in bundles and only occasionally run singly, free of Schwann cell investment (Taxi, 1965; Lane and Rhodin, 1964; Rogers and Burnstock, 1966b). The closest approach of intramural nerves to muscle cells in the taenia coli of the guinea pig is about 1000 Å and in a combined analysis of electrophysiological and fine structural studies, it was suggested that the effective synaptic cleft in the gut might be at least 3000 Å (Bennett and Rogers, 1967). However, in the circular muscle coat of the gut, there are many examples of closer (200 Å) apposition of nerve and muscle membranes (Rogers and Burnstock, 1966b; Thaemert, 1963, 1966; Nagasawa and Mito, 1967; and Fig. 2b).

*References pp. 402–404*

### POST-SYNAPTIC STRUCTURE

A number of authors have examined the question of post-synaptic specialisation of smooth muscle membranes in the regions of closest apposition with terminal varicosities, but usually no increase in membrane thickening or density has been seen (Richardson, 1962; Merrillees et al., 1963; Lane and Rhodin, 1964; Nagasawa and Mito, 1967; Taxi, 1969).

An elongated sac of endoplasmic reticulum (sub-synaptic cysternae) has been noted in the vas deferens (Fig. 2a and Richardson, 1962; Merrillees, et al., 1963; Lane and Rhodin, 1964), but since this is not a consistent feature of all areas of close apposition, it is still not certain that it can be regarded as a feature of autonomic post-synaptic specialisation. Similarly, aggregations of micropinocytotic vesicles are often seen in post-synaptic regions in the gut (Fig. 2b), but again this is not a consistent feature.

### 'INTRACELLULAR' NERVE TERMINALS

In some organs, notably the rat and mouse vas deferens, nerve profiles were occasionally observed within deep grooves in smooth muscle cells (Richardson, 1962; Lane and Rhodin, 1964; Taxi, 1965). More recently, with improved methods of preservation of granular vesicles, including the use of short-term injection of 5- and 6-hydroxydopamine (Tranzer and Thoenen, 1968b; Furness et al., 1970a; Bennett et al., 1970), it has been shown that considerable numbers of both adrenergic and cholinergic axons penetrate and perhaps terminate deep inside smooth muscle cells (Fig. 2c, and Watanabe, 1969; Furness and Iwayama, 1971). Varicosities containing abundant vesicles are often characteristically in close apposition to the nucleus and are enveloped by the perinuclear organelles. The functional significance of this extraordinary finding is not known, but their inaccessibility may partly explain the difficulty in altering neuromuscular responses with various autonomic blocking and potentiating drugs (Holman, 1970).

### MULTIAXONAL JUNCTIONS

Groups of 4 to 7 axons have been shown to be in close apposition (150–200 Å) with single muscle cells in the small intestine of mammals where they were termed 'multiterminal synapses' (Brettschneider, 1962) and of toad where they were called 'multiaxonal junctions' (Rogers and Burnstock, 1966b). This is illustrated in Fig. 2b. It is not known whether each axon profile that comes into contact with a single muscle cell represents a different axon from separate neurones or whether they are branches of one axon. However, junction potentials resulting from stimulation of different nerves have been recorded recently from single cells in the guinea pig and bird gut, although coupling of activity between neighbouring muscle cells complicates the interpretation (Furness, 1969; Bennett, 1970).

The terminal regions of adrenergic and cholinergic nerves are often closely associated within the same Schwann process (Thoenen et al., 1966; Thaemert, 1966; Iwayama, *et al.*, 1970). The concept that there is a cholinergic link in the adrenergic transmission process (Burn and Rand, 1959) has been discussed at some length (Ferry, 1966; Burn and Rand, 1965; Campbell, 1970). The close association of adrenergic and cholinergic terminals has been proposed recently (Burn, 1968) as a morphological basis for this theory.

### INTRA-AXONAL FEATURES OF DIFFERENT AUTONOMIC NERVES

A diagrammatic representation of the essential intra-axonal features of the main nerve types is presented in Fig. 3.

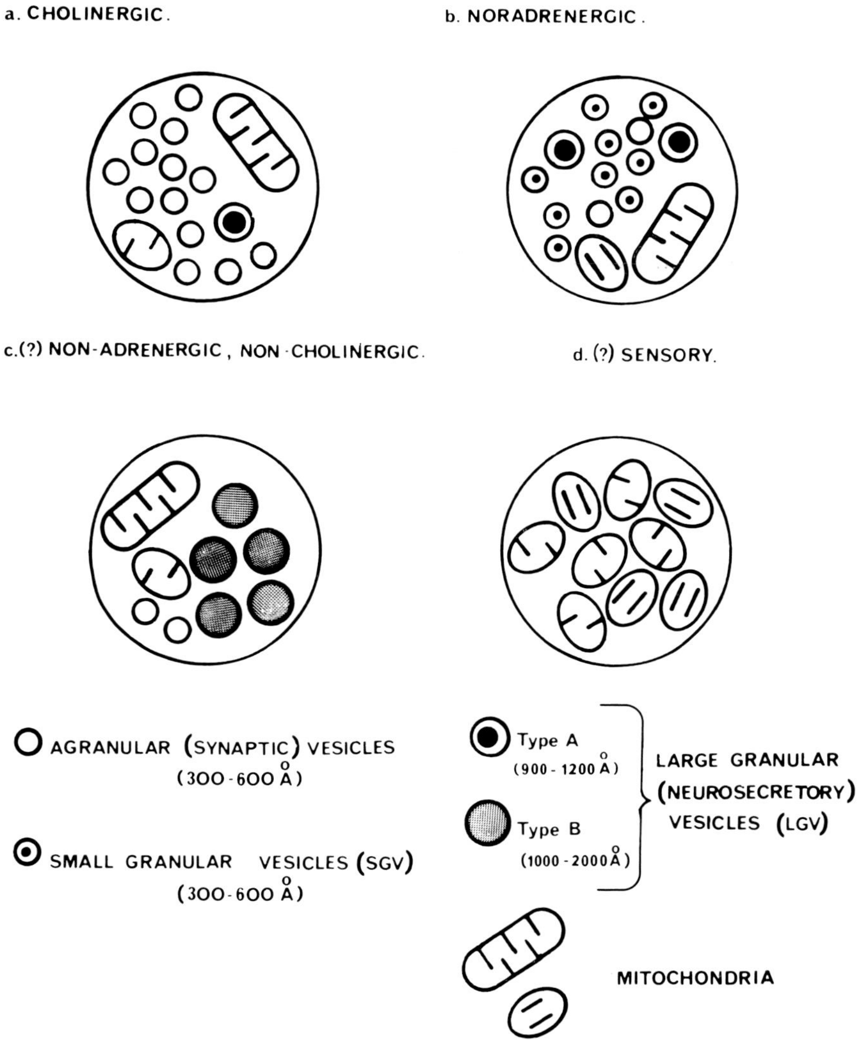

**Fig. 3.** Diagrammatic representation of sections through the terminal varicosities of autonomic nerves. For explanation see text.

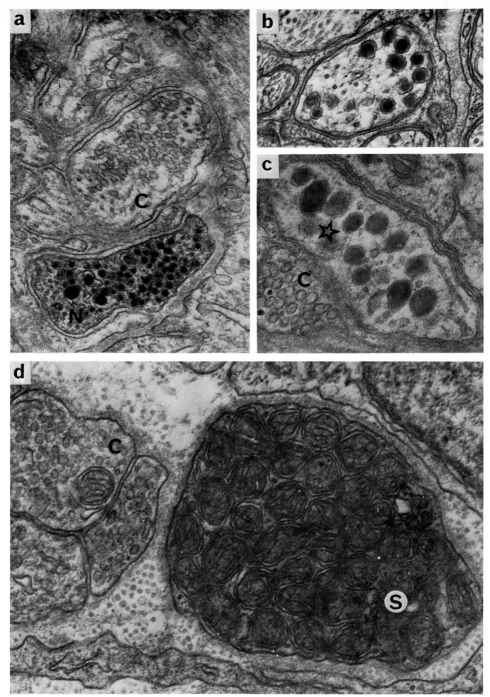

Fig. 4. Intra-axonal structure of different autonomic nerves: (a) Cholinergic (C) and noradrenergic (N) nerve profiles in the circular muscle coat of the vas deferens of a rat treated for 30 min with 5-OHDA (50 mg/kg). Note that *both* small and large-granular vesicles in the adrenergic profile have taken up the drug, but not the agranular or large-granular vesicles in the cholinergic profile. Osmium fixation. × 38000. (b) Adrenergic axon profile in Auerbach's plexus of chicken gizzard. In this case large granular vesicles (which take up 5- and 6-OHDA) are predominant. Note halo between intra-vesicular, granular and limiting vesicle membrane. Osmium fixation. × 42000. (c) Non-adrenergic, non-cholinergic axon profile (asterisk) in large intestine of toad, treated for 45 min with 6-OHDA (100 mg/kg). The large-granular vesicles (characterised by granulation *throughout* the vesicle) contained in these nerves do not take up 6-OHDA. Note also the cholinergic nerve profile (C). Glutaral-dehyde–osmium fixation. × 48000. (d) Nerve profile (S) probably representing the terminal portion of a sensory nerve fibre in the mucosa of the finch ureter. Note the aggregation of small mitochondria, absence of vesicles and Schwann cell investment. The other axons (C) are probably cholinergic. Osmium fixation. × 48000. (d, courtesy of Dr. Yasuo Uehara, Zoology Department, University of Melbourne.)

*Cholinergic nerves*

It is generally accepted that profiles containing predominantly *small agranular vesicles* (300–600 Å) represent cholinergic nerves (De Robertis and Bennett, 1955; Whittaker *et al.*, 1964; Grillo, 1966; Burnstock and Robinson, 1967; and Fig. 4a, d). A few *large-granular vesicles* (900–1200 Å) are usually also present; they do not take up catecholamines, 5- or 6- hydroxydopamine (OHDA) (Tranzer *et al.*, 1969; Bennett *et al.*, 1970) and their function is not known.

*Adrenergic nerves*

Considerable evidence has accumulated that nerves containing noradrenaline are characterised by the predominance of *small-granular vesicles* (300–600 Å) with a dense core (see Grillo, 1966; Burnstock and Robinson, 1967; Farrell, 1968; Hökfelt, 1968; Taxi, 1969; Geffen and Livett, 1971; and Figs. 2a, c; 4a). Some large-granular vesicles (900–1200 Å) are also present. However in this case, there is evidence that they are also capable of taking up and storing catecholamines (Tranzer and Thoenen, 1968a, b; Hökfelt, 1968; Bennett *et al.*, 1970; Furness *et al.*, 1970a), although they are relatively resistant to depletion by reserpine (Bloom and Barrnett, 1966; Bondareff and Gordon, 1966; Clementi *et al.*, 1966; Hökfelt, 1966). It seems more likely that the low percentage of small agranular vesicles present in varicosities of adrenergic nerves represent 'empty' small-granular vesicles rather than providing evidence for the cholinergic link hypothesis (Burn and Rand, 1959) since drug treatment leading to increase in levels of noradrenaline in the nerves is associated with a decrease in the percentage of agranular vesicles (Thoenen *et al.*, 1966; Van Orden *et al.*, 1966; Tranzer *et al.*, 1969).

While fixation of the tissue with potassium permanganate readily preserves the granules within vesicles in adrenergic nerves, other fixatives do not always do so (Richardson, 1966; Hökfelt and Nilsson, 1965; Hökfelt and Jonsson, 1968; Tranzer *et al.*, 1969). An important observation has been made recently in our laboratory (Iwayama and Furness, 1971) that incubation of the tissue in Krebs' solution prior to fixation in osmium or glutaraldehyde gives consistent preservation of granules. This method may be of particular value in studies of the action of drugs on intra-axonal stores of catecholamines (see below).

In birds, some adrenergic profiles contain predominantly large granular vesicles and take up 6-OHDA (Bennett *et al.*, 1971 and Fig. 4 b) and are therefore presumably adrenergic. Similar adrenergic profiles have been found in reptiles (Baumgarten and Braak, 1968).

*Non-adrenergic, non-cholinergic (purinergic) nerves*

The existence of non-adrenergic inhibitory nerves in the gut has been established with both pharmacological (Burnstock *et al.*, 1966; Campbell, 1966; Martinson, 1965; Day and Warren, 1968) and electrophysiological (Burnstock *et al.*, 1963b, 1964; Bennett *et al.*, 1966; Bülbring and Tomita, 1967; Kuriyama *et al.*, 1967) methods, and evidence has been presented that ATP or some related purine nucleotide is the neuro-transmitter substance released from these nerves (Burnstock *et al.*, 1970a), which have been tentatively termed 'purinergic' (Burnstock, 1971). In a recent study of the fine structural features of the non-adrenergic inhibitory nerves which supply the toad lung, it has been shown that axon profiles containing predominantly large-granular vesicles (1000–2000 Å) (characterised by the absence of an electron-opaque halo between the granular core and the boundary membrane) remain in the lung as do non-adrenergic inhibitory responses following degeneration of adrenergic inhibitory nerves with 6-OHDA (Robinson *et al.*, 1971). These profiles are identical with those seen in the toad intestine (Fig. 4c; Rogers and Burnstock, 1966b) which also contains non-adrenergic, non-cholinergic autonomic nerves (see Burnstock, 1969). A study of the fine structure of nerve profiles in the highly localised and concentrated Auerbach's plexus of the avian gizzard has been made (Bennett and Cobb, 1969; Bennett *et al.*, 1971). Cholinergic, adrenergic and non-adrenergic inhibitory nerves have been identified in this plexus by physiological means (Bennett, 1969) and two types of profile containing predominantly large-granular vesicles demonstrated (Bennett *et al.*, 1970b). The large-granular vesicles in one type of profile are characterised by a size range of 900–1200 Å with a dense granular core and a light halo between the granule and the membrane (Fig. 4b); these vesicles are associated with catecholamines and take up 6-OHDA (Bennett *et al.*, 1970). The other type of profile contains granular vesicles which are usually larger (1000–2000 Å), do not have a clear halo between the granule and boundary membrane and are closely comparable to those described for non-adrenergic inhibitory nerves in the toad lung and intestine.

*5-Hydroxytryptamine-containing nerves*

A specific cytochemical method for the localisation of 5-HT at the ultrastructural level has been developed (Tranzer and Thoenen, 1967a; Etcheverry and Zieher, 1968a, b) and, together with the use of *p*-chlorophenylalanine as a depletor of 5-HT, small-granular vesicles (400–600 Å) have been shown to be associated with 5-HT in autono-mic nerve terminals in the pineal gland (Bloom and Giarman, 1967). These results suggest that both 5-HT and catecholamines are normally contained within small-granular vesicles in pineal nerves, but whether the two amines are stored in the same or different vesicles is not known. In either case, the 5-HT contained in the intrapineal portions of the sympathetic nerves cannot be regarded as true autonomic transmitter substance, since it is synthesised *outside* the nerves in the pineal parenchymal cells and merely taken up and stored by the nerves (Zweig and Axelrod, 1969).

*Sensory nerves*

In view of the many sensory nerves which are known to supply most autonomically innervated tissues, it is surprising that these profiles have not previously been recog-nised.

Axon profiles which are quite different from those characteristic of cholinergic and adrenergic nerves, have been observed in a variety of tissues, including vas deferens (Merrillees, 1968), pial artery (Hagen and Wittkowski, 1969), rat anterior cerebral artery (Burnstock *et al.*, 1970c), bird ureter (Uehara and Burnstock, 1971) and cat bladder (Campbell and Uehara, personal communication). They contain few, if any, vesicles and are packed with small, oval mitochondria with characteristically only two cristae seen in transverse sections; such a profile in the ureter of the finch is shown in Fig. 4d. It should be pointed out that mitochondria of this kind are often also seen in adrenergic and cholinergic nerve profiles. In the rat cerebral artery, these profiles have been traced back by serial sampling to myelinated nerve fibres, suggesting that they may represent sensory nerves (Burnstock *et al.*, 1970c), a feature which has also been demonstrated in a longitudinal section by Hagen and Wittkowski, 1969.

*Non-nervous profiles in smooth muscle*

Apart from the nerve types described above, a number of other profiles are sometimes found in close relation to smooth muscle. These include sections through:

*(1) Chromaffin or 'chromaffin-type' cells.* These cells are characterised by many large membrane-bound granules, comparable to those seen in the adrenal medulla (see Elfvin, 1965). The granules in dopamine-containing cells described in many tissues in ruminants (Hebb *et al.*, 1968), often show a substructure made up of 150-Å granules (Burnstock *et al.*, 1970c).

*(2) 'Interstitial' cells.* These are found particularly in the gut and their status was in doubt for many years, until ultrastructural studies showed clearly that they were probably fibroblast-like cells and/or macrophages (Richardson, 1960; Rogers and Burnstock, 1966a). They usually partially envelop bundles of axons, Schwann cell processes and sometimes form close relationships to muscle cells; but their function is still not known.

*(3) Muscle cell intrusions and Schwann cells.* Occasionally sections through Schwann cell processes unaccompanied by nerves are seen in close relation to muscle cells. Intrusions of processes of one smooth muscle into its neighbour are characteristic of many tissues (Merrillees *et al.*, 1963; Thaemert, 1963). These profiles are often relatively free of organelles, incuding myofilaments, and therefore difficult to identify. The use of 5- or 6-OHDA as a marker for sympathetic nerves is often a useful way of distinguishing these nerves from muscle or Schwann cell profiles (see Figs. 2a, c; 4a).

### EFFECT OF DRUGS ON ADRENERGIC NERVES

The acute and chronic actions of a large number of drugs on the fine structure of sympathetic nerves has been reported (see Van Orden *et al.*, 1966; Burnstock and Robinson, 1967; Tranzer *et al.*, 1969; Hökfelt, 1968; Geffen and Livett, 1971). In these studies the main observations were of alterations in the number and proportion of granular vesicles. This approach, because of the problem of obtaining reliable control values with the fixation procedures available, has been largely disappointing and inconclusive. In this report, discussion will be confined to changes in fine structure produced by only two drugs, 6-OHDA and guanacline, which do not involve vesicle counts.

## 6-OHDA

6-OHDA depletes the catecholamines from sympathetically innervated tissues (Porter *et al.*, 1963; Laverty *et al.*, 1965; Porter *et al.*, 1965). More recently, it has been shown that, within one hour of injection of the drug, there is a marked increase in the density of cores of both large and small intra-axonal vesicles in sympathetic nerves (Bennett *et al.*, 1970a; Furness *et al.*, 1970a); by 24 hours, if the concentration of injected drug is sufficient, there is specific degeneration of adrenergic nerve terminals (Tranzer and Thoenen, 1967b, 1968a; Thoenen and Tranzer, 1968; Malmfors and Sachs, 1968).

There has been a recent analysis of the mechanism of action of 6-OHDA in producing these changes (Bennett *et al.*, 1970a; Furness *et al.*, 1970a). The first sign of nerve damage is seen at 1–2 hours, consisting of electron transparency of the axoplasm and a decrease in number of organelles. From 2–10 h, the axoplasm becomes generally electron dense, reminiscent of the appearance of nerves following surgical denervation (Birks *et al.*, 1960; Taxi, 1965; Pluchino *et al.*, 1970; Roth and Richardson, 1969; Iwayama, 1970) and is accompanied by failure of neuromuscular transmission (Furness *et al.*, 1970a). While entry of 6-OHDA into vesicles occurs, the important factor in degeneration appears to be the extragranular (axoplasmic) concentration of the drug in the nerve. Damage to the membrane could account for the potentiation of packaged release of noradrenaline (measured as spontaneous junction potentials) which is known to occur under these conditions (Furness *et al.*, 1970a), and lead to degeneration of the nerve.

## Guanacline

Guanacline (*N*-2-guanedinoethyl-4-methyl-1,2,3,6-tetrahydropyridine sulphate) has catecholamine-depleting and adrenergic-blocking actions similar to guanethidine (Kroneberg *et al.*, 1967; Schümann and Philippu, 1968). It has been used in the treatment of hypertension (Gross *et al.*, 1965), but it was reported that postural hypotension persists in humans even several months after withdrawal of therapy (Dawborn *et al.*, 1969). In a recent ultrastructural and histochemical study of sympathetic neurones both during and after cessation of chronic treatment of rats with guanacline (5 mg/kg/day), it has been shown that a massive deposition of lipoprotein granules (comparable to 'ageing pigment') is produced (Burnstock *et al.*, 1971). This persists for up to at least 12 weeks following cessation of treatment. No comparable changes were observed in animals treated with the same dose of guanethidine.

### SUMMARY

(1)  A general model of the autonomic neuromuscular junction has been proposed,

based on both structural and physiological data. It takes into account the spread of activity between neighbouring smooth muscle cells via nexus and 'en passage' release of transmitter from varicosities in extensive terminal regions of the nerves.

(2)   Nexus between smooth muscle cells grown in tissue cultures suggest that they are an inherent feature of smooth muscle and do not depend on innervation by nerves. Similarly, varicosities appear in tissue cultures of nerves, which suggests that they are a genetically determined feature of axons and are not induced by the organs they innervate. Nerve profiles in close apposition to muscle are described in joint cultures of nerves and smooth muscle.

(3)   The synaptic cleft is difficult to define precisely at autonomic neuromuscular junctions: close approaches of nerve and muscle membranes in the vas deferens and circular muscle coat of the intestine are of the order of 200 Å, but transmitter released from up to 1200 Å appears to be effective; in most arteries the minimum neuromuscular separation is of the order of 800 Å and the functional cleft appears to be about $1\mu$. Other preparations show intermediate separations.

(4)   No consistent post-synaptic specialisation of muscle membranes has been seen at autonomic neuromuscular junctions. However, subsynaptic cysternae are often seen in muscle in the vas deferens, and aggregations of micropinocytotic vesicles in the muscle beneath terminal axons in gut and some blood vessels are also common.

(5)   Terminal varicosities penetrate deep inside some smooth muscle cells of the vas deferens, sometimes in close relation to perinuclear organelles; the significance of this finding is unknown.

(6)   Multiaxonal junctions with single smooth muscle cells, particularly in the circular muscle coat of the intestine, have been described and the close relationship of terminal regions of some adrenergic and cholinergic nerves discussed.

(7)   The intra-axonal features of different nerves have been described. *Cholinergic axons* contain a predominance of small (300–600 Å) agranular vesicles, and a small proportion of large (900–1200 Å) granular vesicles of unknown function.

*Adrenergic axons* contain a predominance of small (300–600 Å) granular vesicles, but some large (900–1200 Å) granular vesicles (which also take up monoamines) and small agranular vesicles (which probably represent 'empty' small granular vesicles) are also present. Some adrenergic profiles in birds and reptiles contain predominantly large (900–1200 Å) granular vesicles.

*Non-adrenergic, non-cholinergic autonomic axons* in gut and lung contain a predominance of large (1000–2000 Å) granular vesicles, which, unlike those described in adrenergic and cholinergic nerves, are completely filled with granular material. Some small agranular vesicles are usually also present.

Some nerve profiles, which probably represent *sensory nerves*, are characterised by large numbers of small, oval mitochondria and few, if any, vesicles.

(8)   Non-nervous profiles in close relation to smooth muscles have also been described, including chromaffin and 'chromaffin-type' cells, 'interstitial cells', and Schwann cells.

(9)   Ultrastructural changes produced in sympathetic nerves by various drugs have been discussed. *5- and 6-OHDA* displace noradrenaline from small- and large-granular vesicles within 1 hour of injection. When the concentration of 6-OHDA reaches a

critical concentration in the axoplasm, membrane damage seems to occur that may lead to the structural changes associated with degeneration of the terminal regions of the nerves, which are comparable to those seen following surgical denervation. Chronic treatment with the anti-hypertensive drug, *guanacline*, causes massive deposition of lipoprotein granules in sympathetic neurones, which is long-lasting and perhaps irreversible.

## REFERENCES

BAUMGARTEN, H. G. AND BRAAK, H. (1968) *Z. Zellforsch.*, **86**, 574–602.

BELL, C. (1969) *Circulation Res.*, **24**, 61–70.

BENNETT, M. R. AND BURNSTOCK, G. (1968) *Handbook of Physiology, Section 6. Alimentary Canal, IV. Motility*, Publ. American Physiological Society, Washington, pp. 1709–1732.

BENNETT, M. R. AND MERRILLEES, N. C .R. (1966) *J. Physiol.*, **185**, 520–535.

BENNETT, M. R. AND ROGERS, D. C. (1967) *J. Cell Biol.*, **33**, 573–596.

BENNETT, M., BURNSTOCK, G. AND HOLMAN, M. E. (1966) *J. Physiol.*, **182**, 541–558.

BENNETT, T. (1969) *J. Physiol.*, **204**, 669–686.

BENNETT, T. (1970) *Comp. Biochem. Physiol.*, **32**, 669–680.

BENNETT, T., BURNSTOCK, G., COBB, J. L. S. AND MALMFORS, T. (1970) *Brit. J. Pharmacol.*, **38**, 802–809.

BENNETT, T. AND COBB, J. L. S. (1969) *Z. Zellforsch.*, **99**, 109–120.

BENNETT, T., COBB, J. L. S. AND MALMFORS, T. (1971) Experimental studies on Auerbach's plexus, with particular reference to the adrenergic component, To be published.

BIRKS, R., HUXLEY, H. E. AND KATZ, B. (1960) *J. Physiol.*, **150**, 134–144.

BLOOM, F. E. AND BARRNETT, R. J. (1966) *Nature*, **210**, 599–601.

BLOOM, F. E. AND GIARMAN, N. J. (1967) *Anat. Rec.*, **157**, 351.

BONDAREFF, W. AND GORDON, B. (1966) *J. Pharmacol. Exp. Therap.*, **153**, 42–47.

BRETTSCHNEIDER, H. (1962) *Z. Mikroskop.-Anat. Forsch.*, **683**, 333–360.

BÜLBRING, E. AND TOMITA, T. (1967) *J. Physiol.*, **189**, 299–315.

BURN, J. H., (1968) In WOLSTENHOLME AND O'CONNOR (Eds.), *Adrenergic Neurotransmission Cibu Foundation Study Group No. 33*, Churchill, London, p. 39 in: Discussion of the mechanism of the release of noradrenaline.

BURN, J. H. AND RAND, M. J. (1959) *Nature*, **184**, 163–165.

BURN, J. H. AND RAND, M. J. (1965) *Ann. Rev. Pharmacol.*, **5**, 163–182.

BURNSTOCK, G. (1968) *Proc. 24th Intern. Congr. Physiol. Sci.*, Washington, **6**, 7–8.

BURNSTOCK, G. (1969) *Pharmacol. Rev.*, **21**, 247–324.

BURNSTOCK, G. (1970) In BRADING, JONES AND TOMITE (Eds.), *Smooth Muscle*, Edward Arnold Publ. Ltd. London, pp. 1–69.

BURNSTOCK, G. (1971) *Nature*, **229**, 282–283.

BURNSTOCK, G., DOYLE, A. E., GANNON, B. J., GERKINS, J. F., IWAYAMA, T. AND MASHFORD, M. L. (1971) *Europ. J. Pharmacol.*, **13**, 175–187.

BURNSTOCK, G., CAMPBELL, G., BENNETT, M. AND HOLMAN, M. E. (1963b) *Nature*, **200**, 581–582.

BURNSTOCK, G., CAMPBELL, G., BENNETT, M. AND HOLMAN, M. E. (1964) *Intern. J. Neuropharmacol.*, **3**, 163–166.

BURNSTOCK, G., CAMPBELL, G. AND RAND, M. J. (1966) *J. Physiol.*, **182**, 504–526.

BURNSTOCK, G., CAMPBELL, G., SATCHELL, D. G. AND SMYTHE, A. (1970a) *Brit. J. Pharmacol.*, **40**, 668–688.

BURNSTOCK, G., CAMPBELL, G. R., UEHARA, Y., FURNESS, J. B. AND MALMFORS, T. (1970b) *Proc. Austr. Physiol. Pharmacol. Soc.*, **May 1970**, **1**, 70–71P.

BURNSTOCK, G., GANNON, B. AND IWAYAMA, T., (1970c) *Circulation Res.*, **27** (Suppl. II), S-24.

BURNSTOCK, G., HOLMAN, M. E. AND PROSSER, C. L. (1963a) *Physiol. Rev.*, **43**, 482–527.

BURNSTOCK, G. AND ROBINSON, P. M. (1967) *Circulation Res.*, **21**, Suppl. 3, 43–55.

CAMPBELL, G. (1966) *J. Physiol.*, **185**, 600–612.

CAMPBELL, G. (1970) In BRADING, JONES AND TOMITE (Eds.), *Smooth Muscle* Edward Arnold Publ. Ltd., London, pp. 451–495.

CAMPBELL, G. R., UEHARA, Y., MARK, G. AND BURNSTOCK, G. (1971) *J. Cell Biol.*, **49**, 21–34.

CLEMENTI, F., MANTEGAZZA, P. AND BOTTURI, M. (1966) *Intern. J. Neuropharmacol.*, **5**, 281–285.

DAWBORN, J. K., DOYLE, A. E., EBRINGER, A., HOWQUA, J., JERUMS, G., JOHNSTON, C. I., MASHFORD, M. L. AND PARKIN, J. D. (1969) *Pharmacol. Clin.*, **2**, 1–5.

DAY, M. D. AND WARREN, P. R. (1968) *Brit. J. Pharmacol.*, **32**, 227–240.

DE ROBERTIS, E. AND BENNETT, H. S. (1955) *J. Biophys. Biochem. Cytol.*, **1**, 47–65.

DEWEY, M. M. AND BARR, L. (1962) *Science*, **137**, 670–672.

ELFVIN, L. G. (1965) *J. Ultrastruct. Res.*, **12**, 263–286.

ETCHEVERRY, G. J. AND ZIEHER, L. M. (1968a) *J. Histochem. Cytochem.*, **16**, 162–171.

ETCHEVERRY, G. J. AND ZIEHER, L. M. (1968b) *Z. Zellforsch.*, **86**, 393–400.

FARRELL, K. E. (1968) *Nature*, **217**, 279–281.

FERRY, C. B. (1966) *Physiol. Rev.*, **46**, 420–456.

FURNESS, J. B. (1969) *J. Physiol.*, **205**, 549–562.

FURNESS, J. B. (1970) *Pflügers Arch. Ges. Physiol.*, **314**, 1–13.

FURNESS, J. AND BURNSTOCK, G. (1969) *Comp. Biochem. Physiol.*, **31**, 337–345.

FURNESS, J. B., CAMPBELL, G. R., GILLARD, S. M., MALMFORS, T. AND BURNSTOCK, G. (1970a) *J. Pharmacol. Exp. Therap.*, **174**, 111–122.

FURNESS, J. B. AND IWAYAMA, T. (1970) *Z. Zellforsch.*, **113**, 259–270.

FURNESS, J. B., MCLEAN, J. R. AND BURNSTOCK, G. (1970b) *Develop. Biol.*, **21**, 491–505.

GEFFEN, L. B. AND LIVETT, B. G. (1971) *Physiol. Rev.*, **51**, 98–157.

GRAINGER, F., JAMES, D. W. AND TRESMAN, R. L. (1968) *Z. Zellforsch.*, **90**, 53–67.

GRILLO, M. A. (1966) *Pharmacol. Rev.*, **18**, 387–399.

GROSS, W., BRACHARZ, H., AND LAAS, H. (1965) In *Hochdruckforschung Fortschritte auf dem Gebiete der Inneren Medizin*, **11**, *Symposium held in Freiburg i. Br., July 18 and 19, 1964*, Georg Thieme Verlag, Stuttgart.

HAGEN, E. AND WITTKOWSKI, W. (1969) *Z. Zellforsch.*, **95**, 429–444.

HEBB, C., KÁSA, P. AND MANN, S. (1968) *Histochemical Journal*, **1**, 166–175.

HILLARP, N. A. (1946) M.D. Thesis, *Acta Anat.*, **2**, Suppl. 4, 1–153.

HÖKFELT, T. (1966) *Experientia*, **22**, 56.

HÖKFELT, T. (1968) *Z. Zellforsch.*, **91**, 1–74.

HÖKFELT, T. AND JONSSON, G. (1968) *Histochemie*, **16**, 45–67.

HÖKFELT, T. AND NILSSON, O. (1965) *Z. Zellforsch.*, **66**, 848–853.

HOLMAN, M. E. (1970) In E. BÜLBRING (Ed.), *Smooth Muscle*, Edward Arnold Publ. Ltd., London.

IWAYAMA, T. (1970) *Z. Zellforsch.*, **109**, 465–480.

IWAYAMA, T. AND FURNESS, J. B. (1971) *J. Cell Biol.*, **48**, 699–703.

IWAYAMA, T., FURNESS, J. B. AND BURNSTOCK, G. (1970) *Circulation Res.*, **26**, 635–646.

KRONEBERG, G., SCHLOSSMANN, K. AND STOEPEL, K. (1967) *Arzneimittel Forsch.*, **17**, 199–207.

KURIYAMA, H., OSA, T. AND TOIDA, N. (1967) *J. Physiol.*, **191**, 257–270.

LANE, B. P. AND RHODIN, J. A. G. (1964) *J. Ultrastruct. Res.*, **10**, 470–488.

LAVERTY, R., SHARMAN, D. F. AND VOGT, M. (1965) *Brit. J. Pharmacol.*, **24**, 549–560.

MALMFORS, T. (1965) *Acta Physiol. Scand.*, **64**, (Suppl. 248), 1–93.

MALMFORS, T. AND SACHS, CH. (1968) *Europ. J. Pharmacol.*, **3**, 89–92.

MARTINSON, J. (1965) *Acta Physiol. Scand.*, **64**, 453–462.

MERRILLEES, N. C. R. (1968) *J. Cell Biol.*, **37**, 794–817.

MERRILLEES, N., BURNSTOCK, G. AND HOLMAN, M. E. (1963) *J. Cell Biol.*, **19**, 529–550.

NAGASAWA, J. AND MITO, S. (1967) *Tohoku J. Exp. Med.*, **91**, 277–293.

NORBERG, K.-A. AND HAMBERGER, B. (1964) *Acta Physiol. Scand.*, **63**, Suppl. 238, 1–42.

PLUCHINO, S., VAN ORDEN III, L. S., DRASKOCZY, P. R., LANGER, S. Z. AND TRENDELENBURG, V. (1970) *J. Pharmacol. Exp. Therap.*, **172**, 77–90.

PORTER, C. C., TOTARO, J. A. AND BURCIN, A. (1965) *J. Pharmacol. Exp. Therap.*, **150**, 17–22.

PORTER, C. C., TOTARO, J. A. AND STONE, C. A. (1963) *J. Pharmacol. Exp. Therap.*, **140**, 308–316.

READ, J. B. AND BURNSTOCK, G. (1970) *Develop. Biol.*, **22**, 513–534.

RICHARDSON, K. C. (1960) *J. Anat.*, **94**, 457–472.

RICHARDSON, K. C. (1962) *J. Anat.*, **96**, 427–442.

RICHARDSON, K. C. (1966) *Nature*, **210**, 756.

ROBERTSON, J. D. (1962) In *Ultrastructure and Metabolism of the Nervous System*, **40**, 94–158.

ROBINSON, P. M. (1969) *J. Cell Biol.*, **41**, 462–476.

ROBINSON, P. M., McLEAN, J. R. AND BURNSTOCK, G. (1970) *J. Pharmacol. Exp. Therap.*, in press.
ROGERS, D. AND BURNSTOCK, G. (1966 a); *J. Comp. Neurol.*, **126**, 255–284.
ROGERS, D. AND BURNSTOCK, G. (1966 b) *J. Comp. Neurol.*, **126**, 625–652.
ROTH, C. D. AND RICHARDSON, K. C. (1969) *Amer. J. Anat.*, **124**, 341–360.
SCHÜMANN, H. J. AND PHILIPPU, A. (1968) *Arzneimittel-Forsch.*, **18**, 1571–1574.
TAXI, J. (1965) *Naturelles Zoologie*, 12e série, **VII**, 413–674.
TAXI, J. (1969) *Progr. Brain Res.*, **31**, 5–20.
THAEMERT, J. C. (1963) *J. Cell Biol.*, **16**, 361–377.
THAEMERT, J. C. (1966) *J. Cell Biol.*, **28**, 37–49.
THOENEN, H. AND TRANZER, J. P. (1968) *Arch. Exp. Pathol. Pharmakol.*, **261**, 271–288.
THOENEN, H., TRANZER, J. P., HÜRLIMANN, A. AND HAEFELY, W. (1966) *Helv. Physiol. Pharmacol. Acta*, **24**, 229–246.
TRANZER, J. P. AND THOENEN, H. (1967a) *Experientia*, **23**, 743–745.
TRANZER, J. P. AND THOENEN, H. (1967 b) *Naunyn-Schmiedebergs Arch. Pharmakol. Exp. Pathol.*, **257**, 343.
TRANZER, J. P. AND THOENEN, H. (1968 a) *Experientia*, **24**, 155–156.
TRANZER, J. P. AND THOENEN, H. (1968 b) *Experientia*, **24**, 484–486.
TRANZER, J. P., THOENEN, H., SNIPES, R. L. AND RICHARDS, J. G. (1969) *Progr. Brain Res.*, **31**, 33–46.
UEHARA, Y. AND BURNSTOCK, G. (1971) *Z. Zellforsch.*, submitted.
VAN ORDEN, L. S. III, BLOOM, F. E., BARRNETT, R. J. AND GIARMAN, N. J. (1966) *J. Pharmacol. Exp. Therap.*, **154**, 185–199.
WATANABE, H. (1969) *Acta Anat. Nippon*, **44**, 189–202.
WHITTAKER, V. P., MICHAELSON, I. A. AND KIRKLAND, R. J. A. (1964) *Biochem. J.*, **90**, 293–303.
YAMAUCHI, A. AND BURNSTOCK, G. (1969 a) *J. Anat.*, **104**, 1–15.
YAMAUCHI, A. AND BURNSTOCK, G. (1969 b) *J. Anat.*, **104**, 17–32.
ZWEIG, M. AND AXELROD, J. (1969) *J. Neurobiol.*, **1**, 87–97.

# On the Vegetative Cardiac Innervation

T. H. SCHIEBLER AND J. WINCKLER

*Department of Anatomy, University of Würzburg (Germany)*

## INTRODUCTION

In mammals the heart is among those organs which abound in vegetative innervation. This has long been a well-known fact and it is therefore not surprising that the number of relevant investigations is immense. The topic of the vegetative cardiac innervation recently acquired new importance with the introduction of methods for the differential demonstration of ortho- and parasympathetic fibres. To begin with I would like to give you a short review of the principles of cardiac innervation as presently known. I will then move on to more detailed problems. The keynote of this paper will be to scrutinize our current conception of the regulatory mechanisms of cardiac function.

Figs. 1–3 give an impression of the subepicardial and subendocardial plexus. These two plexus are located in the connective tissue between the myocardium and the innermost and outermost cardiac surface respectively (Ehinger *et al.*, 1968; Winckler, 1969 a). The plexus are found in the atrium as well as in the ventricles. Fig. 1 shows the andrenergic part of the subepicardial plexus in the atrium of a rat. You will observe a dense network of strongly fluorescent preterminal and terminal fibres. Fig. 2 shows a sector of the subendocardial plexus. Compared with the subepicardial plexus the density of nerve fibres is significantly lower here. However this finding can not be generalized since in guinea pigs, for example, the density of subendocardial nerve fibres almost equals that of the subepicardial ones. Finally Fig. 3 shows the cholinergic sector of the subendocardial plexus of the ventricle of the rat, as demonstrated by means of the acetylcholinesterase reaction. The fact that these fibres give the impression of being much plumper than they appear to be with the catecholamine technique is due to the fact that the acetylcholinesterase reaction for light microscopy also demonstrates Schwann's sheath in which in some parts several neurites are embedded.

From the plexus just mentioned nerve fibres together with arteries extend into the myocardium. In Fig. 4 you see a branch of a rat coronary artery which is closely enveloped by adrenergic nerve fibres. Only a few of these nerve fibres serve for the innervation of the blood vessels, the majority only follow the track of the vessels (Winckler, 1970). The same applies to cholinergic nerves (Fig. 5).

Within the cardiac musculature exists a wide-meshed intramural network of terminal fibres, which, in most cases however, take a course independent of that of the capillaries (Fig. 6). Frequently, terminal fibres traverse muscle fibres. As for the actual

*References p. 413*

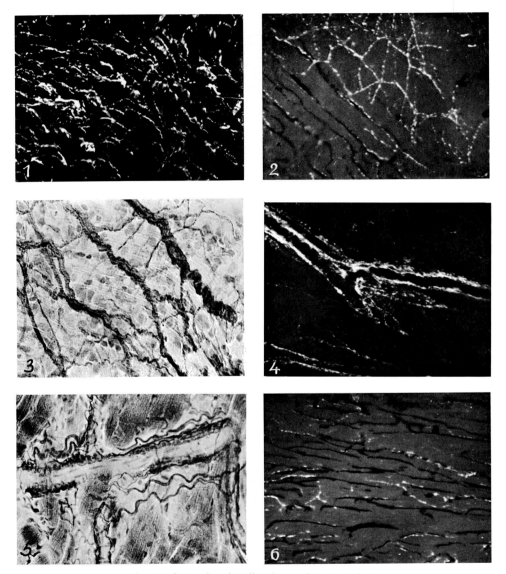

Fig. 1. Adrenergic epicardial plexus of the rat atrium.

Fig. 2. Section through myo- and endocardium of the rat ventricle. India-ink injection of the capillaries. Fluorescence of adrenergic myocardial nerves and endocardial plexus.

Fig. 3. Acetylcholinesterase reaction (Karnovsky, 1964) of the endocardial plexus of the guinea pig ventricle. High magnification.

Fig. 4. Myocardial artery of the rat ventricle. Beside adrenergic terminals just between adventitia and media there are numerous nerves that run for some distance more or less parallel to the vessel.

Fig. 5. Same as in Fig. 4. Acetylcholinesterase reaction.

Fig. 6. Adrenergic nerve terminals and India-ink injected capillaries of the rat ventricular myocardium.

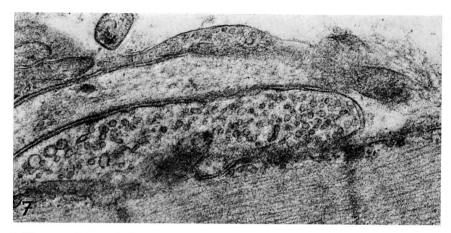

Fig. 7. Electron-microscopic demonstration of a myoneural junction in the ventricle of the pigeon (Photograph by Dr. R. Gossrau).

innervation of the cardiac muscle fibres, it has to be said that it is relatively unusual to observe myoneural connections in which the distance between membranes is approximately 200 Å (Fig. 7) (Hadek and Talso, 1967; Novi, 1968; Thaemert, 1969). In the majority of cases we will only find synapses 'en distance' which are located in the region of varicosities. The concentration of amines in the varicosities was found to be much higher than that in the fibrous parts (Dahlström, 1967). To conclude the general part of my paper I would like to add that all the vegetative ganglion cells on and in the heart are cholinergic ones, at least in all species investigated using histochemical techniques for catecholamines (Ehinger et al., 1968; Winckler, 1969 a; Dahlström et al., 1965).

### SPECIALIZED PROBLEMS OF THE VEGETATIVE CARDIAC INNERVATION

To start with I would like to mention the ontogenetic development (Winckler, 1969 a; Schiebler and Heene, 1968; Friedman et al., 1968). In all species so far investigated it was found, that transmitters in nerves are only seen during a relatively late developmental phase. In rats it is the second half of the third week of life, in guinea pigs approximately the 50th embryonic day. In the beginning we observe comparatively thick nerve fibres in the atrium which in many cases are connected to branches of the coronary arteries. The terminal network in the cardiac musculature can be demonstrated at a slightly later point.

It is quite remarkable that the region of the conducting system belongs to those cardiac regions which are densely innervated at a very early stage. In contrast to these findings which were established in the mammalian heart by histochemical methods, catecholamines have been demonstrated by biochemical methods in chickens on the third day of egg incubation (Ignarro and Shideman, 1968). I must admit however that in this case I would much rather rely on histochemical methods since they exclude errors, due to preparative mistakes. The importance of the findings which were

established in this evolutionary investigation seems to lie in the fact, that in the
'life story' of the heart, there is quite obviously a period during which nerve fibres can
be demonstrated by impregnation (Fukutake, 1925), but that these nerve fibres do not
seem to contain any histochemically demonstrable transmitters. It has to be assumed
that these nerves are incapable of functioning. Nevertheless, even during this period
the heart is fully operative. In this context I would like to refer to the conducting
system, bearing in mind the fact that the heart shows synchronized contractions a
long time before a specific conducting system can be demonstrated (Goerttler, 1963).
The question remains open as to whether the heart, during the period where the
innervation is not yet fully operating, can be adjusted to special circulatory situations.
This, however, is a purely academic problem, since it seems improbable that embryonic
heart will ever have to meet such requirements. Nevertheless we know that catecholamines are already produced in the suprarenals in early fetal life and that the fetal
myocardial cells are sensitive to norepinephrine and later to epinephrine, too (Bernard
and Gargouil, 1967).

### BEHAVIOUR OF VASCULAR AND MYOCARDIAL NERVES UNDER DIFFERENT CONDITIONS

The first item to be clarified is whether the vascular nerves merely accompany the
coronary arteries or are needed for the actual vascular innervation (Winckler, 1970;
Ehinger and Falck, 1966). This question is of great consequence since the regulation
of the coronary circulation is of crucial importance for cardiac action. According to
our findings obtained in rats and guinea-pigs, both possibilities under discussion are
observed in the mammalian heart. We are under the impression that in rats the
innervation of the vascular system proper is only slightly developed. Apart from
terminal fibres which obviously use the adventitial connective tissue merely as
'conducting track', we did in fact observe nerves which adhere closely to the adventitia–media boundary zone; these fibres, however, proceed only in exceptional cases in
a circular fashion and with the development of plexus-like formations. Apart from this
we repeatedly observed terminal fibres which deviate from a close vascular connection
and penetrate into the connective tissue and into the myocardium. This means that we
are dealing with fibres which innervate the vascular musculature as well as the
myocardium.

The situation which I just described is slightly different in the guinea pig. Apart
from nerve fibres which first approach the media and then proceed in the opposite
direction, we observe nerve plexus in the region of the adventitia–media zone, which
seem to be exclusively destined for the innervation of the vascular musculature. In
this region coronary vessels of varying size are enveloped in a basket-work-like
fashion. It seems as if the vascular innervation of the guinea pig heart is regulated in a
much more sophisticated way than is the case in the rat.

One observation seems of particular interest, namely that the nerves in the vicinity
of vessels under experimental stress seem to react differently from myocardial nerves.
Fig. 8 was taken from the ventricular myocardium of a rat which, four hours before

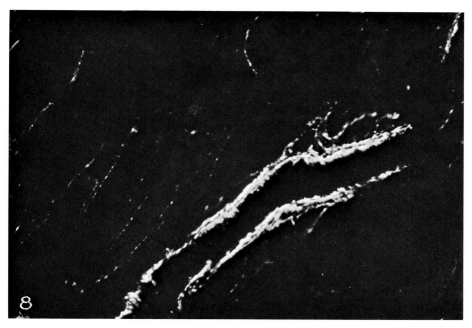

Fig. 8. Ventricular myocardium of the rat. Following premedication with Pertofran (Geigy) —25 mg/kg i.p. 4 h before sacrifice there is a decrease in fluorescence of myocardial terminals while the intensity of fluorescence of adrenergic nerves around the artery seems not to be diminished.

being sacrificed, was given an intraperitoneal injection of 25 mg/kg Pertofran — a drug which resembles cocaine in its action. The nerve fibres which are close to vessels show an almost unchanged fluorescence, whereas the myocardial nerves are only just visible (Winckler, 1969 b). The picture resembles in several respects the pictures which were obtained following the administration of Segontin — hibernation type of myocardial innervation (Nielsen and Owman, 1967). The effect is even more marked if the animals are subjected to physical stress in addition to the treatment with Pertofran (Winckler, 1969 b). It is noteworthy that the adrenergic nerves of the atrium, the epicardial and endocardial plexus, as well as conducting system (fig. 9) react like vascular nerves. This shows that there is a distinct difference in the reaction of myocardial nerves to stress.

The question is raised of how meaningful this observation is. We tend to hold a sceptical view since only at low concentrations of catecholamines are changes of concentration accompanied by an almost linear change in the intensity of the fluorescence; if, however, the substrate concentration is high, this linear relationship does not hold to the same extent (Olson *et al.*, 1968). We must however take into consideration that the initial situation in the myocardial nerves differs from that of the vessels, so that in myocardial nerves in which the initial concentration of catecholamines is lower anyhow, the reserves of catecholamines are exhausted much more quickly than those of the vascular nerves and the nerves of the atrium. Finally it seems very likely that perfusion plays an important part (Blakeley and Brown, 1966;

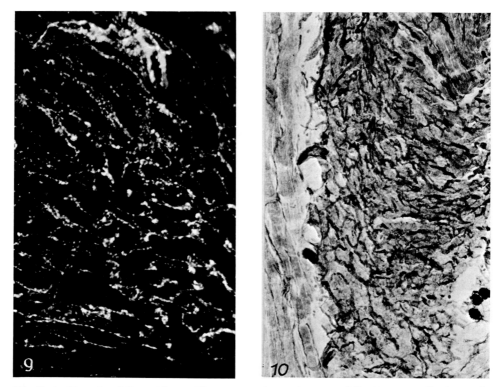

Fig. 9. A. V. node of the rat heart. Fluorescent adrenergic nerves following premedication as in Fig. 8. Note the density of adrenergic fibres and the fact that the drug has not diminished the intensity of specific fluorescence of the varicosities.

Fig. 10. Sinus node. Rat. Acetylcholinesterase reaction.

Peiper *et al.*, 1966) insofar as in the ventricular myocardium the decrease in concentration of the secreted transmitters through the blood is of much greater importance than in other areas. Nevertheless the possibility cannot be excluded that under stress vascular and myocardial nerves secrete their transmitters in different quantities.

## MYOCARDIAL INNERVATION

In discussing this topic, I wish to deal mainly with the pattern of innervation. As is well known, some animals show distinct differences in the innervation of the various cardiac regions, differences which are either not observed at all in other animals or which are much less striking (Ehinger *et al.*, 1968; Winckler, 1969a; Dahlström *et al.*, 1965; Schiebler and Heene, 1968; Angelakos *et al.*, 1963; Nielsen and Owman, 1968). It is not necessary that adrenergic and cholinergic innervation inevitably work in parallel. Let us take the rat as an example: it is known that in this animal the adrenergic atrial innervation exceeds the ventricular one; only a relatively poor ventricular myocardial adrenergic plexus is to be seen. As far as the cholinergic nerves are concerned, they are not present in the ventricular myocardium apart from regions which are in the vicinity of large vessels.

In the guinea pig a different picture is observed from that in the rat in that some areas of the ventricular myocardium show just as many adrenergic terminal fibres as the atrium. It is not a rare observation in guinea pigs that small bundles of muscle fibres are surrounded in a circular fashion by adrenergic terminal fibres. In cats the ventricular nnervation is even more marked than in the guinea pig, whereas according to Nielsen and Owman (1968) in hibernating animals the vascular innervation of the ventricles dominates by far.

I feel that it is not incorrect to assume that these characteristic differences in the pattern of innervation between the various species have an effect on the function and extent of the control which the sympathicus exerts on the heart. So, in some species, there might be a more or less important direct neuronal control of the myocardium, while in others this control is an indirect one: only the coronary arteries are innervated and thereby the efficiency of the heart is regulated. It is surprising however that there is in all species a high density of adrenergic innervation in the atria, *i.e.* in those cardiac regions which show less musculature than the ventricles and which do less work. We have considered whether the density of nerves in the atria is somehow connected with the regulation of the tonus of the atrial wall. This could mean a neuronal control of the atrial volume which in turn regulates the magnitude of the cardiac stroke volume (Starling's 'Law').

### Vegetative innervation

At this point the question arises of how the vegetative innervation of the heart and the conducting system are balanced (Schiebler and Doerr, 1963). Thorough investigations prove that no structure of the heart shows an innervation which is as dense as that of the specific musculature (Ehinger *et al.*, 1968; Winckler, 1969a, b; Dahlström *et al.*, 1965; Schiebler and Heene, 1968; Nielsen and Owman, 1968). Fig. 9 shows catecholamine fluorescence of the A.V. node of a rat. There is a large number of preterminal and terminal fibres. Fig. 10 shows an acetylcholinesterase preparation of the sinus node. We see the same pattern in the other parts of the conducting system.

These findings seem to be of great importance. We would like to look upon the conducting system as the essential target organ of the vegetative cardiac innervation. The specific musculature is the only trigger for synchronized positive or negative chronotropic regulatory stimuli to the heart. All other possibilities of the vegetative nervous system mentioned above as influencing heart action seem to be of secondary importance. The role of ventricular innervation especially seems to be of minor importance since in some species, as for example in hibernating animals, the ventricular nerves are exclusively vascular nerves (Nielsen and Owman, 1968). It is quite possible that the neurotransmitters have no specific effect whatever on the ventricles if one disregards the general positive metabolic effect of the catecholamines.

Since this short exposition has shown that many facets of the rôle of vegetative myocardial innervation remain to be elucidated, it becomes an even more pressing

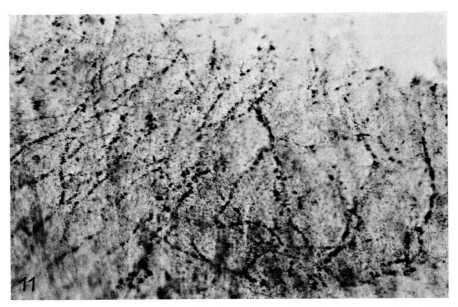

Fig. 11. Adrenergic plexus of the tricuspid valve of the rat. Stripping film autoradiography of a freeze-dried postfixed cryostat section (Winckler and Hempel, 1971) following the injection of 500 mC/kg DL-DOPA — ($a$, $\beta$ — T$_2$) (specific activity 7700 mC/11 mole) 6 h before sacrifice. Exposition 10 days. Note the pronounced uptake of tritiated DOPA into the varicosities.

problem in those regions of vegetative cardiac innervation where dense nerve plexus are seen and musculature or blood vessels are absent. I refer particularly to the plexus on the cardiac valves (Ehinger *et al.*, 1968; Winckler, 1969 a; Lipp and Rodin, 1968 a, b). I would like to avoid descriptive details and discuss instead Lipp's view (1968 b) that the vegetative nerves which are found in the region of the valves do not have any function as far as innervation goes, but that on the contrary they have the ability to diffuse transmitters into the blood stream and/or to reabsorb them from the blood stream (Braunwald *et al.*, 1964). To investigate this question we injected rats with radioactive DOPA. Fig. 11 shows the autoradiogram of the valve plexus of an animal following the administration of DOPA. The activity in the valve plexus is particularly bound to the varicosities. These terminal fibres have taken up more DOPA than the terminal fibres in the myocardium or other organs such as intestine or spleen. These investigations were only very recently started so I feel that conclusions are not yet justified. It is conceivable however that under physiological conditions a diffuse 'secretion' and absorption of transmitters takes place.

CONCLUSION

In a subject which has been as thoroughly investigated as vegetative cardiac inner-vation, completeness cannot be the object of any exposition. We consider the problem of vegetative cardiac innervation with some scepticism: we think that the mere presence of a large number of vegetative nerves in the heart can not be assumed to mean that they play a prominent rôle in cardiac action. The species-specific differences are too obvious and the fact remains that during development the heart works over a long period without possessing any nerves that are fully functioning. Apart from this we know that transmitters, at least the catecholamines, have effects (*e.g.* metabolic) that far exceed their function in neuronal transmission.

## REFERENCES

ANGELAKOS, E. T., FUXE, K. AND TORCHIANA, M. L. (1963) *Acta Physiol. Scand.*, **59**, 184.
BERNARD C. AND GARGOUIL, L. M. (1967) *C.R. Soc. Biol.*, **161**, 2600.
BLAKELEY, A. G. H. AND BROWN, G. L. (1966) In U. S. VON EULER, S. ROSELL AND B. UVNÄS (Eds.), *Mechanisms of Release of Biogenic Amines*, Pergamon Press, Oxford–London–Edinburgh, p. 185.
BRAUNWALD, E., HARRISON, D. C. AND CHIDSEY, C. A. (1964) *Amer. J. Med.*, **36** 1.
DAHLSTRÖM, A., FUXE, K., MYA-TU, M. AND ZETTERSTRÖM, B. E. M. (1965) *Am. J. Physiol.*, **209**, 689.
DAHLSTRÖM, A. (1967) *Naunyn-Schmiedebergs Arch. Pharm. Exp. Pathol.*, **257**, 93.
EHINGER, B. AND FALCK, B. (1966) *Bibl. Anat. (Basel)*, **8**, 35.
EHINGER, B., FALCK, B., PERSSON, H. AND SPORRONG, B. (1968) *Histochemie*, **16**, 197.
FRIEDMAN, W. F., POOL, P. E., JACOBOWITZ, D., SEAGREN, S. C. AND BRAUNWALD, E. (1968) *Circulation Res.*, **23**, 165.
FUKUTAKE, K. (1925) *Z. Anat. Entwickl.-Gesch.*, **76**, 592.
GOERTTLER, K. (1963) In: W. BARGMANN UND W. DOERR, (Hrsg.), *Das Herz des Menschen*, Thieme, Stuttgart, p. 71.
HADEK, R. AND TALSO, P. J. (1967) *J. Ultrastruct. Res.*, **17**, 257.
IGNARRO, L. J. AND SHIDEMAN, F. E. (1968) *J. Pharm. Exp. Therap.*, **159**, 38.
LIPP, W. AND RODIN, M. (1968a) *Anat. Anz.* **121**, *Erg.-H.* 83.
LIPP, W. AND RODIN, M. (1968b) *Acta Anat.*, **69**, 312.
NIELSEN, K. C. AND OWMAN, CH. (1967) *Experientia*, **23**, 203.
NIELSEN, K. C. AND OWMAN, CH. (1968) *Acta Physiol. Scand., Suppl.* **316**.
NOVI, A. N. (1968) *Anat. Rec.*, **160**, 123.
OLSON, L., HAMBERGER, B., JOHNSON, G. AND MALMFORS, T. (1968) *Histochemie*, **15**, 38.
PEIPER, U., OHNHAUS, H. AND BRETTSCHNEIDER, E. E. (1966) *Pflügers Arch. Ges. Physiol.*, **209**, 362.
SCHIEBLER, T. H. AND DOERR, W. (1963) In: W. BARGMANN UND W. DOERR, (Hrsg.), *Das Herz des Menschen*, Thieme, Stuttgart, p. 165.
SCHIEBLER, T. H. AND HEENE, R. (1968) *Histochemie*, **14**, 328.
THAEMERT, J. C. (1969) *Anat. Rec.*, **163**, 575.
WINCKLER, J. (1969a) *Z. Zellforsch.*, **98**, 106.
WINCKLER, J. (1969b) *Z. Zellforsch.*, **101**, 380.
WINCKLER, J. (1970) *Anat. Anz.* **126**, *Erg.-H.* in press.
WINCKLER, J. AND HEMPEL, K. (1971) *Histochemie*, (in preparation).

# Innervation of Bull Retractor Penis Muscle and Peripheral Autonomic Mechanism of Erection

E. KLINGE AND P. POHTO

*Department of Pharmacology, University of Helsinki (Finland)*

The peripheral autonomic nervous mechanisms that regulate the entrance of blood into the penile erectile tissue are poorly understood and they have been the object of little interest among present-day histochemists. To the authors' knowledge there are only a few descriptions of adrenergic nerve fibres (Eränkö, 1967; Baumgarten *et al.*, 1969; Klinge and Penttilä, 1969) and of the localization of cholinesterases (Klinge and Penttilä, 1969; Grieten and Gerebtzoff, 1957) in the cavernous bodies of some species. At least since the painstaking investigations of Langley and Anderson (1895), however, here has been certain evidence suggesting that the sympathetic nervous system contributes to the maintenance of a continuous constriction of the penile arteries and thus prevents filling of the cavernous sinusoids. The experiments of the same authors also indicate that in dogs and cats the muscles of the penile arteries are subjected to a similar nervous control as the retractor penis muscle which is probably continuously contracted, being relaxed only coincidently with penile erection. The understanding of the nervous mechanism of relaxation of these muscles has encountered serious obstacles, although it was demonstrated more than a hundred years ago that they can be relaxed by electrical stimulation of the pelvic nerve (Eckhard, 1863).

In the following presentation the function of the efferent nerve fibres of the bull retractor penis muscle, *i.e.* of the excitatory and inhibitory fibres, and the possible peripheral autonomic mechanism of erection will be considered partly on the basis of the authors' own studies and partly on the basis of the literature. The afferent nerve fibres are beyond the scope of this consideration.

## EXCITATORY FIBRES

In the whole muscle the smooth cells are embraced by numerous fine branches of postganglionic adrenergic nerve fibres (Klinge *et al.*, 1970). The large amount of these characteristically coiled and frequently anastomosing fibres is reflected by a high content of noradrenaline (3.8 $\mu$g/g) in this muscle, which probably is devoid of adrenaline (Klinge, 1970 a). If the nervous supply is analogous to that of the retractor penis of the dog and the cat, the bulk of the motor fibres reach the muscle by way of the pudic nerve, probably originating from the paravertebral ganglia at the sacral level. A minor part runs down along the hypogastric nerve *via* the pelvic plexus (Langley and Anderson, 1895).

Within the muscle the adrenergic nerve fibres did not exhibit ganglionic synapses, nor were any non-neuronal monoamine cells observed (Klinge *et al.*, 1970). It is known that adrenergic neurons with a presumably intermittent activity form ganglionic synapses close to their target organs or within their walls, as those supplying the vasa deferentia, the seminal vesicles or the prostate (Sjöstrand, 1965). Certain studies indicate that the short adrenergic postganglionic neurons of the internal accessory male genital organs differ from the ordinary long neurons with respect to the storage and release mechanism of the transmitter substance (Sjöstrand and Swedin, 1968; Stjärne and Lishajko, 1966). So far it is not known whether the adrenergic nerves of the bull retractor penis muscle are linked by ganglionic synapses located in the close vicinity of the muscle or not. But the obviously continuous activity of these nerves rather suggests that they represent long postganglionic neurons. This assumption requires further evidence but is it indirectly supported by the observation that a high concentration of hexamethonium does not inhibit the contractions of the cavernous bodies of the rabbit penis induced by stimulation of the pudic nerve (Hukovic and Bubic, 1967). It is also possible that the neurons running to the retractor penis muscle by way of the hypogastric nerve do not have a ganglionic synapse in the pelvic (cavernous) plexus, contrary to the possibility illustrated in Fig. 1.

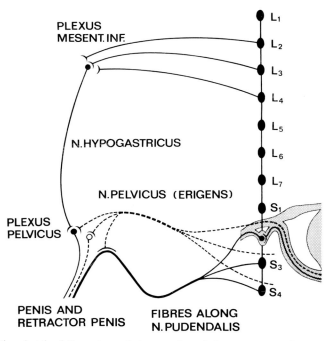

Fig. 1. A tentative sketch of the autonomic innervation of the retractor penis muscle and the penile artery of the bull. The solid lines represent the adrenergic system and the dotted lines the cholinergic system. The possible interactions of these systems are considered in the text.

Strips of the bull retractor penis muscle suspended in Tyrode solution are vigorously contracted by low concentrations of noradrenaline or adrenaline (Klinge, 1970 c). Under these conditions phenoxybenzamine has a $pA_2$ value against noradrenaline of 9.41, which shows a high blocking capacity (Birmingham and Szolcsányi, 1965). Erection of the penis in humans or relaxation of the retractor penis muscle in dogs (Dale, 1906) can not be produced by $a$-adrenergic blocking agents. It is generally accepted that phenoxybenzamine and other $a$-receptor blocking drugs are effective against injected noradrenaline and also against noradrenaline released by electrical nerve stimulation. But it is not well understood to what extent they influence the normal sympathetic tone maintained in various vascular areas of healthy subjects by the physiological release of noradrenaline from long postganglionic neurons. It is also conceivable that in the areas under consideration there is a strong sympathetic activity with a high concentration of the transmitter substance at the receptor sites. This is not necessarily identical with the situation where the sympathetic tone alone would be responsible for the continuous constriction of the penile artery and for the contraction of the retractor penis muscle. Of all the substances examined, bradykinin exerts the highest contracting power on the bull retractor penis muscle *in vitro* (Klinge, 1970 c), but it is difficult to assign any physiological role to bradykinin in this connection. So far no drugs have been described which administered intra-arterially would be able to induce a full erection of the canine penis (Dorr and Brody, 1967). The effects of sympathectomy on penile erection in man have been critically considered by Whitelaw and Smithwick (1951).

There is no definite evidence that acetylcholine would bring about the release of noradrenaline from motor nerve endings in the bull retractor penis muscle. Possibly, however, the cholinergic link hypothesis (Burn and Rand, 1959) might be valid, since the muscle contains considerable amounts (1.6 $\mu$g/g) of acetylcholine (Klinge, 1970 b) and the localization of acetylcholinesterase in light microscopic studies shows a certain correspondence to that of noradrenaline (Klinge *et al.*, 1970). It has been demonstrated that physostigmine intensifies the contractions of the dog retractor penis muscle produced by stimulation of the pudic nerve (Armitage and Burn, 1967).

### INHIBITORY FIBRES

It is generally agreed that erection of the penis in dogs, cats and rabbits can be evoked by stimulation of the pelvic nerve. The erection is always accompanied by a simultaneous relaxation of the retractor penis muscle which constitutes a prerequisite of erection in dogs and cats, while the rabbit lacks this muscle (Langley and Anderson, 1895). Also in bulls the straightening of the penis is impossible without a coincident relaxation of the retractor penis muscle (Klinge, 1969). But there is a great deal of disagreement regarding the presence of erectile fibres in the hypogastric nerve. Concerning dogs, cats and rabbits the negative position is held by Langley and Anderson (1895), Semans and Langworthy (1938) and many others, but the positive view has several supporters (Bacq, 1935; Root and Bard, 1947; Thielen *et al.*, 1969) as well. The problem has to be regarded as unsolved, its settlement being hampered by

*References p. 421*

several factors, such as an aberrant course of nerves and the influence of various reflex patterns. We have found no information about bulls on this point. It also remains to be solved whether the hypogastric nerve carries motor adrenergic fibres to pelvic arteries other than the penile artery. An activation of such fibres during erection might increase the penile blood flow.

Physostigmine increases the enlargement of the penis in dogs (Bacq, 1935; Henderson and Roepke, 1933) and rabbits (Hukovic and Bubic, 1967) induced by stimulation of the pelvic nerve. This strongly suggests a cholinergic mechanism. Nevertheless, atropine does not abolish the effect of the stimulation (Dorr and Brody, 1967; Goldenberg, 1965). Neither is it influenced by $\beta$-adrenergic blockade (Luduena and Grigas, 1966), probably being prevented only by ganglionic blocking agents (Langley and Andersson, 1895; Dorr and Brody, 1967; Henderson and Roepke, 1933; Goldenberg, 1965; Von Anrep and Cybulski, 1884; Spina, 1897). This suggests the existence of a ganglionic synapse in the pelvic nerve. Erectile impotence is rarely if at all caused in humans by drugs having a pure antimuscarinic activity, whereas it may be encountered as a side effect when ganglionic blocking agents are used (Goodman and Gilman, 1965).

It is reasonable to suppose that a local interruption or decrease of the adrenergic activity is required before relaxation of the retractor penis muscle and penile erection can take place. It is also plausible that a cholinergic mechanism is responsible for, or at least contributes to, such an interruption. In bulls the retractor penis muscle contains as much acetylcholine as the duodenum (Klinge, 1970 b). But when strips of the muscle are suspended in Tyrode solution no dose-dependent response of any kind to acetylcholine can be obtained (Klinge, 1970 c). This could indicate a scarcity or an absence of acetylcholine receptors in the muscle cells, the major part of the acetylcholine activity being confined to the nervous tissue.

In a mammalian tissue like the retractor penis muscle there probably is a high degree of correspondence between the localizations of acetylcholine and acetylcholinesterase. In this muscle of the bull the bulk of acetylcholinesterase was found in nerve fibres, and the light-microscopic studies further pointed to a certain correspondence between its localization and that of noradrenaline (Klinge et al., 1970). It could not be determined whether they were located in the same nerve fibre or in concominant fibres, but it was difficult to escape the conclusion that acetylcholine may influence the function of postganglionic adrenergic axons. The same conclusion might also be drawn from light-microscopic studies of other mammalian tissues (Eränkö and Härkönen, 1964; Eränkö and Räisänen, 1965; Ehinger and Falck, 1965; Jacobowitz and Koelle, 1965).

On the basis of the criteria described above the theory is put forward that cholinergic impulses conducted mainly along the pelvic nerves transiently reduce the activity in the postganglionic adrenergic nerves running in the penile artery and its branches and in the retractor penis muscle. A consequence of this would be relaxation of the retractor penis muscle with coincident erection of the penis. In Fig. 1 there are illustrated some hypotheses of the morphology of the synapses between the pelvic nerves and the adrenergic nerves concerned. The synapses could be ganglionic, ganglionic-like or

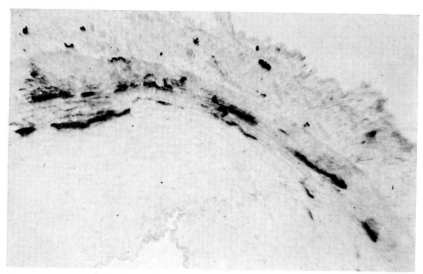

Fig. 2. Transverse section of bull penile artery 5 cm proximal to the point where it divides into the arteriae dorsalis and profunda penis. Acetylcholinesterase staining, incubation time 18 h, 20 μm, × 150.

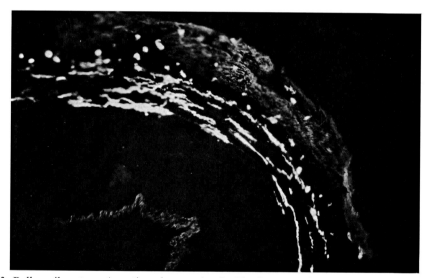

Fig. 3. Bull penile artery. A section close to that in Fig. 2. Formaldehyde-induced catecholamine fluorescence, 20 μm, × 100. The thick muscular wall is supplied by a dense adrenergic innervation.

postganglionic axo-axonal. With our present knowledge the existence of the last type mentioned would probably be the easiest to defend.

Applying a theory of Burn and Rand (1965) it may be assumed that an excess of acetylcholine released from the erectile fibres at high impulse frequencies would induce a continuous depolarization in the axonal membrane of the adrenergic neurons. Some recent investigations indicate that high concentrations of acetylcholine in certain

*References p. 421*

conditions reduce the effect of stimulation of postganglionic sympathetic nerves (Malik and Ling, 1969; Löffelholz and Muscholl, 1969). So far there is no convincing evidence of the cholinergic mechanism suggested here for relaxation of the bull retractor penis muscle and for penile erection. But it seems likely that the true mechanism includes a cholinergic inhibitory influence upon the function of postganglionic adrenergic neurons.

OTHER ASPECTS

It is well known that especially the vascular morphology of the penis exhibits wide species differences (Klinge, 1969; Kiss, 1921; Deysach, 1939; Conti, 1952; Watson, 1964). The vascular mechanisms of erection in bulls (Klinge, 1969; Lewis *et al.*, 1968; Watson, 1964) probably differ considerably from those in many smaller mammalian species (Dorr and Brody, 1967; Christensen, 1954; Newman *et al.*, 1964; Hart and Kitchell, 1966). This does not imply that the basic principles of the peripheral autonomic nervous mechanisms of erection show as high a degree of variation.

In Figs. 2 and 3 there is seen the particularly thick muscular wall in two close sections of the bull penile artery. The localization of the acetylcholinesterase-positive bundles of circular nerve fibres show some rough correspondence to noradrenaline fluorescence, although the latter seems to be more widespread. This may only indicate, however, that the technique used for induction of the monoamine fluorescence (Eränkö, 1967; Klinge *et al.*, 1970) is more sensitive than the method employed for staining cholinesterases (Karnovsky and Roots, 1964; Klinge *et al.*, 1970). The responses to drugs obtained at perfusion of the bull penile artery (Penttilä and Klinge, 1966; Penttilä, 1966) closely resemble those seen on stimulation of the isolated bull retractor penis muscle (Klinge, 1970 c).

Finally there may be substances not generally attributed to the function of the peripheral part of the autonomic nervous system that could exert an influence upon the degree of constriction of the penile artery. Such substances are, for instance, vasopressin and oxytocin. Intravenous injection of rather small doses of vasopressin or large doses of oxytocin induce a moderate engorgement of the penis in dogs (Holmquist and Olin, 1969), and large doses of these posterior pituitary hormones relax the bull retractor penis muscle *in vitro* (Klinge, 1970 c). It further has been demonstrated that intravenous administration of synthetic oxytocin to male rabbits increases their willingness to copulate (Fjellström *et al.*, 1968). These experiments indicate, but do not conclusively establish, that the posterior pituitary hormones may have some role in the physiological mechanism of erection. So far there is no precise suggestion for the locus and mode of their action. Low concentrations of the prostaglandins $E_1$ and $E_2$, on the other hand, considerably reduce the effect of postganglionic stimulation of adrenergic nerves on the guinea pig vas deferens (Euler and Hedquist, 1969) and the perfused rabbit heart (Wennmalm and Hedquist, 1970; Hedquist *et al.*, 1970). It is by no means certain that the prostaglandins are not involved in the physiological erection of the penis although intra-aortic administration of the prostaglandin E-217 failed to produce signs of erection in the canine penis (Dorr and Brody, 1967).

REFERENCES

ARMITAGE, A. K. AND BURN, J. H. (1967) *Brit. J. Pharmacol.*, **29**, 218.
BACQ, Z. M. (1935) *Arch. Intern. Physiol.*, **40**, 311.
BAUMGARTEN, H. G., FALCK, B. AND LANGE, W. (1969) *Z. Zellforsch.*, **95**, 58.
BIRMINGHAM, A. T. AND SZOLCSÁNYI, J. (1965) *J. Pharmacol.*, **17**, 449.
BURN, J. H. AND RAND, M. J. (1965) *Ann. Rev. Pharmacol.*, **5**, 163.
BURN, J. H. AND RAND, M. J. (1959) *Nature*, **184**, 163.
CHRISTENSEN, G. C. (1954) *Amer. J. Anat.*, **95**, 227.
CONTI, G. (1952) *Acta Anat.*, **14**, 217.
DALE, H. H. (1906) *J. Physiol.*, **34**, 163.
DORR, L. D. AND BRODY, M. J. (1967) *Amer. J. Physiol.*, **213**, 1526.
DEYSACH, L. J. (1939) *Amer. J. Anat.*, **64**, 111.
ECKHARD, C. (1863) *Beitr. zur Anat. Physiol. v. C. Eckhard*, III Band, Giessen.
EHINGER, B. AND FALCK, B. (1965) *Life Sci.*, **4**, 2097.
ERÄNKÖ, O. (1967) *Ann. Rev. Pharmacol.*, **1**, 203.
ERÄNKÖ, O. (1967) *J. Roy, Microscop. Soc.*, **87**, 259 .
ERÄNKÖ, O. AND HÄRKÖNEN, M. (1964) *Acta Physiol. Scand.*, **61**, 299.
ERÄNKÖ, O. AND RÄISÄNEN, L. (1965) *Acta Physiol. Scand.*, **63**, 505.
FJELLSTRÖM, D.KIHLSTRÖM J. E. AND MELIN, P., (1968) *J. Reprod. Fertil.*, **17**, 207.
GOLDENBERG, M. M. (1965) *Pharmacologist*, **7**, 158.
GOODMAN, L. S. AND GILMAN, A. (1965) *The Pharmacological Basis of Therapeutics*, The Macmillan
    Company, New York, p. 536.
GRIETEN, J. AND GEREBTZOFF, M.-A. (1956) *Ann. Histochim.* **2**, 127.
HART, B. L. AND KITCHELL, R. L. (1966) *Amer. J. Physiol.*, **210**, 257.
HEDQVIST, P., STJÄRNE, L. AND WENNMALM, Å. (1970) *Acta Physiol. Scand.*, **79**, 139.
HENDERSON, V. E. AND ROEPKE, M. H. (1933) *Amer. J. Physiol.*, **106**, 441.
HOLMQUIST, B. AND OLIN, T. (1969) *Scand. J. Urol. Nephrol.*, **3**, 291.
HUKOVIC, S. AND BUBIC, I. (1967) *Pathol.-Biol.*, **15**, 153.
JACOBOWITZ, D. AND KOELLE, G. B. (1965) *J. Pharmacol. exp. Therap.*, **148**, 225.
KARNOVSKY, M. J. AND ROOTS, L. (1964) *J. Histochem. Cytochem.*, **12**, 219.
KISS, F. G. (1921) *Z. Anat. Entwickl.-Gesch.*, **61**, 455.
KLINGE, E. (1969) *M.D. Thesis*, University of Helsinki.
KLINGE, E. (1970a) *Acta. Physiol. Scand.*, **78**, 103.
KLINGE, E. (1970b) *Acta Physiol. Scand.*, **78**, 159.
KLINGE, E. (1970c) *Acta Physiol. Scand.*, **78**, 280.
KLINGE, E. AND PENTTILÄ, O. (1969) *Ann. Med. exp. Fenn*, **47**, 17.
KLINGE, E. POHTO, P. AND SOLATUNTURI, E. (1970) *Acta Physiol. Scand.*, **78**, 110.
LANGLEY, J. N. AND ANDERSON, H. K. (1895) *J. Physiol.*, **19**, 85.
LEWIS, J. E. WALKER, D. F. BECKETT S. D. AND VACHON, (1968) *J. Reprod. Fertil.*, **17**, 155.
LÖFFELHOLZ, K. AND MUSCHOLL, E. (1969) *Naunyn-Schmiedeberg's Arch. Pharmakol.*, **265**, 1.
LUDUENA, F. P. AND GRIGAS, E. O. (1966) *Amer. J. Physiol.*, **210**, 435.
MALIK, K. U. AND LING, G. M. (1969) *Circulation. Res.*, **25**, 1.
NEWMAN, H. F. NORTHRUP, J. D. AND DEVLIN, J. (1964) *Invest. Urol.*, **1**, 350.
PENTTILÄ, O. AND KLINGE, E. (1966) *Acta Physiol. Scand.*, **68**, Suppl. 277, p. 159.
PENTTILÄ, O. (1966) *Ann. Med. exp. Fenn.*, **44** Suppl. 9.
ROOT, W. S. AND BARD, P. (1947) *Amer. J. Physiol.*, **151**, 80.
SEMANS, J. H. AND LANGWORTHY, O. R. (1938) *J. Urol.*, **40**, 836.
SJÖSTRAND, N. O. (1965) *Acta Physiol. Scand.*, **65**, Suppl. 257.
SJÖSTRAND, N. O. AND SWEDIN, G. (1968) *Acta Physiol. Scand.*, **72**, 370.
SPINA, A. (1897) *Wien. Med. Blätter*, **20**, 210.
STJÄRNE, L. AND LISHAJKO, F. (1966) *J. Neurochem.*, **13**, 1213.
THIELEN, P., RENDERS, M. AND RECTEM, D. (1969) *Arch. Intern. Physiol.*, **77**, 340.
ANREP, B. v. AND CYBULSKI, N. (1884) *St. Petersb. Med. Wochschr.*, **20**, 215.
EULER, U. S. v. AND HEDQVIST, P. (1969) *Acta Physiol. Scand.*, **77**, 510.
WATSON, J. W. (1964) *Nature*, **204**, 95.
WENNMALM, Å. AND HEDQVIST, P. (1970) *Life Sci.*, **9**, 931.
WHITELAW, G. P. AND SMITHWICK, R. H. (1951) *New Engl. J. Med.*, **245**, 121.

# Observations on the Nerve Terminals in the Neural Lobe of the Hypophysis of the Rat

LEENA RECHARDT

*Department of Anatomy, University of Helsinki, Helsinki (Finland)*

## INTRODUCTION

The main innervation of the neural lobe of the hypophysis of the rat is supplied by two paired hypothalamic nuclei, the supraoptic and paraventricular nuclei (Bargmann, 1954). Their axonal nerve fibres, which end in the pericapillary spaces of the neural lobe, contain large neurosecretory granules measuring over 1000 Å in diameter. These granules carry the neurohypophyseal hormones to be liberated into blood stream. The number of granules decreases under various stress situations, as for example in the axonal nerve fibers of dehydrated animals (Reinhardt *et al.*, 1969). The same neurosecretory endings also contain clear vesicles of the same size and appearance as real presynaptic endings, which function in synaptic transmission (Palay, 1957; De Robertis, 1962). Recently, Cannata and Tramezzani (1969) reported four types of nerve endings in the neural lobe of the rat. The differentiation was based on the distribution of several types of granules and vesicles in individual nerve endings.

Evidence is accumulating which indicates that the release of the neurohypophyseal hormones of mammals is under cholinergic and adrenergic control. Acetylcholine, cholineacetyltransferase and acetylcholinesterase, which are the essential components required in cholinergic transmission are all biochemically determined in this hormone-secreting organ (LaBella and Shin, 1968; Lederis and Livingston, 1968). As far as we know, however, there is no postsynaptic site in the neural lobe, although the reported findings suggest the presence of real cholinergic neurons.

At the light-microscopic level there are differing reports as to the presence of histochemically detectable cholinesterase activity. The differences are obviously due to the relatively low level of activity, to differences in the techniques used, and the use of different animal species. One of the earliest demonstrations of cholinesterase activity in the neural lobe of the cat was reported by Koelle and Geesey in 1961. They found low enzymatic activity, which was hard to localize at the light microscopic level in any definite structures.

With the specific fluorescence technique it has been possible to demonstrate a relatively rich network of fluorescent fibres. These observations suggest aminergic innervation of the neural lobe of the rat (Björklund, 1968). Some fluorescent fibers, possibly of sympathetic origin, were earlier localized around blood vessels (Fuxe, 1964; Dahlström and Fuxe, 1966).

*References p. 431*

On the basis of biochemical assays the amines in the neural lobe were mainly dopamine, but noradrenaline and 5-hydroxytryptamine were also found in lower concentrations (Björklund, 1968).

The distribution and localization of these possible 'transmitter' substances in the neurosecretory endings have not yet been determined. In the present paper an electron-microscopic cholinesterase technique was applied in addition to some morphological studies in order to identify different nerve endings in the neural lobe.

## MATERIAL AND METHODS

Adult male albino rats of the Sprague–Dawley strain weighing about 250 g were used. For ultrastructural studies two kinds of fixatives were employed: 2.5% purified glutaraldehyde in 0.1 M phosphate buffer, and 2–3% potassium permanganate in 0.1 M phosphate buffer (Richardson, 1964). These fixatives were perfused *via* the left ventricle under chloral hydrate anaesthesia and artificial respiration by cannulating the trachea. Combined fixative including 3.5% formaldehyde prepared from paraform-aldehyde powder and 1% purified glutaraldehyde in 0.1 M phosphate buffer was used in the enzyme studies (Karnovsky, 1965). Postfixation with $OsO_4$, embedding and poststaining with lead citrate (Reynolds, 1963) were performed in the regular manner. Ultra-thin sections in which histochemical reactions were carried out were examined unstained.

Cholinesterases were demonstrated using the thiocholine-based technique of Gomori-Koelle (Koelle, 1951) and its modification (Karnovsky and Roots, 1964) at the fine structure level. In this modification copper ferrocyanide forms the end product, and in order to reduce the crystal size a further modification was made as suggested by Kokko *et al.* (1969). The substrates were acetylthiocholine iodide and butyrylthiocholine iodide (Fluka AG., Buchs), and the studies incorporated the specific inhibitors iso-OMPA $10^{-5}$ and $10^{-6}$ M (L.Light & Co. Ltd., Colnbrook, England), 284 C51 $10^{-5}$ M (Wellcome Research Laboratories, England) and eserine $10^{-5}$ M.

Serpasil$^R$ (Ciba) was given 5 mg/kg i.p. on three consecutive days before the animal was sacrificed.

## RESULTS

Three types of nerve endings were observed in electron micrographs: (1) Large nerve endings which contained only neurosecretory granules of variable electron density; (2) smaller endings which, in addition, contained clear synaptic-like vesicles of 400–500 Å size; and (3) a third type of nerve ending containing dense-cored vesicles of 800–1400 Å size with clear synaptic-like vesicles .Type 1 and 2 endings formed the main part of the nervous network around the capillaries and pituicytes. Type 3 endings were scarce and were scattered in the network of the terminal bulbs. They were not seen more often near capillaries. In Fig. 1 we can see all three types in the same electron micrograph. Large dense-cored vesicles did not disappear after reserpine treatment. This finding is illustrated in Fig. 2.

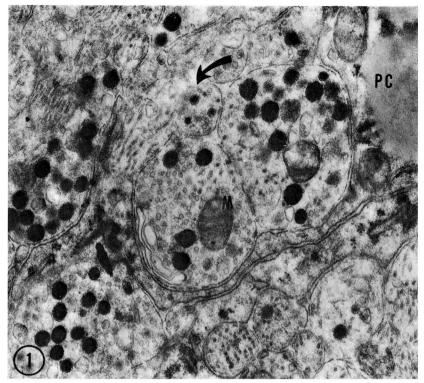

Fig. 1. Large neurosecretory granules are seen in other nerve endings except in the one indicated by an arrow. In this nerve terminal three large dense-cored vesicles are observed. Glutaraldehyde and $OsO_4$ fixation. Lead citrate poststaining. M = mitochondrion; PC = pericapillary space. × 2800.

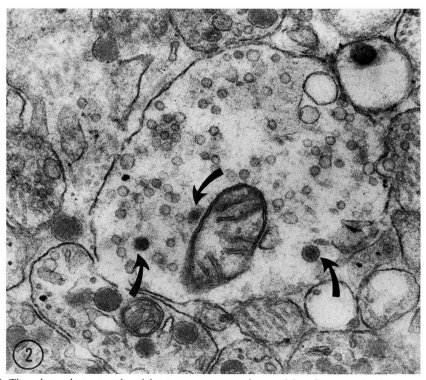

Fig. 2. Three large dense-cored vesicles are seen among clear vesicles after reserpine treatment. No large neurosecretory granules are visible in this type of nerve ending. Specimen was prepared as in Fig. 1. × 4600.

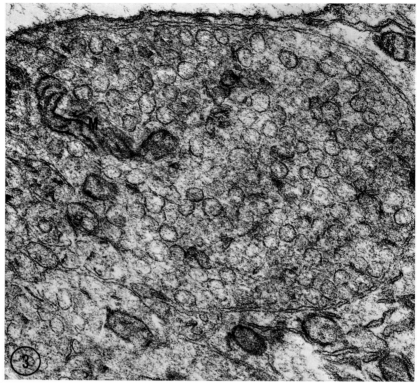

Fig. 3. Neurosecretory granules which fill a large nerve ending have lost their electron-dense granular core. 2% potassium permanganate fixation. No poststaining. × 15 000.

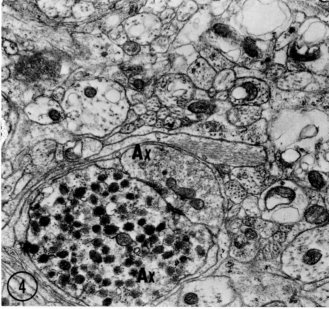

Fig. 4. An axo-axonal synaptic contact is seen in the area of the supraoptic nucleus of the hypo-thalamus. Specimen was prepared as in Fig. 1. Ax = axon. × 18 000.

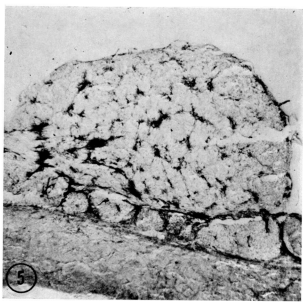

Fig. 5. A light-microscopic view of the neural and intermediate lobes of the hypophysis of the rat. In the lower part of the picture a part of the anterior lobe is also seen. In the neural lobe a network of fibres which show reaction product of the cholinesterase reaction is observed. In the intermediate lobe the positive fibres encircle larger cell groups. Fixation in formaldehyde–glutaraldehyde mixture. Incubation in Gomori–Koelle's medium for 8 h. Acetylthiocholine as a substrate and iso-OMPA $10^{-6}$ M as an inhibitor. × 100.

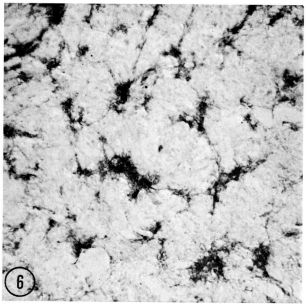

Fig. 6. A light-microscopic view with higher magnification of the cholinesterase reaction. Cholinesterase-positive fibres are observed to accumulate in the neighborhood of blood vessels. Specimen was prepared as in Fig. 5. ×300.

References p. 431

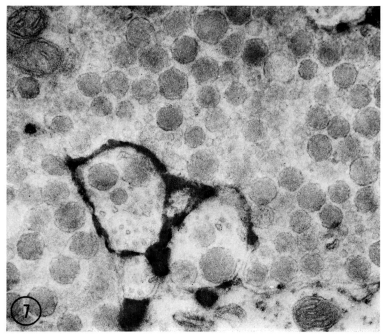

Fig. 7. Electron-microscopic view of acetylcholinesterase activity in the neural lobe of the hypo-physis of the rat. Reaction product is localized around three small nerve endings. These are surrounded by larger neurosecretory endings which show no reaction product in their axon membranes. The specimen was fixed with glutaraldehyde–formaldehyde perfusion; incubated in Karnovsky–Roots' medium for 1 h. Acetylthiocholine as a substrate and iso-OMPA $10^{-5}$ M as an inhibitor. Refixed in $OsO_4$. No poststaining. $\times$ 30 000.

So far no small dense-cored vesicles have been found in potassium permanganate-fixed specimens. After this fixation procedure large neurosecretory granules were empty as the protein moiety had possibly been washed out as seen in Fig. 3.

Special attention was given to the matter of finding synaptic contacts on axonal bulbs or pituicytes, however none were found. In the hypothalamic area, where the neurosecretory axons have just grown out from their neuronal bodies, axo-axonal synapses were observed. An axo-axonal synapse is seen in Fig. 4.

### Cholinesterase activity

At the light-microscopic level both the Gomori–Koelle method and its Karnovsky–Roots modification gave the same results. With acetylthiocholine as a substrate and iso-OMPA $10^{-6}$ M as an inhibitor for non-specific cholinesterase it was possible to demonstrate a specific acetylcholinesterase activity. The reaction product was shown in delicate and coarser fibres in the neural lobe as well as in the intermediate lobe (Fig. 5). With higher magnification in Fig. 6 the positively stained fibres are localized in the neighborhood of blood vessels. When butyrylthiocholine was used as a substrate and 284 C51 $10^{-5}$ M as an inhibitor no activity was detected even with prolonged incubation times (16 hours in Gomori–Koelle's medium).

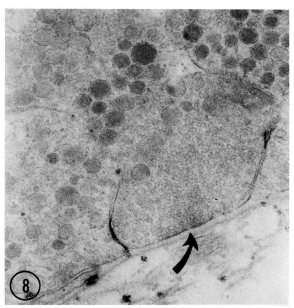

Fig. 8. Reaction product is seen only in some parts of the axon membrane of the neurosecretory ending. Observe the large number of clear vesicles and a faint synaptic-like thickening indicated by an arrow. Procedures as in Fig. 7. × 28 000.

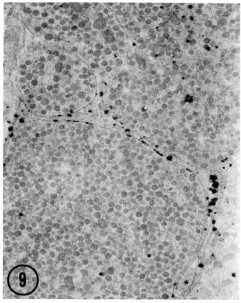

Fig. 9. In this picture large neurosecretory endings show some reaction product in their axon membranes. Usually they were devoid of any activity. No activity is observed inside the axons and in the neurosecretory granules. Procedures as in Fig. 7. × 6 200.

At the fine-structure level the end-product of the cholinesterase reaction, copper ferrocyanide, was localized as a fine crystalline precipitate in the membranes of the smaller nerve endings. These endings contained clear synaptic-like vesicles. In Fig.7 two nerve terminals with reaction product are surrounded by larger negative-looking nerve terminals. These positive fibres were found near a capillary and its pericapillary space. The reaction product was also localized in some fibres as a discontinuous line as seen in Fig. 8. The nerve ending in this picture seems to be crowded with clear vesicles and a faint synaptic-like thickening was observed. Larger nerve terminals which contained only neurosecretory granules were mainly devoid of activity but sometimes a faint reaction product was localized in their membranes as seen in Fig. 9.

Pituicytes were negative. There was some randomly scattered reaction product in the capillaries without any special localization. When butyrylthiocholine with 284 C51 was used in the incubation medium, no positive-reacting nerve fibres were detected. Eserine $10^{-5}$ M in the incubation medium inhibited the enzymatic reaction although some randomly scattered crystals were seen.

### DISCUSSION

On the basis of morphological studies it seems obvious that different types of nerve endings exist in the neural lobe of the rat. Knowles (1965) reported two separate nerve fibre systems in fishes. He suggested that the fibres without large neurosecretory granules might be involved in the release of the hormones. Lederis and Livingston (1968) could demonstrate biochemically that in the rabbit a portion of the acetylcholine activity was in endings other than those containing hormones. By using acetyl-cholinesterase techniques at the fine-structure level we have been able to elucidate further the differences between the different nerve endings. Acetylcholinesterase activity was mainly localized around the small-diameter nerve endings which contained clear synaptic-like vesicles believed to be the site of acetylcholine (Gerschenfeld *et al.*, 1960; Lederis and Livingston, 1968). In addition, reaction product resulting from enzymatic activity was found to be located around the endings which contained both small clear vesicles and neurosecretory granules. Thus it was not possible to identify only one type of acetylcholinesterase-positive fibres. Acetylcholinesterase reaction was, however, correlated with the presence of small clear vesicles in the nerve terminals. The large end bulbs crowded with neurosecretory granules were essentially devoid of reaction product.

Nerve endings with small dense-cored vesicles generally believed to contain amines were not found with the techniques used. Large dense-cored vesicles which were observed among the clear ones did not respond to reserpinization and obviously are not the site of amines demonstrated by fluorescence microscope by Björklund (1968). It is possible that the clear vesicles in the neural lobe as in the median eminence of the rat are the site of amines (Hökfelt, 1967). Because acetylcholinesterase is localized around these endings, which may also contain amines, the situation is the same as in the pineal body of the rat in which acetylcholinesterase-positive fibres with small dense-cored vesicles were recently demonstrated (Eränkö *et al.*, 1970).

No real synaptic contacts were observed in the neural lobe. Because axo-axonal synapses were found in the hypothalamic area (Rechardt, 1969), the neurosecretory fibres seem to be influenced at that level by direct nervous stimuli.

The functions of acetylcholine and acetylcholinesterase in the neural lobe are not fully understood. According to Koelle, acetylcholine is involved in the release of another transmitter substance, in this case the hormones to be liberated from the neurosecretory granules (see *e.g.* Koelle, 1969). Acetylcholine might also stimulate the release of amines or unknown transmitter substances yet unidentified. On the other hand, it has been suggested that acetylcholinesterase is not necessarily needed to destroy acetylcholine (see Lederis and Livingston, 1969; Cottle and Silver, 1970). In the neural lobe the function of acetylcholinesterase in the permeability changes of the membranes of neurosecretory endings and the blood vessels would be well adapted.

## REFERENCES

BARGMANN, W., (1954); *Das Zwischenhirn-Hypophysensystem*, Springer-Verlag, Berlin–Göttingen–Heidelberg.

BJÖRKLUND, A. (1968); *Z. Zellforsch.*, **89**, 573–589.

BJÖRKLUND, A., FALCK, B., HROMEK, F., OWMAN, CH. AND WEST, K. A., (1970); *Brain Res.*, **17**, 1–23.

CANNATA, M. A. AND TRAMEZZANI, J. A. (1969); *Experientia*, **25**, 1281–1282.

COTTLE, M. K. W. AND SILVER, A., (1970); *Z. Zellforsch.*, **103**, 570–588.

DAHLSTRÖM, A. AND FUXE, K. (1966); *Acta Endocrinol.*, **51**, 301–314.

DE ROBERTIS, E., (1962); Ultrastructure and function in some neurosecretory systems. In H. HELLER AND R. B. CLARK, (Eds.), *Neurosecretion*, No. **12**, Academic Press, London and New York, pp. 3–20.

ERÄNKÖ, O., RECHARDT, L., ERÄNKÖ, L. AND CUNNINGHAM, A. (1970); *Histochem. J.*, in press.

FUXE, K., (1964); *Z. Zellforsch.* **61**, 710–724.

GERSCHENFELD, H. M., TRAMEZZANI, J. H. AND DE ROBERTIS, E., (1960); *Endocrinology*, **66**, 741–762.

HÖKFELT, T. (1967); *Brain Res.*, **5**, 121–123.

KARNOVSKY, M. J. (1965); *J. Cell Biol.*, **27**, 137–138 A.

KARNOVSKY, M. J. AND ROOTS, L., (1964); *J. Histochem. Cytochem.*, **12**, 219–221.

KNOWLES, F. (1965); *Arch. Anat. Microscop. Morphol. Exp.*, **54**, 343–358.

KOELLE, G. B. (1951); *J. Pharmacol. Exp. Therap.*, **103**, 153–171.

KOELLE, G. B. (1969); *Federation Proc.*, **28**, 95–100.

KOELLE, G. B. AND GEESEY, C. N., (1961); Localization of acetylcholinesterase in the neurohypophysis and its functional implications. *Proc. Soc. Exp. Biol.*, **106**, 625–628.

KOKKO, A. MAUTNER, H. G., AND BARRNETT, R. J., (1969); *J. Histochem. Cytochem.*, **17**, 625–640.

LABELLA, F. S. AND SHIN, S., (1968); *J. Neurochem.*, **15**, 335–342.

LEDERIS, K. AND LIVINGSTON, A., (1968); In *Proc. Physiol. Soc., J. Physiol.*, **196**, 34–36P.

LEDERIS, K. AND LIVINGSTON, A., (1969); *J. Physiol.*, **201**, 695–709.

PALAY, S. L., (1957); The fine structure of the neurohypophysis. In WAELSCH, H. (Ed.), *Ultrastructure and Cellular Chemistry of Neural Tissues*, (*Progress in Neurobiology*, Vol. **2**, KOREY S. R. AND NURNBERGER, J. I. (Ed.), Hoeber, New York, pp. 31–49.

RECHARDT, L., (1969); *Acta Physiol. Scand.*, Suppl. **329**, 1–79.

REINHARDT, H. F. HENNING, L. CH. AND ROHR, H. P., (1969); *Z. Zellforsch.*, **102**, 182–192.

REYNOLDS, E. S. (1963); *J. Cell Biol.*, **17**, 208–212.

RICHARDSON, K. C. (1964); *Amer. J. Anat.*, **114**, 173–206.

# The Postnatal Development of Monoamines and Cholinesterases in the Paracervical Ganglion of the Rat Uterus

LASSE KANERVA

*Department of Anatomy, University of Helsinki, Siltavuorenpenger 20*
*Helsinki 17 ( Finland)*

## INTRODUCTION

The first critical and one of the most detailed descriptions of the innervation of the female internal genital organs is that by Frankenhäuser (1867). Langley and Andersson (1894–1896) correlated the work of previous investigators and presented their own experiments in a series of papers in 1894–1896. These studies form the basis of modern descriptions of these nerves in laboratory animals and in man. Other important contributions are contained in the reviews of Davis (1933), Krantz (1959), Reynolds (1965), Sjöberg (1967) and Marshall (1970).

It is now generally acknowledged that the preganglionic fibres of the pelvic adrenergic nerves may synapse with their postganglionic neurons in a variety of locations including the lumbar vertebral ganglia, the inferior mesenteric ganglia, ganglia in the pelvic plexus and ganglia in or near the pelvic viscera. Utilizing fluorescence histochemical techniques, morphological evidence for the presence of adrenergic ganglia peripheral to the inferior mesenteric ganglia has recently been obtained, and it has been shown that adrenergic and cholinergic ganglion cells are found in the utero-vaginal junction (Owman *et al.*, 1966; Rosengren and Sjöberg, 1967; Owman and Sjöberg, 1967; Sjöberg, 1967, 1968; Kanerva, 1970).

The peripheral adrenergic neurons in or near the pelvic viscera have been termed 'short adrenergic neurons' by Owman and Sjöstrand (1965) to distinguish them from the 'long adrenergic neurons' arising in the vertebral and inferior mesenteric ganglia. The short neurons are believed to represent a special type of ganglion cell resembling in location the cholinergic (parasympathetic) ganglia. Thus far they have been found in the urogenital tract of the male as well as of the female.

The 'short' neurons are both functionally and anatomically different from the 'long' adrenergic neurons. Firstly, the noradrenaline-containing granules have a much slower rate of spontaneous release of noradrenaline than granules isolated from the splenic nerves (Euler and Lishajko, 1966; Stjärne and Lishajko, 1966). Secondly, after a single injection of reserpine, the noradrenaline concentration in the uterine adrenergic nerves of the rabbit declines at a much slower rate than in the adrenergic

*References pp. 443–444*

nerves in the heart and spleen (Nilsson, 1964). Thirdly, during the first stage of pregnancy there is a prominent increase in the noradrenaline content in the uterus. A marked increase was also registered in the uterus after treatment of non-pregnant rabbits with $17\beta$-estradiol. The increased noradrenaline content manifested itself as an increased number of adrenergic nerves with a clearly visible fluorescence. This might represent a further functional parameter distinguishing 'short adrenergic neurons' from ordinary 'long adrenergic neurons' (Sjöberg, 1967).

In addition to adrenergic ganglion cells and their peripheral neurons, another type of catecholamine-containing cell has been found within or close to the paracervical ganglion (Owman and Sjöberg, 1966; Rosengren and Sjöberg, 1967; Sjöberg, 1968; Kanerva, 1971). These cells were first described in the superior cervical ganglion (Eränkö and Härkönen, 1963, 1965a, b; Norberg and Hamberger, 1964; Jacobowitz and Woodward, 1968) then in other ganglia such as the ganglia of the urogenital tract of different male mammals (Owman and Sjöstrand, 1965), the intrapancreatic ganglion (Alm *et al.*, 1967) and the heart ganglia (Jacobowitz, 1967). The identity of these cells, first called 'small, intensely fluorescent cells' (SIF cells) by Eränkö and Härkönen (1965), is not fully understood; they possess properties similar to both 'chromaffin cells' and nerve cells. In microspectrofluorometric studies Norberg *et al.* (1966) demonstrated that SIF cells store a primary catecholamine in the rat ganglia. They could not however decide whether this amine was noradrenaline or dopamine. Recently Björklund *et al.* (1968) have differentiated these two primary catecholamines by means of microspectrofluorometry. According to Björklund *et al.* (1970) the SIF cells in the sympathetic chain ganglia of the pig, the cat and the rat contain dopamine, while Eränkö and Eränkö (1971) have found noradrenaline in the SIF cells of the superior cervical ganglion of the rat.

Electron microscopically small ganglion cells which structurally resemble the 'chromaffin' cells of the carotid and aortic bodies and the adrenal medulla have also been found in the superior cervical ganglion (Grillo, 1966; Siegrist *et al.*, 1968; Williams and Palay, 1969; Matthews and Raisman, 1969), in the inferior mesenteric ganglion (Elfvin, 1968) and in the paracervical ganglion (Kanerva, 1971).

The functional significance of these cells is not known, but there are many hypotheses as to their function. From electrophysiological studies carried out on sympathetic ganglia of rabbits and turtles, Eccles and Libet (1961) formed the opinion that the preganglionic stimulation causes the 'chromaffin cell' (in fact the small, intensely fluorescent cell?) to liberate adrenaline, and this, after diffusing to a site on a ganglion cell, hyperpolarizes it and so modifies its response to preganglionic signals. From morphological considerations, Williams and Palay (1969) classified the small granule-containing cells (electron microscopically) as interneurons which receive and transmit impulses from preganglionic sympathetic fibres to small nerve processes within the ganglion. According to these authors, the function may be to provide negative feed-back to the ganglionic neurons, thus limiting their dependence on direct signals from the preganglionic neuron. Siegrist *et al.* (1968) also suggested that these cells play an important part in the control of inhibitory transmission through the ganglion, but also supported a possible endocrine function which had been proposed by Eränkö and

Härkönen (1965 b) in the small cells of the superior cervical ganglion. Finally, Terä-väinen (1970) has presented a new hypothesis as to the function of the small, intensely fluorescent cells in the paracervical ganglia, according to which these cells could induce uterine contractions humorally by mediating biogenic monoamines under hormonal (estrogen) control.

It has been known for some time that stimulation of the hypogastric nerves causes the uterus to contract or to relax depending upon the appropriate species and the endocrine state of the individual (*cf.* Marshall, 1970), but the precise role of the adrenergic nerves, when stimulated at physiological frequencies, in the functional activity of the uterus has not been identified. On the other hand, most of the electro-physiological work using stimulation of the parasympathetic nerves has failed to cause action potentials in the uterus (*e.g.* Bower, 1966). However, some reports have also appeared favouring the parasympathetic nervous system control of the uterine function. After experiments including nerve section, electrical and pharmacological nerve stimulation and acetylcholine depletion, Shabanah *et al.* (1964) reported an important role for the parasympathetic system in myometrial activity and blood flow. Mustonen and Teräväinen (1971) studied the fine structure of synapses in the para-cervical ganglion and observed degenerative nerve endings to the ganglion cells after both sympathectomy and parasympathectomy. The results were interpreted as indicating both sympathetic and parasympathetic innervation of the ganglion cells sending their axons to the uterus.

The first attempt at solving the cholinergic part of the neurons of the paracervical ganglion was made by Mäkelä and Grönroos (1959), who were able to distinguish within the ganglion both acetylcholinesterase-containing neurons and neurons devoid of AChE activity. According to Teräväinen and Mustonen (1970) about one fifth of the ganglion cells exhibit an intense cytoplasmic acetylcholinesterase (AChE) activity. It was suggested that these cells were cholinergic. The rest of the ganglion cells contained moderate to weak AChE activity. In some of these cells, about one third of the ganglion cells, AChE-containing nerves and sites presumed to be synapses were observed in the region of their cell membrane. These ganglion cells were also presumed to be cholinergic and to receive cholinergic synapses. A minor part of the cholinergic neurons according to Teräväinen and Mustonen (1970), were surrounded by intensely fluorescent nerves and were thus hypothesized to be innervated by adrener-gic, presumably inhibitory nerves. The 'chromaffin cells' did not exhibit AChE activity. Non-specific cholinesterases (ns-ChE) were mainly localized in the glial cells around the nerves, the ganglion cells and the 'chromaffin cells'.

The purpose of this paper is to study the developmental aspects of this interesting ganglion, using the formaldehyde-induced fluorescence method (Eränkö, 1955, 1967; Falck, *et al.*, 1962) for histochemical demonstration of catecholamines and the copper thiocholine method (Koelle, 1951; Gomori, 1952) for localization of cholinesterases.

An abstract has previously been published (Kanerva, 1970).

## MATERIAL AND METHODS

### Cholinesterase histochemistry

Rats of different ages were used. The ages and number of rats per group were: 0 days, 5; 1 day, 5; 2 days, 3; 5 days, 3; 10 days, 3; 15 days, 3; 20 days, 3; 22 days, 3; 24 days, 3; 26 days, 3; 28 days, 3; 30 days, 3; 35 days, 3; 40 days, 3; 60 days, 3; 90 days or older, 15. The animals were killed by a blow on the head. The caudal part of the uterus and the paracervical ganglia were quickly excised and immediately fixed at 4° for 6 h in a solution containing 3.5% neutralized formaldehyde and 1% $CaCl_2$, followed by washing for 12–16 h in 0.1 M phosphate buffer at pH 7.4 at 4°. The specimens were sectioned frozen at 15–20 $\mu$m, and while still frozen, placed on slides, allowed to melt, and carried through the various steps on the slides. Acetylcholinesterase (AChE) activity was demonstrated with acetylthiocholine iodide (Fluka AG, Buchs) as a substrate and $10^{-5}$ M iso-OMPA (tetra-isopropylpyrophosphoramide: L. Light & Co., Ltd., Colnbrook) in the incubation solution to inhibit any other (non-specific) cholinesterase activity (ns-ChE). The method used was based on the Gomori variation (1952) of the Koelle (1951) technique. Butyrylthiocholine iodide (Fluka AG., Buchs) was used to demonstrate ns-ChE activity with $10^{-5}$ M 284 C51 in the incubation solution for the inhibition of AChE activity. Preincubation for 30 min with the inhibitor was used in the experiment after which period the substrates used were added. The specimens were incubated for 16 h in all the experiments. The inhibitory effect was assured by using both iso-OMPA and 284 C51 simultaneously in the incubation solution with acetylthiocholine substrate. These were negative.

### Fluorescence histochemistry

Rats (Sprague–Dawley) of different ages were used. The ages and number of rats per group were: 0 days (newborn), 10; 1 day, 5; 2 days, 5; 5 days, 10; 10 days, 5; 15 days, 5; 20 days, 5; 25 days, 5; 30 days, 5; 60 days, 5; 90 days or older, 20. The animals were killed by a blow on the head. The paracervical ganglia of both sides of the uterus were rapidly removed together with a small piece of parametrium and immediately cut into small blocks. The formaldehyde-induced fluorescence method was used for the histochemical demonstration of biogenic amines as described previously from this laboratory (Eränkö, 1967). Small blocks of tissue were rapidly frozen in propane cooled by liquid nitrogen, freeze-dried *in vacuo* in a desiccator containing phosphorus pentoxide for 7 days at —45° C, treated with gaseous formaldehyde, previously equilibrated with 40% relative humidity, for $\frac{1}{2}$ h at 40° C and $\frac{1}{2}$ h at 80° C. The specimens were embedded in paraffin wax and sectioned serially. Fluorescence microscopy was carried out using deparaffinized sections mounted in xylene. A Wild microscope was employed featuring a HBO-200 mercury lamp and Schott BG 38, 12 and two OG 1 filters.

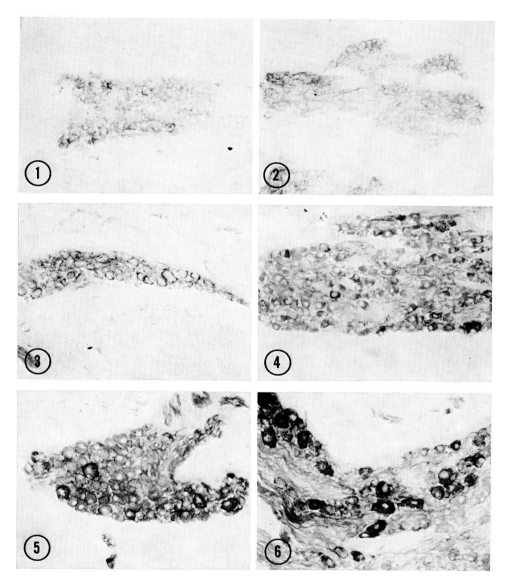

Figs. 1–6. AChE activity in cells of the developing paracervical ganglion of the rat uterus. (× 170) Fig. 1. Newborn rat. Weak AChE activity in the periphery of the cells. Fig. 2. 5-day-old rat. The same localization as in the newborn. Fig. 3. 10-day-old rat. Stronger activity in the ganglion cell membrane and weak activity in the cytoplasm. Fig. 4. 20-day-old rat. A marked increase in the AChE activity of the cytoplasm. Fig. 5. 24-day-old rat. The ganglion cells with stronger AChE activity are surrounded by AChE-containing nerves, and positive sites presumed to be synapses are observed in the region of their cell membrane. Fig. 6. 30-day-old rat. The same appearance as in the adult rat. About one fifth to one third of the cells exhibit intense cytoplasmic AChE activity.

*Cholinesterases*

*Acetylcholinesterase*

The ganglia were localized close to the utero-vaginal junction on either side of the cervix. Each was composed of one larger mass of ganglion cells and sometimes two or more smaller paraganglia. Weak acetylcholinesterase (AChE) activity was observed in the ganglion cells of the newborn rat (Fig. 1). The activity was concentrated in the periphery of the cells. This gave the ganglion a honeycomb appearance. The AChE activity of the ganglion remained at the same low level in 1-, 2- and 5-day- (see Fig. 2 for 5-day-old specimen). The cells grew in size and the AChE activity became stronger. In 10-day-old rats (Fig. 3), the activity in the cell membrane and around the cells was stronger and some weak activity could also be seen in the cytoplasm. After this the activity increased in the cytoplasm. In the ganglion of 20-day-old rats fairly high activity was seen in all the ganglion cells (Fig. 4). Some of the ganglion cells showed slightly stronger activity than the other cells. The difference between the activity in the individual cells became much clearer during the next ten days. In the 24-day-old rats (Fig. 5) the cells with the strongest AChE activity could be seen to be surrounded by a strong cholinergic nerve net. The nerve net around the cells with moderate activity showed weaker activity. In 30-day-old rats (Fig. 6), the paracervical ganglion had the same appearance as in the adult rat, but the activity became even stronger with age. About one fifth to one third of the cells exhibited intense cytoplasmic AChE activity. These cells were large and received AChE-containing nerves. The rest of the ganglion cells showed moderate to weak AChE activity. No 'chromaffin cells' could be distinguished with certainty.

*Non-specific cholinesterase*

In the paracervical ganglion of the newborn rat (Fig. 7) the distribution of non-specific cholinesterases (ns-ChE) was very much the same as the distribution of AChE, *i.e.* in the periphery of the cells. The same localization was seen in the ganglia of the 1-, 2-, 5- and 10-day-old rats (see Fig. 8 for 2-day-old specimen) but the activity became stronger than the AChE activity and it became apparent that it was situated in the intercellular tissue containing satellite cells, Schwann cells, pre- and postganglionic axons, dendrites and capillaries. In 15-day-old rats (Fig. 9) this was already clear, and a very weak activity could also be found in the cytoplasm. After this there was a great increase in the activity of the ns-ChE in the interstitial tissue. All the ganglion cells were surrounded by strong ns-ChE activity. The adult pattern was already visible at the age of 20 days (Fig. 10, 22 days), but the activity became even stronger and the ganglion cells grew considerably in size (Fig. 11, 28 days and Fig. 12, adult rat).

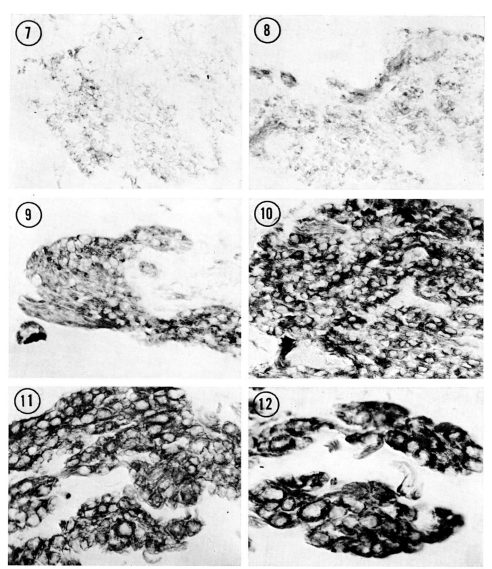

Figs. 7–12. Non-specific cholinesterase activity in a cell of the developing paracervical ganglion of the rat uterus. ($\times$ 170) Fig. 7. Newborn rat, and Fig. 8, 2-day-old rat. The distribution of ns-ChE is reminiscent of the distribution of AChE in the same age group. Fig. 9. 15-day-old rat. Ns-ChE is localized in the interstitial tissue. Weak activity can be seen in the cytoplasm of the cells. Fig. 10. 22-day-old rat. Relatively strong activity in the interstitial tissue. Fig. 11. 28-day-old rat, and Fig. 12, adult rat. The localization remains the same during later development, but activity increases.

## Catecholamines

The ganglion consisted of two kinds of cells exhibiting specific formaldehyde-induced fluorescence: cells with a relatively weak greenish fluorescence and small cells with an intense yellowish fluorescence (SIF cells). Even at birth these two different kinds of

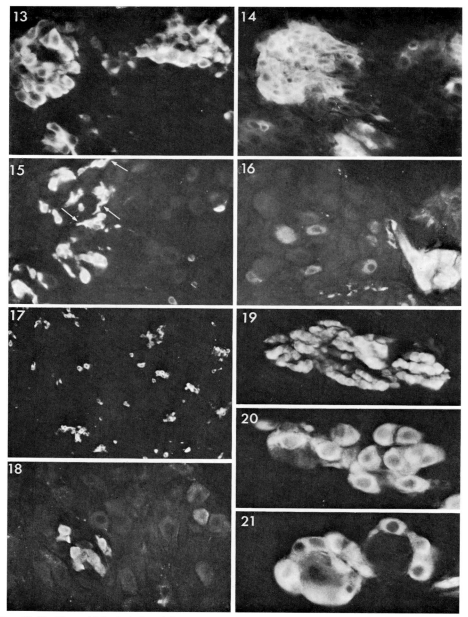

Figs. 13–21. Formaldehyde-induced fluorescence in the paracervical ganglion of the rat uterus. Fig. 13. Newborn rat. Clusters of small, intensely yellowish fluorescing cells. The weak fluorescence in the ganglion cells cannot be seen because when exposed to UV-light it rapidly faded away. × 600. Fig. 14. 5-day-old rat. A big cluster of small, intensely fluorescing cells. The immature ganglion cells can be seen showing weak fluorescence. × 900. Fig. 15. 15-day-old rat. SIF cells among and around ganglion cells. The SIF cells are seen to send processes (arrows). Some of the ganglion cells are devoid of fluorescence, while others show moderate fluorescence. × 300. Fig. 16. 30-day-old rat. A big cluster of SIF cells on one edge of the ganglion. The ganglion cells show slightly stronger fluorescence than in the previous figure. The intensity varies between individual cells. × 300.

Figs. 17–21. Adult rat. Fig. 17. Large amounts of SIF cells in small clusters or singly in the ganglion. The background appears black because of underexposure to avoid overexposure of the SIF cells. × 200. Fig. 18. The ganglion cells show moderate or weak fluorescence. Some autofluorescent granules are seen in some of the ganglion cells. In the center, SIF cells. × 300. Fig. 19. A big group of SIF cells in the connective tissue outside the ganglion. × 300. Fig. 20. SIF cells at a higher magnification in the ganglion. × 900. Fig. 21. Two ganglion cells surrounded by SIF cells. One of the ganglion cells shows fluorescence. The other is devoid of fluorescence. × 900.

cells could be differentiated (Fig. 13). Great numbers of SIF cells were seen in the paracervical ganglion. These cells were often arranged in big clusters with more than fifty cells in a single section. The non-fluorescent nucleus was surrounded by a narrow ring of intensely fluorescent cytoplasm. These cells were also seen in small clusters (Fig. 17), standing alone (Fig. 17), around blood vessels, around weakly green'sh fluorescent (ganglion) cells (Fig. 21), in nerve bundles near the ganglion and also outside the ganglion in the connective tissue (Fig. 19). They were mostly round, but sometimes they were found to send out processes measuring 5–10 microns. The diameter of these cells was about 5–10 microns.

The ganglion cells with the weak greenish fluorescence made up the major part of the ganglion. In newborn rats the green fluorescence rapidly faded away when exposed to ultraviolet light. The intensity of the fluorescence was the same in all these cells, which were tightly packed together and had an immature appearance. These cells also had little cytoplasm. The diameter of the ganglion cell nucleus was 6–8 microns and the diameter of the whole cell 7–9 microns. The same appearance was seen in the 1-, 2- and 5-day-old (Fig. 14) ganglia. In the 5-day-old ganglion the greenish fluorescence did not fade away as quickly as in the newborn, suggesting a rise in catecholamine concentration. In 10-day-old rats differences were seen in the fluorescence intensity of individual cells. This was seen more clearly in 15-day-old rats (Fig. 15). The ganglion cells had increased in size, the cytoplasm in particular having become more prominent. The nucleus measured about 10 microns and the whole cell 15–17 microns in diameter. However, the intensely fluorescent cells remained small. The localization remained the same as in the newborn, but more separate cells were seen and these more often had a short process. In 20-, 25- and 30-day-old rats (Fig. 16) the picture was essentially the same. In the adult rat big clusters of small, intensely fluorescent cells were seldom seen. Figs. 17–21 show typical localizations of small, intensely fluorescent cells in the adult rat.

No granules with autofluorescence could be seen in the ganglion cells of the young rats. In 30-day-old rats some yellow autofluorescent granules could occasionally be found and the amount greatly increased with age, being highest in the oldest rat studied (one year). The granules were evenly d'spersed throughout the cell cytoplasm.

## DISCUSSION

Development of cholinesterase activity in the ganglia has been studied relatively little using histochemical methods. Light microscopy has been used to study this development in the dorsal root ganglion of the chicken (Strumia and Baima-Bollone, 1964) and of the rat (Kalina and Wolman, 1970), and electron microscopy in the dorsal root ganglion of the rabbit and the human fetus (Tennyson et al., 1968). An abstract has appeared from our laboratory concerning the development of the superior cervical ganglion (Eränkö, L., 1970).

Strumia and Baima-Bollone (1964) found a positive AChE reaction in the spinal ganglia of the chick embryo at the 4th incubation day. During the following 19 days a rise in intensity took place in the ganglia, However, immediately before and after hatching, there were few intensely reacting neurons and later the reaction was weak or wholly negative. The development of the dorsal root ganglion of the rat, reported to exhibit a positive AChE reaction by Kokko (1965), was studied by Kalina and Wolman (1970). Relatively high enzymatic activity was already seen in the 18-day-old fetus. No difference could be found between individual cells. Ns-ChE showed a weak diffuse reaction in all cells. With maturation the ganglion cells differentiated into 'light' (mostly large) and 'dark' (mostly small) cells. The differentiation was accompanied by higher AChE activity in the small than in the large neurons. With ns-ChE, maturation of the cells was accompanied by loss of activity in perikarya and increased activity in axons and satellite cells.

The cholinergic part of the uterine innervation has been presumed to be sympathetic because no action potentials have been observed after stimulation of the sacral parasympathetic nerves (Bowei, 1966; Theobald, 1968; see also INTRODUCTION).

Non-specific cholinesterase activity has been reported to be intense in the superior cervical ganglion (Eränkö, L., 1970) and moderate in the sensory ganglia (Kalina and Wolman, 1970) in almost all cells of newborn rats, weakening later and becoming limited to glial elements. In the present study, the ns-ChE activity was very low in the paracervical ganglion at birth, but gradually the glial elements showed a strong ns-ChE reaction. The ns-ChE activity might also have been higher in the cells of the paracervical ganglia, but the peak would have been before birth.

Using electron microscopy the development of cholinesterase activity has been studied in the neural tube and dorsal root ganglion of the rabbit embryo and human fetus (Tennyson et al., 1968). The enzyme appeared very early in development, just before the onset of morphological differentiation of the neuroblast. Activity appeared first in the nuclear envelope of a few scattered cells in the neural tube (10 days gestation). It was then found in the endoplasmic reticulum, particularly as differentiation proceeded. Shortly thereafter the enzyme could be found in cells migrating from the neural crest to form the dorsal root ganglion. No enzyme activity appeared in the satellite cells until later in development, when the neuroblasts differentiated into immature neurons. Neurons and axons of a human fetus of three month's gestation contained a high amount of cholinesterase activity in locations similar to those in the rabbit fetus. Tennyson's results (1968) concentrate on the young prenatal rabbit embryo and cannot be correlated with the observations obtained in this paper. An investigation of the ultrastructural localization of the cholinesterases in the paracervical ganglion and the superior cervical ganglion is in progress in our laboratory.

The development of the superior cervical ganglion using the formaldehyde-induced fluorescence method has been studied in our laboratory (Eränkö, L., 1970, a personal communication). Many of the developmental features of the paracervical ganglion described in this paper are the same. A gradual increase in the weakly greenish fluorescing cells can be seen, as well as great amounts of SIF cells. The localization of the SIF cells is partly the same in these two ganglia; they can be found around blood vessels, around ganglion cells and in nerve bundles near the ganglion. However, in the paracervical ganglion of the newborn rat the SIF cells were arranged in clusters containing more than fifty cells seen in a single section, and the impression was that the number of cells in the clusters became smaller with age. This is different from the case of the superior cervical ganglion (Eränkö, L., 1970, a personal communication) where the number of cells in the clusters increased with age. In the adult sympathetic chain ganglia of the pig and the cat, the SIF cells have been found to contain dopamine (Björklund et al., 1970). It has also been noted that the cervical part of the rat uterus contains an 'unexpectedly high amount of dopamine' (Swedin and Brundin, 1968). This might be due to the paracervical ganglia having been included in the piece of cervix studied. But it is not known what catecholamine these small, intensely fluorescent cells contain in the younger rat, nor is it known whether all these intensely fluorescent cells are of the same cell type. That they are not is suggested by divergent observations of Björklund et al. (1970), who report the presence of dopamine, and Eränkö and Eränkö (1971), who found noradrenaline. This is of interest in view of our preliminary ultrastructural observations of the paracervical ganglion in the newborn rat suggesting the presence of more than one kind of cell type containing many large dense-cored vesicles. Some of the small, intensely fluorescent cells might also be sympathico-blasts. Wechsler and Schmekel (1967) studied the ultrastructure of the sympathetic and spinal ganglion in developing chicks. They found a vast number of large dense-cored vesicles (600–1200 Å) already present in the 4½-day-old chicken embryo. In the 3-, 4- and 7-week-old chicks the dense-cored vesicles were not seen as often as in the embryo. In the rat embryo, there are a vast number of small, intensely fluorescent cells in the sympathetic chain (Hervonen and Kanerva, unpublished observation). These could correspond to the cells seen electron microscopically in the chicken embryo.

The ganglion and satellite cells could not be distinguished under the fluorescence microscope in the paracervical ganglion of the newborn rat. On the contrary, all the cells with a weak greenish fluorescence seemed to be identical, as did the satellite cells. Perhaps the satellite cells also contain catecholamines at this stage. The catecholamines might be localized in part in the soluble pool (Eränkö and Härkönen, 1963; Euler and Lishajko, 1965) in the ganglion cells of the newborn rat. This would explain why most cells on electron microscopic examination do not contain dense-cored vesicles in the paracervical ganglion of young rats (unpublished observation) and why diffusion artefacts were frequently obtained in freeze-dried ganglia of young animals.

In the ganglion of the 10-day-old rat and more clearly later during development, some of the ganglion cells began to show stronger fluorescence. The satellite cells remained small and were devoid of fluorescence. The SIF cells always exhibited strong fluorescence, and the impression was that the cells showing moderate fluorescence developed from the weakly fluorescent cells and not from the intensely fluorescent cells in which the fluorescence intensity ought to have diminished considerably. In this case the hypothesis that some of the small, intensely fluorescent cells were sympathicoblasts would be wrong.

## REFERENCES

ALM, P., CEGRELL, L., EHINGER, B. AND FALCK, B. (1967) Z. Zellforsch., **83**, 178–186.
BOWER, E. (1966) J. Physiol., **183**, 748–767.

444                              L. KANERVA

BJÖRKLUND, A., EHINGER, B. AND FALCK, B. (1968) *J. Histochem. Cytochem.* **16**, 263–270.
BJÖRKLUND, A., CEGRELL, L., FALCK, B., RITZEN, M. AND ROSENGREN, E. (1970) *Acta Physiol. Scand.* **78**, 334–338.
DAVIS, A. A. (1933) *J. Obstet. Gynaecol. Brit. Empire*, **40**, 481–497.
ECCLES, R. M. AND LIBET, B. (1961) *J. Physiol.*, **157**, 484–503.
ELFVIN, L.-G. ,(1968); *J. Ultrastruct. Res.*, **22**, 37–44.
ERÄNKÖ, L. (1970) *IX Intern. Congr. of Anatomists, Leningrad*, p. 36.
ERÄNKÖ, O. (1955) *Acta Endocrinol.*, **18**, 174–179.
ERÄNKÖ, O. (1967) *J. Roy. Microscop. Soc.*, **87**, 1–18.
ERÄNKÖ, O. AND ERÄNKÖ, L. (1971) *Progr. Brain Res.*, this volume, p. 39.
ERÄNKÖ, O. AND HÄRKÖNEN, M. (1963) *Acta Physiol. Scand.*, **58**, 285–286.
ERÄNKÖ, O. AND HÄRKÖNEN, M. (1965a) *Acta Physiol. Scand.*, **63**, 411–412.
ERÄNKÖ, O. AND HÄRKÖNEN, M. (1965b) *Acta Physiol. Scand.*, **63**, 511–512.
EULER, U. S. VON, AND LISHAJKO, F. (1965) *Nature*, **205**, 179–180.
EULER, U. S. VON, AND LISHAJKO, F. (1966) *Life Sci.*, **5**, 687–691.
FALCK, B., HILLARP, N.-Å., THIEME, G. AND TORP, A. (1962) *J. Histochem. Cytochem.*, **10**, 348–354.
FRANKENHÄUSER, F. (1867) *Die Nerven der Gebärmutter und ihre Endigung in glatten Muskelfasern, Mauke, Jena*, pp. 1–82.
GOMORI, G. (1952) *Microscopic Histochemistry*, Chicago University Press, Chicago.
GRILLO, M. (1966) *Pharmacol. Rev.*, **18**, 387–399.
JACOBOWITZ, D. (1967) *J. Pharmacol. Exp. Therap.*, **158**, 227–240.
JACOBOWITZ, D. AND WOODWARD, J. (1968) *J. Pharmacol. Exp. Therap.*, **162**, 213–226.
KALINA, M. AND WOLMAN, M. (1970) *Histochemie*, **22**, 100–108.
KANERVA, L. (1970) *Scand. J. Clin. Lab. Invest.*, *Suppl.* **113**, 18.
KANERVA, L. (1971) *Scand. J. Clin. Lab. Invest.*, *Suppl.* **116**, 65.
KOELLE, G. B. (1951) *J. Pharmacol. Exp. Therap.*, **103**, 153–171.
KOKKO, A (1965) *Acta Physiol. Scand.*, **66**, *Suppl.* **261**, 1–76.
KRANTZ, K. E. (1959) *Ann. N.Y. Acad. Sci.*, **75**, 770–784.
LANGLEY, J. N. AND ANDERSON, H. K. (1895a) *J. Physiol.*, **19**, 122–130.
LANGLEY, J. N. AND ANDERSON, H. K. (1895b) *J. Physiol.*, **19**, 131–139.
LANGLEY, J N AND ANDERSON, H K. (1896b) *J. Physiol.*, **20**, 372–406.
MARSHALL, J. M. (1970) *Ergeb. Physiol.*, **62**, 6–67.
MATTHEWS, M. AND RAISMAN, G. (1969) *J. Anat.*, **105**, 255–282.
MÄKELÄ, S. AND GRÖNROOS, M. (1959) *Ann. Med. Exp. Fenn.*, **37**, 407–413.
NILSSON, O. (1964) *Experientia*, **20**, 679.
NORBERG, K.-A. AND HAMBERGER, B. (1964) *Acta Physiol. Scand.*, **63**, *Suppl.* **238**.
NORBERG, K.-A., RITZÉN, M. AND UNGERSTEDT, U. (1966) *Acta Physiol. Scand.*, **67**, 260–270.
OWMAN, CH., ROSENGREN, E. AND SJÖBERG, N.-O. (1966) *Life Sci.*, **5**, 1389–1396.
OWMAN, CH., ROSENGREN, E. AND SJÖBERG, N.-O. (1967) *Obstet. Gynecol.*, **30**, 763–773.
OWMAN, CH. AND SJÖBERG, N.-O. (1966) *Z. Zellforsch.*, **74**, 182–197.
OWMAN, CH. AND SJÖBERG, N.-O. (1967) *Life Sci.*, **6**, 2549–2556.
OWMAN, CH. AND SJÖSTRAND, N. O. (1965) *Z. Zellforsch.*, **66**, 300–320.
REYNOLDS, S. M. R. (1965) *Physiology of the Uterus*, 2nd ed. Hafner Publ. Co., New York.
ROSENGREN, E. AND SJÖBERG, N.-O. (1967) *Amer. J. Anat.*, **121**, 271–284.
SHABANAH, E., TOTH, A. AND MAUGHAN, G. M. (1964) *Amer. J. Obstet. Gynecol.*, **89**, 860–880.
SIEGRIST, G., DOLIVO, M., DUNANT, Y., FOROGLOU-KERAMEUS, C. AND RIBAUPIERRE, FR. (1968) *J. Ultrastruct. Res.*, **25**, 381–407.
SJÖBERG, N.-O. (1967) *Acta Physiol. Scand.*, *Suppl.* **305**, 5–26.
SJÖBERG, N.-O. (1968) *Acta Endocrinol.*, **57**, 405–413.
STJÄRNE, L. AND LISHAJKO, F. (1966) *J. Neurochem.*, **13** 1213–1216.
STRUMIA, E. AND BAIMA-BOLLONE, P. L. (1964) *Acta Anat.*, **57**, 281–293.
SWEDIN, G. AND BRUNDIN, J. O. (1968) *Experientia*, **24**, 1015–1016.
TENNYSON, V. M., BRZIN, M. AND DUFFY, P. (1968) In LAJTHA, A. AND FORD, D. H. (Eds.), *Progr. Brain Res.*, Vol. 29, Elsevier, Amsterdam-New York, p. 41–61.
TERÄVÄINEN, H., (1970) personal communication.
THEOBALD, G. W. (1968) *Clin. Obstet. Gynec.*, **11**, 15–33.
WECHSLER, W. AND SCHMEKEL, L. (1967) *Acta Neuroveg.*, **30**, 427–444.
WILLIAMS, T. H. AND PALAY, S. L. (1969) *Brain Res.*, **15**, 17–34.

# On the Innervation and Differentiation of Human Fetal Chromaffin Tissue

A. HERVONEN

*Department of Anatomy, University of Helsinki, Siltavuorenpenger, Helsinki (Finland)*

## REVIEW OF THE LITERATURE

Though the adrenal medulla has been studied in detail by many investigators, the extra-adrenal chromaffin tissue (EACT) has been largely neglected. The endocrine function of adrenal chromaffin tissue is well known and the secretory responses of it to various nervous or chemical stimuli have been extensively studied. The functional role of EACT, however, is still obscure.

The preganglionic nature of adrenal medullary innervation is generally accepted (for references see Coupland, 1965). Furthermore, all workers who have attempted to ascertain the origin of adrenal nerve fibres by degeneration experiments have observed the persistence of some intrinsic nerve fibres after section of all visible extrinsic nerves. Neurones can invariably be found, using cholinesterase techniques, in the adrenal glands of all common laboratory animals and man, according to Coupland (1965). The nature of these neurones is not understood.

Zuckerkandl (1901, 1912) did not find any evidence of innervation of EACT in his classic paraganglion study. By the use of methylene blue staining, however, Pines (1924) demonstrated unmyelinated fibres in EACT of the cat. Iwanow (1932) stated that the nerve supply of EACT was sparse, inconstant and different from the rich innervation of IACT. Kofmann (1935) concluded that the nerve plexuses associated with EACT in dog, cat, rabbit and man were similar to those in corresponding adrenal medulla. The problem was approached experimentally by Hollinshead (1936, 1937), whose findings indicate that EACT receives a preganglionic sympathetic innervation. Muscholl and Vogt (1964) performed stimulation experiments on intraganglionic chromaffin tissue and found no evidence of functional innervation. Brundin (1966) was not able to find EACT response to stimulus mediated via the splanchnic nerves, and he supported the opinion of previous authors that the paraganglia (EACT) probably lack a functional innervation.

Acetylcholinesterase-positive fibres were found in the human fetal EACT by Hervonen (1967). Coupland and Weakley (1968, 1970) studied the development of

Abbreviations: AChE — acetylcholinesterase, CC — Chromaffin cell, ns.ChE — nonspecific cholinesterase, EACT — extra-adrenal chromaffin tissue, FIF — formaldehyde-induced fluorescence. IACT — intra-adrenal chromaffin tissue, PSC — primitive sympathetic cell.

*References p. 454*

rabbit chromaffin tissue by electron microscope. Nerve fibres were found in the EACT, but no typical nerve endings could be demonstrated. Virágh and Korényi-Both (1967) and Battaglia (1969) made no comments on the innervation of EACT in their electron-microscopic papers.

To date no evidence of functional innervation of EACT is available, though a nerve supply of it can invariably be demonstrated.

In the present paper a larger study on the development of human fetal chromaffin tissue (Hervonen, 1971) is summarized. The results concerning the innervation of both EACT and IACT correlated with the differentiation of these tissues are presented.

## MATERIAL AND METHODS

All material was obtained from legal interruptions of pregnancy performed by laparotomy. The total number of fetuses processed was 172, the age distribution being from the 5th to the 24th week of pregnancy. Specimens for each of the three methods were prepared from the same fetus if possible. Thus three identical series were obtained. With special arrangements the handling of the fetus could be started within 1–2 min after disconnection of fetoplacental circulation.

Formaldehyde-induced fluorescence was demonstrated following the general rules presented by Eränkö (1967). Numerous variations of the method were used. The drying temperature was –33– –40°C, drying time from 1–6 days. The exposure to formaldehyde vapour lasted 15–180 min and temperatures between 60–80°C were used. Embedding in both paraffin and epon or epon–araldite was used. The drying vacuum was $10^{-3}$–$10^{-5}$.

For cholinesterases the Gomori (1952) modification of the Koelle (1951) technique was used. Adrenal slices and pieces of EACT were fixed in 3.5% calcium–formalin for 6–12 h at 4°C. For demonstration of AChE acetylthiocholine iodide was used as substrate and $10^{-5}$ M iso-OMPA (M-tetra-isopropylpyrophosphoramide) as a specific inhibitor for ns.ChE. For demonstration of ns.ChE butyrylthiocholine was used as substrate and $10^{-5}$ M 284 C 51 (,15-bis-4-allyldimethylammoniumphenyl pentan-3-one di-iodide) to inhibit AChE.

For electron microscopy both immersion and perfusion fixation were used. The umbilical vein was connected with the perfusion apparatus and the pressure was adjusted to 30–40 cm $H_2O$. Perfusion time was 10–15 min and the fixation was further prolonged by immersion of small prepared pieces of tissue. The main fixation fluid was 2.5% glutaraldehyde in 0.1 M phosphate buffer with 0.3 M sucrose. The pH was adjusted to 7.0. Postfixation with 1% $OsO_4$ in the same buffer was used. The epon or epon–araldite-embedded specimens were sectioned with LKB Ultrotome and viewed and photographed with Philips EM 200 and 300.

## RESULTS

### *Development of formaldehyde-induced fluorescence (FIF)*

The first green specific FIF appeared in para-aortic collections of differentiating PSC

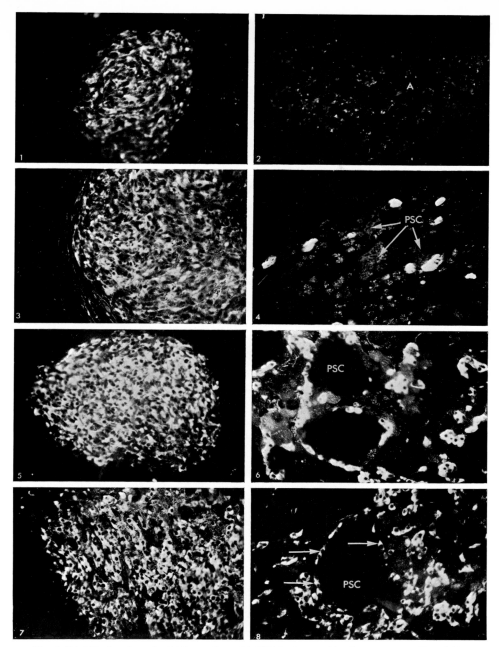

Fig. 1. EACT of an 8-week-old fetus. Greenish FIF is observed in almost every cell. × 240.

Fig. 2. Adrenal cortex of the same fetus. Mainly non-specific fluorescence could be seen. × 240.

Fig. 3. EACT of a 10-week-old fetus. Yellow highly fluorescing cells could be seen between weaker green FIF. × 240.

Fig. 4. Adrenal gland of 11-week-old fetus. Three groups or PSC in the centre. The paper is over-exposed for demonstrating the weak green FIF of PSC groups. Brightly yellow fluorescing clusters of chromaffin cells are seen scattering among the cortical cells. × 240.

Fig. 5. A compact small cluster of EACT of a 12-week-old fetus. Bright yellow FIF is seen all over the tissue. × 280.

Fig. 6. The premedullary area of a 12-week-old fetus. Two groups of PSC surrounded by chromaffin cells. × 280.

Fig. 7. The main para-aortic body of a 15-week-old fetus. Columns of brightly yellow fluorescing chromaffin cells can be observed between the capillaries. × 280.

Fig. 8. An adrenal group of primitive sympathetic cells. Note the intracapsular chromaffin cells indicated by the arrows. The picture is underexposed for clearer demonstration of chromaffin cells and thus the weak FIF of PSC is not visible. × 280.

at 7 weeks. Only solitary weakly fluorescing cells could be noticed. During the follow-ing three weeks there was a rapid intensification of the FIF. At 10 weeks, all the cells of EACT exhibited FIF of varying intensity (Fig. 3). In the 9-week fetus the first fluores-cing cells could be found within the adrenal cortical tissue (Fig. 2). Thus the spreading of FIF with increasing age occurred towards the adrenals.

The intensity of FIF in EACT increased rapidly and at 10 weeks yellow fluores-cence could be seen in several cells (Fig. 3). At the same time small groups of highly fluorescing cells could be found scattered in the adrenal cortex. Weak green FIF could also be observed in the invading groups of PSC (Fig. 4).

After the twelfth week only brightly yellow FIF could be seen in EACT (Fig. 5). Intra-adrenally a rapid increase of the number of brightly yellow fluorescing cells was taking place. Instead of small ovoid or round clusters, columnar organization of cells became general. A typical organization of fluorescing cells also developed after the 12th week. The groups of PSC which exhibited weak green FIF were gradually surrounded by a circle of chromaffin cells. These cells appeared inside the connective tissue capsule of PSC-groups (Figs. 6 and 8) forming a surrounding rim, and they were never seen in the central areas of PSC groups.

The final cellular organization in the present material appeared to be the following.

In EACT only columns of yellow highly fluorescing cells could be observed (Fig. 7). No differences in the intensity of the FIF could be demonstrated. In the sympathetic ganglion tissue weak green fluorescence of the developing neurones was found after the fourth month of development. No fluorescing fibres were seen in EACT.

Intra-adrenally two kinds of fluorescing cells were visible (Fig. 8). (1) The clusters and columns of highly yellow fluorescing chromaffin cells formed a premedullary area where the proportion of cortical tissue decreases. Numerous large groups of PSC were found in this area and were invariably surrounded by a chain of 'intra-capsular' chromaffin cells. (2) After the 12th week of development a specific FIF was found in the groups of PSC. During the period studied the intensity of this FIF re-mained weak and rapid fading made it difficult to documentate.

### The cholinesterases

Acetylcholinesterase activity was found in the preaortic primitive sympathetic plexus of a 7-week-old fetus. Fine AChE-positive fibres were seen to reach adrenal medullary elements. Within 2 weeks the amount of the fibres invading adrenal tissue rapidly increased and they were also found in the central area of the gland. After the 9th week of development a fine anastomosing network of AChE-positive fibres could be found and activity was also observed between the PSC in groups along the coarser nerves (Figs. 9, 11). All groups of PSC were in contact with nerve fibres.

The primitive sympathetic plexus was the site of the most intense activity during the whole development studied, and the EACT was completely negative until the 10th week. During the eleventh week of development fine AChE-positive fibres were observed to penetrate the most superficial layers of the main para-aortic body (Fig. 13).

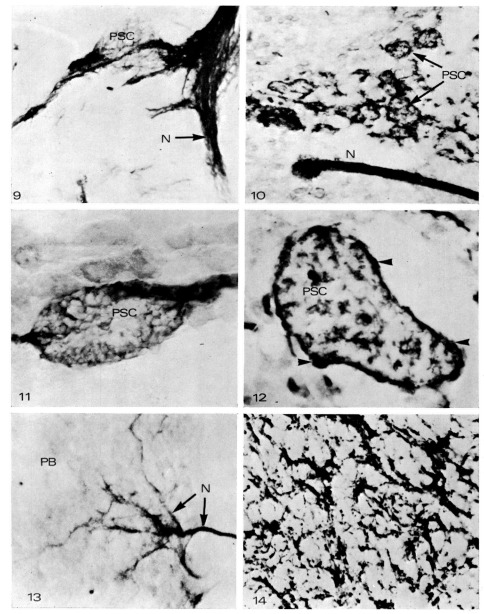

Fig. 9. AChE-positive nerve fibres in the adrenal medulla of 9-week-old fetus. Note the fine fibres of activity between the PSC. × 250.

Fig. 10. Ns.ChE in the premedullary area of a 15-week-old fetus. The groups of PSC are surrounded by a rim of activity and short streaks of activity are scattered between them. × 70.

Fig. 11. AChE activity in a group of PSC in a 15-week-old fetus. Fine positive fibres can be noticed between PSC. × 330.

Fig. 12. Ns.ChE activity in the PSC group of the same adrenal as in Figs. 10 and 11. A surrounding rim of activity can be observed. Possible cytoplasmic activities are indicated with arrows. × 300.

Fig. 13. AChE in the main para-aortic body (EACT) of 12-week-old fetus. Branching fine nerve fibres could be found in the superficial layers of para-aortic body (PB). × 330.

Fig. 14. Ns.ChE activity in EACT of 12-week-old fetus. Strong intercellular network of activity. × 400.

After this age a fine network of AChE activity was a constant finding in the main para-aortic body.

Nonspecific cholinesterase activity appeared during the 8th week of development in EACT. Only intercellular streaks were seen. After the 12th week a continuous network of strong ns.ChE activity was always found (Fig. 14). No cytoplasmic activity was found even after longer incubations.

The first activity observed intra-adrenally appeared during 7th–8th weeks, and was in the form of coarse streaks directed towards the centre of the cortex. Finer fibres and streaks scattered around the premedullary area also appeared rapidly. However, no anastomosing network was found before the condensation of the medullary area started at the 12th week. With longer incubations cytoplasmic activity could be seen in small groups of cells which were probably maturing chromaffin cells. After the 10th week of development a peculiar organization of the ns.ChE activity was noticed. The groups of PSC were regularly surrounded by a rim of strong activity (Figs. 10, 12). Cytoplasmic activity was also observed along the borders of these groups. This activity is probably due, at least in part to the 'intracapsular chromaffin cells' and the connective tissue capsule of PSC groups.

*Electron microscopy*

The development of synaptic contacts to chromaffin cells and the differentiation of sympathetic elements are summarized here.

Bundles of axons were frequently found between the cells of EACT after the 10th week of development. Though the axons were often in contact with chromaffin cells and on the walls of venous sinuses, no typical axon terminals with synaptic vesicles could be found regularly. A few dense-cored vesicles (mean diameter ca. 900 Å) were found in these nerves. Occasionally, an axon terminal with synaptic vesicles (mean diameter ca. 420 Å) could be found, but no contact with chromaffin cells could be demonstrated.

After the 7th week of development nerve trunks could be regularly found in adrenal tissue. Before the age of 10 weeks only rather coarse bundles were found, with groups of primitive sympathetic cells along their course. Very soon, however, solitary axons were observed to be in contact with both chromaffin cells and cells in the centre of PSC groups. Synapses could be regularly found on the adrenal medullary cells after the 12th week of development. Axon terminals could be observed in three different localizations:

(1) Synapses on chromaffin cells in solitary groups. Both in the centre and on the periphery of a group of CC similar synapses were noticed. Empty vesicles and dense-cored vesicles were regularly found in the terminals.

(2) Synapses on the intracapsular chromaffin cells. The PSC groups were surrounded by a layer of fibroblasts and collagen fibres (Fig. 18). With increasing age this capsule became thicker and almost continuous around the whole group. After the age of ten weeks chromaffin cells, morphologically similar to those already existing outside the

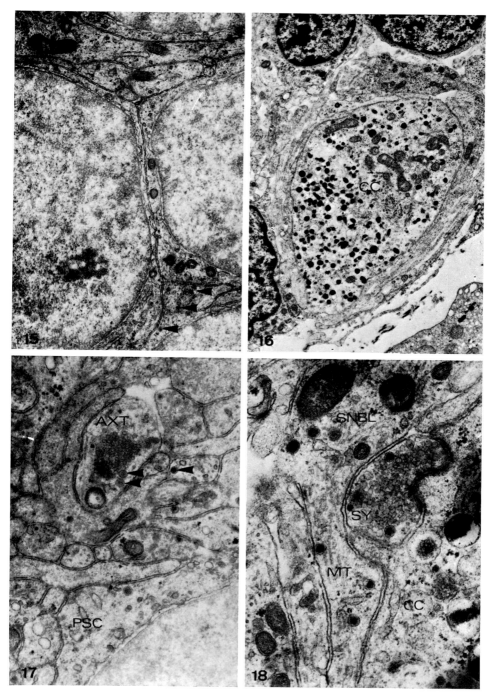

Fig. 15. PSC of a 10-week-old fetus. Cytoplasmic processes and dense-cored vesicles (mean diameter ca. 980 Å) can be observed. × 29 000.

Fig. 16. An intracapsular chromaffin cell in the adrenals of a 12-week-old fetus surrounded by the cytoplasmic processes of PSC. A thin layer of connective tissue separates the cortical tissue from the PSC group. × 8100.

Fig. 17. An axon terminal (AXT) in the middle of a PSC group in the adrenals of 12-week-old fetus. Dense-cored vesicles (mean diameter ca. 940 Å) are indicated with arrows. × 21 000.

Fig. 18. A synapse (SY) on the inner surface of an intracapsular chromaffin cell (CC) in the adrenals of 12-week-old fetus. Processes of sympathetic neuroblast (SNBL) with microtubules (MT) and dense-cored vesicles can be observed. × 36 400.

capsule, appeared inside it (Fig. 16). At the same time several changes in the cytoplasm of PSC could be seen. Some PSC acquire characteristics of a developing sympathetic neurone and are thus called sympathetic neuroblasts. Amounts of cellular processes were formed and dense-cored vesicles (mean diameter 980 Å) could be found in the cytoplasm. The intracapsular chromaffin cells were surrounded by the cellular processes of sympathetic neuroblasts and after the 12th week synapses were seen on them. The origin of the processes forming these synapses is not clear, but to the author it seems probable that they came from developing sympathetic neuroblasts in the centre of the PSC groups.

(3) Axon terminals and synaptic contacts on the surface of the sympathetic neuroblasts or surrounded by their cellular processes were frequently seen (Fig. 17). With glutaraldehyde fixation no difference in the structure or size of the vesicles could be found between different localizations of axon terminals.

### DISCUSSION

#### *Extra-adrenal chromaffin tissue*

The first FIF appeared in EACT of a 7-week-old fetus. The light-microscopic studies of Coupland (1952) indicate that at this stage of development only phaeochromoblasts (an intermediate cell type between PSC and mature CC) could be found. Thus this immature precursor of chromaffin cell already contains catecholamines, indicating that the metabolic differentiation probably started already during the 7th week of fetal life.

Axons and some occasional axon terminals were found in EACT. However, no typical synaptic contacts could be found in any age-group studied, whereas synapses were regularly found in adrenal medullary chromaffin tissue after the 12th week. Similar findings were made by Coupland and Weakley (1968, 1970) in rabbit chromaffin tissue. The present results support the opinion of previous authors (Muscholl and Vogt, 1964; Brundin, 1966) that EACT probably lack a functional innervation, at least during the first two-thirds of fetal development.

Although the possibility of endocrine-active EACT has been neglected by several authors, it is apparent that it possesses features indicating this kind of function, as pointed out by West *et al.* (1953) and Hunter *et al.* (1952, 1953). The EACT is known to contain relatively larger amounts of catecholamines than the adrenal chromaffin tissue, (Niemineva and Pekkarinen (1952); West *et al.* (1953); Genneser and v. Studnitz (1969)), the amine being predominantly noradrenaline. The possibility of humoral regulation of EACT has been pointed out by Muscholl and Vogt (1963), Coupland (1965) and Winckler (1969). It is suggested that if the human fetal EACT is operative, its function is regulated by some as yet unknown humoral stimulus. Further, the possibility that the main product released is a biologically active compound other than catecholamine, possibly a polypeptide, should be considered.

## Intra-adrenal chromaffin tissue

The growth of preganglionic nerve fibres into human fetal adrenal glands and the migration of PSC along them have been extensively studied by Iwanow (1925); Keene *et al.* (1927); Iwanow (1932); Coupland (1952); Ito (1959) and Boyd (1960). From all these studies it is apparent that chromaffin cells differentiate from elements which are initially associated with the primitive sympathetic plexus. The PSC are generally accepted as the common origin for both chromaffin tissue and sympathetic neurones. In the human fetal adrenal medulla large amounts of PSC persist up to the full term. Since neurones are a constant feature of the human adrenal medulla it is apparent that a part of the fetal PSC would differentiate to sympathetic neuroblasts instead of chromaffin cells. This process of differentiation has not been studied in detail before.

Synaptic contacts between chromaffin cells and axons branching from thicker bundles were seen regularly after the 12th week of pregnancy. At the same time features of sympathetic neuroblasts could be observed in some cells of larger groups of PSC. Axon terminals were found between sympathetic neuroblasts. The sympathetic line cells formed a tight network of cellular processes, which also surrounded the intracapsular chromaffin cells. Synapses were frequently found on these CC. With increasing age the amount of cellular processes and preganglionic axons greatly increased within the PSC groups.

In a separate investigation the microcirculation of fetal chromaffin tissue has been studied (Hervonen, 1971). The PSC groups are surrounded by venous sinuses but even in the largest groups of PSC, no kind of blood channels could be found. Considering the size of these groups it is apparent that the supply of humoral or other agents carried by the blood must be poor in the central areas. In other words, the surface layer of PSC is more readily subjected to various chemical stimuli.

On the other hand, it is generally known according to Villee (1969), that from the end of the third month of pregnancy the human fetal adrenal cortex is capable of forming the steroid nucleus and converting cholesterol to pregnenolone and thence to dehydroepiandrosterone. Thus, cortisone and hydrocortisone are produced by the fetal adrenal cortex. Further, it is evident that these two steroids are strong inducers of new enzymatic activity in embryonic tissue, according to Moscona and Piddington (1967). Lempinen (1964) showed that administration of hydrocortisone to post-natal rat prevented the disappearance of EACT and even induced the appearance of new chromaffin cells. Eränkö *et al.* (1966) for the first time found direct evidence of the effect of cortical hormone on the methylation of noradrenaline into adrenaline in chromaffin cells of rat fetuses, and this effect was confirmed by Coupland and Mac-Dougall (1966) in noradrenaline-storing cells cultivated *in vitro*.

It is generally accepted that the adrenal cortical hormones exert an effect on the latest stage of differentiation of chromaffin cells. On the basis of the present results it is further suggested that the primary differentiation of PSC to chromaffin cells intra-adrenally is also dependent on the concentration of cortical hormones. The lack of this effect would cause the development of sympathetic neuroblast, as is the case in the centre of PSC groups. Those PSC which are in good contact with the circulation, or in direct contact with adrenal cortical cells, differentiate to chromaffin cells. The relative ease with which cortical hormones can pass from the mother to the fetus is supposed to maintain concentrations high enough to cause the maturation of chromaffin cells in tissues where the vascular supply is efficient, as in EACT.

In the adrenal medulla the sympathetic neurones develop within the PSC groups. Evidence has been found that the processes of these cells possibly form synaptic contacts with the 'intracapsular chromaffin cells'. Thus, some chromaffin cells might later have a functional postganglionic innervation.

## REFERENCES

BATTAGLIA, G. (1969) *Z. Zellforsch.*, **99**, 529–537.
BOYD, J. D. (1960) In: *Adrenergic Mechanisms*, Churchill, London, p. 63–82.
BRUNDIN, T. (1966) *Acta Physiol. Scand.*, **70**, Suppl. 290.
COUPLAND, R. E. (1952) *J. Anat.*, **86**, 357–372.
COUPLAND, R. E. (1963) *J. Anat.*, **97**, 141–142.
COUPLAND, R. E. (1965) In: *The Natural History of the Chromaffin Cell*, Longmans, London.
COUPLAND, R. E. AND MACDOUGALL, J. D. B. (1966) *J. Endocrinol.*, **36**, 317–324.
COUPLAND, R. E. AND WEAKLEY, B. S. (1968) *J. Anat.*, **102**, 425–455.
COUPLAND, R. E. AND WEAKLEY, B. S. (1970) *J. Anat.*, **106**, 2, 213–231.
ERÄNKÖ, O. (1967) *J. Roy. Microscop. Soc.*, **87**, 259–276.
ERÄNKÖ, O., LEMPINEN, M. AND RÄISÄNEN, L. (1966) *Acta Physiol. Scand.*, **66**, 253–254.
GOMORI, H. G. (1952) *Microscopic Histochemistry*, Univ. Chicago Press, 169–171.
GENNESER, G. AND STUDNITZ, W. v. (1969) *Scand. J. Clin. Lab. Invest.*, **24**, 2, 169–171.
HERVONEN, A. (1967) *Scand. J. Clin. Lab. Invest.*, *Suppl. 95*, 77.
HERVONEN, A. (1970) *Scand. J. Clin. Lab. Invest.*, *Suppl. 113*, 18.
HERVONEN, A. (1971) *Acta Physiol. Scand.*, *Suppl. 368*.
HOLLINSHEAD, W. H. (1936) *J. Comp. Neurol.*, **64**, 449–467.
HOLLINSHEAD, W. H. (1937) *J. Comp. Neurol.*, **67**, 133–143.
HUNTER, R. B., MacGREGOR, A. R., SHEPHERD, D. M. AND WEST, G. B. (1952) *J. Physiol.*, **118**, 11P–12P.
HUNTER, R. B., MacGREGOR, A. R., SHEPHERD, D. M. AND WEST, G. B. (1953) *J. Pharmacol. (Lond.)*, **5**, 407.
ITO, I. (1959) *Arch. Histol. Jap.*, **17**, 279–294.
IWANOW, G. (1925) *Z. Anat. Entwickl. Gesch.*, **77**, 234–244.
IWANOW, G. (1932) *Z. Anat. Entwickl. Geshh.*, **29**, 87–280.
KEENE, M. F. AND HEWER, E. E. (1927) *J. Anat.*, **61**, 302–324.
KOELLE, G. B. (1951) *J. Pharmacol. exp. Ther.*, **103**, 153–171.
KOFMANN, U. (1935) *Z. Anat.*, **105**, 305–315.
LEMPINEN, M. (1964) *Acta Physiol. Scand.*, **62**, 1–91.
MOSCONA, A. A. AND PIDDINGTON, R. (1967) *Science*, **158**, 496–497.
MUSCHOLL, E. AND VOGT, M. (1963) *Brit. J. Pharmac. Chemother.*, **22**, 193–203.
NIEMINEVA, K. AND PEKKARINEN, A. (1952) *Ann. Med. exp. Fenn.*, **30**, 274–286.
PINES, L. (1924) *Arch. Psychiat. Nervenkr.*, **70**, 636–647.
SHEPHERD, D. M. AND WEST, G. B. (1951) *Brit. J. Pharmacol.*, **6**, 665–672.
SHEPHERD, D. M. AND WEST, G. B. (1952) *Nature*, **170**, 42–43.
VILLEE, D. B. (1969) *New Engl. J. Med.*, **28**, 241–270.
VIRACH, S. AND KORENYI-BOTH, A. (1967) *Acta Biol. Hung.*, **18**, 167–169.
WEST, G. B., SHEPHERD, D. M. AND HUNTER, R. B. (1951) *Lancet*, ii, 966–969.
WEST, G. B., SHEPHERD, D. M., HUNTER, R. B. AND MacGREGOR, A. R. (1953) *Clin. Sci.*, **12**, 317–325.
WINCKLER, J. (1969) *Z. Zellforsch.*, **96**, 490–494.
ZUCKERKANDL, E. (1901) *Anat. Anz.*, **15**, 97–107.
ZUCKERKANDL, E. (1912) In N. KEIBEL AND MALL (Eds.), *Manual of Human Embryology*, Lippincott, Philadelphia, **2**, 157–179.

# Localization of Acid Phosphatase in the Adrenal Medulla of the Albino Rat

R. E. COUPLAND, LUCIA MASTROLIA* AND BRENDA S. WEAKLEY**

*Department of Human Morphology, University of Nottingham (U.K.)*

Histochemical evidence of differences in the acid phosphatase content of chromaffin cells of the rat adrenal medulla was provided by Eränkö (1952) using the Gomori method for light microscopy. Small islands of non-reactive elements were noted in formal-fixed tissues, while the majority of the cells gave a strongly positive cytoplasmic reaction. Subsequently, the same worker (1955) demonstrated that the apparently non-reactive islands were composed of noradrenaline-storing cells, while the strongly reactive areas were comprised of cells which store adrenaline. The different reactions of adrenaline-storing (A) cells and noradrenaline-storing (N) cells for acid phosphatase is, however, now known to be species specific, being evident in the albino rat but not in mouse (Eränkö, 1955), bovine (Hillarp and Falck, 1956), man, pig and rabbit (Coupland, 1965 a).

By comparison with the strong generalised cytoplasmic reaction for acid phosphatase observed in the A cells the N cells appear at first sight to be unreactive and were so considered initially. However, more refined methods have made it apparent that a fine particulate reaction does occur within the N cells in rats and in both A and N cells in other forms with a frequency and distribution suggesting the possibility that the reaction may be associated with lysosomes. Biochemical and electron histochemical evidence for the occurrence of acid phosphatase in lysosomes of the bovine adrenal medulla was provided by the work of Smith and Winkler (1966), and Bradbury *et al.*, (1966).

The strongly positive cytoplasmic reaction of adrenaline-storing cells of the rat adrenal medulla was investigated by Benedeczky (1967) using electron histochemical techniques. He described a positive reaction in 'microbodies' said to be distinct from chromaffin granules. He also observed a diffuse deposit within Golgi lamellae but reported a negative reaction in chromaffin granules and mitochondria. In comparison with this latter worker Holtzman and Dominitz reported (1968) the presence of acid phosphatase in secretory granules and Golgi apparatus of the adrenal chromaffin cells in the rat, but made no reference to any difference in reactivity of A and N cells.

In the present work which has extended over some three years and concerning which a preliminary report has already been published (1968), the acid phosphatase reaction

---

* Present address: Instituto di Zoologia, Dell'Universita, Viale Regina Elena 324 Roma (7).
** Present address: Department of Anatomy, University of Dundee.

*References pp. 463–464*

of the rat adrenal medulla has been observed after various periods of incubation in Gomori type media and the results correlated with biochemical findings relating to the localization of the enzyme in supernatant and particulate fractions of the adrenal medulla.

## METHODS

### *Electron microscopy*

Adrenal glands were removed from the male 250–300 g Sprague–Dawley rats within 1 min of sacrifice by decapitation. Slices of glands were fixed in ice-cold 4% glutaraldehyde buffered to pH 7.4 with 0.1 M sodium cacodylate for $2\frac{1}{2}$ h. They were then washed at least overnight in ice-cold 0.1 M cacodylate containing 0.22 M sucrose.

Frozen sections 25–50 m$\mu$ thick were incubated in a Gomori type medium for acid phosphatase (0.3% sodium-$\beta$-glycerophosphate in 0.1 M acetate buffer pH 5 containing 0.12% lead nitrate) at room temperature or 37°C for 10, 20 or 30 min. Sections were then washed for 15 min in three changes of acetate buffer, post-fixed in 1% osmium tetroxide (Caulfield, 1958), rinsed briefly and then dehydrated in ethanol prior to embedding in araldite. Sections were prepared using a Cambridge–Huxley microtome and mounted on grids. Some were stained with lead citrate (Reynolds, 1963), and 1% uranyl acetate; others were examined unstained with an AEI 6B electron microscope. Some frozen sections, after incubation, were treated with dilute ammonium sulphide solution, and examined with the light microscope.

Control sections were incubated in the absence of substrate and in the presence of 0.2 M sodium fluoride.

### *Enzyme assay*

Groups of 12 animals were sacrificed and the adrenal medullae enucleated and placed in ice-cold 0.3 M sucrose. The tissues were then homogenised in a Potter–Elvehjem homogeniser having a clearance between the glass mortar and Teflon pestle of 0.08 mm. The pestle was passed slowly up and down four times, care being taken to avoid producing cavitation within the fluid. The homogenate was then subjected to the procedure of Smith and Winkler (1967) which involves the preparation of a large-granule fraction followed by the layering in tubes of a suspension of large-granule fraction in 0.3 M sucrose over 7.5 ml of ice-cold 1.6 M sucrose solution. The tubes were centrifuged for $66 \times 10^5$ g/min in an A-40 rotor of the Spinco ultracentrifuge. Layers 1–5 were identified by naked eye examination, but because of the small amount of material present within the tubes, it was extremely difficult to separate layers 3, 4, and 5 from each other satisfactorily. In consequence, and also as a result of the electron histochemical findings, it was decided that the supernatant of the large-granule fraction should be removed and assayed separately and that the particulate deposit should be pooled to represent total particulate fractions.

Acid phosphatase was estimated using a Boehringer kit (Catalogue No. 15988

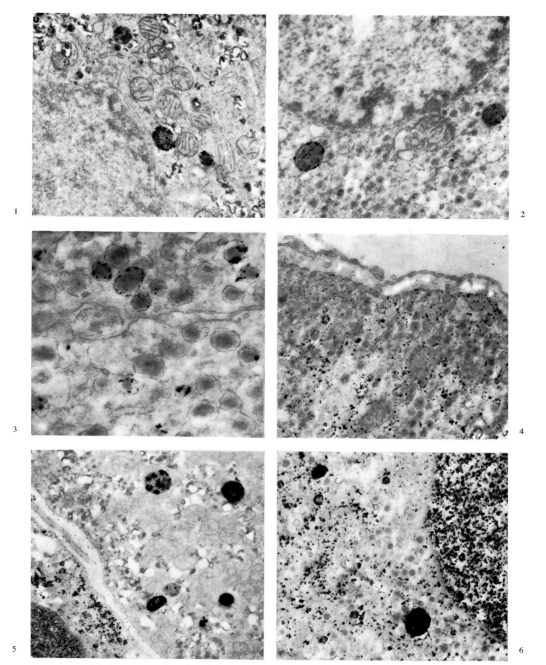

All tissues were incubated in a Gomori-type medium for acid phosphatase.
Fig. 1. Noradrenaline-storing chromaffin cell incubated at room temperature for 10 min. Note particulate deposit over periphery of lysosomes. × 13600.
Fig. 2. Adrenaline-storing cell after 10 min incubation at room temperature. Reaction in lysosomes and occasional granules. × 10400.
Fig. 3. Adrenaline-storing cells after 10 min incubation at room temperature showing reaction products on and adjacent to the external limiting membranes of chromaffin granules. × 53000.
Fig. 4. Adrenaline-storing cell lying adjacent to blood capillary (above). Incubated for 20 min at room temperature. Note more extensive deposit of reaction products in association with chromaffin cel granules. × 13600.
Fig. 5. Noradrenaline-storing cell (above right) showing acid phosphatase reaction confined to lysosomes and adrenaline-storing cell (below left) showing more diffuse cytoplasmic reaction and deposits over nucleus after 30 min incubation at room temperature. × 10000.
Fig. 6. Adrenaline-storing cell showing deposits over lysosomes, granules and nucleus after 30 min incubation at room temperature. × 10400.

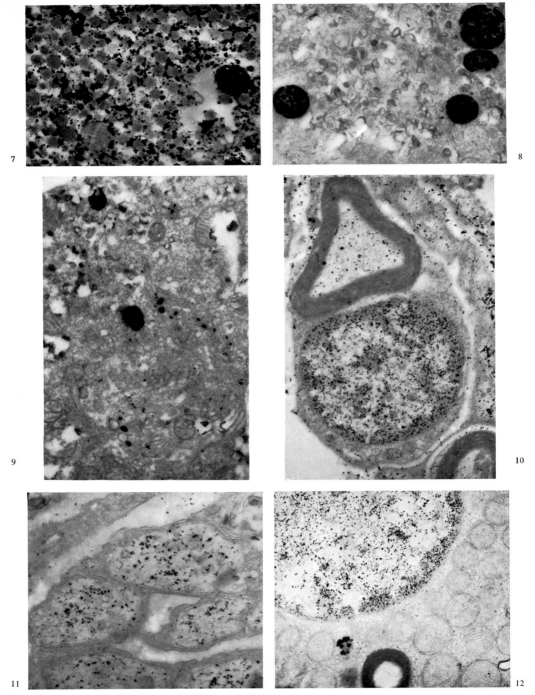

Fig. 7. Adrenaline-storing cell showing reaction throughout lysosome and on and around the periphery of storage granules after 30 min incubation at 37°. × 20800.

Fig. 8. Noradrenaline-storing cell showing reaction in lysosomes only after 30 min incubation at 37° × 20800.

Fig. 9. Noradrenaline-storing cell after 30 min incubation at room temperature showing reaction deposits within vesicles of the Golgi complex and in adjacent lysosomes. × 14400.

Fig. 10. Tissue incubated 30 min at 37°. Fine reaction deposits over connective tissue cell processes and Schwann cell, especially over the nucleus, and over axoplasm. Little deposit over myelin. × 13 000.

Fig. 11. Tissue incubated 30 min at 37° showing deposits over contents of axon and over amorphous intercellular substance. × 16800.

Fig. 12. Reaction deposits over lysosomes of adreno-cortical cell with fine deposit over nuclear chromatin after 30 min incubation at room temperature. Very fine generalized deposits may also be noted within the cytosol. × 10400.

TS.AA) Triton X-100 being added to the buffer solution to a concentration of 0.1 %
in order to lyse membrane-bound elements.

RESULTS

*Electron histochemical*

Unstained sections were most useful for localizing the reaction products on or within
cell organelles and inclusions. No difficulty was encountered in identifying A and N
cells owing to the relative symmetry of the contents of A granules and their finely
granular moderate electron density. In contrast N granules appear as empty shells or
contain eccentric deposits of homogeneously high electron density.

Incubation for 10 min at room temperature results in a particulate deposit of
reaction products over the peripheral parts of lysosomes of chromaffin cells. The
reaction is always on or internal to the limiting membrane of these structures (Figs.
1 and 2). After the same incubation time A cells showed reaction products on and
immediately adjacent to the limiting membrane of membrane-bound granules, which
in size and appearance are identical with typical A chromaffin granules (Figs. 3 and 4).
In N cells only lysosomes react after 10 min incubation and this state of affairs is
observed in cortical cells, Schwann cells and macrophages.

After 20–30 min incubation the reaction product is deposited on or external to the
peripheral membrane of all A granules, the deposit being more extensive in relation
to some than to other granules (Figs. 4, 6 and 7). There is no size difference, however,
between those which react strongly and those which have a weak reaction. Even after
20–30 min N granules fail to react (Figs. 5 and 8) though widespread and possibly
non-specific deposits are visible over other cells. After 30 min the perigranular cytosol
in A cells shows a heavy deposit of reaction products which may occupy almost the
whole of the cytosol between individual chromaffin granules and organelles.

After 20 min incubation a positive acid phosphatase reaction is evident within the
Golgi membranes in both A and N cells. This is most clearly defined in the N cells
(Fig. 9), probably as a result of the absence of reaction products within the cytosol.
Deposits within the Golgi membranes increase in size as the periphery of the zone is
approached and immediately external to the region typical lysosomes are usually seen.
The lysosomal reaction is strong after both 20 and 30 min incubation, and deposits
cover the granular contents of these organelles. No deposit is observed in the cytosol
adjacent to Golgi complex or lysosomes after either 20 or 30 min incubation. After
incubation for 20–30 min a fine particulate deposit is observed over the nuclei of all
cell types including A and N cells, and is heaviest over chromatin material. This latter
reaction is considered to be non-specific. Since the phenomenon is not evident in
sections treated with sodium fluoride it is probably due to acid phosphatase active
however, and probably due to diffusion of reaction products from reactive cytoplasmic
organelles, with subsequent binding to chromatin.

After 20–30 min incubation islands of cortical cells within the adrenal medulla show
a fine particulate deposit over all nuclei; this is once again most intense over chro-

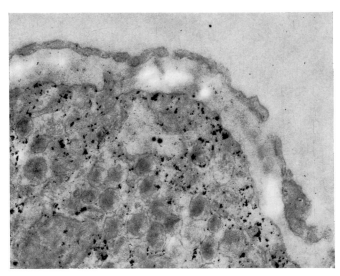

Fig. 13. Adrenaline-storing cell lying adjacent to blood vessel showing fine particulate deposit over membranes of chromaffin granules and on or internal to the plasma after 10 min incubation at room temperature. × 39000.

matin (Fig. 12). Cytoplasmic reaction is mainly confined to lysosomes, but in some instances a fine particulate deposit is also observed in the cytosol after incubation for 20 min or more. A fine particulate deposit is also observed over both cellular and amorphous intercellular connective tissue elements in 20 and 30 min specimens (Figs. 10 and 11). These fine diffuse deposits may represent non-specific reactions. After 20 min incubation fine particulate reaction deposits are also observed over profiles of both myelinated and unmyelinated axons but are not apparently associated with definite organelles or inclusions (Figs. 10 and 11). Little reaction occurs over myelin sheaths (Fig. 10).

In addition to the reaction observed within the cytoplasm of adrenaline-storing cells, after 10 min and longer incubation times some reaction deposits are also associated with the plasma membrane of these cells. Other cell types do not show this reaction. After 20 min incubation it is difficult to determine whether the reaction product lying on or internal to the plasma membrane of A cells is associated with the plasma membrane or with adjacent chromaffin granules (Figs. 13 and 14).

Sections incubated in medium free from substrate or in the presence of 0.2 M sodium fluoride showed no evidence of reaction.

*Biochemical results*

The results are summarised in Table 1. In three separate preparations little enzyme activity occurs in the supernatant fraction, while strong activity is observed in the particulate fraction.

It would seem likely that the relatively low level of enzyme activity within the supernatant is due to inadvertant damage to organelles or inclusions during processing

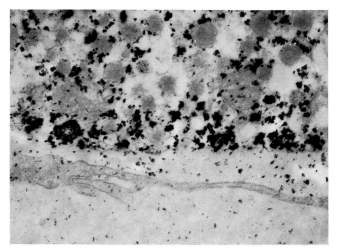

Fig. 14. Adrenaline-storing cell incubated 30 min at 37° Note heavy reaction around chromaffin granules and on and adjacent to plasma membrane of chromaffin cell. Endothelial cell shows no reaction. × 40000.

TABLE 1

ACID PHOSPHATASE ACTIVITY IN ARBITRARY UNITS OF SUPERNATANT AND PARTICULATE
FRACTIONS PREPARED FROM HOMOGENATES OF RAT ADRENAL MEDULLA

| Supernatant | Particulate |
|---|---|
| 0.35 | 19.11 |
| 0.38 | 12.00 |
| 0.62 | 23.83 |

with consequent release of small amounts of acid phosphatase, and that all or most of this activity is normally associated with cell particles.

DISCUSSION

Cell centrifugation and assay indicates that in the adrenal medulla acid phosphatase is largely or completely confined to the particulate fractions of cells. This finding is in accord with the results obtained by electron histochemistry after incubation for only 10 min. At this time a reaction is observed over lysosomes of all cell types present within the adrenal medulla, and also over the peripheral membrane of granules which in size and morphology are identical with A granules, and are considered to be these elements by the writers. After only 10 min incubation the reaction within the lysosome is largely confined to the periphery of the structure, and the deposit lies on or within the peripheral limiting membrane. The reaction product associated with A granules in these short incubation experiments is deposited directly on the external limiting membrane or immediately adjacent to it.

In tissues incubated for 20 min and longer a more diffuse reaction occurs within the lysosome and may extend across the whole of the contents of this organelle. It does not, however, extend into the adjacent cytosol. In contrast with this finding, the reaction product associated with A granules is observed overlying the membrane and extending into the adjacent cytosol. This phenomenon could be accounted for if acid phosphatase existed within the cytosol as well as in cell particles, but this state of affairs is ruled out by the biochemical findings. More likely explanations are, therefore, that the reaction products pass peripherally, either because the active centre of a membrane-associated enzyme is directed externally, or because the reaction products, *viz*. phosphate ions, of an enzyme which shows no polarization diffuse outwards from the granules rather than move internally, possibly as a result of some chemical or physical barrier to internal movement. Since the granules contain high concentrations of adenosine triphosphate, the latter is a distinct possibility, but the former could only be excluded experimentally. Whatever the explanation of the localization of the reaction product in relation to adrenaline-storing chromaffin granules, the results are in direct contrast not only with the reaction of lysosomes, but also of Golgi membranes, since in both these cases the lead deposit occurs on or entirely within the external limiting membrane.

It is of interest to note that N granules give a negative acid phosphatase reaction in all preparations irrespective of incubation time. It is also of interest that the reaction of the A granules themselves is not uniform, and that some react more strongly than others as revealed by the accumulation of reaction products around the periphery of some of the granules. There is no evidence to support the suggestion of Benedeczky (1967) that the acid phosphatase reaction occurs in 'microbodies' which are distinct from chromaffin granules since, as indicated above, the reactive but non-lysosomal granules within the A cells resemble typical adrenaline-storing granules in both size and morphology — hence it is unnecessary to invoke the presence of an element, the 'microbody' which has not previously been identified within chromaffin cells.

In preparations incubated for 10 min at room temperature, particulate deposits are occasionally observed on or contiguous with plasma membranes of A cells, but not on other cell types. This may be interpreted as evidence in favour of exocytosis as a method of granule discharge since, if the limiting membrane of the granule fuses with the plasma membrane prior to discharge of granule contents, the enzyme may persist for a time in its new site. In tissues incubated for longer periods more abundant reaction deposits are observed on or adjacent to the plasma membrane of A cells, but since these are often closely related to reactive A granules it is impossible to determine whether the deposit resulted from enzyme associated with granule or with plasma membrane.

As noted above and in contrast with changes associated with A granules, reaction products associated with lysosomes and Golgi membranes accumulate within the membrane of the organelles, and show no tendency to diffuse to the periphery. This difference could result from the active centre of the enzyme being directed to the interior, to charge differences on the two sides of the membranes, or to the relative impermeability of the membrane to the phosphate ions. The latter would seem unlikely.

The occurrence of the reaction product entirely within the Golgi membranes and on, or external to, chromaffin granule membranes would suggest that these two membranes are not structurally identical. Indeed, from the point of view of distribution of acid phosphatase within the limiting membrane, lysosomes and the Golgi complex have apparently more in common than chromaffin granules and the Golgi complex. The possibility that some granular material membrane bound within the region of the Golgi complex may represent a stage in lysosome formation in chromaffin cells has been previously suggested (Coupland, 1965 b). This suggestion is supported by the current observations that the volume of reaction product within the membranes increases towards the periphery of the Golgi region and that typical lysosomes may be identified around the periphery of this zone. These observations, together with the observation that minute amounts of primary amine (possibly noradrenaline) may be identified within some small Golgi vesicles (Coupland and Weakley, 1968, 1970) is in keeping with the view that in a secretory cell the Golgi complex is concerned with both the elaboration of secretory products and lysosome formation (Smith and Farquhar, 1966).

The metabolic significance of the high content of acid phosphatase within adrenaline-storing chromaffin cells in the albino rat is difficult to evaluate. Since it is species specific the findings are probably not of prime importance in terms of synthesis, storage, or secretion of catecholamines. More probably the phenomenon represents a chemical and metabolic consequence of a genetic change during phylogeny which resulted in the protein components of the external membrane of the adrenaline-storing granule containing acid phoshatase. Although the evidence for the occasional occurrence of acid phosphatase in secretory granules has occasionally been obtained (Smith and Farquhar, 1966; Biempica and Moutes, 1965) the association is unusual.

The presence of reaction products within the axoplasm of adrenal medullary nerve fibres is of interest even if, as suggested by many workers, it is non-specific so far as acid phosphatase is concerned (Adams, 1965). Under certain circumstances the deposit does afford a means of clearly demonstrating the presence of neurons and their processes (Coupland, 1965 a).

ACKNOWLEDGEMENT

This work was supported by a grant (to R.E.C.) from the Medical Research Council, for which the authors are most grateful.

REFERENCES

ADAMS, C. W. M. (1965) *Neurohistochemistry*, Elsevier, Amsterdam, p. 405.
BENEDECZKY, I. (1967) *Nature* **214**, 1243–1244.
BIEMPICA, L. AND MOUTES, L. F. (1965) *Amer. J. Anat.*, **117**, 47–72.
BRADBURY, S., SMITH, A. D. AND WINKLER, H. (1966) *Experientia*, **22**, 142–143.

CAULFIELD, J. B. (1958) *J. Biophys. Biochem. Cytol.*, **2**, 357–372.

COUPLAND, R. E., (1965a) *The Natural History of the Chromaffin Cell*, Longmans. London, pp. 20, 202.

COUPLAND, R. E. (1965b) *J. Anat.*, **99**, 231–254.

COUPLAND, R. E., MASTROLIA, LUCIA AND WEAKLEY, BRENDA S. (1968) *J. Anat.*, **103**, 582.

COUPLAND, R. E. AND WEAKLEY, BRENDA S. (1968) *J. Anat.*, **102**, 425–455.

COUPLAND, R. E. AND WEAKLEY, BRENDA S. (1970) *J. Anat.*, **106**, 213–231.

ERÄNKÖ, O. (1952) *Acta Anat.*, **16**, *Suppl. 17*, 1–60.

ERÄNKÖ, O. (1955) *Ann. Med. Exp. Biol. Fenna₂i*, **33**, 278–290.

HILLARP, N.-Å. AND FALCK, B. (1956) *Acta Endocrinol.*, **22**, 95–106.

HOLTZMAN, E. AND DOMINITZ, R. (1968) *J. Histochem. Cytochem.*, **16**, 320–336.

REYNOLDS, E. S. (1963) *J. Cell Biol.*, **17**, 208–212.

SMITH, A. D. AND WINKLER, H. (1966) *J. Physiol.*, **183**, 179–188.

SMITH, R. E. AND FARQUHAR, M. G. (1966) *J. Cell Biol.*, **31**, 319.

SMITH, A. D. AND WINKLER, H. (1967) *Biochem. J.*, **103**, 480–482.

# VII. EXPERIMENTAL HISTOCHEMISTRY OF AUTONOMIC INNERVATION

# Sympathetic Reinnervation of Anterior Chamber Transplants

TORBJÖRN MALMFORS AND LARS OLSON

*Department of Histology, Karonlinska Institutet, Stockholm (Sweden)*

The sympathetic innervation apparatus constitutes a widespread 3-dimensional plexus of nerve terminals in most organs. It is involved in a multitude of important regulatory autonomic functions. Almost any kind of injury to the body will inevitably include axotomy of a number of postganglionic sympathetic axons and consequently at least partial sympathetic denervation of a certain region. Modern techniques of surgery and transplantations thus produce large sympathetically denervated areas. Reinnervation of such areas in the adult animal then becomes one of the necessities for re-establishment of proper function of the denervated tissues.

In our studies of the growth characteristics of the sympathetic adrenergic nerves special attention has been paid to the problem of morphological and functional reinnervation of denervated tissues in adult animals. A model system using tissue transplantations to the anterior chamber of the eye has been used (see Fig. 1 and Olson and Malmfors, 1970). The present paper will summarize some of our results, for a more detailed description the reader is referred to Olson and Malmfors (1970) and to Malmfors *et al.* (1970).

## METHODS

Albino rats and guinea pigs were mostly used. Small pieces of tissues were prepared

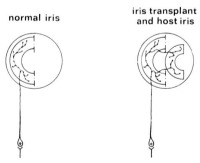

normal iris

iris transplant
and host iris

Fig. 1. Schematic representation of the intraocular transplantation experiments. Left: Normal animal. The cell body of an adrenergic neuron is located in the superior cervical ganglion. Its nerve terminals innervate the iris (only one half of the iris is shown). Right: Iris transplantation. The iris of one eye is transferred to the anterior chamber of the other eye. The original plexus of nerves in the transplant degenerates. New nerves grow over from the iris of the host eye, where they are formed by collateral sprouting, to the transplant (from Olson and Malmfors, 1970, with permission of the publisher).

*References p. 473*

and transplanted by means of a fine pipette to the anterior chamber of the eye through a small slit in the cornea. Operations were performed under sterile conditions using a dissection microscope (Olson and Malmfors, 1970). The adrenergic nerves were studied by the histochemical fluorescence technique of Falck and Hillarp (Falck *et al.*, 1962; see also Corrodi and Jonsson, 1967) often in combination with [$^3$H]-noradrenaline uptake studies (Olson *et al.*, 1968). This made it possible to quantitatively follow the reinnervation in iris transplants. Re-establishment of neuromuscular transmission was monitored by studying contractions of transplanted smooth muscle strips *in vitro* (Malmfors *et al.*, 1970).

*Histochemistry of reinnervation*

The distribution and transmitter pharmacology of the adrenergic ground plexus in the albino rat iris is well known (Malmfors 1965; Jonsson *et al.*, 1969) and this organ was therefore used for the initial reinnervation experiments.

When an iris is autologously transplanted to the contralateral eye all intrinsic nerves degenerate. No fluorescent nerve fibres can be detected in the transplant two days postoperatively. However, already after four days, the first new fluorescent fibres are seen arborizing in the transplant. At this time vascular connections between the iris of the recipient eye and the transplant also begin to form. The subsequent reinnervation of the iris transplant is a fairly rapid process, leading to a normal density of nerves within one month (Figs. 1, 2).

Moreover, the morphology of the newly formed ground plexus is essentially the same as in a normal iris. The nerve terminals run two or more together in each strand of the plexus and show the typical regularly spaced varicosities which are supposed to be sites of transmitter release (Malmfors, 1965).

The iris transplantation experiments thus offer a unique possibility to quantitate the growth rates at the cellular level. Such a quantification has been carried out (Fig. 3) and made it possible to study different factors influencing the growth in order to obtain information about the mechanisms of growth and growth regulation.

The type of nerve growth demonstrated in the iris transplantation experiments is probably best described as collateral sprouting (see Murray and Thompson, 1957). The intact adrenergic nerves in the iris of the host eye responds to the demands of the denervated transplant and extend their field of innervation to include also the new iris. Concomitantly to the reinnervation of the transplant a certain hyperinnervation of the host iris is always noted, indicating that the same factor that causes nerves to grow over to the transplant affects also the plexus of the host iris.

A series of experiments similar to the one described above and other types including transplantation of sympathetic ganglia to the anterior chamber (Olson and Malmfors, 1970) permits the following conclusions concerning growth of sympathetic nerves in the adult rat:

1. The sympathetic adrenergic neuron has marked capacities for growth in the adult individual both following axotomy close to the cell body an in the form of collateral sprouting. A certain neuron can easily at least double its innervation area.

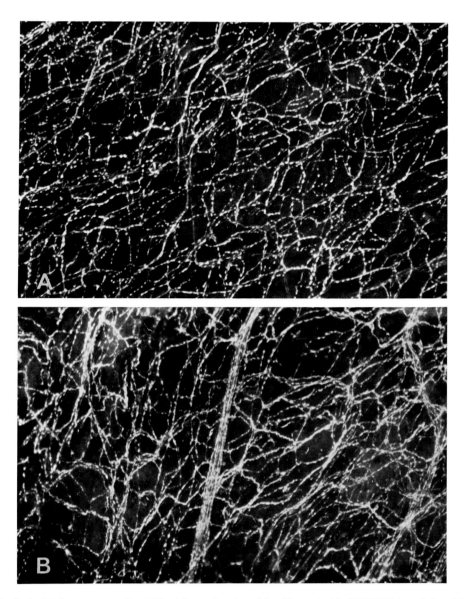

Fig. 2. A, Iris from a normal rat. The iris was incubated for 30 min in $10^{-7}$M [$^3$H]NA and rinsed in amine-free buffer for 10 min. It was then prepared as a whole mount, air dried, reacted with para-formaldehyde gas and photographed in the fluorescence microscope. The adrenergic ground plexus with its varicose nerve terminals is seen. $\times$ 225.

B, Iris transplant prepared as in A. The photograph demonstrates the amount of newly formed adrenergic nerves present in the transplant two weeks after transplantation. The ground plexus is similar to that in A, although more irregular and with a larger number of axon bundles. $\times$ 225 (from Olson and Malmfors, 1970, with permission of the publisher).

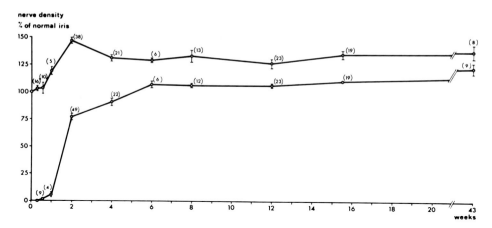

Fig. 3. Time course of reinnervation of irides autologously transplanted to the anterior chamber and the effect on the host irides as observed in the fluorescence microscope. The density of the nerve plexus after different times was estimated on coded slides as per cent of the density in normal irides. At each point the mean ± s.e.m. is given. Number of observations within brackets. Upper curve: Host irides. Lower curve: Iris transplants. The first few fluorescent fibres were found in the transplants after four days (seven out of nine transplants). The irides were incubated *in vitro* in [³H]noradrenaline as described in Fig. 2 A prior to preparation for fluorescence microscopy. Subsequent radioactivity determination yielded growth curves which were similar to the ones illustrated (from Olson and Malmfors, 1970, with permission of the publisher).

2. Growth is specific in the sense that nerves will grow only to locations in the transplant where they are normally present (certain qualitative and quantitative exceptions to this statement do, however, occur).

3. Growth is unspecific in the sense that any neuron of the sympathetic nervous system seems to be able to reinnervate any denervated effector organ.

4. Growth is stimulated by the presence of a sympathetically denervated tissue. Degenerating nerves are not the stimulating agent.

5. The new nerves possess essentially normal transmitter mechanisms as soon as they are being formed. Interference with the adrenergic transmission or transmitter mechanisms does not alter the growth.

### Re-establishment of neuromuscular transmission

The presence of varicose, fluorescent nerve terminals with normal transmitter mechanisms, that is normal uptake, retention and release of noradrenaline, indicates that functional neurotransmission is also re-established between the ingrown nerve and the effector cells of the transplants. In order to test this hypothesis, various smooth muscle transplants were tried where contractile responses could be measured *in vitro* after reinnervation.

Return of neuromuscular transmission could be demonstrated *in vitro* in small strips of the rat vas deferens and the portal vein by recording the contractions following

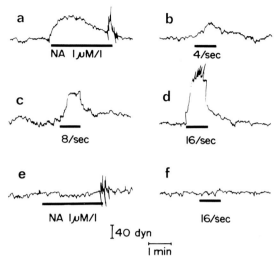

Fig. 4. Contractions recorded isometrically *in vitro* from a rat vas deferens transplant which had been situated in the anterior chamber for 13 months. a: The effect of noradrenaline added to the bath. b, c, and d: The effect of electrical field stimulation. e: Inhibition of the noradrenaline effect by alpha-adrenergic blockade. f: Inhibition of the effect of electrical field stimulation by alpha-adrenergic blockade. $10^{-6}$M phenoxybenzamine was used in e and f. Rapid pen movements following noradrenaline in the bath are rinsing artefacts (from Olson and Malmfors, 1970, with permission of the publisher).

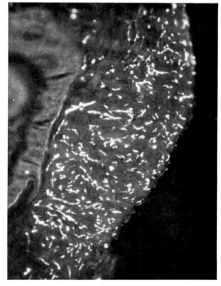

Fig. 5. Vas deferens transplant from the rat after 3 weeks in the anterior chamber. The smooth muscle bundles of the transplant are richly supplied with a new plexus of adrenergic nerves. Fluorescence photomicrograph of 8 $\mu$ section. $\times$ 185 (from Olson and Malmfors, 1970, with permission of the publisher).

electrical field stimulation. These responses were inhibited by $\alpha$-adrenergic blockade (Fig. 4). The tested muscle strips were found to be well reinnervated (Fig. 5).

In order to follow more closely the time courses of the functional recovery and the appearance of the receptor tissue similar experiments were carried out on guinea pig vas deferens, where larger transplants can be used. During the first four weeks after transplantation, no mechanical response was observed in the transplanted strip of the guinea pig vas deferens in spite of the presence of adrenergic nerves (Malmfors et al., 1970). As there was also a poor response to added NA it seems reasonable to assume that the failure was due to improper function of the effector cells. This hypothesis was confirmed by ultrastructural studies which showed that the smooth muscle cells of the vas deferens transplant underwent marked changes after the transplantation. During the first week there was a massive degeneration of muscle cells. This was followed by a progressive regeneration of the smooth muscle cells and after 4 weeks they started to form bundles again. After 6 weeks, nerve-mediated responses could be obtained. There was a gradual development of the force of the contraction and 14 weeks after transplantation a few transplants showed the same amplitude of response as a corresponding strip directly prepared from the vas deferens. However, the transplant had a somewhat steeper frequency response curve than the control and showed fatigue somewhat faster. Furthermore, the transplants did not start to contract until 2–3 sec after the start of the stimulation while the controls contracted within 0.2–0.5 sec. The significance of this difference is unclear. Those transplants which responded to nerve stimulation also responded to added NA. At some occasions the cervical sympathetic trunk was stimulated before the preparation of the transplant and contraction of the transplant could then be observed in vivo.

Subsequent fluorescence histochemical studies of the transplants after the in vitro experiments revealed that there was no close correlation between the number of nerves and the mechanical response during the first four weeks after the transplantation. During the first two weeks there were a lot of nerves located to the periphery but later also among the bundles of the smooth muscle cells. However, even if small areas in some of the guinea pig vas deferens transplants had the same density of adrenergic nerves as normally, no transplant showed normal nerve density throughout the whole strip within 14 weeks, which was the longest time studied. A few transplants which showed a very good mechanical response after 14 weeks, in fact, had a very sparse innervation. It is therefore obvious that the mechanical response is more dependent upon the effector cells than upon the number of nerves.

## COMMENTS

The intraocular transplantation technique, first used in combination with the Falck–Hillarp fluorescence method by Owman 1964, has proved to be an excellent tool for studies of adrenergic nerve growth mechanisms. Our transplantation experiments (Malmfors and Olson 1967, Olson and Malmfors 1970, Malmforse, t al., 1970) have clearly demonstrated that the adrenergic nerves possess very efficient growth mechanisms also in the adult animal. Reinnervation of transplanted tissues is a specific and rapid process leading to a morphologically normal pattern of nerves that restores adrenergic neurotransmission in the transplants.

As pointed out above, some general conclusions concerning regeneration and reinnervation in the adrenergic nervous system have already been obtained. Many interesting and important questions remain, however, to be answered. It was for instance noted that a slight infection of the host iris enhanced the hyperinnervation observed there following transplantation. The reason for this effect is obscure. Since pharmacological blockade of the adrenergic receptors seemed to have very small effects on growth and since the presence of degenerating nerves was not necessary for growth, the interest is focused on the plexus of Schwann cells. Electron microscopy has demonstrated that the newly formed nerves are enclosed in the Schwann cells both in the vas deferens transplants (Malmfors *et al.*, 1970) and following iris and ganglion transplantations (Hökfelt and Olson, unpublished observations). It seems thus probable that it is the Schwann cell plexus that is responsible for the structural organization of the newly formed nerve plexuses, but the Schwann cells might, of course, play a more active part in the reinnervation process.

ACKNOWLEDGEMENT

Supported by the Swedish Medical Research Council (B70-14X-711-05B and B71-14X-3185-01), Svenska Livförsäkringsbolags nämnd för medicinsk forskning, Olli and Elof Ericssons Stiftelse and Stiftelsen Therese och Johan Anderssons Mine.

REFERENCES

CORRODI, H. AND JONSSON, G. (1967) *J. Histochem. Cytochem.*, **15**, 65–78.
FALCK, B., HILLARP, N.-Å., THIEME, G. AND TORP, A. (1962) *J. Histochem. Cytochem.*, **10**, 348–354.
JONSSON, G., HAMBERGER, B., MALMFORS, T. AND SACHS, CH. (1969) *Europ. J. Pharmacol.*, **8**, 58–72.
MALMFORS, T. (1965) *Acta Physiol. Scand.*, **64**, *Suppl. 248*, 1–93.
MALMFORS, T., FURNESS, I. B., CAMPBELL, G. R. AND BURNSTOCK, G. (1970) *J. Cell Biol.*, in press.
MALMFORS, T. AND OLSON, L. (1967) *Acta Physiol. Scand.*, **71**, 401–402.
MURRAY, J. G. AND THOMPSON, J. W. (1957) *J. Physiol.*, **135**, 133–162.
OLSON, L., HAMBERGER, B., JONSSON, G. AND MALMFORS, T. (1968) *Histochemie*, **15**, 38–45.
OLSON, L. AND MALMFORS, T. (1970) *Acta Physiol. Scand.*, *Suppl. 348*, 1–112.
OWMAN, CH. (1964) *Intern. J. Neuropharmacol.*, **2**, 105–112.

# Changes in Autonomic Nerves of Salivary Glands on Degeneration and Regeneration

J. R. GARRETT

*Department of Oral Pathology, The Dental School, King's College Hospital Medical School, London, S.E.5 (U.K.)*

The nerves of the major salivary glands are convenient for studying the changes that occur after *post-ganglionic* denervations. The sympathetic nerve trunk to the submandibular gland of the cat is readily identifiable and can be traced from the superior cervical ganglion to the artery of the gland. Post-ganglionic parasympathetic nerves for the parotid gland run in the auriculo-temporal nerve. These nerve supplies are virtually pure in the old-fashioned sense of the post-ganglionic divisions of the sympathetic and parasympathetic systems, as will become evident from the text. Being paired they allow an experimental control in the same animal. The physiological events which occur after these denervations have been extensively studied by Professor Nils Emmelin and his colleagues in Lund (see Emmelin, 1965, 1967a, b, 1968a, b) and this affords functional data against which to assess results. In brief the nerves to the glands normally leak subliminal amounts of neurotransmitter, in the absence of nerve impulses, and at a certain period after section of the post-ganglionic nerves the leakage increases and may even cause an overt secretion — *degeneration secretion* — which continues for a limited time. Thereafter the secretory cells show a gradually increasing sensitivity to autonomimetic drugs which can not be solely explained on the basis that the normal mechanisms for removal of the transmitter are reduced. The onset of the degeneration activation has an inverse relationship with the length of nerve that has to degenerate for any one organ but there are big differences in the timings of the events in different species and in different organs of the same species.

In the present paper the ultrastructural and histochemical events which occur in the non-myelinated nerves of the glands after *post-ganglionic* denervations will be considered and related, as far as possible, to the physiological phenomena. The long-term changes, usually after preventing reinnervation from the natural source, will also be mentioned.

## POST-GANGLIONIC PARASYMPATHETIC DENERVATION

### Changes in terminal nerves of the parotid gland

After removal of the auriculo-temporal nerve distinctive ultrastructural changes are found for a time in terminal parasympathetic nerves of the parotid gland of the cat.

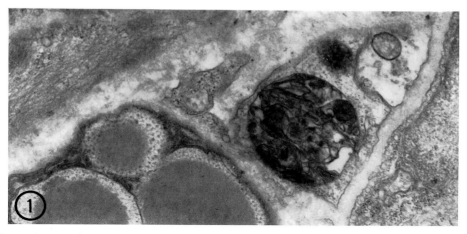

Fig. 1. Electron micrograph of a parotid gland showing osmiophilic degenerative changes in an axon 48 hours after avulsion of the auriculo-temporal nerve. × 27500.

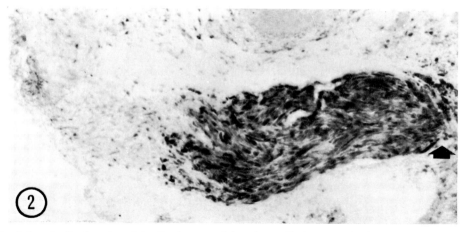

Fig. 2. Longitudinal section of the distal stump of the submandibular sympathetic trunk 48 hours after sectioning at site marked (↑) showing increased activity of non-specific esterase in fusiform axonal swellings. × 80.

Few of these changes are seen by 24 h; they are more frequent at 48 h; and can occasionally be seen 4 days afterwards (Garrett, 1966 d). A variety of changes are seen at any one time and each is associated with increased osmiophilia: sometimes a granular osmiophilic structure is seen within an axon; other axons are loaded with organelles which are losing their definition and becoming generally darker; and some whole axons have a granular osmiophilic appearance (see Fig. 1). Many axons appear to be going through a state of dissolution with cytoplasmic structures scattered about in dark clumps. There is little swelling of the axons and burst ones have not been seen, but instead they soon lose their mes-axon and become incorporated within the Schwann cell cytoplasm. In addition dense laminated bodies are seen in some Schwann cells. The above changes are possibly maximal some time after 48 h and thereafter the nerves rapidly disappear. The changes are very irregular in their general distribution. Serial sections indicate that they also occur irregularly along individual axons and thus it is not possible to be certain that a relatively normal looking axon is not disintegrating somewhere out of the plane of the section. The osmiophilic changes, however, are readily recognisable and give a clear indication that such axons have come from the nerve supply which has been interrupted. Similar changes have recently been described in the iris of the rat after ciliary ganglionectomy by Roth and Richardson (1969).

These events have begun before the occurrence of the degeneration secretion, which starts about 28 h after section of the auriculo-temporal nerve, but in the main they lag behind, for degeneration secretion is often maximal after about 36–40 h and has usually ceased by 56 h (Emmelin, 1968 b). It may be that vesicles accumulate prior to degeneration secretion but this is very difficult to ascertain because of the discontinuous arrangement of the vesicles and the irregular occurrence of the degenerative changes. It is considered that the leakage of transmitter occurs whilst the axolemmal membrane is intact rather than when the axon disrupts, for the disruption occurs by incorporation into the Schwann cell and not by bursting outwards. This is supported by the finding of Emmelin and Strömblad (1958) that degeneration secretion was abolished by cocaine in doses which did not interfere with the effects of intravenous acetylcholine, and it was suggested that the cocaine was inhibiting the release of acetylcholine from the axons. Thus leakage probably precedes the stage of increased osmiophilia. How then does one explain the fact that some osmiophilic degenerative features are seen prior to degeneration secretion? It is likely that the leakage of transmitter is sporadic and at widely separate sites in the early and late stages of the degeneration process and is not then sufficient to induce an overt secretion; the secretion only becomes detectable when the events are more frequent and widespread.

Histochemically the cholinergic nerves in the parotid gland of the cat show strong acetylcholinesterase (AChE) activity and weaker less extensive non-specific cholinesterase (ChE) activity (Garrett, 1966 a) and the latter possibly represents activity in Schwann cells. After avulsion of the auriculo-temporal nerve no change in either cholinesterase activity was detectable at 48 h, but thereafter there was a fairly rapid extensive loss which reached a peak from the 6th to 8th day (Garrett, 1966 c). However, some AChE-positive nerves always persisted, even after superior cervical ganglionectomy as well. These changes are very similar to those detected by Strömblad (1957) using a manometric method. Nordenfelt (1963, 1964) found a more rapid and more complete loss of choline acetyltransferase after post-ganglionic parasympathetic denervation of the parotid, but a small activity always persisted and probably related to the remaining cholinergic nerves that had not been destroyed by the denervation. The loss of choline acetyltransferase begins at a similar time to, or even precedes, the increased leakage of the acetylcholine which causes the degeneration secretion, whereas the AChE loss occurs afterwards, possibly when the degenerating axon is being incorporated into the Schwann cell. There is an accompanying loss of ChE which, if it be from the Schwann cells, would indicate that its presence in the Schwann cell has a functional connection with normal axonal activity. This loss of ChE contrasts with the increase that occurs in the Schwann cells of the rat after degeneration of motor nerves (Eränkö and Teräväinen, 1967).

In time a gradually progressive reinnervation by AChE-positive nerves occurs irregularly throughout the gland (Garrett, 1966 c) and it was attributed to collateral sprouting by the intact nerves from uncharted sources, but it was not known if any restoration of function occurred. More recently attention has been directed to the post-ganglionic parasympathetic innervation of the parotid gland in dogs (Emmelin, et al., 1968; Garrett and Holmberg, 1970a, b), for the functional changes of dener-vation can be ascertained more readily in the dog. It has been found that all of the parasympathetic nerves do not course throughout the whole of the anatomically defined auriculo-temporal nerve. Most, if not all, of the nerves appear to pass through the third branch of the trigeminal nerve, some twigs passing via the artery alongside (Holmberg, 1970). The parotid gland of the dog contains a more dense innervation by AChE-positive nerves than that of the cat but the sequence of events after post-ganglionic parasympathetic denervation is similar to that described for the cat. Associated with the reinnervation that occurs in time there is some return of reflex secretion and a corresponding decrease in the sensitivity of the cells to parasym-pathomimetic drugs. Thus it would appear that if any cholinergic nerves remain in the gland they can give rise to collateral sprouts which can establish a functional activity. Since this occurs with cholinergic nerves does it also occur with adrenergic nerves? Simple post-ganglionic parasympathectomy of the parotid glands in dogs does not cause any detectable change in the adrenergic nerves at any stage after the denervation as viewed by formaldehyde-induced fluorescence (Garrett and Holmberg, 1970 b). Thus there does not appear to be any replacement of lost cholinergic nerves by adrenergic nerves.

### POST-GANGLIONIC SYMPATHETIC DENERVATION

#### A. Changes in terminal nerves of the submandibular gland

Twenty-four hours after excision of the superior cervical ganglion in the cat little or no change is evident in the formaldehyde-induced fluorescent appearance of adrenergic nerves within the submandibular gland, but they are all lost by about 48 h and show no sign of reappearance 1 year later (Garrett, 1970 a). The time sequence for the loss of fluorescence by the nerves is similar to that in the nictitating membrane of the cat (Van Orden et al., 1967), but is much slower than the loss of noradrenaline in the submandibular gland of the rat (Benmiloud and Euler, 1963) or of fluorescent nerves in the iris of the rat (Malmfors and Sachs, 1965).

Simple section of the sympathetic trunk to the submandibular gland causes an almost complete loss of fluorescing nerves within the submandibular gland, and confiirms that most of the sympathetic supply for the gland travels by way of this nerve trunk.

No changes were detected in terminal nerves of the gland by cholinesterase staining at any stage after sympathectomy (Garrett, 1966 c), and this agrees with the mano-metric findings of Strömblad (1957). Some changes did occur, however, in the cholinesterase reactions of the main sympathetic trunks within the gland and will be mentioned in the next section.

At the ultrastructural level sympathetic axons of the submandibular gland showed degenerative changes after sympathectomy which were similar in appearance and time sequence to those described above in the parotid after parasympathectomy (Garrett, 1966 d): few osmiophilic appearances indicative of degeneration were seen by 24 h; they were much more plentiful at 48 h; and they could occasionally be seen 4 days afterwards. In the absence of the use of specific fixation to demonstrate catecholamine-containing vesicles no comment was possible about the timing of their fate. Similar osmiophilic degenerative changes were found by Van Orden et al. (1967) in the nictitating membrane of the cat after excision of the superior cervical ganglion, being infrequent at 24 h but common 48 h afterwards. These workers used glutaraldehyde fixation and found that loss of granular vesicles preceded the osmiophilic changes. More recently Roth and Richardson (1969) have described identical osmiophilic degenerative changes in the iris of the rat after superior cervical ganglionectomy, but the time sequence was more rapid and these appearances ceased to be detected within 48 h. Van Orden et al. (1967) found degranulation of the vesicles to be the first detectable change and it corresponded in time to degeneration contraction of the nictitating membrane, but at this stage the axons showed no loss of fluorescence, and this was thus attributed to extravesicular noradrenaline. Loss of fluorescence occurred mainly during the phase of cessation of degeneration contraction and as this proceeded the osmiophilic changes increased. Sympathetic degeneration secretion, when present in the cat, lags behind degeneration contraction of the nictitating membrane (Emmelin, 1968 a), but no attempt at correlation between the secretory events and the morphological histochemical changes has yet been made.

## B. *Changes in the sympathetic trunk on the submandibular artery*

The part of the trunk examined was always at a distance from the site of transection, which was usually by superior cervical ganglionectomy and occasionally by simple section of the trunk proximal to the submandibular artery. All the experiments were performed on cats.

A moderate degree of formaldehyde-induced fluorescence occurs in the normal trunk but it is much weaker 24 h after ganglionectomy, although the arterial nerves still show strong fluorescence, and it is lost by 48 h (Garrett, 1969).

Cholinesterase histochemistry of the sympathetic trunks shows a distinctive pattern of weak fine fibre-like AChE activity, which is probably axonal, and a coarser denser band-like ChE activity, which is probably in the Schwann cells. This pattern is very different from that in post-ganglionic parasympathetic trunks, which exhibit a stronger AChE than ChE activity, and the latter is always more positive than that in the sympathetic trunks (Garrett, 1966 a). After sympathectomy the activity of both enzymes is gradually lost in a patchy manner from about 2 days onwards and the process is complete after 8 to 12 days (Garrett, 1969, 1970 a). The loss of ChE, presumably from the Schwann cells, lags a little behind that of AChE and its loss implies

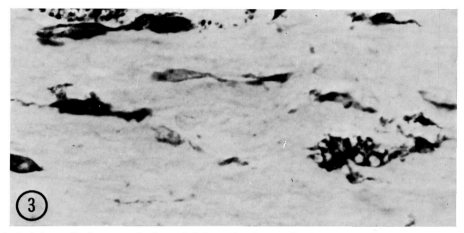

Fig. 3. Submandibular sympathetic trunk 8 days after decentralisation showing cells with strong non-specific esterase activity, one of which has a vesiculated appearance. × 640.

some functional connection with normal axonal activity, and again contrasts with the increased activity in Schwann cells of motor nerves in the rat after denervation (Eränkö and Teräväinen, 1967). The nerve trunks do not disappear, and in time there is a gradual re-emergence of cholinesterase activity with a reverse in the staining intensities of the 2 enzymes so that AChE now shows the stronger reaction, thus giving features more like parasympathetic nerves. The process has started by about the 16th day and within 2 months the reaction has become quite strong and does not increase much more up to 1 year. It always has an irregular distribution with some negative areas in the trunk and never becomes as strong as in the main parasympathetic trunks. In the 3 to 8-week period sections of the nerve close to the gland showed stronger activity than those taken nearer the origin of the artery. The re-emergence of activity still occurred when measures were taken to prevent any reinnervation from the stump end, and similar changes have even been observed in the sympathetic trunks within the gland 21 days after total removal of the submandibular artery as well as the superior cervical ganglion. These results, and the finding by Nordenfelt (1965) that an increase in choline acetyltransferase occurs in the submandibular gland of the cat after superior cervical ganglionectomy, are taken to indicate that collateral sprouting from cholinergic post-ganglionic parasympathetic nerves has occurred and progressed in a retrograde manner down the sympathetic trunks.

Other enzymes have also been studied histochemically in the submandibular sympathetic trunk of the cat after superior cervical ganglionectomy (Garrett, 1970 a). Non-specific esterase, demonstrated by an azo-dye method, gives a faint diffuse reaction in the normal trunk. Shortly after sympathectomy, scattered strongly stained spindly cells are seen, reaching a peak in intensity of stain and numbers between the 4th to the 8th post-operative days; thereafter the staining gradually diminishes and eventually returns to a more normal appearance. This activity is E600 sensitive but Mipafox resistant. Only a certain number of cells develop this activity, and since electron microscopy does not reveal the migration of new cells into the trunk it is wondered whether the cells are reactive fibroblasts. However by 8 days occasional vacuolated positive cells are seen (Fig. 3) resembling some of the Schwann cells (described later), but if Schwann cells are included in this group of strongly stained cells they represent only a percentage of the total population of Schwann cells. Little acid phosphatase activity is detectable in the normal sympathetic trunks; faint perinuclear activity is just visible in Schwann cells by an azo-dye method. After sympathectomy some increase in this activity occurs up to about the 16th day but it is never very remarkable and no strongly positive cells are found in the trunk. Although a strong monoamine oxidase activity has been found in the neurones of the superior cervical ganglion of the cat by Giacobini and Kerpel-Fronius (1970) it is almost undetectable in the submandibular sympathetic trunk and it was not possible to recognise any change after superior cervical ganglionectomy.

Ultrastructurally the non-myelinated axons in the submandibular sympathetic trunk cut transversely (Fig. 4) show an orderly appearance and are arranged singly or in small groups with an investing Schwann cell (Garrett, 1966 b). Their diameter varies somewhat but most are between 1.5–2 $\mu$. The axoplasm contains numerous tubules, some filaments, mitochondria, and vesicles, few of which contain a dense-cored granule. Collagen is present between the Schwann-axon bundles and scattered fibroblasts are also seen. After removal of the superior cervical ganglion (Garrett, 1966 and 1970 a) little change is noticed by 24 h apart from an occasional swollen axon with less dense cytoplasm. By 48 h the axoplasm in most axons has lost its structure and has a faint amorphous appearance. Any mitochondria left are losing their definition but do not show increased osmiophilia. Many axons are now very small as if compressed but a few are rather distended and vacuolated (Fig. 5). In contrast with the terminal nerves little or no features of increased osmiophilia occur in the axons. The Schwann cells look somewhat reactive, with the endoplasmic reticulum and ribosomes more pronounced than usual. The fibroblasts often look more reactive and appear packed with organelles. No inflammatory cells are seen in this part of the trunk at any stage after ganglionectomy. By four days the process is more complete and every non-myelinated axon is altered. Many have already disappeared and left basement membrane envelopes which are either empty or contain processes of Schwann cells. Similar basement membrane envelopes have been found in somatic nerve degeneration (Nathaniel and Pease, 1963 a, b; Thomas, 1964). Most of the axonal remains are now small and appear to be in the process of being absorbed into the Schwann cell. Some axons are still distended and these particularly show fragmentation of the axoplasmic membrane. Few axonal remains are seen after eight days and the process is virtually complete by about the 12th day (Fig. 6). At this time numerous basement membrane envelopes are seen and the basement membrane around most Schwann cells lies in loose folds. In the 8–12 day period some of the Schwann cells exhibit a peculiar vesiculated appearance (see Fig. 6). Holtzman and Novikoff (1965) have recognised similar 'transformed' Schwann cells in degenerating somatic nerves and associated the change with digestive processes.

From about this time onwards axons begin to reappear and these presumably give

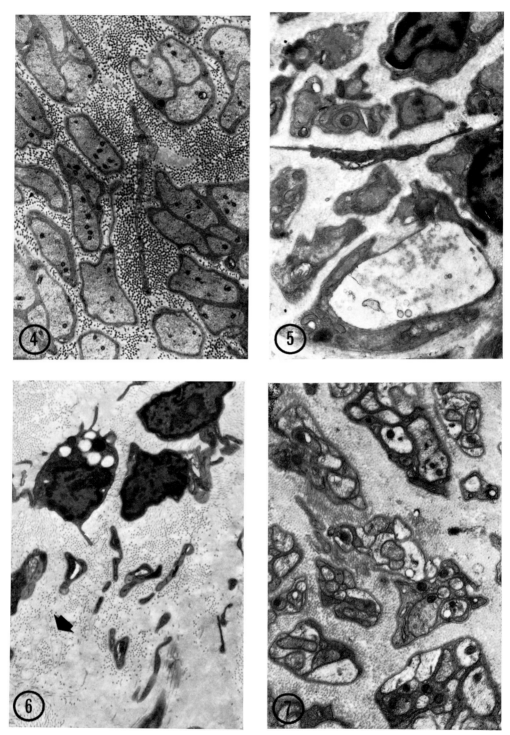

Figs. 4–7. Electron micrographs of submandibular sympathetic trunks. 4. Normal control. × 9500.
5. Two days after superior cervical ganglionectomy showing loss of axoplasmic structure. Most axons
are now small but one is dilated. × 9500. 6. Twelve days after superior cervical ganglionectomy
showing loss of axons. Basement membrane envelopes are present (↑) and also a vesiculated Schwann
cell. × 6500. 7. One year after superior cervical ganglionectomy showing numerous irregular Schwann-
axon bundles. × 13 500.

rise to the cholinesterase appearances described above. Occasionally axons containing numerous organelles are seen in the early stages and these possibly represent growing ends of new axons. By 21 days a fair number of axons are seen and a large number are present at the end of a year (Fig. 7). Although the axons appear normal they are generally smaller than in the control trunk; often there are more axons per Schwann cell, and the overall profile is more irregular than normal. In fact many of the nerves look more like nerves in a peripheral tissue rather than those in transit in a nerve trunk. Empty basement membrane envelopes have been seen 4 months after ganglionectomy, which shows that their chemical constituents are not readily broken down in this situation. It also indicates that some sites of previous nerves are not reinnervated, and in fact the trunk never contains so many non-myelinated Schwann-axon bundles so closely packed as in the control and this accounts for the somewhat patchy cholinesterase staining. As discussed above these nerves are thought to have arisen by collateral sprouting within the gland from post-ganglionic parasympathetic nerves which have grown out along the trunk in a retrograde manner.

*C. Changes in the submandibular sympathetic trunk immediately distal to the site of transection*

This has been studied after 2, 8 and 12 days in cats (Garrett, 1970 a). At 2 days the stumps were not ligatured but at subsequent times they were ligatured for identification purposes.

The ultrastructural changes found after 2 days were similar to those found after 24 h by Kapeller and Mayor (1969) in splenic and hypogastric nerves just distal to a ligature. There was gross swelling of some, but not all, axons in any one section. The swollen axons were densely laden with osmiophilic organelles including numerous mitochondria, and neurofilamentous material could often be seen interspersed between the organelles. Sites of rupture have been observed in transverse sections (Fig. 8) and the extruded material was not bounded by a limiting membrane. The other axons mostly showed amorphous contents but neurofilaments and tubules were still present in some of them. Kapeller and Mayor (1969) found that all axons were distended adjacent to a ligature and the axonal variation in the present observations may be due to the sections not being immediately adjacent to the site of transection. However, from the light-microscopical appearance (see below) it would appear that the axonal swellings are discontinuous and do not all continue to the cut end of the stump. Thus it is possible that many of the non-swollen axons were in fact connected to a swelling somewhere out of the plane of the section, either above or below. The associated Schwann cells showed reactive changes with prominence of the endoplasmic reticulum and some dense bodies were seen in their cytoplasm.

By the twelfth day most of the axonal swellings had disappeared, and although some still persisted, their contents were mainly less dense than at 2 days. Occasional sites showed where a burst had previously occurred but by this time the extruded material was bounded by Schwann cells (Fig. 9). The stump was very cellular and composed mostly of Schwann cells that looked very reactive and nearly all contained

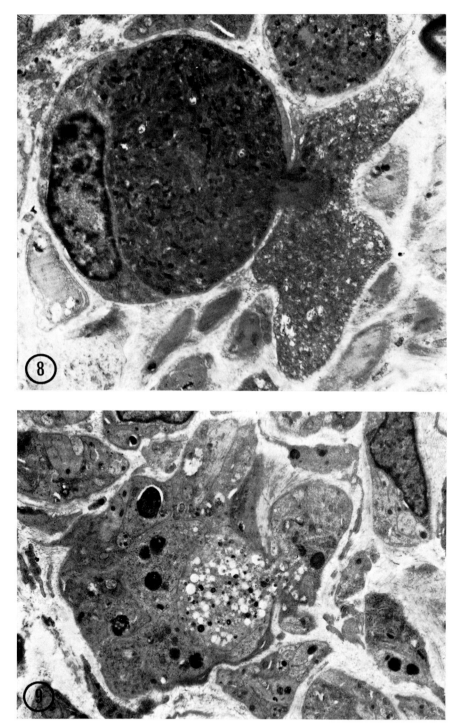

Figs. 8 and 9. Electron micrographs of the distal stumps of submandibular sympathetic trunks near the site of transection. 8. Two days after sectioning showing a very swollen organelle-loaded axon, which has burst in one small place. The extruded contents is loosing its structure and is not bounded by a limiting membrane. × 8000. 9. Twelve days after sectioning showing the remains of a swollen axon which has previously burst. There is less structure in the contents than at 2 days and it is now completely surrounded by Schwann cells, many of which contain conspicuous dense bodies. × 5000.

dense bodies. This contrasts with the more empty appearance of the trunk at a distance from the transection. It would seem that most of the digestion is done by the Schwann cells, but in the 12-day specimen an inflamed vessel was seen with inflammatory cells migrating into the stump and so some of the final mopping up may be done by these cells in this situation.

The light-microscopical material was sectioned longitudinally and after 2 days the non-ligatured distal stump showed a distinct swelling for about 2–3 mm composed largely of discontinuous fusiform swellings of axons. This zone showed remarkable histochemical activity and the fusiform swellings gave very strong acid phosphatase and non-specific esterase reactions (Fig. 2). They even showed an accumulation of amine oxidase which, as aforesaid, is not readily detectable in the normal trunk. Large accumulations of acid phosphatase and esterase have been demonstrated light microscopically in the distal stump of the sciatic nerve close to the site of transection by Gould and Holt (1961) and the electron-microscopical localization of acid phosphatase in such a preparation has been described by Holtzman and Novikoff (1965). Kreutzberg (1963) showed that there was also an accumulation of oxidative enzymes in the distal stump of a somatic nerve near the site of transection and recently Banks et al. (1969) detected an increase in cytochrome oxidase in the most proximal part of the distal stump of a transected adrenergic nerve trunk.

The cholinesterases showed a very different change. AChE was almost totally lost from the distal stump 48 h after section whereas the nerves at some distance from the swollen stump still showed activity. This contrasts with the accumulation of AChE demonstrated on the distal side of a ligature in somatic nerves by Zelená and Lubińska (1962). The ChE activity was now seen in strands separated in a lattice-like manner by the non-reactive axonal swellings which indicated that the activity is in the Schwann cells.

The histochemical activities in the distal stump decreased with time and at 12 days not many fusiform swellings were found. Non-specific esterase-positive cells were seen at 8 and 12 days and by 12 days the acid phosphatase activity was largely found in Schwann cells, which showed most activity towards the tip. At 8 and 12 days occasional inflammatory cells containing strong acid phosphatase activity were also seen near the tip.

The cause of the dramatic formation of organelle-loaded swellings of axons just distal to the site of transection has been discussed by Kapeller and Mayor (1969) who, though favouring a view that the organelles have come from more distal parts, consider they are the result of a reactive change rather than reflecting an aspect of normal retrograde axoplasmic flow as suggested by Lubińska (1964). How has this movement come about? Some of it may be by natural active forces within the axon, whatever they may be, but it is possible that physical forces acting on the axon from without, principally by the Schwann cell, may play some part. Rhythmic contractions of Schwann cells have been observed in culture by Pomerat (1959). Kapeller and Mayor (1969) have shown that development of these swellings has already occurred by 24 h but, as mentioned above, very few of the more peripheral parts of the nerve show detectable change at this time. It would seem that interruption of the nerves causes a weakness of the nearby axoplasmic membrane and thus any pressure on the nerves will be translocated to this part and induce a swelling that can not be contained by the Schwann cells. However, on a purely physical basis it is difficult to explain why the swellings contain such a high percentage of mitochondria and other organelles. Nevertheless in some of the swellings one can see neurofilamentous material in amongst the organelles, which supports the idea that some of the movement may be by pressure on the axons. Such pressure may explain why most of the axons further along the trunk become collapsed prior to dissolution; the swellings in this situation being the consequence of weaknesses in the axonal wall which allow local distension by migrating axonal contents and by imbibition of extra-cellular fluid.

### D. The reinnervation capabilities of the sympathetic nerves

It is well known that adrenergic nerves have a great capacity for reinnervation and this may even occur from one structure to another, such as in tissues transplanted to the anterior chamber of the eye in rats (Malmfors and Olson, 1967) and in cats (Jacobowitz and Laties, 1970). The reformation of adrenergic axons in the sciatic nerve after interruption of the nerve has recently been studied in rats (Olson, 1969). However, as shown above, removal of the superior cervical ganglion in cats leads to a replacement of the nerves by sprouting from the parasympathetic nerves which even grow down the sympathetic trunk itself. This process is a fairly rapid one and therefore it seemed possible that such sprouting might impair any natural innervation by adrenergic axons growing along the cut nerves.

To test this possibility the submandibular sympathetic trunk of a cat was sectioned proximal to the submandibular artery and the ends repositioned. The results were compared with the effects of superior cervical ganglionectomy performed on the opposite side at the same time (Garrett, 1970 b). A biopsy of the submandibular gland taken after 8 days from the side on which simple section of the trunk had been performed showed an almost complete loss of adrenergic nerves within the gland, thus confirming the efficacy of the denervation. After 2 months tissues from both sides were removed. Those from the side of the ganglionectomy remained totally devoid of adrenergic nerves. But the submandibular gland from the side of simple section of the nerve trunk now showed some reinnervation by adrenergic nerves, and the trunk itself also showed a patchy fluorescence distal to the original lesion, which indicates that some of the reinnervation probably came along this channel as well as by any sprouting from nerves left intact by the original manoeuvre.

Examination of the trunks on the submandibular artery for cholinesterases showed the usual changes on the side of the superior cervical ganglionectomy, with the nerves now giving a strong AChE reaction and a slightly weaker one for ChE. The trunks on the side of simple section were totally different and gave a uniform weak AChE reaction and a slightly stronger one for ChE, features similar to normal sympathetic trunks. Therefore, after simple section of the trunk, sprouting by cholinergic nerves down the trunk either did not occur, or if it did, the nerves subsequently regressed and did not interfere with adrenergic reinnervation.

This implies that after denervation the presence of some adrenergic nerves exerts a restraining force on parasympathetic sprouting. What this force is and how it operates is a matter for speculation. Furthermore, taken in conjunction with the results of parasympathetic denervation in the parotid, it indicates that there are other forces acting to restore a normal innervation should any nerves of the appropriate division of the autonomic system remain, the modus operandi of which again affords great scope for speculation.

## CONCLUSIONS

The early changes of degeneration in post-ganglionic autonomic nerves after decentralisation are dramatic near the site of section and in the terminal axons but rather passive in the territory between. Wherever the site, the axons are finally lost by digestion in the accompanying Schwann cells and both axons and Schwann cells lose their cholinesterase activities. Any remaining nerves have a great capacity for inducing reinnervation, which, in the total absence of the appropriate autonomic division, may be taken over to some extent by the other division, but if any of the appropriate nerves remain a great effort is exerted to re-establish normal innervation. The factors inducing and controlling these changes are not known.

## REFERENCES

BANKS, P., MANGNALL, D. AND MAYOR, D. (1969) *J. Physiol.*, **200**, 745–762.
BENMILOUD, M. AND EULER, U. S. V. (1963) *Acta Physiol. Scand.*, **59**, 34–42.
EMMELIN, N. (1965) *Experientia*, **21**, 57–65.
EMMELIN, N. (1967 a) In: L. H. SCHNEYER AND C. A. SCHNEYER (Eds.), *Secretory Mechanisms of Salivary Glands*, Academic Press, New York, pp. 127–140.
EMMELIN, N. (1967 b) In: C. F. CODE (Ed.), *Handbook of Physiology — Section 6 — Alimentary Canal*, Vol. II, *Secretion*, American Physiological Society, Washington, pp. 595–632.
EMMELIN, N. (1968 a) *Experientia*, **24**, 44–45.
EMMELIN, N. (1968 b) *J. Physiol.*, **195**, 407–418.
EMMELIN, N., GARRETT, J. R. AND HOLMBERG, J. (1968) *Experientia*, **24**, 460–461.
EMMELIN, N. AND STRÖMBLAD, B. C. R. (1958) *J. Physiol.*, **143**, 506–514.
ERÄNKÖ, O. AND TERÄVÄINEN, H. (1967) *J. Neurochem.*, **14**, 947–954.
GARRETT, J. R. (1966 a) *J. Roy. Microscop. Soc.*, **85**, 135–148.
GARRETT, J. R. (1966 b) *J. Roy. Microscop. Soc.*, **85**, 149–162.
GARRETT, J. R. (1966 c) *J. Roy. Microscop. Soc.*, **86**, 1–13.
GARRETT, J. R. (1966 d) *J. Roy. Microscop. Soc.*, **86**, 15–31.
GARRETT, J. R. (1969) *J. Physiol.*, **202**, 34 P.
GARRETT, J. R. (1970 a) in preparation.
GARRETT, J. R. (1970 b) unpublished observations.
GARRETT, J. R. AND HOLMBERG, J. (1970 a) *J. Physiol.*, **209**, 19–20P.
GARRETT, J. R. AND HOLMBERG, J. (1970b) unpublished observations.
GIACOBINI, E. AND KERPEL-FRONIUS, S. (1970) *Acta Physiol. Scand.*, **78**, 522–528.
GOULD, R. P. AND HOLT, S. J. (1961) In: *Cytology of the Nervous System*, Proc. Anatomical Soc. Taylor Francis, London, p. 45–48.
HOLMBERG, J. (1970) unpublished observation.
HOLTZMAN, E. AND NOVIKOFF, A. B. (1965) *J. Cell Biol.*, **27**, 651–669.
JACOBOWITZ, D. AND LATIES, M. (1970) *Endocrinology*, **86**, 921–924.
KAPELLER, K. AND MAYOR, D. (1969) *Proc. Roy. Soc. London, B.*, **172**, 53–63.

KREUTZBERG, G. (1963) *Naturwissenschaften*, **50**, 96.

LUBIŃSKA, L. (1964) In: M. SINGER AND J. P. SCHADÉ (Eds.), *Mechanisms of Neural Regeneration, Progress in Brain Research, Vol. 13*, Elsevier, Amsterdam, London, New York, pp. 1–71.

MALMFORS, T. AND OLSON, L. (1967) *Acta Physiol. Scand.*, **71**, 401–402.

MALMFORS, T. AND SACHS, C. (1965) *Acta Physiol. Scand.*, **64**, 211–223.

NATHANIEL, E. J. H. AND PEASE, D. C. (1963 a) *J. Ultrastruct. Res.*, **9**, 511–532.

NATHANIEL, E. J. H. AND PEASE, D. C. (1963 b) *J. Ultrastruct. Res.*, **9**, 533–549.

NORDENFELT, I. (1963) *Quart. J. Exp. Physiol.*, **48**, 67–79.

NORDENFELT, I. (1964) *Quart. J. Exp. Physiol.*, **49**, 103–111.

NORDENFELT, I. (1965) *Quart. J. Exp. Physiol.*, **50**, 57–61.

OLSON, L. (1969) *Histochemie*, **17**, 349–367.

POMERAT, C. M. (1959) *Science*, **130**, 1759–1760.

ROTH, C. D. AND RICHARDSON, K. C. (1969) *Amer. J. Anat.*, **124**, 341–360.

STRÖMBLAD, B. C. R. (1957) *Acta Physiol. Scand.*, **41**, 118–138.

THOMAS, P. K. (1964) *J. Anat.*, **98**, 175–182.

VAN ORDEN, L. S., BENSCH, K. G., LANGER, S. Z. AND TRENDELENBURG, U. (1967) *J. Pharmacol. Exp. Therap.*, **157**, 274–283.

ZELENÁ, J. AND LUBIŃSKA, L. (1962) *Physiol. Bohemoslov.*, **11**, 261–268.

# Noradrenaline Transport in Sympathetic Nerves

D. MAYOR, P. BANKS, D. R. TOMLINSON AND ROSANNE GRIGAS

*Departments of Human Biology and Anatomy and Biochemistry, University of Sheffield (U.K.)*

## INTRODUCTION

It is now well established that dense cored, or granular, vesicles containing noradrenaline are synthesized in the cell bodies of noradrenergic neurones and subsequently transported down the axons to the varicose terminal network. This sequence of events has been deduced mainly from the results of experiments carried out *in vivo* on constricted post-ganglionic sympathetic nerves (see Dahlström, 1971b).

At the present time little is known about the processes responsible for the movement of noradrenaline-containing vesicles along axons. Some features of the mechanism should become apparent if it were possible to examine the effects of various metabolic inhibitors on the movement of noradrenaline and granular vesicles in noradrenergic nerves. Such experiments, however, are likely to yield ambiguous results if carried out *in vivo*.

This paper will describe a recently developed technique for studying the transport of noradrenaline and granular vesicles *in vitro* and will compare the results with those obtained previously in these laboratories using *in vivo* techniques.

## METHODS

Under nembutal anaesthesia cat hypogastric nerves were constricted with a fine silk ligature, which was left in place, about 3 cm distal to the inferior mesenteric ganglion. The nerves from this ganglion accompanying the inferior mesenteric artery, which will be collectively referred to as 'colonic' nerves, were also ligated as far from the ganglion as possible.

### In vivo experiments

In these the abdomen was closed in layers and the animal was allowed to survive for periods up to 4 days after operation. Some animals were treated with the monoamine oxidase inhibitor Iproniazid (iproniazid phosphate, 'Marsilid' Roche Products Ltd.), 30 mg/kg in sterile saline intraperitoneally, immediately after operation and at 16-hourly intervals until death. Other animals received a single dose of Reserpine ('Serpasil' Ciba) 5 mg/kg intraperitoneally, 16 h before death. Further details of the operation are given elsewhere (see Kapeller and Mayor, 1967, 1969a).

## In vitro experiments

After ligating the post-ganglionic nerves as indicated above, the pre-ganglionic nerves were also ligated. The various nerves and the inferior mesenteric ganglion were then freed of mesenteric tissue, excised *en bloc* and suspended on a glass pipette in a large diameter test-tube (see Banks, 1970) containing Eagles Minimal Essential tissue culture medium with added antibiotics. A mixture of 95 % oxygen and 5 % carbon dioxide was bubbled through the medium via the glass pipette to which the preparation was attached. The test-tube was kept at 37° in a thermostatically controlled water bath.

In some of these experiments iproniazid, 100 mg/l, reserpine, 10 mg/l, or the mitotic inhibitors colchicine (Colchicine, B.D.H.) 1 or 10 mg/l (*i.e.* $2.5 \times 10^{-6}$M or $2.5 \times 10^{-5}$M) or vinblastine sulphate (Vilbe, Lilly) 1 or 10 mg/l (*i.e.* $1.1 \times 10^{-6}$M or $1.1 \times 10^{-5}$M) were added to the incubation medium at the start of the experiment. The preparations were maintained *in vitro* for periods up to 48 h.

Isolated pieces of somatic nerves which contain some post-ganglionic noradrenergic nerves have also been studied *in vitro*. Hypogastric nerves were considered unsuitable because they sometimes contain aberrant noradrenergic neuronal cell bodies or ectopic chromaffin cells both of which may make the noradrenaline content of small pieces of nerve misleadingly high (see Banks *et al.*, 1969 b). Therefore, for the studies on isolated nerve trunks, 6 to 8-cm lengths of the medial popliteal (tibial) nerves from which the connective tissue had been removed were suspended in the incubation medium for 10 h after ligating each end tightly.

At the end of the experiments *in vivo* and *in vitro* the nerves were placed on a dry card and the regions adjacent to the constrictions were cut into 0.8 mm long segments (see Fig. 1) which were used for either electron microscopy or noradrenaline estimations. In general the colonic nerves were used for microscopy after fixation in osmium tetroxide buffered to pH 7.4 with veronal acetate buffer and the hypogastric nerves were used for the noradrenaline estimations using the fluorimetric method of Häggendal (1963) described previously (Banks *et al.*, 1969 b).

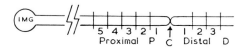

Fig. 1. Diagrammatic representation of the segmentation Proximal (P) and Distal (D) to the constriction (C) on the hypogastric/colonic nerves used for the biochemical analysis and electron microscopy. IMG is the inferior mesenteric ganglion. Each segment was 0.8 mm long. Only the proximal segments from the experiments *in vitro* were used.

## RESULTS

### Electron microscopy

The ultrastructural details of non-myelinated post-ganglionic noradrenergic nerves under normal conditions and after constriction *in vivo* have already been described,

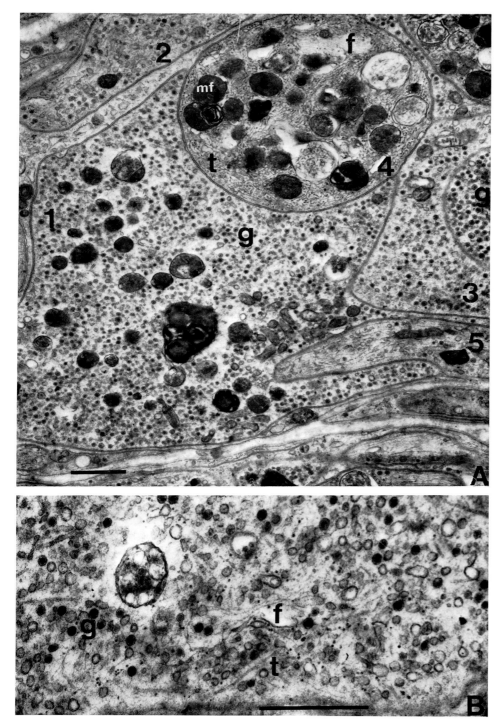

Fig. 2. Electron micrographs from the middle of segment P1, about 0.5 mm proximal to the site of the constriction. Cat colonic nerve maintained *in vitro* for 48 h. Tissue fixed in 1% buffered osmium tetroxide and section stained with lead citrate. Micron markers = 1 $\mu$.

A. Shows the accumulation of granular vesicles (g) and myelin figures (mf) in swollen axons 1–4. Axon 4 contains a dense network of fine tubules (t) and filaments (f). More typical microtubules can be seen in the less swollen axon 5. × 15 000.

B. Illustrates the contents of a swollen axon at higher magnification. Granular vesicles, (g), agranular vesicles, short lengths of microtubules (t) and filamentous structures (f). × 30 000.

(see Kapeller and Mayor, 1967, 1969 a, 1969 b). These will only be briefly described here for comparions with the nerves *in vitro* and with particular respect to the accumulation of granular vesicles and the appearances of microtubules (neurotubules).

Normal noradrenergic axons fixed in osmium tetroxide alone and stained only with lead citrate exhibit a faint longitudinal striation due to the presence of intra-axonal fine tubules, morphologically similar to cytoplasmic microtubules seen in other cells, and also to fine filamentous structures. Typical catecholamine-containing granular vesicles are rarely seen even in relatively long lengths of these axons cut longitudinally.

After constriction of these axons *in vivo* there was a rapid accumulation of granular vesicles proximal, but not distal to the lesion in axons which became progressively more swollen. This accumulation was most marked in the first 1 mm of nerve immediately adjacent to the constriction but as time progressed a significant accumulation of these organelles was seen up to 3 mm above the lesion. The morphology and configuration of the microtubules could not be established clearly in the more swollen axons where they were overshadowed by the accumulation of other organelles and by degenerative changes. At slightly more proximal levels and in the less swollen axons the microtubules were more electron dense and therefore more conspicuous than in normal axons.

Following treatment of the animals with iproniazid there were more granular vesicles accumulating above the constriction *in vivo* than after operation alone. After reserpine treatment they were almost completely absent from the constricted axons (Banks *et al.*, 1969 a).

After 24 to 48 h incubation *in vitro* the ultrastructural pattern in segments P1 (Figs. 2A and 2B) and P2 were generally indistinguishable from those seen in the experiments *in vivo*. Bearing in mind the pathological changes induced by the ligation procedure and the subsequent incubation *in vitro* the ultrastructure of the axons was remarkably well preserved. Granular vesicles and other organelles, *e.g.* mitochondria and myelin figures, or dense bodies, accumulated in many axons. Microtubules were more prominent in the less swollen axons as was also the case *in vivo*. However, the degree of axonal swelling and the overall density of the packing of the accumulating organelles seemed to be less marked *in vitro* than *in vivo*. This could possibly be due to a decreased rate of proximo-distal movement of axoplasm from the cell bodies incubated under abnormal conditions which had also had their pre-ganglionic input severed.

Initial observations on the ganglion/nerve preparations incubated *in vitro* in the presence of either iproniazid or reserpine have revealed ultrastructural features identical with those seen previously in experiments *in vivo* by Banks *et al.* (1969 a). It appears therefore that the accumulation of granular vesicles and the changes in the microtubules seen in preparations incubated *in vitro* for 48 h are comparable with those seen *in vivo* over the same period of time.

When colchicine was added to the incubation medium the most striking ultrastructural changes so far identified proximal to the site of constriction were 1. the absence of any significant accumulation of granular vesicles, 2. swelling of the axons immediately above the constriction was less common and not as marked and 3. mi-

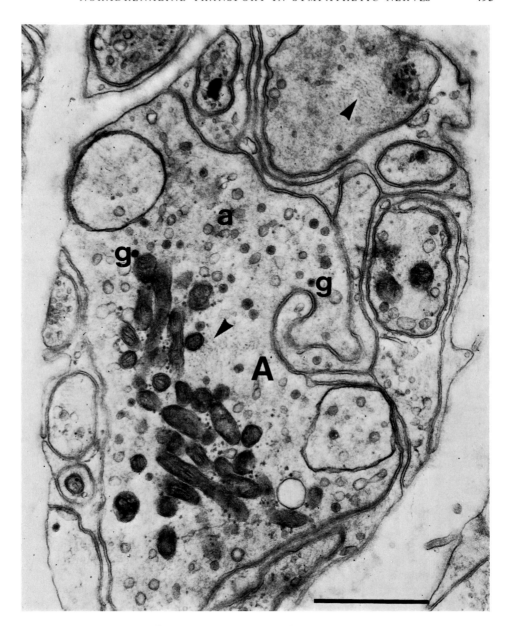

Fig. 3. Electron micrograph from the 0.5 mm portion of segment P1 immediately proximal to the constriction. Cat colonic nerve maintained *in vitro* for 48 h with added colchicine 10 mg/l. Group of non-myelinated axons cut transversely. Many contain few organelles and are approximately normal in diameter. Axon A is considerably swollen and contains a small accumulation of mitochondria and a few granular vesicles (g) and several agranular vesicles (a). Remains of microtubules, arrowed, can be seen. Note the absence of an accumulation of granular vesicles like that seen in Fig. 2. × 30 500. Micron marker = 1 μ.

TABLE 1

NORADRENALINE CONTENT OF SEGMENTS P1 + P2 + P3 (see Figure 1) FROM A SINGLE
CONSTRICTED CAT HYPOGASTRIC NERVE AFTER TREATMENT WITH IPRONIAZID AND
RESERPINE *in vivo*

Noradrenaline content of 1 segment of normal nerve was 0.01 ± 0.004 nmoles.

| Drug | nmoles Noradrenaline/nerve (Means ± S.D.) | |
| --- | --- | --- |
| | 24 h | 48 h |
| None | 0.24 ± 0.03 | 0.48 |
| Iproniazid 30 mg/kg | 0.36 | 1.91 |
| Reserpine 5 mg/kg | 0.0 | 0.0 |

TABLE 2

THE EFFECT OF IPRONIAZID AND RESERPINE ON THE NORADRENALINE CONTENT OF SEG-
MENTS P1 + P2 + P3 (see Figure 1) FROM A SINGLE CONSTRICTED CAT HYPOGASTRIC NERVE
FOLLOWING INCUBATION OF THE GANGLION/NERVE PREPARATION *in vitro*

1 segment of normal nerve *in vivo* contains 0.01 ± 0.004 nmoles noradrenaline.

| Drug | nmoles Noradrenaline/nerve (Means ± S.D.) | |
| --- | --- | --- |
| | 24 h | 48 h |
| None | 0.19 ± 0.03 | 0.35 ± 0.02 |
| Iproniazid 100 mg/l | 0.3 ± 0.07 | 0.63 |
| Reserpine 10 mg/l | 0.0 | 0.0 |

crotubules were subjectively less conspicuous and less numerous compared with
nerves incubated *in vitro* without this drug (Fig. 3). Further experiments to elucidate
the nature of any other changes in the microtubules due to mitotic inhibitors are in
progress.

*Biochemistry*

*Constricted hypogastric nerves in vivo*

There is very little noradrenaline detectable in normal cat hypogastric nerves;
single 0.8 mm segments contain 0.01 ± 0.004 (S.D.) nmoles noradrenaline per
single segment (Banks *et al.*, 1969 b). During the first 4 days after operation there
was a linear increase in the amount of noradrenaline accumulating in the first three
segments (*i.e.* P1 + P2 + P3) immediately proximal to the constriction.

The administration of iproniazid produced a three to four fold increase in the
amount of noradrenaline accumulating during the first 48 h after constriction. When
reserpine was given 16 h before death no noradrenaline could be detected 48 h after
the original ligation operation (Banks *et al.*, 1969 a). These results have been confirmed and amplified in subsequent experiments (Table 1).

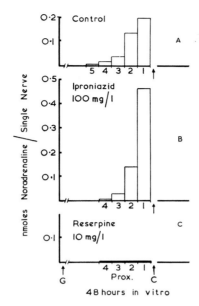

Fig. 4. Histograms illustrating the distribution of noradrenaline in constricted cat hypogastric nerves maintained *in vitro* for 48 h. The site of the constriction is indicated by the vertical arrows (C), G indicates the position of the inferior mesenteric ganglion. Each individual segment was 0.8 mm long (see Fig. 1).
A, after ligation only. B, after ligation and the addition of iproniazid (100 mg/l) to the incubation medium. C, after ligation and the addition of reserpine (10 mg/l) to the incubation medium.

*Constricted hypogastric nerves/inferior mesenteric ganglion preparation in vitro*

In these preparations there was a similar linear increase in the noradrenaline content of the first three segments immediately proximal to the site of constriction during the first 48 h after incubation. Although the absolute amounts of noradrenaline *in vitro* (Table 2 and Fig. 4) were slightly less than those found in experiments *in vivo* (Table 1) the pattern of transmitter accumulation was similar in both instances.

When iproniazid was added to the incubation medium there was a 2 fold increase in the amount of noradrenaline accumulating above the constriction during the 48 h incubation. When reserpine was added to the medium, no noradrenaline could be detected in the constricted nerves as seen in the histogram in Fig. 4 and in Table 2. These results are comparable with those from experiments *in vivo* (see Table 1).

Thus despite the fact that the pre-ganglionic nerves have been transected and the inferior mesenteric ganglion/ligated hypogastric nerve preparation had been maintained in an artificial environment, the production, movement and accumulation of granular vesicles in the preparations is similar to that seen in constricted nerves *in vivo*.

*Effects of mitotic inhibitors on the accumulation of noradrenaline in constricted hypogastric nerves/inferior mesenteric ganglion in vitro*

After adding colchicine or vinblastine to the incubation medium there was a very marked reduction in the amount of noradrenaline accumulating above a constriction

*References p. 498*

TABLE 3

EFFECTS OF COLCHICINE AND VINBLASTINE ON THE NORADRENALINE CONTENT OF SEG-
MENTS P1 + P2 + P3 (see Figure 1) OF A SINGLE CONSTRICTED CAT HYPOGASTRIC NERVE
FOLLOWING INCUBATION OF THE GANGLION/NERVE PREPARATION *in vitro*

1 segment of normal nerve *in vitro* contains 0.01 ± 0.004 nmoles noradrenaline.

| Drug | nmoles Noradrenaline/nerve (Mean ± S.D.) | |
|---|---|---|
| | 48 h | 24 h |
| None | 0.19 ± 0.03 | 0.35 ± 0.02 |
| Colchicine 1 mg/l | — | 0.22 ± 0.10 |
| Colchicine 10 mg/l | 0.05 ± 0.01 | 0.08 ± 0.05 |
| Vinblastine 1 mg/l | 0.10 ± 0.003 | 0.10 ± 0.01 |

(Table 3). Preliminary experiments *in vitro* have indicated that neither colchicine nor vinblastine cause the granules to lose their content of noradrenaline. Therefore, it would appear that they may act by either inhibiting the production of noradrenaline-laden granular vesicles in the neuronal cell body or by inhibiting the mechanism responsible for the axonal transport of granular vesicles.

*Movement of noradrenaline in isolated nerve trunks in vitro*

In the 6–8-cm pieces of the medial popliteal nerve maintained *in vitro* for 10 h, 0.029 ± 0.007 (S.D.) nmoles noradrenaline were found to accumulate immediately above the distal constriction. This confirms previous observations that noradrenaline, and presumably granular vesicles, continue to move in a predominantly proximo-distal direction in noradrenergic nerves without the influence of the neuronal cell bodies (Dahlström, 1967; Mayor and Kapeller, 1967; Banks *et al.*, 1969 b).

The addition of colchicine (10 mg/l) to the Eagles medium did not reduce the amount of noradrenaline accumulating immediately above the distal constriction during 10 h incubation. This failure of colchicine to inhibit the movement of nora-drenaline in isolated pieces of nerve during this period may be a consequence of either a long induction period before the effects of the drug are manifest or of a slow rate of penetration of the drug into the nerve. Further experiments to clarify these questions are in progress.

DISCUSSION

These experiments have shown that it is possible to study the movement of granular vesicles and bound noradrenaline in post-ganglionic noradrenergic nerves *in vitro* and that the results are comparable with those obtained from experiments *in vivo*, at least during the first 2 days after constricting the nerves. Furthermore, the effects of certain drugs on the accumulation of noradrenaline in constricted noradrenergic nerves were identical in comparable experiments performed *in vivo* and *in vitro*.

Since the movement of noradrenaline can occur in isolated segments of nerve both *in vivo* (Banks *et al.*, 1969 b; Dahlström, 1967, 1971 a; Mayor and Kapeller, 1967) and *in vitro*, the cell bodies giving rise to the isolated axons are not essential for the movement, although they are necessary for the continued production of granular vesicles. Furthermore, since the pre-ganglionic nerves were cut in the preparations *in vitro*, it is clear that stimulation from this source is not essential for the output of granular vesicles and noradrenaline from the cell bodies of post-ganglionic sympathetic neurones. However, such stimuli may regulate the rate of production of granular vesicles by these cells.

The rate of the proximo-distal movement of noradrenaline, and therefore presumably of the granular vesicles, in constricted cat hypogastric nerves *in vivo* has been estimated to be of the order of 2 mm per hour. While it may be slightly slower in the experiments *in vitro* it is still faster than the slow proximo-distal movement of axoplasm and proteins in myelinated axons described by other authors (see Banks *et al.*, 1969 b for references). This raises the question of the mechanism underlying the relatively rapid transportation system for noradrenaline in non-myelinated axons.

The involvement of axonal microtubules (neurotubules) in the translocation of granular vesicles has been suggested from the inhibitory effect which large doses of colchicine and vinblastine have on the movement of noradrenaline *in vivo* (Dahlström, 1968, 1971 a; Hökfelt and Dahlström, 1970). A similar inhibition of noradrenaline transport has now been observed in constricted noradrenergic nerves attached to their ganglion incubated *in vitro* with very low doses of colchicine and vinblastine.

Although in these and previous studies (Kapeller and Mayor, 1969 a, b), axonal microtubules ('fine tubules') were more prominent and apparently more numerous after axonal constriction, no particular relationship has so far been seen between granular vesicles and microtubules. However, this alone does not exclude the possibility that microtubules are involved in the transport of granular vesicles.

Hökfelt and Dahlström (1971), using permanganate or aldehyde followed by osmium tetroxide fixation for electron microscopy, suggested that there was a transformation of microtubules to neurofilaments (*sic*) in sympathetic nerves after the local application of colchicine and vinblastine in high concentrations. Except for the fact that microtubules were less obvious and possibly reduced in number, we have not found any alterations in their ultrastructure in the osmium-fixed material so far examined which could be unequivocally attributed to the low doses of colchicine used in the present experiments *in vitro*.

At the present time, therefore, the evidence for the involvement of microtubules in the proximo-distal movement of granular vesicles in noradrenergic nerves is indirect and of necessity incomplete. However, the possibility receives some further support from the present experiments on sympathetic ganglion–nerve preparations maintained *in vitro*.

### ACKNOWLEDGEMENTS

We are grateful to Professors R. Barer and W. Bartley for the facilities of their Departments. This work has been supported by grants from the Wellcome Trust, Smith,

Kline and French Foundation, S.R.C. and M.R.C. which we gratefully acknowledge. We wish to thank Mr. T. Owen and Mrs. M. M. Hollingsworth for their expert technical assistance. We thank Roche Products Ltd., and Ciba for generous supplies of Iproniazid and Reserpine respectively. D.R.T. is in receipt of a post-graduate research grant from the Wellcome Trust.

SUMMARY

Preparations for the study of noradrenaline transport *in vitro* in constricted noradrenergic nerves are described and compared with previous experiments on constricted noradrenergic nerves carried out *in vivo*.

Colchicine and vinblastine in low concentrations inhibit the proximo-distal movement of noradrenaline and granular vesicles in cat hypogastric nerves attached to the inferior mesenteric ganglion *in vitro*.

The possible implication of microtubules in the transport of noradrenaline storage granules is considered.

REFERENCES

BANKS, P. (1970) *Biochem. J.*, **118**, 813–818.
BANKS, P., KAPELLER, K. AND MAYOR, D. (1969 a) *Brit. J. Pharmacol.*, **37**, 10–18.
BANKS, P., MANGNALL, D. AND MAYOR, D. (1969 b) *J. Physiol.*, **200**, 745–762.
DAHLSTRÖM, A. (1967) *Acta Physiol. Scand.*, **69**, 158–166.
DAHLSTRÖM, A. (1968) *Europ. J. Pharmacol.*, **5**, 111–113.
DAHLSTRÖM, A. (1971a) *Acta Physiol. Scand.*, Suppl., **357**, 6.
DAHLSTRÖM, A. (1971b) *Phil. Trans. Roy. Soc. London B*, **261**, 325–358.
HÄGGENDAL, J. (1963) *Acta Physiol. Scand.*, **59**, 242–254.
HÖKFELT, T. AND DAHLSTRÖM, A. (1970) *Acta Physiol. Scand. Suppl.*, **357**, 10–11.
KAPELLER, K. AND MAYOR, D. (1967) *Proc. Roy. Soc. London, B*, **167**, 282–292.
KAPELLER, K. AND MAYOR, D. (1969 a) *Proc. Roy. Soc. London, B.*, **172**, 39–51.
KAPELLER, K. AND MAYOR, D. (1969 b) *Proc. Roy. Soc. London, B*, **172**, 53–63.
MAYOR, D. AND KAPELLER, K. (1967) *J. Roy. Microscop. Soc.*, **87**, 277–294.

# Studies on the Sympathetic Neurone *in vitro*

J. D. LEVER AND R. PRESLEY

*Department of Anatomy, University College, Cardiff (U.K.)*

It has already been shown (Murray and Stout, 1947; Levi-Montalcini and Angeletti, 1963; England and Goldstein, 1969) that axonal growth and elongation can occur in cultures of dissociated sympathetic neurones.

This communication presents a fine-structural and light-microscopical study of chick sympathetic ganglion explants maintained *in vitro*.

## MATERIALS AND METHODS

Paravertebral sympathetic ganglia were dissected aseptically from chick embryos at developmental stages 35, 36, 37 (Hamburger and Hamilton, 1951), transferred to growth medium and further subdivided into pieces 0.1–0.5 mm diameter. After two washes in fresh medium, pieces were then contained in a further 0.5 ml of growth medium. By means of a Pasteur pipette medium plus pieces were then transferred to the surface of 8 × 35 mm Melinex 0 strips (300 gauge, ICI) individually contained in Leighton tubes. The atmosphere in the tubes was replaced by humidified 5% $CO_2$ in air prior to sealing and the cultures were incubated at 37° C.

Nerve growth medium consisted of 4 parts Medium 199 (Wellcome) containing penicillin 200 U/ml and streptomycin 100 $\mu$g/ml; 1 part chick embryo extract (Flow); 1 part foetal bovine serum (Flow). This medium was centrifuged at 600 $g$ for 30 min, passed through a sterile Millipore (G.S.) filter, equilibrated with 5% $CO_2$ in air and the pH adjusted to 7.2.

Cultures were observed at 37°C by means of an inverted phase contrast microscope and after 7–14 days of culture were prepared as follows:

*1. For the chromaffin reaction* (4 cultures). Melinex strips were washed in Dulbecco's phosphate-buffered saline (pH 7.2) at 4°C, fixed in 5% glutaraldehyde and processed by the method of Jones (1967).

*2. For the formol-fluorescence demonstration of catecholamines* (4 cultures). After washing in Hanks B.S.S. at 37°C cultures were dried, formol-gassed by the method of Spriggs *et al.* (1966) and examined by fluorescence microscopy.

*3. For electron microscopy* (2 cultures). Cultures were fixed in 4% glutaraldehyde at 4°C for 3 h, washed overnight in cacodylate buffer (pH 7.2) and post-fixed in 1% osmium tetroxide for 30 min. Following graded ethanol dehydration specimens were araldite-embedded (culture surface up) in a shallow flat polythene dish. Throughout these manoeuvres the Melinex strips were transferred from one reagent to another.

Araldite blocks containing the cultures were trimmed down to the edges of the contained Melinex strips by means of a hacksaw. These strips were then detached from blocks leaving cultures at the araldite surface. Blocks were then positioned, culture face upwards, in polythene dishes and covered by a further layer of araldite for final embedding. Cultures were orientated under the dissecting microscope and after suitable trimming by hacksaw were attached by quick-setting araldite to the surface of conventional plastic blocks fitting the microtome chuck.

Cultures were fine sectioned at cellular, axonal and terminal levels with respect to the neurone.

## OBSERVATIONS

By the third day of incubation it was observed that successful cultures were attached to the Melinex and exhibited centrifugal outgrowths.

### Light microscopic appearances

After 4 days *in vitro*, explants were surrounded by fringes of polymorphic fibroblasts. In successful nerve cultures these fringe areas also exhibited a reticulum of axonal processes (Fig. 1). Two days later nerve cells with typical axonal processes were discernible peripheral to the explants, (Figs. 3 and 4). Bundling and linear deployment of axons were features of older (2-weeks) cultures (Fig. 2).

At all stages of axon growth, terminal expansions were seen at axon extremities.

After 4, 6, 8 and 13 days of growth, cultures exhibited fluorescence (in u.v. light) characteristic of catecholamines, following formaldehyde gassing. This fluorescence was very intense in the primary explant, in which discrete fluorescent cells could be seen. In addition many of the cells and cell processes peripheral to the explant were also fluorescent (Fig. 3). After fluorescent study, toluidine blue staining of the same cultures enabled positive cell identification (Fig. 4): formerly fluorescent neurones were found to be more basophilic than adventitial elements.

In cultures processed for the chromaffin reaction, the explant was strongly chromaffin-positive, while the peripheral elements consisted of chromaffin-negative fibroblasts and chromaffin-positive neurones (with axonal processes) which showed cytoplasmic chromaffin colouration but no chromaffin granules.

### Electron microscopic appearances

A typical culture studied was approximately 1 mm in length and (to the naked eye) was composed of an almost spherical proximal portion (ca. 0.3 mm d), a rectilinear intermediate portion (0.1 mm wide) and an expanded distal portion (ca. 0.2 mm wide). Fine sections were taken at right angles to the long axis of the culture progressing from terminal to proximal levels.

It was clear that (i) the proximal part of the culture consisted of parenchymal cell bodies, axonal and dendritic processes with no supporting elements (Fig. 5), (ii) the

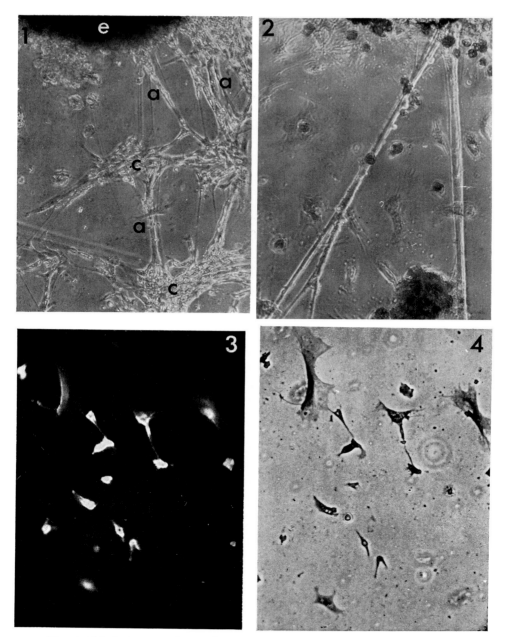

Figs. 1–14 inclusive are cultures of chick embryonic paravertebral ganglion explants.
Figs. 5–14 are all electron micrographs of 14-day cultures.
Fig. 1. Living 6-day culture. Note explant (e) peripheral cell clusters (c) and axonal processes (a): phase contrast micrograph. × 175.
Fig. 2. Axonal outgrowths in 14 day culture: phase contrast micrograph. × 175.
Figs. 3 & 4. Neurones at the periphery of a 6-day culture. In Fig. 3, cells and cell processes show specific fluorescence for catecholamines: compare with Fig. 4 in which same cells were subsequently stained by toluidine blue. Fig. 3 — fluorescence micrograph after formol gassing: magnification × 175.

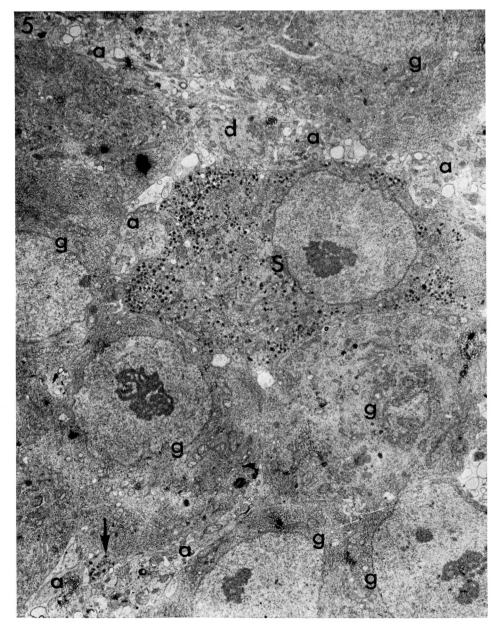

Fig. 5. Cell field from proximal portion of culture. Note ganglion cells (g): granulated ('small') cell
( S) and process of similar cell (↓); dendritic process (d): axon profiles (a): × 6000.

intermediate portion (Fig. 12) consisted exclusively of axons and axon terminals
(without supporting elements), (iii) the distal portion consisted of axon terminals with
occasional fibroblasts associated (Fig. 13). The total axon count progressively dimin-

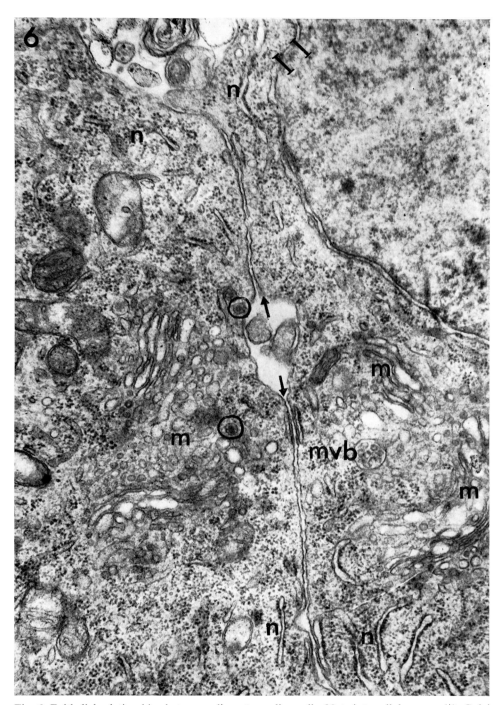

Fig. 6. Epithelial relationships between adjacent ganglion cells. Note intercellular space (↓): Golgi membranes (m) with dense-cored vesicles (◯): Nissl substance (n): nucleopores (I): multivesicular body (mvb): × 35 000.

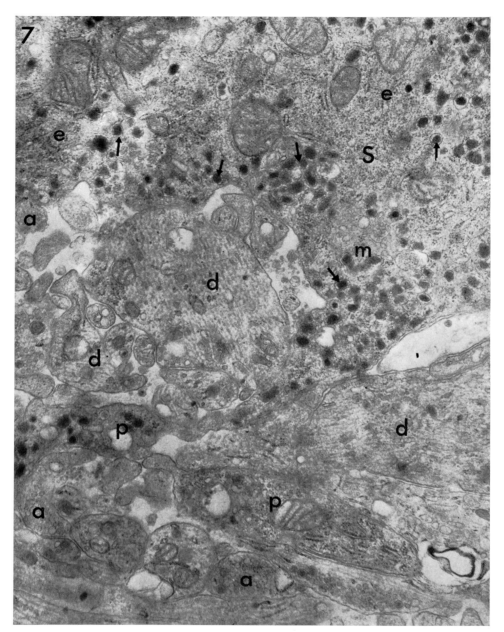

Fig. 7. Field from proximal portion of culture. Note granulated ('small') cell (S): small cell processes (p): membrane-bound granules (↓), granular endoplasmic reticulum (e) and Golgi membranes (m) all in small cell body: ganglion cell dendrites (d): axon profiles (a): × 24 000.

ished from proximal to distal along the intermediate part of the culture thus confirming the termination of some axons short of the distal part of the culture.

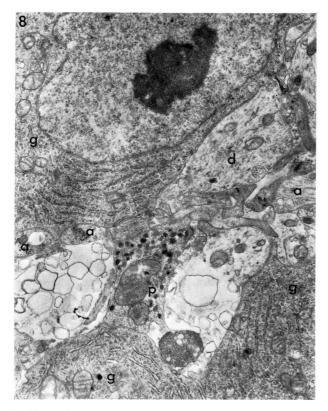

Fig. 8. Variegated field, proximal portion of culture. Note portions of three ganglion cells (g) with profuse Nissl substance: 'small' cell process (p): dendritic (d) and axonal (a) processes: × 21 000.

*The ganglion cells*

Without any satellite cell covering, nerve cell surfaces were either closely applied to one another — epithelial fashion (Fig. 6); directly related, across narrow (200 Å) spaces, to surrounding naked axonal processes (Fig. 8); in contact with the bodies or processes of rarely occurring cells containing numerous membrane-bound dense granules (see Figs. 5, 7 and 8); or were completely uncovered, at least in part. The deployment of cellular and axonal constituents within the proximal portion of the culture appeared to be random.

All the ganglion cells presented a fine-structural appearance typical of neurones in a state of high cellular activity (Figs. 6 and 8), *viz.* large nucleolus; numerous nucleo-pores; cytoplasmic polyribosomal clusters in plenty; typical Nissl collections of granular endoplasmic reticulum; numerous individual Golgi clusters — each fairly circumscribed — scattered about the cell; polymorphic mitochondria disposed in relation to ribosomes and Nissl collections. Besides these well-known neuronal features it was observed that the cultured ganglion cells also contained: occasional membrane-bound dense-cored vesicles — 1000 Å d — not only in the Golgi region, but also elsewhere in the cytoplasm (Fig. 6); agranular portions of the endoplasmic reticulum;

neuro- or microtubules (ca. 200 Å wide) dispersed through the cytoplasm; lysosomes.

What appeared to be dendritic processes were encountered in profile and in ganglion cell connection, in the proximal portion of the culture (Figs. 5, 8 and 9). These processes, with a high neurotubular content, akin to that in axons, were distinguishable from axons by their possession of ribosomes and Nissl elements. Fig. 9 shows what may well be a synaptic relationship between an axonal process and such a dendrite: it can be seen that the axonal microvesicles are polarised towards an electron-dense area of the axonal plasma membrane which is opposed to a comparably dense area of dendritic plasma membrane across an interval measuring some 200 Å.

### The ('small') granulated cells

Of rare occurrence, these cells were seen in small epithelial clusters intermingled with ganglion cells and axons in the proximal portion of the culture (Fig. 5). Polymorphic in shape, they send out cell processes usually loaded with numbers of large (1600 Å d) membrane-bound dense granules. By their granule size (Fig. 7) they can be distinguished from both the axonal and dendritic processes of ganglion cells. In the bodies of these granulated cells, besides an abundance of the specific granules (already referred to) there is evidence which suggests that these granules are formed within the Golgi sacs (Fig. 7) and further evidence, in the shape of an extensive granular endoplasmic reticulum and many ribosomes, which indicates a high level of metabolic activity.

### The axons

Axons were deployed differently in the three main portions of the culture. Proximally they were closely applied to one another in decussating bundles between and around the ganglion cells (Figs. 5, 8 and 9). In the intermediate part of the culture they were loosely grouped in parallel, so that in cross section their profiles were nearly circular (Fig. 12). Distally this bundling was not apparent and terminal axons were not only expanded (see below) but dispersed over a wider front.

Axolemmal surfaces were completely devoid of any cellular or material covering except distally where occasional axon–fibroblast contacts were observed. These infrequent junctions had a 'peg-socket' appearance in section, the axons apparently indenting the surface of the fibroblasts. Some thickening and increased electron density of opposed plasma membranes was observed at these peg-socket junctions and also at some situations where axon terminals were directly juxtaposed to each other.

From several short series of electron micrographs it was apparent that axons were not only beaded terminally but exhibited periodic beadings and narrowings proximal to their actual terminations (Figs. 9, 10, 11 and 14).

### The axoplasm

Two distinct, axially orientated, membrane-bound systems were observed in axons at all levels: (i) *the neurotubules* — 200–250 Å in diameter grouped in parallel for the most part and seen to best advantage in the narrower portions of the axons (Figs.

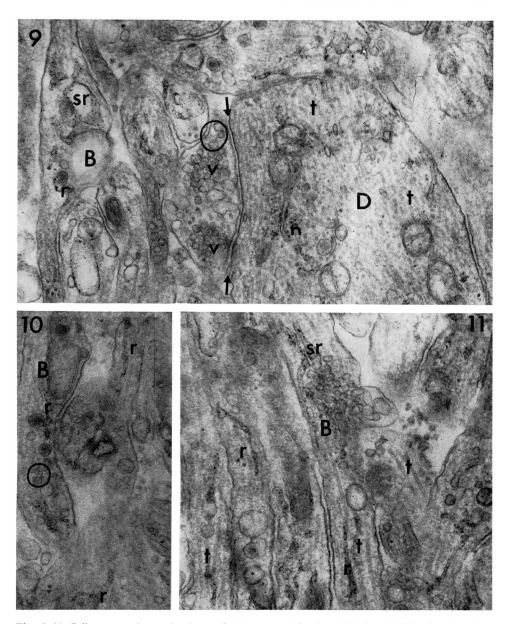

Figs. 9–11. Cell processes in proximal part of culture: magnifications, Fig. 9 × 42 000, Figs. 10 and 11 × 50 000. Note dendritic process (D) of ganglion cell showing neurotubules (t) and Nissl substance (n): axo-dendritic synapse (↓), with accumulation of presynaptic vesicles (v) and increased density of synaptic membranes at one point. Axon beadings (B) may contain 500-Å diameter lucent vesicles (Fig. 11) or lucent vesicles and dense-cored (1000 Å diameter) vesicles (Figs. 9 and 10). Note axonal neurotubules (t): intervesicular connections (○): agranular reticulum (r) with stippled content and saccular dilatations (sr).

11 and 12); (ii) *agranular reticulum* — in places running parallel with the neurotubules and of similar cross-sectional diameter (Figs. 9, 10, 11 and 12), but also lying obliquely across the neurotubules and exhibiting saccular dilatations (Figs. 9 and 11), some measuring more than 2000 Å: this agranular reticulum was clearly identifiable by a content of finely stippled electron-dense material comparable to that seen within lysosomes in the same axons (Fig. 12).

The aforementioned axon beadings were often characterised by the presence of mitochondria and always by clusters of axoplasmic vesicles — however it must be added that the distribution of both these inclusions was not exclusive to the beadings. It was clear that some beadings contained numbers of small relatively lucent vesicles (500 Å or less d) clustered around and possibly in connection with, neurotubules (Fig. 11). Other beadings contained a mixed axoplasmic population of: large, (600–1300 Å d), vesicles, many with a dense core and small (500 Å d) vesicles only a minority of which had an obvious material content (*i.e.* a dense core): and mitochondria (Fig. 14).

The following membrane connections have been seen, principally within axon enlargements at their actual terminations, but also in beaded and (rarely in) narrower parts of the axons proximal to their terminations: (i) *intervesicular connections* — direct membranous continuity between small (500 Å d) vesicles themselves and between small vesicles and large (600–1300 Å d) dense-cored vesicles (Figs. 9, 10, 13 and 14): (ii) mitochondrio-vesicular connections (Fig. 14).

In addition to the inclusions and organelles already mentioned typical lysosomes and multivesicular bodies were encountered at all axonal levels (Figs. 6, 12 and 14). Multivesicular bodies sometimes measured more than 2000 Å in width and contained, besides small (500 Å d) vesicles, variable amounts of a speckled dense material akin to that found within the lysosomes — a fact which suggests a lysosomal identity for these bodies.

### DISCUSSION

This work provides unequivocal evidence of the successful maintenance of embryonic autonomic neurones *in vitro* and of axonal growth from them. Furthermore, since these neurones and their processes show u.v. fluorescence characteristic of catecholamines after formol gassing, their adrenergic nature is most likely. In support of this is the finding that the majority of the cells in the explant exhibit a chromaffin-positive colouration.

Fine-structural evidence — the presence of many nucleopores, polyribosomes and much Nissl material — suggested that cultured neurones were highly active, a state compatible with their protein-forming role during axon growth and with their simultaneous production of catecholamines. The finding of large (600–1000 Å d) dense-cored vesicles in the ganglion cell body and at all axonal levels and the presence of small vesicles (500 Å d) — some of them dense-cored — in axon beadings and terminals would certainly be compatible with an adrenergic identity for these neurones.

Only one type of ganglion cell has been described in this study but there remains the possibility of another — possibly an interneurone. This is suggested by the finding of

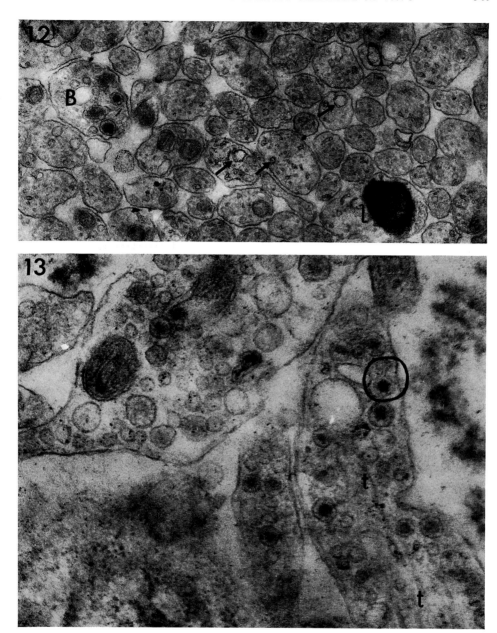

Fig. 12. Axon cross sections in intermediate portion of culture. Note: axon beading (B) with content of dense-cored and lucent vesicles; stippled agranular reticulum (↑) alongside neurotubules (compare Fig. 11); lysosome (l). Axons are not supported by Schwann cells: × 42 000.

Fig. 13. Expanded axon terminals in distal part of culture. Note axoplasmic accumulation of dense-cored and lucent vesicles: intervesicular connection (○); neurotubules (t); mitochondria. × 80 000.

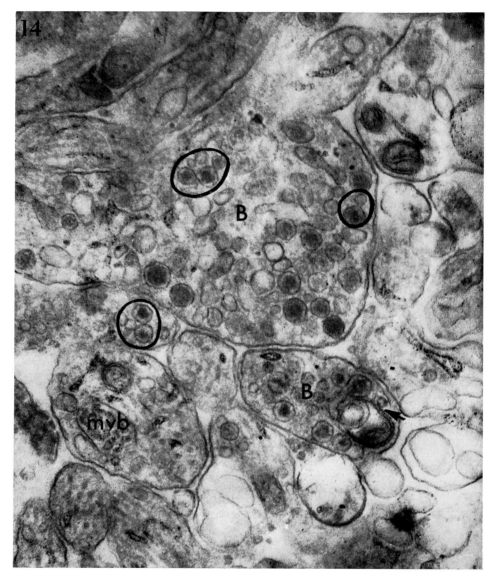

Fig. 14. En passage axon beadings (B) proximal to their terminations. Note 'terminal' features, *viz.*
dense-cored and lucent vesicle accumulations. Note also intervesicular (○) and mitochondrio-vesicular (↑) connections; multivesicular body (mvb). × 60 000.

an axo-dendritic synapse (Fig. 9): it could be argued in the circumstances that axons
preganglionic to neurones (or their dendrites) of the explant must themselves be
derived from explanted cells since they could not have had a spinal cord origin (and
survived — in this experiment). It is most likely that the heavily granulated cells
occurring in small rare clusters correspond to the 'small' cells reported in sympathetic

ganglia by Matthews and Raisman (1969). Their nature and significance forms the subject of further enquiry.

Certainly no Schwann or other supporting elements have been encountered in our cultures either in relation to the neurone cell bodies or their processes — and this is remarkable. Conceivably this situation would lend itself (in a negative sense) to further study of the role of the Schwann cell.

It is pertinent to compare the form and arrangement of axons observed in culture with that of proven adrenergic vasomotor axons *in vivo* (Lever *et al.*, 1965 and 1968). Both exhibit beaded expansions not only at their actual terminations but also proximally along their preterminal course. It has been suggested that *in vivo*, these beadings are en passage terminal areas for humoral release. The comparison between *in vivo* and *in vitro* adrenergic terminals can be carried further. In both, there are concentrations of large and small dense-cored and lucent vesicles as well as mitochondria. In both situations intervesicular and vesico-mitochondrial membrane connections are found (Spriggs *et al.*, 1967).

It would seem that an agranular (endoplasmic) reticulum extends from the perikaryon along the axon. In cultured preparations this system was very readily identified in its axonal extent because of its content of dense finely stippled material resembling closely that found in typical lysosomes and in some of the multivesicular bodies seen scattered along the axon. That this reticulum bears large saccular specialisations also with a stippled content might suggest (i) an origin for axonal lysosomes and (ii) that the reticulum is the means of conveyance from cell to axon of various hydrolytic enzymes.

The possibilities for further study which are suggested by the maintenance and growth of sympathetic neurones *in vitro* and their successful treatment by formol fluorescence histochemical and autoradiographic techniques are manifold.

### ACKNOWLEDGEMENTS

This work is in part supported by the Medical Research Council. One of us (J.D.L.) acknowledges permanent loan of a Siemens electron microscope from the Wellcome Trust. We are most grateful to Miss Caroline Ivens, Mrs. G. Howells and Miss G. Westlake for skilled assistance and to Mr. P. Hire for photographic help.

### SUMMARY

Chick embryonic paravertebral sympathetic ganglia were cultured for periods up to 14 days. Catecholamines demonstrated by a formol-fluorescence technique were detected in explanted cells and in outlying neurones and their axonal processes. Electron microscopy revealed: numbers of typical ganglion cells and a few granulated ('small') cells, both unsupported by adventitial elements: axo-dendritic synapses. Axonal outgrowths from ganglion cells exhibited preterminal narrowings and beadings, were unsupported by Schwann cells and extended peripherally to terminal expansions. In these terminal expansions and in the more proximal beadings concentrations of dense-cored and 'ucent vesicles and of mitochondria were found. A small number of dense-cored vesicles was invariably found in the perikaryon of the ganglion cells.

## REFERENCES

ENGLAND, J. M. AND GOLDSTEIN, M. N. (1969) *J. Cell. Sci.*, **4**, 677.
HAMBURGER, V. AND HAMILTON, H. V. (1951) *J. Morphol.*, **88**, 49.
JONES, P. A. (1967) *Stain Technol.*, **42**, 1.
LEVER, J. D., GRAHAM, J. D. P., IRVINE, G. AND CHICK, W. J. (1965) *J. Anat.*, **99**, 299.
LEVER, J. D., SPRIGGS, T. L. B. AND GRAHAM, J. D. P. (1968) *J. Anat.*, **103**, 15.
LEVI-MONTALCINI, R. AND ANGELETTI, P. V. (1963) *Develop. Biol.*, **7**, 653.
MATTHEWS, M. R. AND RAISMAN, E. (1969) *J. Anat.*, **105**, 255.
MURRAY, M. R. AND STOUT, A. P. (1947) *Amer. J. Anat.*, **80**, 225.
SPRIGGS, T. L. B., LEVER, J. D., REES, P. M. AND GRAHAM, J. D. P. (1966) *Stain Technol.*, **41**, 323.
SPRIGGS, T. L. B., LEVER, J. D. AND GRAHAM, J. D. P. (1967) *J. Microsc.*, **6**, 425.

# Evidence for the Nervous Control of Secretion in the Ciliary Processes

RISTO UUSITALO AND ARTO PALKAMA*

*Department of Anatomy, Eye Research Laboratory, University of Helsinki (Finland)*

The intraocular pressure (IOP) is regulated mainly by the inflow of the aqueous humo in the ciliary processes and by the outflow in the angle of the anterior chamber. These two structures of the eye are innervated both by adrenergic and cholinergic fibers (Laties and Jacobowitz, 1966). Furthermore it is well known that the ciliary processes contain a denser nervous network than the angle area of the anterior chamber (Ehinger, 1966).

On the basis of this rich innervation of the ciliary processes it has often been assumed that the secretion of the aqueous humor and thus also IOP would be under nervous control. So far, however, no direct correlation has been established. It has been found that adrenergic denervation causes a transient decrease of IOP, possibly due to increased outflow (Treister and Bárány, 1970). Similarly adrenergic stimulation causes a drop in IOP which is supposed to reflect relaxation of the smooth muscles in the orbit (Greaves and Perkins, 1952). When cholinergic fibres were stimulated, a rise in IOP was demonstrated which would be due to contraction of extraocular muscles (Davson, 1956).

In previous work we have presented evidence that secretion of aqueous humor and thus also IOP may indeed be directly controlled by autonomic nerves of the eye (Palkama and Uusitalo, 1969). After cholinergic denervation we observed an inhibition of the histochemically demonstrable NaK–ATPase activity in the ciliary processes of the rabbit (Palkama and Uusitalo, 1969). This enzyme is generally assumed to be responsible for the pumping of sodium into the posterior chamber. Demonstration of this 'pump' enzyme activity was based on a new modification of the original Wachstein–Meisel (1957) method, and is believed to be specific for the demonstration of NaK–ATPase in its membrane-bound localization. The enzyme is activated by sodium and potassium and is inhibited by ouabain (Palkama and Uusitalo, 1970). However, because quantification in histochemistry can easily give false results, we performed both quantitative determination of NaK–ATPase activity in the ciliary body and IOP measurements following different types of denervations.

Both adrenergic and/or cholinergic denervations of the rabbit eye have been

* The present study has been supported by a grant from the National Research Council for Medical Sciences, Finland, to one of us (A.P.). This work has also been supported by Star, Ltd., Pharmaceutical Manufacturers, Tampere, Finland.

*References p. 521*

performed. The ocular tension, inflow and resistance of outflow was also measured. In addition to the aforementioned quantitative determinations the NaK–ATPase activity in the ciliary body was demonstrated histochemically and measured fluorometrically. The success of the different denervations was checked.

MATERIAL AND METHODS

The material consisted of 58 male albino rabbits weighing 1–3 kg. The animals were divided into three groups according to the type of denervation.

*Group 1* was subjected under thiomebul sodium anesthesia to dissect on of the ciliary nerves around the optic nerve. These nerves contained both adrenergic and cholinergic fibers. Thus it was possible to cause a combined adrenergic and cholinergic denervation of the ciliary body. The operation is not easy to perform, but after some experience it is reproducible. The details of the operative technique will be published soon elsewhere. Special care has to be paid not to damage the long posterior ciliary arteries which supply the ciliary body.

*Group 2* contained rabbits, the right superior cervical ganglion of which had been d ssected under thiomebul sodium anesthesia.

*Group 3.* The parasympathetic nerves running along the oculomotor nerve were coagulated electrically by using a stereotaxic technique. The fibres were coagulated intracranially before the oculomotor nerve enters the orbital fissure.

IOP was measured manometrically 1, 2, 5 or 30 days after the different operations by using the cannulation technique with Swema SP 230 pressure transducer in conjunction with a recorder (Metrohm E 478). A fine needle (outer diameter 0.47 mm) with an opening at the side of the shaft was introduced into the anterior chamber. The inflow and the resistance of the outflow were calculated after intraocular infusion of saline with a known speed and amount from a reservoir. The calculations were made according to formulas given by Sears and Bárány (1960).

The success of the denervations was checked histochemically by demonstrating the adrenergic and cholinergic nerves in the ciliary bodies of both eyes. The adrenergic fibers were demonstrated either with the fluorescence technique in freeze-dried specimens after paraformaldehyde gassing (Eränkö, 1967) or by studying $KMnO_4$-fixed (3 %) sections with the electron microscope. The cholinergic fibres were demonstrated with a modified thiocholine technique both with light and electron microscopes (Palkama, 1965).

NaK–ATPase activity in the ciliary processes was shown histochemically with a modified Wachstein–Meisel technique according to a procedure reported recently by the present authors (Palkama and Uusitalo, 1970). The biochemical NaK–ATPase analyses were made fluorometrically by using a kinetic enzymatic technique which proceeds according to the following reaction:

$$ATP \xrightarrow{ATPase} ADP + Pi + PEP \xrightarrow{PK} ATP + Pyr + NADH \xrightarrow{LDH} Lac + NAD^+$$

The detailed procedure used in this assay will be published elsewhere with M. Härkönen in the near future.

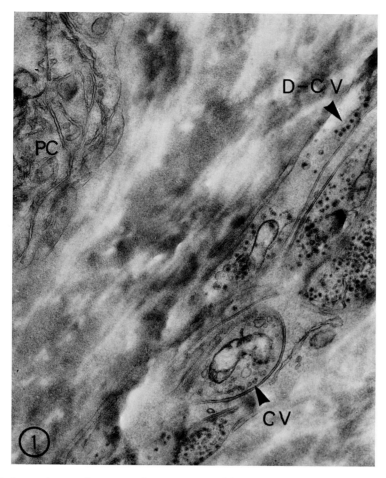

Fig. 1. Electron micrograph representing axons containing both dense-cored (D-CV) and clear vesicles (CV) in the stromal area of the rabbit ciliary process. The specimen has been fixed in 3 % KMnO₄. Two layers of epithelial cells cover the process; the pigmented (outer) cell (PC) is visible. × 20 000.

In the analysis of the changes in IOP, inflow and outflow resistance as well as in the studies concerning ATPase activity, the right (operated) eye was compared with the left (control) eye. The statistical analyses were made according to the matched paired $t$-test (Richterich, 1968).

In group 3, where some damage could also have occurred in the left oculomotor nerve, the fellow (left) eye was not considered to be a reliable control. In this group the right (operated) eye was compared with the left eyes of the other groups. The statistical analyses in the study of group 3 were made according to De Jonge's (1964) test.

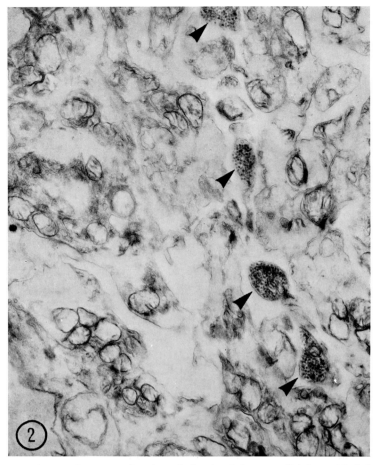

Fig. 2. Electron micrograph representing the apical pole of the two adjoining epithelial cells. With KMnO₄ fixation axons containing dense-cored granules are visible. The intimate association of the epithelial cells and nerves is readily observed. × 8000.


## RESULTS

In the normal (left) eye the distribution of fluorescent fibres was bound to the stromal area of the ciliary processes. No clear-cut fluorescent fibres were seen to penetrate the external limiting membrane and to run around the secretory cells. On the other hand when viewing KMnO₄-fixed sections in the electron microscope, axons containing dense-cored vesicles were seen between the epithelial cells and thus inside the external limiting membrane (Figs. 2 and 3). Although the number of these fibers was small, it seems that the secreting cells are in close direct contact with the nerve fibres. No fibres with empty vesicles in this area were seen, although outside the external limiting membrane dense-cored and empty vesicles containing nerve fibers were observed running in close contact with each other (Fig. 1). On the basis of our earlier

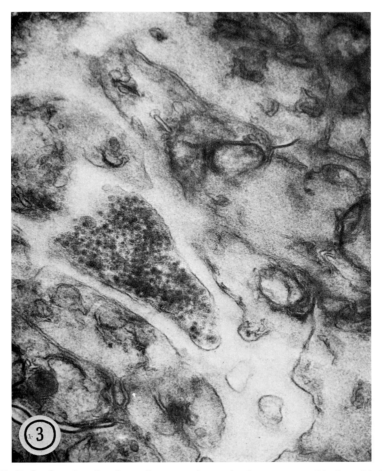

Fig. 3. KMnO₄-fixed section showing a dense-cored axon in close contact with the epithelial cells of the ciliary process. × 50 000.

findings and present observations the structure of the ciliary process can be schematically illustrated as presented in Fig. 4.

After dissection of the right superior cervical ganglion, the number of fluorescent fibres in the right ciliary body was strongly decreased one day after the operation. From two days onwards all the fluorescent fibres were destroyed in the body, whereas in the contralateral side the nerves remained intact.

Dissection of the ciliary nerves caused a clear reduction of both the adrenergic and cholinergic fibres on the ipsilateral side. However, it was seldom possible to obtain a total destruction of both nerve systems.

Stereotaxic operations caused an increase of the cholinesterase activity in the proximal end and a decrease of the enzyme activity in the distal end of the coagulation area of the oculomotor nerve. In the ciliary processes no changes were observed either in the

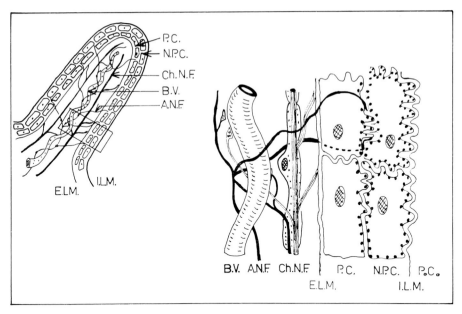

Fig. 4. Schematic illustration of the structure of the ciliary process. E.L.M. = external limiting membrane; B.V. = blood vessel; A.N.F. = adrenergic nerve fiber (which contains dense-cored granules); Ch. N.F. = cholinergic nerve fiber (contains clear vesicles); P.C. = pigmented (outer) epithelial cell; N.P.C. = non-pigmented (inner) epithelial cell; $P_oC_o$ = posterior chamber of the eye. Note that the adrenergic-like nerves penetrate the external limiting membrane and come into close contact with the epithelial cells. The site of NaK–ATPase activity in the epithelial cells is in the apical membranes, being especially concentrated in the region of the tight junctions, the apical complexes. Activity is also visible in the basal parts of the non-pigmented (inner) cells.

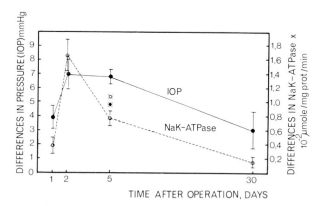

Fig. 5. Effect of dissection of the right ciliary nerves on the intraocular pressure (IOP) and NaK–ATPase activity in the ciliary body-iris. The curves represent the difference mean between the left (control) and right (operated) eye. The decreased IOP and NaK-ATPase activity in the right eye is significant ($p < 0.01$) 5 days after operation. The circles enclosed by squares represent corresponding difference means (■ = IOP, ▣ = NaK-ATPase), 5 days after electrocoagulation of the cholinergic nerves of the right eye. The decrease of IOP and NaK-ATPase activity was significant ($p < 0.01$) in the operated eye.

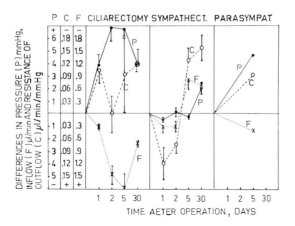

Fig. 6. Effect of dissection of the ciliary nerves, superior cervical ganglion or electrocoagulation of the parasympathetic nerves attached to the oculomotor nerve on intraocular pressure (P), inflow (F) and resistance of outflow (C). The curves represent the mean difference between the left (control) and right (operated) eye. The decrease of intraocular pressure in the right eye is significant ($p < 0.01$) after ciliarectomy and parasympathectomy, but not after sympathectomy. See text.

cholinergic or in the adrenergic fibres. This is evidently due to the fact that the cholinergic fibres in the ciliary body are postganglionic neurons.

The intraocular pressure was measured in the 36 control eyes and found to be 18.9 mm Hg. When studying the mean difference between the left and right eye, IOP was decreased in the operated eye after dissection of the ciliary nerves or coagulation of the cholinergic fibers (Figs. 5 and 6). The mean difference between the control and operated eye was 6.9 mm Hg in ciliarectomized rabbits two days after the operation. Five days after the operation the difference was 6.8 mm Hg ($p < 0.001$). Thirty days after the operation the difference was 4.1 mm Hg, a difference which is not statistically significant. After parasympathetic denervation (5 days after the operation) the difference in IOP was 4.8 mm Hg, which was a significant change ($p < 0.01$).

After sympathectomy, on the contrary, IOP was not significantly changed. Thirty days after the operation the decrease was most marked, being not more than 2.1 mm Hg (Fig. 6).

The decreased IOP in the operated eye after ciliarectomy was accompanied by decreased inflow (Fig. 6). This change was statistically almost significant ($p < 0.05$). On the other hand the decreased resistance of outflow was not significantly changed (Fig. 6). Similar changes in inflow and outflow were also observed after dissection of parasympathetic fibres, although the changes were not significant. The slight initial rise and the late decrease of IOP after sympathectomy seemed to be caused more by a change in the resistance of outflow than by the inflow rate. Initially the resistance of outflow in group 2 increased as the rate of inflow decreased (Fig. 6). After five days the decreased IOP is accompanied by decreased resistance of outflow and increased inflow rate. The difference in the resistance of outflow at the second and fifth days was almost significant ($p < 0.05$). NaK–ATPase activity in the ciliary body-iris in the

*References p. 521*

normal rabbit was $1.081 \times 10^{-2}$ $\mu$moles/mg prot./min. This activity had significantly ($p < 0.05$) decreased five days after dissection of the ciliary nerves to $0.316 \times 10^{-2}$ $\mu$moles/mg prot./min. (Fig. 5). NaK–ATPase activity had also significantly decreased after dissection of the cholinergic fibers stereotactically ($p < 0.01$). After sympathetic denervation, on the contrary, no significant drop of NaK–ATPase was demonstrated. When comparing the changes of IOP and NaK–ATPase after dissection of the ciliary nerves a clear parallelism can be observed (Fig. 5).

## DISCUSSION AND CONCLUSIONS

On the basis of the present findings it can be noted that the secretory cells seem to be in direct contact with the nerve fibres. It has been claimed that nerve fibres do not penetrate the external limiting membrane (*e.g.* Laties and Jacobowitz, 1966). We find that they do penetrate the external limiting membrane. These nerves contain small dense-cored vesicles. Their electron-microscopic appearance is suggestive of real adrenergic nerves. Thus these nerves would be in close contact both with the blood vessels and secretory cells.

Dissection of the ciliary fibres caused a statistically significant decrease of IOP. This decrease was accompanied by an almost significant decrease of inflow, whereas the resistance of outflow was not changed. On the contrary, adrenergic denervation did not significantly change IOP or inflow. The resistance of outflow was almost significantly changed, although it did not seem to cause a marked change in IOP.

On the basis of these findings we concluded that IOP is partly regulated by a parasympathetic-type system, although the nerves demonstrated around the secretory cells contain dense-core vesicles. This decreased IOP is supposed to be due to decreased inflow rate. At the later stage (30 days after the operation) IOP shows a tendency to change its course. In the operated eye in group 1, IOP increases, whereas in group 2, IOP decreases (Fig. 6). Although these changes of IOP at this later stage were not statistically significant, the increasing IOP in group 1 could be due to increased inflow and the decreasing IOP in group 2 may well reflect a decreased resistance of outflow. However, it must be remembered that some other factors such as the tonus in the extraocular and smooth muscles of the orbit, can play an important additional part in regulating IOP. The present authors (Uusitalo and Palkama, 1970) have recently shown with both the light and electron microscope that NaK–ATPase is localized in the ciliary processes mainly in the apical membranes, and especially in the apical complexes. This activity is significantly decreased after parasympathetic denervation. The decreased NaK–ATPase reaction occurs at the same time as IOP drops, which strongly suggests a functional relationship. Furthermore the inflow at the same time decreased, which would also reflect the decreased enzyme activity.

The manner by which the nerve fibres regulate the function of the secretory cells is still difficult to determine. The fibres described here, which are in close contact with the secretory cells, are electron-microscopically adrenergic. On the other hand, IOP changed after parasympathectomy but not after sympathectomy. This would suggest that cholinergic axons containing empty vesicles are present around the secretory cells. However, we have not yet seen such fibres. It must be also remembered that Burnstock (1970) has recently discovered non-adrenergic nerves which contain ATP as a possible transmitter substance. The nerves around the secretory cells possessing both adrenergic and cholinergic features could possibly represent such a new type of nerve. Whichever of the two (or three) nerve types the fibres discovered represent, the present findings suggest that NaK–ATPase activity in the secretory cells is under the control of nervous regulation.

## SUMMARY

Rabbits were subjected to three different types of denervation:
(1) dissection of the ciliary nerves (adrenergic and cholinergic fibers)
(2) sympathectomy (superior cervical ganglion) (adrenergic nerves) or
(3) electrocoagulation of the parasympathetic fibres running along the oculomotor nerve.

1, 2, 5 or 30 days after the operation the intraocular pressure, inflow and resistance of outflow was measured manometrically both in the operated (right) and control eyes. Thereafter NaK–ATPase in the ciliary body was demonstrated histochemically with both the light and electron microscope and assayed fluorometrically.

According to the results obtained the intraocular pressure decreased after parasympathetic denervation at the same time that inflow and NaK–ATPase activity decreased. Adrenergic denervation did not cause such changes.

The results obtained indicate that the NaK–ATPase activity in the secretory cells of the ciliary body is controlled by parasympathetic nerves. When these nerves have been dissected the decreased enzyme activity causes a significantly decreased inflow, and due to this, a marked drop in intraocular pressure.

## REFERENCES

BURNSTOCK, G., (1970); Personal communication.
DAVSON, H., (1956); *Physiology of the Ocular and Cerebrospinal Fluids*, J. A. Churchill Ltd., London.
DE JONGE, H., (1964); *Inleiding tot de Medische Statistiek. Deel 2.* Verhandeling van het Nederlands Instituut voor Praeventieve Geneeskunde. Leiden, 486–487.
EHINGER, B., (1966); *Acta Physiol. Scand.*, **67**, Suppl. **268**, 1–35.
ERÄNKÖ, O., (1967); *J. Roy Microscop. Soc.*, **87**, 259–276.
GREAVES, D. P. AND PERKINS, E. S., (1952); *Brit. J. Ophthalmol.*, **36**, 258–264.
LATIES, A. M. AND JACOBOWITZ, D., (1966); *Anat. Rec.*, **156**, 383–396.
PALKAMA, A., (1965); *Ann. Med. Exp. Fenniae*, **45**, 295–306.
PALKAMA, A. AND UUSITALO, R., (1969); *Scand. J. Clin. Lab. Invest.*, **23**, Suppl. **108**, 67.
PALKAMA, A. AND UUSITALO, R., (1970); *Ann. Med. Exp. Fenniae*, **48**, 49–55.
RICHTERICH, R., (1968); *Klinische Chemie, Theorie und Praxis*, 2. erweiterte Auflage, S. Karger, Basel–New York.
SEARS, M. L. AND BÁRÁNY, E. H., (1960); *Invest. Ophthalmol.*, **64**, 59–68.
TREISTER, G. AND BÁRÁNY, H., (1970); *Invest. Ophthalmol.*, **9**, 331–342.
UUSITALO, R. AND PALKAMA, A., (1970); *Ann. Med. Exp. Fenniae*, **48**, 84–88.
WACHSTEIN, M. AND MEISEL, E., (1957); *Amer. J. Pathol.*, **27**, 13–23.

# Author Index

Akert, K., 305–317
Athee, L., 269–279
Attila, U., 115–125

Banks, P., 489–498
Barnett, R. J., 319–325
Björklund, A., 63–73
Blaschko, H., 239–242
Bogdanski, D. F., 291–302
Burnstock, G., 389–404
Burt, A. M., 327–335

Coupland, R. E., 455–464
Csillik, B., 377–385

Davis, R., 371–375

Eränkö, L., 39–51
Eränkö, O., 39–51

Faeder, I. R., 103–114
Falck, B., 63–73
Fuxe, K., 127–138

Garrett, J. R., 475–488
Giacobini, E., 243–258
Goldstein, M., 127–138
Gosling, J. A., 77–86
Gray, E. G., 149–160
Grigas, R., 489–498
Gueudet, R., 161–170

Hashimoto, P. H., 207–212
Hervonen, A., 445–454
Hökfelt, T., 87–102, 127–138, 213–222
Hyub Joh, T., 127–138

Iawayama, T., 389–404
Ishii, S., 187–206

Jansson, S.-E., 281–290
Jonsson, G., 53–61

Kanerva, L., 433–444
Kása, P., 337–344
Kawana, E., 305–317
Kekki, M., 115–125
Klinge, E., 415–421
Koelle, G. B., 371–375

Kokko, A., 319–325
Lever, J. D., 499–512
Ljungdahl, Å., 87–102

Machado, A. B. M., 171–185
Malmfors, T., 467–473
Mastrolia, L., 455–464
Masuoka, D. T., 77–86
Mayor, D., 489–498

Nakane, P. K., 139–145

Olson, L., 467–473

Paasonen, M. K., 269–279
Palkama, A., 513–521
Pellegrino de Iraldi, A., 161–170
Placidi, G.-F., 77–86
Ploem, J. S., 27–37
Pohto, P., 415–421
Presley, R., 499–512

Rechardt, L., 423–431
Robinson, P. M., 357–370

Salpeter, M. M., 103–114
Sakharova, A. V., 11–25
Sakharov, D. A., 11–25
Sandri, C., 305–317
Schiebler, T. H., 405–413
Silver, A., 345–355
Smyrl, E. G., 371–375
Solatunturi, E., 269–279
Steveni, U., 63–73
Stjärne, L., 259–267
Suburo, A. M., 161–170

Talanti, S., 115–125
Thoenen, H., 223–236
Tissari, A. H., 291–302
Tomlinson, D. R., 489–498
Tranzer, J. P., 223–236

Uusitalo, R., 513–521

Vogt, M., 1–8

Weakley, B. S., 455–464
Winckler, J., 405–413

# Subject Index

Acetylcholinesterase,
central nervous tissue, *337–344*
demonstration, 188
in autonomic axons, *357–369*
electron microscopy, *357–369*
in autonomic ganglia, *371–374*
electron microscopy, *371–374*
peripheral nervous tissue, *337–344*
spatial relations with acetylcholine-synthesizing system, *377–385*
ultrastructural localization, *337–344*
visualization of activity, 364
Acetylcholine,
release, 357
synthesizing system, *377–385*
Adrenal medulla, *455–463*
comparison with sympathetic nerves,
*259–267*
Adrenergic nerves,
effect of drugs, 399
Adrenergic neurones, *239–242*
Adrenergic transmission mechanism in CNS,
granulated vesicles, *187–205*
minute vesicles, *207–212*
Albino rat, *455–463*
Alcohol treatment, *319–325*
γ-Aminobutyric acid uptake, 87, 91
Anterior chamber transplants,
sympathetic reinnervation, *467–473*
Autonomic
ganglia, *371–374*
nerves, *389–402*
changes, *475–487*
fine-structural identification, *389–402*
intra-axonal features, 395
relation to smooth muscle, *389–402*
neuromuscular junction, 389
Autoradiography, *87–100, 115–125*
combined with fluorescence microscopy,
*87–100*
Axon, *357–369, 506*
autonomic, *357–369*
Axoplasm, 506

Biogenic amines,
metabolism, 272
release, 272
storage, 269
uptake, 272
Biogenic monoamines, *53–60*
formaldehyde fluorescence method, *53–60*
chemistry, 53

quantitation and differentiation, *53–60*
Blood platelet, *269–277*
monoaminergic neuron model, *269–277*
Bull retractor penis muscle, *415–421*
excitatory fibres, 415
inhibitory fibres, 417
innervation, *415–421*

Cardiac innervation,
vegetative, 405
Catecholamines, 161, 239
differentiation, 58, 161
microassay, 188
newly formed *259–267*
preferential secretion, *259–267*
Choline acetyltransferase, *327–335*
histochemical localization, *327–335*
motor end-plate, 339
sciatic nerve, 339
spinal cord, 339
ultrastructural localization, *337–344*
Cholinergic neuron, *377–385*
Cholinesterase, *345–354*, 438, 448
activity, 428
developing nervous system, *345–354*
foetal activity, *337–350*
histochemistry, 436
occurrence during development, 348
postnatal development, *433–443*
role during development, 351
Chromaffin
cells, *239–242*
granules, 315
tissue, *445–454*
extra-adrenal, 452
human fetal, *445–454*
differentiation, *445–454*
innervation, *445–454*
intra-adrenal, 452
Chromogranins, *239–242*
Ciliary processes, 513
nervous control of secretion, *513–521*
CNS, *187–205, 207–212*
of rat, 67, 133
Cryostat thin-section method, 80
L-Cysteine,
35S-labelled, *115–125*
kinetics, *115–125*

Dense contents in synaptic vesicles,
sequential cation binding, *319–325*
Dense-cored vesicles, 312

Differentiation,
   between 5-hydroxytryptamine and catechol-
      amines, *161–169*
      synaptic vesicles, *161–169*
   of monoamines, 58
Distribution
   of granulated vesicles, 188
Dopamine-β-hydroxylase, *127–138*
   rat superior cervical ganglion, 131

Electrolytes, inorganic, *291–301*
Electron microscopy, 450, 456
   localization of acetylcholinesterase, *371–374*
   of sympathetic fibers, *171–184*
Enzyme assay, 456

False adrenergic transmitters,
   amine properties, *227–229*
   functional importance of cellular distri-
      bution, *223–235*
Fluoraldehyde-induced fluorescence, 446
Fluorescence, *27–36*
   histochemistry, 436
   intraneuronal monoamines, 13
   microscopy,
      combined with autoradiography, *87–100*
Fluorescent granule-containing cells,
   small, intensely fluorescent, *39–50*
Formaldehyde
   condensation, 30
   fluorescence, *53–60*
      chemistry, 53
   -induced fluorescence, *27–36*, 446
      colour differentiation, *27–36*
      instrumentation, 28
Formalin solutions, *11–25*
Formation of granular vesicles, *171–184*
Freeze-dried paraffin-embedding method, 78

Ganglion cells, 40, 505
Glutamate uptake,
   the role of sheath cells, *103–113*
Golgi complex, 308
Granular vesicles,
   small, 174, 180, 219
   large, 176, 181, 219
Granulated cells,
   small, 506
Granulated vesicles, *187–205*
Granule-containing cells, *39–50*

Histochemical fluorescence microscopy,
   combined with autoradiography techniques,
      *77–86*
5-Hydroxytryptamine, 161, 281
   differentiation, 58, 161
Hypophysis, *423–431*
Hypothalamic-hypophyseal system of rat,
   *115–125*

Immunohistochemistry, *127–138*
Impulse activity, 247
'Intracellular' nerve terminals, 394
Intraneuronal monoamines, *11–25*, *213–221*
   small and large granular vesicles, 219
   ultrastructural localization, *213–221*
      fixed tissue studies, 215
      test tube experiments, 213
   visualization, *11–25*
Intraocular pressure, *513–521*
Iris
   of rat, 132

Light microscopy,
   acetylcholinesterase, *371–374*
Localization, *77–86*
   of acid phosphatase, *455–463*
   cellular,
      of dopamine-β-hydroxylase, *127–138*
      of phenylethanolamine-N-methyl trans-
         ferase, *127–138*

Mast cell,
   comparison with nervous tissue, 288
   distribution of 5-HT *in vitro*, 283
   isolated granules,
      uptake of 5-HT, 286
   model for uptake and storage of 5-HT,
      *281–289*
   uptake of 5-HT *in vitro*, 281
Microscopic autoradiography
   using [³H]DOPA, 188
Minute vesicles, *207–212*
Monoamines, *63–72*, *433–443*
   fluorophores, *64–67*
   microspectrofluorimetric characterization, 63
   neuronal, in rat CNS, 67
   postnatal development, *433–443*
Multiaxonal junctions, 394
Multivesicular bodies, 308
Myocardial
   innervation, 410
   nerves, 408

Nerve muscle preparations,
   insect, *103–113*
Nerve terminals, *305–317*
Nervous tissue,
   acetylcholinesterase, *337–344*
   choline acetyl transferase, *337–344*
Nervous transmission
   molecular mechanisms, *243–257*
Neural lobe of the rat hypophysis,
   nerve terminals, *423–431*
Neuro-muscular transmission re-establishment,
   470
Neurons,
   cholinergic, 358
   non-cholinergic, 358

transmitter metabolism, 247
Neurosecretory granules, 315
Neurosecretory system
    of rat, *115–125*
Noradrenaline
    transport, *489–498*
    uptake, 87, 90
        CNS, 90
        peripheral nervous system, 90
Norepinephrine
    membrane transport, *291–301*
    metabolism, *291–301*

Osmium tetroxide fixation, *319–325*

Paracervical ganglion, *433–443*
Parotid gland, 475
Peripheral autonomic mechanism of erection,
    *415–421*
    inhibitory fibres, 417
Phenylethanolamine-N-methyl transferase,
    *127–138*
Pineal body of rat,
    granular vesicles, 178
    sympathetic innervation development,   178,
        183
Pineal gland, 163
Pineal innervation in immature rat, 172
Pituitary gland,
    anterior, 141
Plasmalemmal vesicles, 315
Post-synaptic structure,
    in smooth muscle, 394

Quantitation,
    of monoamines, 59

Rat adrenal gland, 128, 136
Reinnervation histochemistry, 468

Salivary glands
    degeneration, *475–487*
    regeneration, *475–487*
Satellite proteins, *239–242*
Sciatic nerve,
    of rat, 132, 137
Secretion in ciliary processes, 513
Sequential cation binding, *319–325*
Serotonin
    membrane transport, *291–301*
    metabolism, *291–301*
Sheath cells, *103–113*
SIF cells,
    see small intensely fluorescent cells, *39–50*
Smooth muscle, *389–402*
Submandibular

artery, 479
gland, 478
Superior cervical ganglion,
    of rat, 131, 137
Sympathetic fibres, *171–184*
Sympathetic ganglion
    of rat, *39–50*
Sympathetic nerves, *489–498*
    comparison with adrenal medulla, *259–267*
    noradrenaline transport,
        constricted hypogastric nerves *in vitro*, 494
        constricted hypogastric nerves *in vivo*, 494
Sympathetic neurone,
    *in vitro* studies, *499–512*
Sympathetic reinnervation,
    anterior chamber transplants, 467
Synapses, *149–159*
    with closed clefts, 155
        receptor cell synapses, 157
    fine structural differentiation, *149–159*
    learning, 158
    with open clefts, 149
        at nodes of Ranvier, 155
        lateral geniculate synapses, 153
        olfactory bulb connections, 154
        presynaptic contacts, 153
        pyramidal and stellate cell contacts, 153
Synaptic cleft, 393
Synaptic connections, 247
Synaptic plasticity, *243–257*
    heterogenous synapses, *251–257*
Synaptic vesicles, 161, 319
    agranular, 307
    dense contents, 319
    origin, 157
Synaptosomes, *291–301*

Thyrotropic cells,
    *in vitro*, *139–144*
Thyrotropin-releasing factor, *139–144*
Transmitter substance, *1–7*
    acetylcholine, 2
    dopamine, 4
    5-hydroxytryptamine, 5
    localization, *1–7*
    noradrenaline, 3

Uterus of rat, *433–443*

Vascular nerves, 408
Vegetative cardiac innervation, *405–413*

Zinc iodide-osmium tetroxide mixture,
    see ZIO, *305–317*
ZIO-positive vesicles, *305–317*
ZIO-negative vesicles, *305–317*